The Fetus as a Patient

Dedication

This book is dedicated to the participants, invited lecturers, and the Board of Directors of
The International Society of the Fetus as a Patient

The Fetus as a Patient

Advances in Diagnosis and Therapy

Edited by
Asim Kurjak and Frank A. Chervenak

Published on behalf of
The International Society of
The Fetus as a Patient

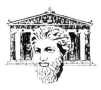

The Parthenon Publishing Group
International Publishers in Medicine, Science & Technology

NEW YORK   LONDON

Published in the UK by
The Parthenon Publishing Group Ltd.
Casterton Hall, Carnforth
Lancs, LA6 2LA, England

Published in the USA by
The Parthenon Publishing Group Inc.
One Blue Hill Plaza
PO Box 1564, Pearl River
New York 10965, USA

Copyright © 1994 The Parthenon Publishing Group Ltd.

British Library Cataloguing in Publication Data
The Fetus as a Patient : Advances in Diagnosis and Therapy
  I. Kurjak, Asim   II. Chervenak, Frank A.
618.3
ISBN 1-85070-558-5

Library of Congress Cataloging-in-Publication Data
The Fetus as a patient : advances in diagnosis and therapy / edited
  by Asim Kurjak and Frank A. Chervenak.
    p. cm.

  Includes bibliographical references and index.
  ISBN 1-85070-558-5
  1. Fetus—Diseases.   2. Fetus—Abnormalities.   3. Fetus—
    Diseases—Diagnosis. I. Kurjak. Asim. II. Chervenak. Frank A.
  [DNLM: 1. Fetal Diseases—ultrasonography. 2. Ultrasonography,
Prenatal.
    3. Fetal Diseases—therapy. WO 209 F4212 1994]
RG626.F468 1994
618.3′2—dc20
DNLM/DLC
for Library of Congress   94-7115
                                                                                                      CIP

No part of this publication may be reproduced in any form
without permission from the publishers except for
the quotation of brief passages for the purposes of review

Typesetting by AMA Graphics Ltd., Preston, England
Printed and bound by T G Hostench S. A., Spain

Contents

List of principal contributors		ix
Preface		xiii

Section 1 Background

1. The central role of the fetus as a patient in defining an ethical standard of care for fetal therapy — 3
   F. A. Chervenak, L. B. McCullough and A. Kurjak

2. Pregnancy outcome of assisted conception techniques — 11
   A. Samueloff and J. G. Schenker

3. Ontogeny of human lymphocytes during intrauterine life — 19
   G. Lucivero, V. Gambatesa, A. Dell'Osso, M. P. Loria, V. D'Addario, N. Tannoia, L. Bonomo and G. Cagnazzo

4. Prenatal and perinatal development of the human cerebral cortex — 35
   I. Kostović and M. Judaš

5. Screening with ultrasound in obstetrics — 57
   G. P. Mandruzzato, G. D'Ottavio and M. A. Rustico

6. Non-directive prenatal genetic counseling — 71
   Z. Papp, E. Tóth-Pál and Cs. Papp

7. The routine fetal examination — 79
   K. Å. Salvesen and S. H. Eik-Nes

8. Fetal brain pathology — 89
   R. N. Laurini

9. Reproductive decisions after genetic counseling of couples at high risk for cystic fibrosis: a perspective from the last two decades — 107
   Z. Papp, M. Németi, Cs. Papp and E. Tóth-Pál

10. Computer applications in fetal medicine — 117
    I. E. Zador, V. Salari and R. J. Sokol

Section 2 New dimensions in fetal and placental imaging

11	Early detection of congenital anomalies using transvaginal ultrasonography M. M. van Zalen-Sprock, J. M. G. van Vugt and H. P. van Geijn	127
12	Three-dimensional ultrasound in obstetrics and gynecology D. Jurković, E. Jauniaux and S. Campbell	135
13	Sonoembryology in the central nervous system H. Takeuchi	141
14	The multifetal pregnancy: sonographic determination of chorionicity and amnionicity in the first and early-second trimesters A. Monteagudo and I. E. Timor-Tritsch	151
15	The first 3 weeks of gestation assessed by transvaginal color Doppler S. Kupešić and A. Kurjak	161
16	The use of transvaginal sonography in the dynamic evaluation of the uterine cervix in pregnancy I. E. Timor-Tritsch, F. Boozarjomehri and A. Monteagudo	175

Section 3 Assessment of the fetal condition

17	High-order multiple pregnancy S. Mashiach, D. S. Seidman and S. Lipitz	183
18	Computerized evaluation of cardiotocography and its clinical role G. P. Mandruzzato, G. S. Dawes and Y. J. Meir	195
19	Universal intrapartum external monitoring and improved outcome K. Maeda	207
20	Domiciliary fetal heart rate monitoring by telephone S. Uzan, T. Harvey, B. Guyot and M. Uzan	213
21	Assessment of fetal well-being with the actocardiogram and fetal response to acoustic and photic stimuli K. Maeda	225
22	The fetal biophysical profile J. M. Carrera, J. Mallafré and M. Torrents	231
23	Intrauterine growth retardation J. M. Carrera and J. Mallafré	251

24	Computerized analysis of fetal heart rate in normal and growth-retarded fetuses D. Arduini, G. Rizzo and C. Romanini	289
25	Fetal hemodynamics in growth retardation G. Rizzo, D. Arduini and C. Romanini	299
26	Advances in neonatology M. Levene	311
27	Amniotic fluid analysis C. P. O'Reilly-Green and M. Y. Divon	317
28	Prenatal diagnosis of skin disease S. Brenner, A. Kurjak, D. Jurković, T. Kobayasi, R. E. Brandsen, H. Matz and U. Marton	359

Section 4 Doppler ultrasound

29	The prenatal assessment of fetal hypoxia S. Campbell, K. Harrington and C. Lees	381
30	The effect of maternal vasoactive agents on uterine and fetal hemodynamics P. Jouppila, J. Räsänen, S. Alahuhta and R. Jouppila	389
31	Assessment of the hypoxic fetus with color Doppler and automated heart-rate analysis N. Montenegro, J. Bernardes and L. Pereira-Leite	399
32	Doppler velocimetry of the great vessels in fetuses with intrauterine growth retardation: correlation with blood biochemistry and perinatal outcome E. Ferrazzi, M. Bellotti, A. M. Marconi, G. D. Orta and G. Pardi	413
33	Doppler velocimetry of the uterine artery and ischemic–hemorrhagic lesions of the placenta G. P. Bulfamante, E. Ferrazzi, A. Barbera, E. Pollina and G. Pardi	419
34	Venous return in the human fetus J. W. Wladimiroff and T. W. A. Huisman	425
35	Early pregnancy hemodynamics assessed by transvaginal color Doppler A. Kurjak, F. A. Chervenak, D. Zudenigo and S. Kupešić	435
36	Doppler velocimetry in monitoring fetal health during late pregnancy K. Maršál, S. Gudmundsson and H. Stale	455
37	Cerebral circulation in the perinatal period K. Maršál, G. Gunnarsson, D. Ley, A. Maesel and R. N. Laurini	477

Section 5 Fetal therapy

38	Aspirin in pregnancy *S. Uzan and B. Haddad*	491
39	Diagnosis and management of immune thrombocytopenias *K. A. Eddleman, J. B. Bussel and F. A. Chervenak*	505
40	Fetal therapy *L. K. McLean and M. S. Golbus*	517
41	Therapeutic strategies in the management of intrauterine growth retardation *R. N. Pollack and M. Y. Divon*	537
	Index	551

List of principal contributors

D. Arduini
Università di Ancona
Via Corridoni 11
60123 Ancona
Italy

S. Brenner
Department of Dermatology
Tel Aviv Medical Center
Tel Aviv
Israel

G. P. Bulfamante
Departments of Pathology and Obstetrics and Gynecology
Ultrasound Center ISBM San Paolo
University of Milan
Via A. di Rudini 8
20142 Milan
Italy

S. Campbell
Department of Obstetrics and Gynaecology
King's College School of Medicine and Dentistry
Denmark Hill
London SE5 8RX
UK

J. M. Carrera
Institut Universitari Dexeus
Paseo Bonanova 67
08017 Barcelona
Spain

F. A. Chervenak
Department of Obstetrics and Gynecology
The New York Hospital
Cornell Medical Center
525 East 68th Street
New York
NY 10021
USA

K. A. Eddleman
Prenatal Diagnosis, Division of Maternal/Fetal Medicine
Department of Obstetrics and Gynecology
The New York Hospital
Cornell Medical Center
525 East 68th Street
New York
NY 10021
USA

E. Ferrazzi
Department of Obstetrics and Gynecology
Ultrasound Center ISBM San Paolo
University of Milan
Via A. di Rudini 8
20142 Milan
Italy

P. Jouppila
Department of Obstetrics and Gynecology
University of Oulu
SF-90220 Oulu
Finland

D. Jurković
Department of Obstetrics and Gynaecology
King's College School of Medicine and Dentistry
Denmark Hill
London SE5 8RX
UK

I. Kostović
Croatian Institute of Brain Research
Medicical School
University of Zagreb
Šalata 3b
41000 Zagreb
Croatia

S. Kupešić
Ultrasonic Institute
Medical School
University of Zagreb
'Sveti Duh' Hospital
Sveti Duh 64
41000 Zagreb
Croatia

A. Kurjak
Ultrasonic Institute
Medical School
University of Zagreb
'Sveti Duh' Hospital
Sveti Duh 64
41000 Zagreb
Croatia

R. N. Laurini
Division of Developmental and Paediatric
    Pathology
Institute of Pathology
University of Lausanne
25 Rue du Bugnon
1011 Lausanne
Switzerland

M. Levene
Academic Unit of Paediatrics and Child
    Health
University of Leeds
D Floor, Clarendon Wing
The General Infirmary
Belmont Grove
Leeds LS2 9NS
UK

G. Lucivero
Department of Gerontology, Geriatrics and
    Metabolic Diseases
2nd University of Naples
Piazza L. Miraglia
80138 Naples
Italy

L. K. McLean
Departments of Obstetrics, Gynecology,
    Reproductive Sciences and Pediatrics
Reproductive Genetics Unit, Room U-262
San Francisco
CA 94143-0720
USA

K. Maeda
Department of Obstetrics and Gynecology
Seirei Hamamatsu General Hospital
Suniyoshi 2-12-12
Hamamatsu 430
Japan

G. P. Mandruzzato
Department of Obstetrics and Gynecology
Istituto per l'Infanzia
Via dell'Istria 65/1
34100 Trieste
Italy

K. Maršál
Department of Obstetrics and Gynecology
University of Lund
Malmö General Hospital
Malmö
Sweden

S. Mashiach
Department of Obstetrics and Gynecology
The Chaim Sheba Medical Center
52621 Tel Hashomer
Israel

A. Monteagudo
Department of Obstetrics and Gynecology
Sloane Hospital for Women
Columbia Presbyterian Medical Center
622 West 168th Street
New York
NY 10032
USA

N. Montenegro
Department of Obstetrics and Gynecology
Hospital de S. João
Faculdade de Medicina do Porto
4200 Porto
Portugal

C. P. O'Reilly-Green
Montefiore Medical Center
The Jack D. Weller Hospital of the Albert
  Einstein College Medical Division
1825 Eastchester Road
Bronx
New York 10461
USA

Z. Papp
Department of Obstetrics and Gynaecology
Semmelweis University Medical School
Baross utca 27
Budapest
Hungary H-1088

R. N. Pollack
Bikur Cholim Hospital
5 Strauss Street
PO Box 492
Jerusalem
Israel

G. Rizzo
Department of Obstetrics and Gynecology
Università di Roma 'Tor Vergata'
Policlinico Nuovo S. Eugenio
P.le Umanesimo 10
00144 Roma
Italy

K. Å. Salvesen
National Center for Fetal Medicine
Department of Gynecology and Obstetrics
Trondheim University Hospital
N-7006 Trondheim
Norway

A. Samueloff
Department of Obstetrics and Gynecology
Hadassah University Hospital
PO Box 12000
Jerusalem
Israel

H. Takeuchi
Department of Obstetrics and Gynecology
Juntendo University Urayasu Hospital
2-1-1 Tomioka
Urayasu-shi 279
Japan

I. E. Timor-Tritsch
Department of Obstetrics and Gynecology
Sloane Hospital for Women
Columbia Presbyterian Medical Center
622 West 168th Street
New York
NY 10032
USA

S. Uzan
Department of Obstetrics and Gynecology
Hôpital Tenon
4 Rue de la Chine
75020 Paris
France

J. W. Wladimiroff
Department of Obstetrics and Gynaecology
Academic Hospital Rotterdam-Dijkzigt
Dr Molewaterplein 40
3015 GD Rotterdam
The Netherlands

I. E. Zador
Department of Obstetrics and Gynecology
Hutzel Hospital
Wayne State University
4707 St Antoine Boulevard
Detroit
MI 48201-1498
USA

M. M. van Zalen-Sprock
Department of Obstetrics and Gynecology
Free University Hospital
PO 7057
1007 MB Amsterdam
The Netherlands

Preface

The concept of 'the fetus as a patient' has recently emerged. It was not long ago that imagining the fetus as a patient would have been considered science fiction, because the medical profession could not treat, or even diagnose, fetal disorders. Due to the efforts of an interdisciplinary group of dedicated investigators, this has dramatically changed, so that today the concept of the fetus as a patient is part of mainstream obstetric care.

This book bears testament to the fetus as a patient. Section 1 presents background information covering important topics such as ethics, assisted conception, embryology, pathology, counseling, and computers. Section 2 emphasizes new developments in the most important dimension of fetal diagnosis – obstetric ultrasound. Section 3 covers a multitude of methods of assessing the fetal condition, while Section 4 describes the explosion of new information in Doppler ultrasound and its many clinical uses. Section 5 describes innovative approaches to fetal therapy.

We emphasize that the purpose of this book is not to cover each and every aspect of 'the fetus as a patient.' Rather, it emphasizes the most current contributions of the Board of Directors of the International Society of the Fetus as a Patient. Future editions of this book will expand the topics covered and explore new areas, for, while the study of the fetus as a patient has come so far, it is still in its infancy.

Asim Kurjak
Frank A. Chervenak

Section 1

Background

The central role of the fetus as a patient in defining an ethical standard of care for fetal therapy

F. A. Chervenak, L. B. McCullough and A. Kurjak

INTRODUCTION

Fetal medicine is now practiced in an era of increasing innovations in fetal therapy. Preimplantation embryos can be sustained *in vitro* and the capacity to manipulate their genetic and gross structures and functions will continue to increase. We are now able to image the fetus from very early in gestation, to obtain fetal tissue for analysis or transplantation, and to treat fetal anomalies. A battery of diagnostic and therapeutic interventions has also been developed for intrapartum management of pregnancy for fetal indications. The chapters in this book bear testimony to the development of fetal medicine. In summary, fetal medicine is increasingly in the position to do for the fetus what other medical fields offer to other patients, to undertake a wide array of diagnostic and therapeutic interventions and to conduct research on new interventions. In other words, the fetus seems just as much a patient as any other individual, save for its being *in utero*[1-6]. As a consequence, references to the fetus as a patient have become commonplace in the literature and practice of fetal medicine[7-14].

The concept and language of the fetus as a patient developed initially as a by-product of technological advances rather than as a result of careful ethical investigation of the concept of the fetus as a patient and its clinical implications. More recently, the concept of the fetus as a patient and its clinical implications have been examined[1,15]. The purpose of this chapter is to set out the concept of the fetus as a patient and to identify its clinical implications for fetal therapy.

MEDICAL ETHICS: AN OVERVIEW

To talk of the fetus as a patient is to use the language and concepts of medical ethics. This is because protecting and promoting the interests of the patient have constituted the foundation for medical ethics since the days of the Hippocratic Oath[16].

In the ancient version of the Oath the physician swore to do what would benefit the sick, while preventing harm to them[16]. In the technical language of ethics, the Oath should be understood in terms of beneficence-based ethical obligations to patients: the physician is to act in such a way as to produce a greater balance of 'goods' over 'harms', as goods and harms are understood from a clinical perspective[17,18]. Over the centuries, the definition of these goods and harms has been clarified on the basis of what medicine as a profession can reasonably claim as its competencies. The authors believe that on this basis, the goods that medicine is competent to achieve are the prevention of premature death, and the prevention, cure, or at least management of disease, injury, handicap, and unnecessary pain and suffering[1,8]. Pain and suffering are sometimes a necessary price to be paid in the attempt to achieve the other goods of medicine. When pain and suffering occur in the absence of achieving those goods, pain and suffering become unnecessary.

Acting on these goods provides concrete meaning to the fundamental ethical obligation of protecting and promoting the interests of patients.

Beneficence-based clinical judgment and ethical obligations were the whole of medical ethics until our own century. Under the influence of United States common law and philosophical ethics, medical ethics has increasingly come to acknowledge and emphasize the importance of the patient's perspective on her interests and what should count as protecting and promoting her interests[1,19]. The patient is certainly able to form her own judgments about her interests on the basis of her own values and express those judgments in value-based preferences. The ethical principle of respect for autonomy translates this fact into autonomy-based ethical obligations: to acknowledge the integrity of the patient's values in her life; to elicit the patient's value-based preferences; and to assist the patient to put her preference(s) into effect.

Following a well-established and respected ethical theory[20], the authors take the view that autonomy-based obligations are theoretically equally weighted with beneficence-based obligations[1,17]. Beneficence-based and autonomy-based obligations are prima facie: the former cannot be thought automatically to override the latter, nor vice versa. This view of beneficence-based and autonomy-based obligations has been defended in the literature of medical[17,18] and obstetric ethics[1,21,22].

The concepts of autonomy-based clinical judgment and ethical obligations and of beneficence-based clinical judgment and ethical obligations provide a framework in terms of which the concept of the fetus as a patient can be articulated and its clinical implications identified in terms of concrete ethical obligations of the physician to the fetus and to the pregnant woman[1,15]. The distinctive feature of fetal therapy is that there are sometimes two patients and ethical obligations on the physician's part to both must be identified and negotiated[1,21].

THE ETHICAL CONCEPT OF THE FETUS AS A PATIENT

One prominent approach to understanding the concept of the fetus as a patient has involved attempts to show whether or not the fetus has independent moral status[23-32]. Independent moral status for the fetus would mean that one or more of the characteristics possessed either in, or of the fetus itself and, therefore, independently of the pregnant woman or any other factor, generate and therefore ground obligations to the fetus on the part of the pregnant woman and her physician.

A wide range of intrinsic characteristics has been considered for this role, e.g., moment of conception, implantation, central nervous system development, quickening, and the moment of birth[33-35]. Given the variability of proposed characteristics, there are many views about when the fetus does or does not acquire independent moral status. Some take the view that the fetus possesses independent moral status from the moment of conception or implantation[36-38]. Others believe that the fetus acquires independent moral status in degrees, thus resulting in 'graded' moral status[30-32]. Still others hold, at least implicitly, that the fetus never has independent moral status so long as it is *in utero*[31].

Despite a voluminous philosophical and theological literature on this subject, there has been no agreement on a single authoritative account of the independent moral status of the fetus[39,40]. This outcome should surprise no one, given the absence of a single methodology that would be authoritative for all of the markedly diverse theological and philosophical schools of thought involved in this centuries-old debate. In the absence of such a methodology, agreement on the independent moral status of the fetus should not be expected. For agreement ever to be possible, intramural and transmural debates about such a final authority within and between theological and philosophical traditions would have to be resolved in a way satisfactory to all. This is an inconceivable event. It is best, therefore, to set aside futile attempts to understand the fetus as a patient in terms of whether or not the fetus possesses independent moral status and turn to an alternative approach. This approach makes it possible to identify ethically distinct senses of the fetus as a patient and their clinical implications. We need to ask not 'Does the fetus have independent moral status?' but, as Warnock puts it, 'How ought we to treat the fetus[41-42]?'

This alternative approach starts with the recognition that being a patient does not require that one possesses independent moral status[29]. Instead, being a patient means that one can benefit from the application of the clinical skills of the physician. Put more precisely, a human being without independent moral status is properly regarded as a patient when the following conditions are met: that a human being is presented to the physician for the purpose of applying clinical interventions that are reliably expected to be efficacious, in that they are reliably expected to result in a greater balance of goods over harms in the future of the human being in question[1,15].

In other words, an individual is considered a patient when a physician has beneficence-based ethical obligations to that individual. There have been some beneficence-based discussions of the fetus as a patient[43,44]. More recently, the senses in which beneficence-based approaches illuminate the concept of the fetus as a patient have been identified[1,15].

We begin as follows: because the independent moral status of the fetus cannot be established, there can be no autonomy-based obligations to the fetus. To clarify the concept of the fetus as a patient, it is, therefore, appropriate to turn to an account of when there are beneficence-based obligations to the fetus.

The authors have argued elsewhere that beneficence-based obligations to the fetus exist when the fetus can achieve independent moral status, which occurs in early childhood[1]. That is, the fetus is a patient when medical interventions, whether diagnostic or therapeutic, reasonably can be expected to result in a greater balance of goods over harms in the future of the fetus, when independent moral status is achieved. The ethical significance of the concept of the fetus as a patient, therefore, depends on links that can be established between the fetus and the ability to later achieve its independent moral status.

THE VIABLE FETUS AS A PATIENT

One such link is viability, establishing a basis for the first ethical sense of the fetus as a patient. Viability, however, cannot be understood as an intrinsic property of the fetus because viability must be understood in terms of both biological and technological factors[40,45,46]. Both factors are required for a viable fetus to exist *ex utero* and thus later achieve its independent moral status. Interestingly, these two factors do not exist as a function of the autonomy of the pregnant woman. When a fetus is viable, i.e., when it is of sufficient maturity so that it can survive into the neonatal period and later achieve independent moral status given the availability of the requisite technological support, then the fetus is a patient[1,47]. Any beneficence-based obligations to the viable fetus must, of course, be negotiated with beneficence-based and autonomy-based obligations to the pregnant woman[21].

Viability thus exists partly as a function of biomedical and technological capacities, which are different in different parts of the world. As a consequence there can, at the present time, be no worldwide uniform gestational age to define viability. In the United States, the authors believe that viability presently occurs at approximately 24 weeks of gestational age[48,49].

THE PREVIABLE FETUS AS A PATIENT

The only possible link between the previable fetus and its ability to later achieve independent moral status is the pregnant women's autonomy, which provides the sole basis for the second ethical sense of the fetus as a patient. Technological factors cannot result in the previable fetus later achieving independent moral status. This is simply what previable means. A link, therefore, between a previable fetus and the later achievement of its independent moral status can be established only by the pregnant woman's decision to confer the status of being a patient on her previable fetus. The previable fetus, therefore, because it cannot reliably be thought to possess independent moral status, has no claim to the status of being a patient independently of the pregnant woman's autonomy. It follows that the pregnant woman is free to withhold, confer, or, having once conferred, withdraw the status of being a patient on or from her previable fetus according to her own values. In other words, the previable fetus is a patient solely as a function of the pregnant woman's autonomy[1,47].

A subset of the second sense of the fetus as a patient includes *in vitro* embryos. It might seem, at first, that the *in vitro* embryo is a patient because such an embryo is presented to the physician. However, for there to be beneficence-based obligations to a human being without independent moral status, it also must be the case that the medical interventions are reliably expected to be efficacious to the future of that human being.

Simply being presented to a physician does not make the *in vitro* embryo a patient. This is because, in terms of beneficence, whether the fetus is a patient depends also on links that can be established between the fetus and its future, i.e., later achieving its independent moral status. Therefore, the 'reasonableness' of medical interventions on the *in vitro* embryo depends on whether that embryo later becomes viable. Otherwise, no benefit of such intervention can meaningfully be said to result. An *in vitro* embryo, therefore, becomes viable only when it survives *in vitro* cell division, transfer, implantation, and subsequent gestation to such a time as it becomes capable of survival.

This process of achieving viability occurs *in vivo* and is therefore entirely dependent on the woman's decision regarding the status of the fetus(es) as a patient, should assisted conception successfully result in the gestation of the previable fetus(es). Whether an *in vitro* embryo will benefit the fetus are both functions of the pregnant woman's decision to withhold, confer, or, having once conferred, withdraw the moral status of being a patient on or from the previable fetus(es) that might result from assisted conception. It therefore is appropriate to regard the *in vitro* embryo as a previable rather than a viable fetus. As a consequence, any *in vitro* embryo(s) should be regarded as a patient only when the woman into whose reproductive tract the embryo(s) will be transferred confers that status[1,47].

In summary, the viable fetus is a patient. The previable fetus including the *in vitro* embryo, is a patient solely as a function of the exercise of the woman's autonomy.

AN ETHICAL STANDARD OF CARE FOR FETAL THERAPY

Whether invasive fetal therapy can be judged to be a standard of care on ethical grounds depends on the clinical implications of the concept of the fetus as a patient. Such fetal therapy must reliably be thought, on the basis of documented clinical experience, to benefit the child that the fetus can become. Recall that the ethical content of this concept is to be understood, not simply in terms of physical accessibility, but also in terms of whether clinical interventions on the fetus are reliably thought to be efficacious, in that they are reliably expected to result in a greater balance of goods over harms for the child the fetus can become.

Satisfying this condition establishes an ethical standard of care for fetal therapy in its initial, beneficence-based sense. This ethical concept of standard of care, however, cannot be completely understood until its autonomy-based dimensions are considered.

The pregnant woman is under no ethical obligation to confer the status of being a patient on her previable fetus simply because there exists a fetal therapy that meets the preceding beneficence-based condition. Whether such therapy is to be judged an ethical standard of care for her fetus is also a function of the pregnant woman's autonomy. Thus, satisfaction of beneficence- and autonomy-based conditions is necessary for fetal therapy to be reliably judged to be an ethical standard of care for previable fetuses.

The same is true for fetal therapy on the viable fetus. Such a fetus is properly judged to be a patient. However, as noted above, beneficence-based obligations to the fetus must be negotiated with beneficence-based and autonomy-based obligations to the pregnant woman. This is because of a factual consideration – fetal therapy necessarily involves physical and, perhaps, mental health risks to the pregnant woman – and an ethical consideration – she is ethically obliged only to accept reasonable risks to herself in order to attempt to benefit her fetus[1,21].

The afore-mentioned information helps to distinguish an ethical from a legal standard of care for fetal therapy. An ethical standard must take account not only of beneficence-based considerations applied to the fetus but also of both beneficence-based and autonomy-based considerations applied to the pregnant woman. A legal standard of care tends to focus on efficacy and safety, which are beneficence-based considerations applied to both the fetus and, perhaps, the pregnant woman. The legal standard of care tends to ignore autonomy-based considerations applied to the pregnant woman. This constitutes the fundamental difference between a legal and an ethical standard of care for fetal therapy.

THERAPY AND EXPERIMENTAL THERAPY FOR THE VIABLE FETAL PATIENT

There is no simple algorithm by which a pregnant woman, or her physician, can reach the judgment that she is obliged to accept risk to herself on behalf of her viable fetus. In the authors' view, such an ethical obligation – which should not be equated automatically with a legal obligation – exists when three criteria are satisfied. The first criterion concerns the outcome of the procedure for the fetus and the child it can become. The other two criteria concern risks of harm for the viable fetus and the child it can become as well as the pregnant woman. The three criteria are the following:

(1) When invasive therapy of the viable fetus has a very high probability of being life-saving or of preventing serious and irreversible disease, injury, or handicap for the fetus and for the child the fetus can become;

(2) When such therapy involves low mortality risk and low or manageable risk of serious disease, injury, or handicap to the viable fetus and the child it can become; and

(3) When the mortality risk to the pregnant woman is very low, and when the risk of disease, injury, or handicap to the pregnant woman is low or manageable[1,15].

The justifications for these criteria are both beneficence- and autonomy-based. When the first two criteria are satisfied there is a clear and substantial net benefit to the viable fetal patient. When the third criterion is satisfied there is no clear and substantial net harm to the pregnant woman. Given the expected net benefit to the viable fetal patient and the low risk of harm to the pregnant woman, the latter are risks she should reasonably be expected to accept[1,21], for example, as in intravascular transfusion for severe isoimmunization. This moral fact shapes how she should exercise her autonomy in response to her beneficence-based fiduciary ethical obligations to her fetus.

Under beneficence- and autonomy-based clinical judgment, therefore, treatment of the viable fetal patient is warranted when these three criteria are satisfied. The burden of ethical proof rests with those who would propose further ethical obligations when one or more of these three criteria cannot be satisfied. This should be a matter of further careful investigation and debate in the ethics of fetal therapy.

When the pregnant woman is ethically obliged to accept fetal therapy of her viable fetal patient, such management is ethically, though not necessarily legally, judged to be a justified ethical standard of care. Any forms of fetal therapy for which an ethical obligation (as defined above) on the part of the pregnant woman to accept them cannot be established must be regarded as experimental. For example, because open abdominal fetal surgery involves significant risks to the fetus and risks that no pregnant woman can be understood, at this time, to be obliged to accept on behalf of an attempt to benefit her viable fetus, all such surgery must, on ethical grounds, be regarded as experimental. This would only change if the risks to the fetus and the pregnant woman of such therapy someday satisfy the three aforementioned criteria.

In the case of the viable fetal patient the physician is ethically justified in recommending fetal therapy. There is a vital role in this process for the exercise of the woman's autonomy in assessing the risks and benefits to herself and to her fetus. These matters should be explained carefully to the pregnant woman. The benefits and risks of both invasive and non-invasive fetal therapy should be explained without bias, in a clear and understandable manner, to the pregnant woman. She should be given time to reflect, to consult with those close to her or other physicians, and to reach her own decision.

How should the physician respond if the pregnant woman rejects fetal therapy of a viable fetus that satisfies an ethically justified standard of care? Certainly, informed consent as an ongoing dialogue with the pregnant woman should be the first response. In undertaking a further response – negotiation, the physician should acknowledge and take into account the pregnant woman's assessment of the risks and benefits of fetal therapy to herself and her fetus. It is justified to go beyond negotiation to respectful persuasion, and perhaps even to an ethics committee, as part of a preventive ethics clinical strategy[50].

Whether resort should be made to legal intervention is a matter of considerable dispute in the literature on the intrapartum management of pregnancy[51-53]. Given the newness of much fetal therapy, especially invasive fetal therapy, and the fact that few forms of such therapy satisfy all three criteria for an ethical standard of care, it is unclear how courts of law might respond. It is also unclear whether resort to legal intervention bodes well for the future development of new experimental forms of fetal therapy.

Experimental therapy (that is, situations in which one or more of the three criteria are not satisfied) of the viable fetus can be offered to the pregnant woman. That is, unlike the case of 'standard of care' therapy, there is no ethical justification to recommend experimental fetal therapy because there is no clear net benefit to the fetus or there is a clear net harm to the pregnant woman. Moreover, experimental therapy can be offered with ethical confidence only if there is a formal, scientifically sound protocol for the research and that protocol has been approved by the appropriate institutional review process. Obviously, discussion of experimental fetal therapy with the pregnant woman should be rigorously non-directive[1,54].

THERAPY AND EXPERIMENTAL THERAPY FOR THE PREVIABLE FETAL PATIENT

There are two subgroups of previable fetuses. The first comprises those upon whom the pregnant woman has conferred the status of being a patient. When she has done so and the three criteria for an ethical standard of fetal therapy are also satisfied, then it is ethically justified to recommended fetal therapy. This situation is directly analogous to informed consent to therapy for the viable fetal patient and the strategies discussed above apply. When one or more of the three criteria are not satisfied, fetal therapy should be regarded as experimental and should only be offered, not recommended, to the pregnant woman.

When the pregnant woman withholds or withdraws the status of being a patient from her previable fetus, all counseling should be non-directive, even when the three criteria for an ethically justified standard of care for fetal therapy are met[1,54]. This is because there is no ethical obligation on the part of the pregnant woman or the physician to regard the previable fetus as a patient. It follows that any discussion of experimental fetal therapy must be strictly non-directive.

CONCLUSION

The authors are aware that some clinicians may take the view that an ethical standard of care for fetal therapy that is based in large part on respect for the pregnant woman's autonomy is unrealistic, because of the strong, perhaps even coercive, psychological pressure pregnant women may experience when confronted with an imperiled pregnancy and the availability of fetal therapy. To the contrary, the authors are well aware of such a phenomenon and have sought to address its main ethical implication, namely, the possible impairment of the exercise of the pregnant woman's autonomy. Indeed, our emphasis on the place and importance of non-directive counseling is meant precisely as the most powerful antidote to such impairment. In other words, there is no reason whatever to believe, and substantial ethical stakes in not acting on the belief, that such self-imposed, psychological pressure is in all cases irreversible and therefore irresistible. Physicians should avoid the unjustified paternalism implicit in such a belief.

References

1. McCullough, L. B. and Chervenak, F. A. (1994). *Ethics in Obstetrics and Gynecology*. (New York: Oxford University Press)
2. Harrison, M. R., Golbus, M. S. and Filly, R. A. (1988). *The Unborn Patient*. (New York: Grune & Stratton)
3. Liley, A. W. (1972). The fetus as a personality. *Aust. N. Zeal. J. Psychiatry*, **6**, 99–105
4. American Academy of Pediatrics Committee on Bioethics (1988). Fetal therapy: ethical considerations. *Pediatrics*, **81**, 898–9
5. American College of Obstetricians and Gynecologists. *Committee on Ethics (1987). Patient Choice: Maternal–Fetal Conflict*. (Washington, D.C.: American College of Obstetricians and Gynecologists)
6. American College of Obstetricians and Gynecologists. *Technical Bulletin (1989). Ethical Decision-making in Obstetrics and Gynecology*. (Washington, D.C.: American College of Obstetricians and Gynecologists)
7. Mahoney, M. J. (1978). Fetal-maternal relationship. In Reich, W. T. (ed.) *Encyclopedia of Bioethics*, pp. 485–94. (New York: Macmillan)
8. Fletcher, J. C. (1981). The fetus as patient: ethical issues. *J. Am. Med. Assoc.*, **246**, 772–3
9. Pritchard, J. A., MacDonald, P. C. and Gant, N. F. (1985). *Williams Obstetrics*, (17th edn.) p. xi. (Norwalk: Appleton-Century-Crofts)
10. Shinn, R. L. (1985). The fetus as patient: a philosophical and ethical perspective. In Milunski, A. and Annas, G. J. (eds.) *Genetics and the Law III*. (New York: Plenum Press)
11. Murray, T. H. (1987). Moral obligations to the not-yet born: the fetus as patient. *Clin. Perinatol.*, **14**, 313–28
12. Mahoney, M. J. (1989). The fetus as patient. *West. J. Med.*, **150**, 517–40
13. Newton, E. R. (1980). The fetus as patient. *Med. Clin. N. Am.*, **73**, 517–40
14. Walters, L. (1986). Ethical issues in intrauterine diagnosis and therapy. *Fetal Ther.*, **1**, 32–7
15. Chervenak, F. A. and McCullough, L. B. (1991). An ethically based standard of care for fetal therapy. *J. Mat. Fetal Investigation*, **1**, 175–80
16. Edelstein, L. (1967). The Hippocratic Oath: text, translation, and interpretation. In Temkin, O. and Temkin, C. L. (eds.). *Ancient Medicine: Selected Papers of Ludwig Edelstein*, pp. 3–63. (Baltimore: The Johns Hopkins Press)
17. Beauchamp, T. L. and Childress, J. F. (1989). *Principles of Biomedical Ethics* (3rd edn.). (New York: Oxford University Press)
18. Beauchamp, T. L. and McCullough, L. B. (1984). *Medical Ethics: The Moral Responsibilities of Physicians*. (Englewood Cliffs: Prentice-Hall)
19. Faden, R. and Beauchamp, T. L. (1986). *History and Theory of Informed Consent*. (New York: Oxford University Press)
20. Ross, W. D. (1930). *The Right and the Good*. (Oxford: Clarendon Press)
21. Chervenak, F. A. and McCullough, L. B. (1985). Perinatal ethics: a practical method of analysis of obligations to mother and fetus. *Obstet. Gynecol.*, **66**, 442–6
22. Field, D. R., Gates, E. A., Creasy, R. K., *et al.* (1988). Maternal brain death during pregnancy: medical and ethical issues. *J. Am. Med. Assoc.*, **260**, 816–22
23. Engelhardt, H. T., Jr. (1986). *The Foundations of Bioethics*. (New York: Oxford University Press)
24. Strong, C. (1987). Ethical conflicts between mother and fetus in obstetrics. *Clin. Perinatol.*, **14**, 313–28
25. Anderson, G. and Strong, C. (1988). The premature breech: cesarean section or trial of labor? *J. Med. Ethics*, **14**, 18–24
26. Ford, N. M. (1988). *When Did I Begin? Conception of the Human Individual in History, Philosophy and Science*. (Cambridge: Cambridge University Press)
27. Strong, C. and Anderson, G. (1989). The moral status of the near-term fetus. *J. Med. Ethics*, **15**, 25–7

28. Fleming, L. (1987). The moral status of the fetus: a reappraisal. *Bioethics*, **1**, 15–34
29. Ruddick, W. and Wilcox, W. (1982). Operating on the fetus. *Hastings Center Rep.*, **12**, 10–4
30. Dunstan, G. R. (1984). The moral status of the human embryo. A tradition recalled. *J. Med. Ethics*, **10**, 38–44
31. Elias, S. and Annas, G. J. (1987). *Reproductive Genetics and the Law*. (Chicago: Year Book Medical Publishers)
32. Evans, M. I., Fletcher, J. C., Zador, I. E., et al. (1988). Selective first-trimester termination in octuplet and quadruplet pregnancies: clinical and ethical issues. *Obstet. Gynecol.*, **71**, 289–96
33. Curran, C. E. (1987). Abortion: contemporary debate in philosophical and religious ethics. In Reich, W. T. (ed.) *Encyclopedia of Bioethics*, pp. 78–26. (New York: Macmillan)
34. Noonan, J. T. (1970). *The Morality of Abortion*. (Cambridge: Harvard University Press)
35. Hellegers, A. E. (1970). Fetal development. *Theological Studies*, **31**, 3–9
36. Noonan, J. T. (1979). *A Private Choice. Abortion in America in the Seventies*. (New York: The Free Press)
37. Bopp, J. (1984). *Restoring the Right to Life: The Human Life Amendment*. (Provo: Brigham Young University)
38. Bopp, J. (1985). *Human Life and Health Care Ethics*. (Frederick: University Publications of America)
39. Callahan, S. and Callahan, D. (1984). *Abortion: Understanding Differences*. (New York: Plenum Press)
40. *Roe vs. Wade*. (1973). 410 US 113
41. Warnock, M. (1987). Do human cells have rights? *Bioethics*, **1**, 1–14
42. Hare, R. M. (1987). An ambiguity in Warnock. *Bioethics*, **1**, 175–8
43. Fletcher, J. C. (1983). Ethics and trends in applied human genetics. *Birth Defects: Original Article Series*, **19**, 143–58
44. Fletcher, J. C. (1984). Ethical considerations. In Harrison, M. R., Golbus, M. S. and Filly, R. A. (eds.) *The Unborn Patient*, pp. 159–170. (New York: Grune & Stratton)
45. Fost, N., Chudwin, D. and Wikker, D. (1980). The limited moral significance of fetal viability. *Hastings Center Rep.*, **10**, 10–3
46. Mahowald, M. (1989). Beyond abortion: refusal of cesarean section. *Bioethics*, **3**, 106–21
47. Chervenak, F. A. and McCullough, L. B. (1990). Does obstetric ethics have any role in the obstetrician's response to the abortion controversy? *Am. J. Obstet. Gynecol.*, **163**, 1425
48. Hack, M. and Fanaroff, A. A. (1989). Outcomes of extremely-low-birth-weight infants between 1982 and 1988. *N. Engl. J. Med.*, **321**, 1642–7
49. Whyte, H. E., Fitzhardinge, P. M., Shennan, A. T., et al. (1993). Extreme immaturity: outcome of 568 pregnancies of 23–26 weeks' gestation. *Obstet. Gynecol.*, **82**, 1–7
50. Chervenak, F. A. and McCullough, L. B. (1990). Clinical guides to preventing ethical conflicts between pregnant women and their physicians. *Am. J. Obstet. Gynecol.*, **162**, 303–7
51. Annas, G. J. (1988). Protecting the liberty of pregnant patients. *N. Engl. J. Med.*, **316**, 1213–4
52. Nelson, L. J. and Milliken, N. (1988). Compelled treatment of the pregnant woman: life, liberty, and law in conflict. *J. Am. Med. Assoc.*, **259**, 1060–6
53. Chervenak, F. A. and McCullough, L. B. (1991). Justified limits on refusing intervention. *Hastings Center Rep.*, **21**, 12–18
54. Chervenak, F. A. and McCullough, L. B. (1991). The fetus as patient: implications for directive versus non-directive counseling for fetal benefit. *Fetal Diagnostic Ther.*, **6**, 93–100

Pregnancy outcome of assisted conception techniques

A. Samueloff and J. G. Schenker

Since the birth of Louise Brown, more than a decade ago[1], tens of thousands of babies have been born worldwide following assisted conception techniques (ACT) such as *in vitro* fertilization and embryo transfer (IVF/ET), gamete intrafallopian transfer (GIFT) and zygote intrafallopian transfer (ZIFT).

The conventional method by which success of any infertility therapy is judged is by pregnancy rate after specified periods of treatment. However, in the final analysis, the most important result for the parents is the likelihood of having a healthy baby. Consideration of the obstetric outcome of ACT is of great importance since controversy exists in the literature whether the methods used are well established or still empirical and how best to evaluate their success rate.

In trying to evaluate the obstetric outcome of ACT, major limitations exist since scattered studies have control groups in their study population and there is a lack of long term follow-up of babies born.

In view of our experience and the data published in the literature, we would like to discuss in this chapter different topics associated with pregnancy outcome such as maternal complications, multiple pregnancy, and complications of late pregnancy.

COMPLICATIONS OF EARLY PREGNANCY

Demographic studies have suggested that in healthy couples the chances of producing one viable offspring is 25–30% in a given menstrual cycle[2,3]. This suggests that fecundity in humans is relatively low or may reflect a high incidence of early pregnancy loss. The incidence of clinical pregnancy in ACT programs is now approaching 25%, a rate comparable to that of maternal conception yet with a high clinical abortion rate (20–38%)[4].

ABORTIONS

The early and continuous β-human chorionic gonadotropin (hCG) monitoring after embryo transfer allowed the detection of very early pregnancy losses, designated biochemical pregnancies or preclinical abortions occurring before any clinical evidence of pregnancy. It is for this reason that Steer and colleagues[5] suggested that the most effective way of diagnosing a viable pregnancy after assisted conception techniques is by detecting a fetal heart at 4–6 weeks' gestation from follicular rupture. This method also minimizes the psychological impact of pregnancy testing for the patient.

The reported incidence of clinical abortion associated with ACT ranges from 19–33.6%[6–13]. The risk is related to gestational age, most abortions occurring in the first trimester.

Several authors have concluded that the incidence of clinical abortion is higher in pregnancies resulting from ACT than with natural conceptions[10,12,14]. Such comparisons may be complicated by the use of different definitions of pregnancy and abortions, by different methods of calculating abortion rate and by failing to take gestational age at the time of abortion into account.

In natural conception, embryo loss may be due to genetic or environmental factors, developmental mechanisms, anatomical anomalies, endocrine imbalance, infectious disease and immunological factors. In ACT the hormonal manipulations may generate genetically incompetent oocytes or may create a hormonal imbalance in the luteal phase. The ACT culture environment and the technique itself may also effect oocyte and/or embryo quality. Finally, advanced maternal age could be a contributing factor. Liu and Rosenwaks[11] in trying to elucidate possible mechanisms of pregnancy loss found two types of hCG secretory patterns in pregnancies resulting in miscarriages, one with normal titers in early pregnancy that fell out of the normal range shortly before abortion (normal doubling time 24.6–43.2 h) and the other with initial and consistently low hCG titers (prolonged doubling > 43.2 h). Others[15] looked at a single hCG value at day 14–16 as a predictor for pregnancy outcome. Additionally, all miscarriages demonstrated a decrease in serum progesterone alone or concomitant with decreasing serum estradiol concentrations indicating insufficient corpus luteum functions.

In the majority of term pregnancies, implantation occurred between day +7 and day +13[11,16]; late implantation resulted in a high incidence of clinical abortions or preclinical abortions.

The incidence of abortion increases with increasing maternal age and when there is a previous adverse obstetrical history[17].

In conclusion, the increased probability of abortion in ACT represents most probably early detection rather than a greater tendency to fetal wastage.

ECTOPIC PREGNANCY

The incidence of ectopic pregnancy has been estimated to range from 0.27–1.29% of diagnosed conceptions, pregnancies or live births[18–20] for women in the normal reproductive age range. The incidence appears to be increasing over the last few decades and has been attributed to increased use of intrauterine contraceptive devices, pelvic inflammatory disease, sterilization and reversal of sterilization.

The risk for ectopic pregnancy following ACT ranges from 3–17%[4,20–24]. The apparently high incidence of ectopic pregnancy in ACT is a serious complication of the procedures that deserves detailed analysis to try to determine the cause. It looks as if the problem is multifactorial and is composed of factors such as accidental direct insertion of the embryos into the tubes, spontaneous migration of the embryos out of the uterine cavity, increasing number of transfers, the large volume of transfer medium, the use of drugs for induction of ovulation, the high levels of estradiol in the preovulatory phase, and finally, tubal damage[12,25,26].

A wide variety of different types of ectopic pregnancy occurring after ACT have been reported in the literature such as unilateral tubal twin implantation, abdominal pregnancies, cervical pregnancies and heterotropic pregnancies, all having a higher rate after ACT compared to spontaneous pregnancies.

It is for this reason that close clinical monitoring after ACT should be maintained for diagnosis and intervention to ensure safety for the mother and to preserve any simultaneous uterine pregnancy.

It is surprising that ectopic pregnancy does not appear to be related to the clinically diagnosed cause of the patient's infertility and furthermore none of the possible causes previously mentioned have been shown directly to cause this high rate of ectopic pregnancy.

FETAL MALFORMATION

In the last years the rate of congenital malformations associated with ACT was carefully studied and was found to be around 2–3%[4,23,27–32]. Even though there are several reports of extremely low and extremely high incidences of congenital malformations[33–35], in general the incidence of congenital and chromosomal malformation in children resulting from ACT was found not to exceed that of the normal population. Factors which could theoretically raise the risk of congenital malformations after IVF have been reviewed by several authors[35–39]. These factors include the relatively advanced age of infertile couples, increasing the risk of some chromosomal abnormalities and mutational events, the underlying causes of infertility, the drugs used to induce ovulation or for luteal phase support and the ACT themselves. Additionally, the induction of chromosomal aberrations, the increase in the rate of fertilization by abnormal spermatozoa, the induction of point mutations and finally the action of physical and chemical teratogens were all mentioned as possible causes for malformation in ACT.

In general, it is agreed that no specific malformations were significantly increased but some authors mention that a higher than expected number of central nervous system, urogenital, limb and chromosomal malformations were observed.

It is important, however, that data collection continues and that the findings from different countries are pooled together in order to finally solve the important issue. ACT made pre-embryo research more feasible and it is believed that more information will be available on this subject in the coming years.

MULTIPLE PREGNANCY

The incidence of naturally occurring multiple births is about 1% for twins, 0.01–0.017% for triplets and a much lower occurrence rate for higher order multiple pregnancy[40–42].

The use of ovulation induction agents and ACT increased the incidence of multiple pregnancies more than 10 times[43,44]. It is reported that the rate of multiple pregnancies in ACT ranges from 4–25%[4,23,43,45–48] with an average rate of 22%, representing the major complication of outcome in ACT, which is prematurity. Since in the majority of cases of ACT, more than one embryo or ovum is transferred, multiple pregnancy is common. It was found that the average number of babies born per delivery correlates with the number of embryos or ova transferred[29], i.e. an average of 1.3 babies are born per delivery when three embryos are transferred and an average of 1.8 babies when eight embryos are transferred. It is for this reason that in the majority of ACT programs not more than two to four embryos or ova are transferred per cycle.

Although the majority of twin pregnancies after ACT are dizygotic, due to multiple embryo transfer, some monozygotic pregnancies have been described[49].

Multifetal pregnancy should be considered as one of the main complications of ACT since it exposes the woman to increased maternal morbidity and is associated with increased perinatal morbidity and mortality.

Patients undergoing ACT commonly belong to the older age group which itself ranks this population 'at risk'. Moreover, multifetal pregnancies are known to be associated with an increased incidence of pre-eclampsia, placenta previa and abruption, premature rupture of the membranes, postpartum hemorrhage and Cesarean section, causing greater morbidity to these patients[4,43,47]. Early and late abortions, stillbirths and perinatal morbidity and mortality due to prematurity represent the main problem of fetuses from multiple pregnancies.

Limited data are available on the fetal outcome of multiple pregnancies[31,43,45–48] and it appears as if fetuses from ACT multifetal pregnancies are doing much better than previous reports regarding multiple pregnancies. The perinatal mortality in singletons, twins and triplets range from 5–23/1000, 20–38.5/1000 and 0–37/1000, respectively, and available data on quadruplets are of no statistical significance since such information is based on case reports.

Our impression is that perinatal mortality has dropped dramatically for multifetal pregnancies resulting from ACT. This is attributed to several factors: firstly, fetuses from multifetal pregnancies born in ACT have benefited from the availability of improved neonatal care when compared to earlier studies. Secondly, although these pregnancies occurred in patients with a fertility problem, the patients are invariably highly motivated and tend to strictly adhere to medical instructions. Their antenatal care would have been intensive and the majority were delivered in perinatal centers with experienced neonatal departments. Thirdly, all these pregnancies were diagnosed early by ultrasound scan and complications were therefore anticipated well in advance (in previous studies up to 20% were undiagnosed) and finally, the mode of delivery for triplets and quadriplets being mainly Cesarean section could contribute to the improvement of perinatal mortality.

In evaluating peripartum events and neonatal outcome from studies on twins, triplets and quadruplets following ACT[31,43,46–48,50,51]. The mean gestational age at delivery was 35.5, 31.8 and 31 weeks, respectively[43] and indeed, 41% of twins are delivered prematurely and the majority of triplets and quadruplets (75–99%) are born premature. As such, there is a proportionally progressive increase in neonatal complications. The mean weight for twins is around 2450 g, for triplets 1700 and quadruplets 1300 g.

Therefore, it is quite obvious that the rate of admissions to neonatal intensive care units of twins, triplets and quadruplets was high – 22.7%, 64.1% and 75%, respectively, and the length of stay was 12, 17.4 and 57.8 days, respectively.

In general, neonatal morbidity as reflected by the percentage of admissions to neonatal intensive care units significantly increased from twins to triplets to quadruplets and was not statistically different from previous non-ACT reported groups[52–55].

Finally, the sex ratio in multifetal pregnancies is comparable with that of naturally occurring ones.

In recent years, there has been an increasing trend toward selective reduction in multiple pregnancies of higher order including triplets and quadruplets arguing that the perinatal mortality and morbidity are lower in the twins[56–58]. The recent data on ACT multiple pregnancies support selective termination for higher order multiple pregnancies, but here is doubt regarding reduction of triplets and quadruplets.

To prevent multifetal pregnancies and their undesired consequences, ovulation induction drugs should be used with caution, and fewer embryos should be transferred in ACT practice. Recently, Nijs and colleagues[59] recommended that in order to reduce the high frequency of multiple gestations, the number of embryos replaced should be limited to a maximum of two.

OBSTETRIC COMPLICATIONS

When evaluating the obstetric complications in ACT and comparing them with the normal population, three factors must be taken into account:

(1) Women who achieve pregnancy after ACT are usually older, and it is well recognized and established[60–62] that older women are more prone to obstetric complications;

(2) A high percentage of the women undergoing ACT suffer from primary infertility and previous adverse pregnancy outcome, factors which are known to increase the obstetric risks; and

(3) Multifetal pregnancy – a very common event in ACT is associated with high rates of maternal complications.

Tan[46] compared the obstetric complications of ACT pregnancies to normally conceived ones and found that the risk for ACT singleton pregnancies as compared to controls (spontaneously conceived) was significantly higher ($p < 0.05$) for having antenatal bleeding, hypertension, placenta previa and fetal growth retardation. Similar results were found by Frydman and co-workers[8]; the reason for the increased incidence of hypertension in his group was thought to be the larger number of primigravidas and the older maternal age in the ACT group. Hill[10] found no increased incidence of hypertension in ACT pregnancies as compared with an obstetric population matched for maternal age, race and date of delivery. Furthermore, his study showed no difference in the incidence of diabetes mellitus, premature rupture of membranes, fetal growth retardation and placenta previa when compared to the control group. Since suitable comparative data are lacking, no conclusions can be drawn about whether ACT has any specific direct effect on obstetric complications.

LABOR AND DELIVERY

When considering fetal presentation in ACT pregnancies, there is an increase in breech presentation ranging from 13.9–16%[8,23,46]. This high incidence is mainly attributed to the high frequency of multiple births and preterm labor.

In most studies reporting the mode of delivery of ACT pregnancy, there is an increase in the Cesarean section rate. In Britain, 49% of deliveries associated with ACT were by Cesarean section[23], and in Australia and New Zealand, 44%[63]. Cohen and colleagues from France[64] reported 46.8% and Andrews and associates from the USA[65] reported a 56% Cesarean section rate. 'True' contributors to this high rate of Cesarean section are probably multifetal pregnancies (which in triplets and higher order reach 98–100% Cesarean section) and pathological lies at birth which are higher in ACT pregnancies. However, it is well accepted that the anxiety surrounding the management of these pregnancies probably influences the decision as to the mode of delivery.

The gestational ages at delivery and the birth weights of the fetuses varied considerably according to the multiplicity of the birth. This difference is in part due to the high proportion of multiple births associated with ACT. However, when singletons and twins are considered separately, the gestational ages are younger. Tan and colleagues[46] reported an overall of 25% preterm deliveries and 14% for singleton opposed to 6% and 7.9% in control pregnancies, respectively. The reason for the high frequency of preterm delivery and additionally low birth weight is unclear. The mean birth weight declines with the number of fetuses but still for singleton ACT babies the mean birth weight is lower (Table 1).

HEALTH OF THE CHILDREN

The available, commonly used indicators for health of the children are perinatal mortality, Apgar score and long-term follow-up.

The overall mortality rates of ACT fetuses from different registries varies from 22.8 to 44.7[29,45,66,67]. This relatively high rate emanated mainly from newborns of multiple pregnancies whereas the perinatal mortality rate for singletons are not significantly different according to standardized rates and ranges from 11–15/1000.

The risk of other adverse parameters on the health of the children increases, as accepted with increasing multiplicity. Summarized by Beral and colleagues[23], mean Apgar score declines with increasing multiplicity and on the other hand the mean stay of babies in special care units and fetal jaundice increases. Comparative data for births conceived naturally are lacking and therefore comparisons are usually done with national registry data with their limitations.

Overall, the sex ratio of ACT pregnancies is similar to 'naturally' conceived babies and ranges from 0.98:1 to 1.1:1 according to various reports.

Finally, no evaluation of the long-term health and development of the children from ACT has yet been performed. Raul-Duval[68] studied the psychomotor development of IVF fetuses as compared to the naturally conceived fetuses and found that in the postpartum, the minor mother–infant relationship problems seemed to be more frequent in IVF pregnancies, but with no statistical differences. At 9 months, the factors related to sleep disturbances in the child and maternal depressive syndromes seemed to be more frequent in pregnancies resulting from IVF than in the controls. At 18 months, these minor disturbances decreased and there were fewer differences across the three groups. This trend was confirmed at 3 years.

Evaluation and interpretation of the findings on ACT pregnancy outcome should be carried out with caution. The patients are older, presumably with a higher income, come from potential parents who may have genetic or medical disorders and they receive special treatments to induce ovulation. However, the most impor-

Table 1 *Results of various studies showing birth weight (g) in assisted conception technique and control pregnancies*

	MRC study[29]	Hill et al.[10]	Tan et al.[46]	Friedler et al.[45]	Frydman et al.[8]	Seoud et al.[43]
Singleton	3151	3431	3123	3044	—	—
Twins	2353	—	2388	2372	3249	2473
Triplets	1836	—	1895	1743	—	1666
Control singleton		3395	3275	3221	3273	—

tant determinant for the success of the pregnancies and the health of the children is the high frequency of multiple births. It is important that data collection continues and that findings from different countries are pooled together in order to properly evaluate pregnancy outcome of ACT.

References

1. Edwards, R. G., Steptoe, P. C. and Purdy, J. M. (1980). Establishing full term human pregnancies using cleaving embryos grown in vitro. Br. J. Obstet. Gynaecol., **87**, 735
2. Sheps, M. C. (1965). An analysis of reproductive patterns in an American isolate. Pop. Stud. (NY), **21**, 65
3. Vessey, M., Doll, R., Petro, R., Johnson, R. and Wiggins, P. (1961). A long term follow-up study of women using different methods of contraception: An interim report. J. Biosoc. Sci. **8**, 373
4. Ezra, Y. and Schenker, J. G. (1993). Appraisal of in vitro fertilization. Eur. J. Obstet. Gynecol. Reprod. Biol., **48**, 127
5. Steer, C., Campbell, S., Davies, M., Mason, B. and Collins, W. (1989). Spontaneous abortion rates after natural and assisted conception. Br. Med. J., **299**, 1317
6. National Perinatal Statistics Unit and the Fertility Society of Australia. (1988). IVF and GIFT Pregnancies Australia and New Zealand, 1987. (Sydney: National Perinatal Statistics Unit (NPSU))
7. Cohen, J., Mayaux, M. J. and Guihard-Moscato, M. L. (1988). Pregnancy outcomes after in vitro fertilization. A collaborative study on 2342 pregnancies. Ann. NY Acad. Sci., **54**, 1
8. Frydman, R., Belaisch-Allart, J., Fries, N., Hazout, A., Glissant, A. and Testart, J. (1986). An obstetric assessment of the first 100 births from the in vitro fertilization program at Clamart, France. Am. J. Obstet. Gynecol., **154**, 550
9. Society for Assisted Reproductive Technology, The American Fertility Society. (1993). Assisted reproductive technology in the United States and Canada: 1991 results from the Society for Assisted Reproductive Technology generated from the American Fertility Society Registry. Fertil. Steril., **59**, 956
10. Hill, G. A., Bryan, S., Herbert, C. M. III, Shah, D. M. and Wentz, A. C. (1990). Complications of pregnancy in infertile couples: Routine versus assisted reproduction. Obstet. Gynecol., **75**, 790
11. Liu, H. and Rosenwaks, Z. (1991). Early pregnancy wastage in IVF (in vitro fertilization) patients. J. In Vitro Fertil. Embryo Transfer, **8**, 72
12. Lancaster, P. A. L. (1988). Outcome of pregnancy. In Wood, C. and Trounson, A. (eds.) Clinical In Vitro Fertilization, p. 81. (Berlin: Springer Verlag)
13. Kol, S., Levron, J., Lewit, M., Drugan, A. and Itskovitz-Eldor, J. (1993). The natural history of multiple pregnancies after assisted reproduction: its spontaneous fetal demise a clinically significant phenomenon? Fertil. Steril., **60**, 127
14. Goldman, J. A., Ashkenazi, J., Ben-David, M., Feldberg, D., Dicker, D. and Voliovitz, I. (1988). First trimester bleeding in clinical IVF pregnancies. Hum. Reprod., **3**, 807
15. Heiner, J. S., Kerin, J. F., Schmidt, L. L. and Jackson, T. C. (1992). Can a single early quantitative human chorionic gonadotropin measurement in an in vitro fertilization–gamete intrafallopian transfer program predict pregnancy outcome? Fertil. Steril., **58**, 373
16. Edmonds, D. K., Lindsay, K. S., Miller, J. F., Williamson, E. and Wood, P. J. (1982). Early embryonic mortality in women. Fertil. Steril., **38**, 447
17. Edwards, R. G. and Steptoe, P. C. (1983). Current status of in vitro fertilization and implantation of human embryo. Lancet, **2**, 1265
18. Barnes, A. B., Wennberg, C. N. and Barnes, B. A. (1983). Ectopic pregnancy: incidence and review of determinant factors. Obstet. Gynaecol., Survey, **38**, 345
19. Rubin, G. L., Peterson, M. B., Dorfman, S. F., Layde, P. M., Maze, J. M., Ory, H. W. and Kope, W. (1983). Ectopic pregnancy in the United States 1970 through 1978. J. Am. Med. Assoc., **249**, 1725
20. Westrom, L., Bengtsson, L. P. H. and Mardh, P. A. (1981). Incidence, trend and risks of ectopic pregnancy in a population of women. Br. Med. J., **282**, 14
21. Guirgis, R. R. and Craft, I. L. (1991). Ectopic pregnancy resulting from gamete intrafallopian transfer and in vitro fertilization. Role of ultrasonography in diagnosis and treatment. J Reprod. Med., **36**, 793
22. Martinez, F., Trounson, A. (1986). An analysis of factors associated with ectopic pregnancy in a human in vitro fertilization program. Fertil. Steril., **45**, 79
23. Beral, V., Doyle, P., Tan, S. L., Mason, B. A. and Campbell, S. (1990). Outcome of pregnancies

resulting from assisted conception. *Br. Med. Bull.* **46**, 753

24. Lopata, A. (1983). Concepts in human *in vitro* fertilization and embryo transfer. *Fertil. Steril.*, **40**, 289
25. Iffy, L. (1976). Reflux theory of ectopic implantation. *Lancet*, **2**, 1091
26. Kerin, J. F., Warnes, G. M., Quinn, P. J., Kirby, C., Seamark, R. F., Jeffrey, R., Matthews, C. D. and Cox, L. W. (1983). Incidence of multiple pregnancy after *in vitro* fertilization and embryo transfer. *Lancet*, **2**, 537–40
27. Sas, M. (1977). Obstetric results and problems after induction of ovulation. Geburtshilfliche Eergebnisse und Probleme nach Ovulatiosinduktion. *Fortschr. Med.*, **212**
28. Wennerholm, U. B., Janson, P. O., Wennergrean, M. and Kjellmer, I. (1991). Pregnancy complications and short-term follow-up of infants born after *in vitro* fertilization and embryo transfer (IVF/ET). *Acta Obstet. Gynecol. Scand.*, **70**, 565
29. Report of the MRC Working Party (1990). Children conceived by *in vitro* fertilization. Births in Great Britain resulting from assisted conception, 1978–1987. *Br. Med. J.*, **300**, 1229
30. Lancaster, P. A. (1985). Obstetric outcome. *Clin. Obstet. Gynecol.*, **12**, 847
31. Rizk, B., Doyle, P., Tan, S. L., Rainsbury, P., Betts, J., Brinsden, P. and Edwards, D. (1991). Perinatal outcome and congenital malformations in *in vitro* fertilization babies from the Bourn-Hallam group. *Hum. Reprod.*, **6**, 1259
32. Simpson, J. L. and Carson, S. A. (1992). Preimplantation genetic diagnosis. *N. Engl. J. Med.*, **327**, 951
33. Plachot, M. (1989). Choosing the right embryo: the challenge of the nineties. *J. In Vitro Fertil Embryo Transfer*, **6**, 193
34. Huang, T. Jr., McNamee, P., Kosasa, T., Silva, J., Hale, R. W., Terada, F., Chun, B. and Morton, C. (1991). Birth of the first babies in Hawaii after conception *in vitro*: experience at the Pacific In-Vitro Fertilization Institute. *Hawaii Med. J.*, **50**, 358
35. Biggers, J. D. (1981). *In vitro* fertilization and embryo transfer in human beings. *N. Engl. J. Med.*, **304**, 336
36. Lancaster, P. (1987). Congenital malformations after *in-vitro* fertilization. *Lancet*, **2**, 1392
37. Schlesselmann, J. J. (1979). How does one assess the risk of abnormalities from human *in-vitro* fertilization: *Am. J. Obstet. Gynecol.* **135**, 135
38. Shoham, Z., Zosmer, A. and Insler, V. (1991). Early miscarriage and fetal malformations after induction of ovulation (by clomiphene citrate and/or human menotropins) *in vitro* fertilization and gamete intrafallopian transfer. *Fertil. Steril.*, **55**, 1
39. Shields, L. E., Serafini, P. C., Schenken, R. S. and Moore, C. M. (1992). Chromosomal analyais of pregnancy losses in patients undergoing assisted reproduction. *J. Assisted Reprod. Genet.*, **9**, 57
40. Spellacy, W. N., Handler, H. and Ferre, C. D. (1990). Case–control study of 1253 twin pregnancies from 1982–1987 perinatal data base. *Obstet. Gynecol.*, **75**, 168
41. Olofsson, P. (1990). Triplet and quadruplet pregnancies – a forthcoming challenge for the 'general obstetrician'. *Eur. J. Obstet. Gynecol. Reprod. Biol.*, **35**, 159
42. Collins, M. S. and Bleyl, J. A. (1990). Seventy-one quadruplet pregnancies. Management and outcome. *Am. J. Obstet. Gynecol.*, **162**, 1384
43. Seoud, M. A. F., Toner, J. P., Kruithoff, C. and Muasher, S. J. (1992). Outcome of twin triplet and quadruplet in *in vitro* fertilization pregnancies: the Norfolk experience. *Fertil. Steril.*, **57**, 815
44. *In vitro* fertilization–embryo transfer (IVF–ET) in the United States. 1989 Results from the IVF-ET Registry. (1991). *Fertil. Steril.*, **55**, 14
45. Friedler, S., Mashiach, S. and Laufer, N. (1992). Births in Israel resulting from *in vitro* fertilization/embryo transfer 1982–1989: National Registry of the Israeli Association for Fertility Research. *Hum. Reprod.*, **7**, 1159
46. Tan, S., Dogle, P., Campbell, S., Beral, V., Rizk, B., Brinsden, P., Mason, B. and Edwards, R. G. (1992). Obstetric outcome of *in vitro* fertilization pregnancies compared with normally conceived pregnancies. *Am. J. Obstet. Gynecol.*, **167**, 778
47. Seoud, M. A. F., Kruithoff, C. and Muasher, S. J. (1991). Outcome of triplet and quadruplet pregnancies resulting from *in vitro* fertilization. *Eur. J. Obstet. Gynecol. Reprod. Biol.*, **41**, 79
48. Kingsland, C. R., Steer, C. V., Pampiglione, J. S., Mason, R. A., Edwards, R. G. and Campbell, S. (1990). Outcome of triplet pregnancies resulting from IVF at Bourn Hallam 1984–1987. *Eur. J. Obstet. Gynecol. Reprod. Biol.*, **34**, 197
49. Yovich, J., Stanger, J. and Gravaug, A. (1984). Monozygotic twins from *in vitro* fertilization. *Fertil. Steril.*, **6**, 833
50. Daw, D. (1978). Triplet pregnancy. *Br. J. Obstet. Gynaecol.*, **85**, 505
51. Leslie, G. I., Brown, J. R., Arnold, J. D. and Saunders, D. M. (1992). *In vitro* fertilization and neonatal ventilator use in a tertiary perinatal center. *Med. J. Aust.*, **156**, 165
52. Kovacs, B. W., Kirschbaum, T. H. and Richard, P. (1989). Twin gestations: I. Antenatal care and complications. *Obstet. Gynecol.*, **74**, 313

53. Newman, R. B., Hamer, C. and Miller, C. (1989). Outpatient triplet management: A contempory review. *Am. J. Obstet. Gynecol.*, **161**, 547
54. Sassoon, D. A., Castro, L. C., Davis, J. L. and Hobel, C. J. (1990). Perinatal outcome in triplet vs. twin gestations. *Obstet. Gynecol.*, **75**, 817
55. Thompson, S. A., Lyons, T. L. and Makowski, E. L. (1987). Outcome of twin gestation at the University of Colorado Health Sciences Centre, 1973–1983. *J. Reprod. Med.*, **32**, 328
56. Lynch, L., Berkowitz, R. L., Chitakara, U. *et al.* (1990). First trimester transabdominal multiple pregnancy reduction: a report of 85 cases. *Obstet. Gynecol.*, **75**, 735
57. Evans, M. I., May, M., Drugan, A. *et al.* (1990). Selective termination: clinical experience and residual risks. *Am. J. Obstet. Gynecol.*, **162**, 1568
58. Evans, M. I., Littmann, L., King, M. and Fletcher, I. C. (1992). Multiple gestation: the role of multifetal pregnancy reduction and selective termination. *Clin. Perinatol.*, **19**, 345
59. Nijs, M., Geerts, L., Van Roosendael, E., Segal-Bertin, G., Vanderzwalman, P. and Schogsman, R. (1993). Prevention of multiple pregnancies in an *in vitro* fertilization program. *Fertil. Steril.*, **59**, 1245
60. Berkowitz, G. S., Skovron, M. L., Lapinski, R. H. and Berkowitz, R. L. (1990). Delayed childbearing and the outcome of pregnancy. *N. Engl. J. Med.*, **322**, 659
61. Cnattingius, S., Forman, M. R., Berendes, H. W. and Isolato, L. (1992). Delayed childbearing and risk of adverse perinatal outcome. *J. Am. Med. Assoc.*, **268**, 886
62. Hansen, J. P. (1986). Older maternal age and pregnancy outcome: a review of the literature. *Obstet. Gynecol. Survey*, **41**, 726
63. National Perinatal Statistics Unit. (1988). *IVF and GIFT Pregnancies, Australia and New Zealand, 1987* (Sydney, Australia: NPSU)
64. Cohen, J., Mayaux, M. J. and Guihar-Moscato, M. L. (1988). Pregnancy outcome after *in vitro* fertilization. *Ann. NY Acad. Sci.*, **54**, 1
65. Andrews, M. C., Muasher, S. J., Levy, D. L., Jones, H. W., Garcia, J. E., Rozenwaks, Z., Jones, G. S. and Acosta, A. A. (1986). An analysis of the obstetric outcome of 125 consecutive pregnancies conceived *in vitro* and resulting in 100 deliveries. *Am. J. Obstet. Gynecol.*, **154**, 848
66. Saunders, D. M. and Lancaster, P. A. L. (1990). Pregnancy rates and perinatal outcome in Australia and New Zealand. In Mashiach, ? *et al.* (eds.) *Advances in Assisted Reproductive Technologies*, p. 1019. (New York: Plenum Press)
67. De Mouzon, J., Bachelot, A., Logerot-Lebrun, H. and le Bureau de FIVNAT. (1990). *Dossier FIVNAT 90. Analyse de resultats 1986–1990.* (Paris: Le Bureau de FIVNAT)
68. Raoul-Duval, A., Bertrand-Servais, M. and Frydman, R. (1993). Comparative prospective study of the psychological development of children born by *in vitro* fertilization and their mothers. *J. Psychosom. Obstet. Gynecol.*, **14**, 117

Ontogeny of human lymphocytes during intrauterine life

G. Lucivero, V. Gambatesa, A. Dell'Osso, M. P. Loria, V. D'Addario, N. Tannoia, L. Bonomo and G. Cagnazzo

INTRODUCTION

Fetal lymphopoiesis

Throughout fetal life, the immune system develops in an environment such as the maternal uterus, that might be considered relatively free of foreign antigens, even if viruses, but not bacteria, can be transmitted through the placenta. The yolk sac, liver and bone marrow are the most relevant sites of hematopoiesis at early stages of embryonal and fetal development. Lymphopoiesis has not been observed in the yolk sac, but during gestation lymphocytes have been detected in the liver at the 6th week, in the thymus and spleen at the 8th, in the lymphatic plexus at the 9th and in lymph nodes at the 11th week[1]. In the 7–9-week-old embryos, lymphocytes have been observed in blood[2], and lymphocyte subsets can be identified in the fetal liver at the 13th week of gestation[3]. The number of fetal lymphocytes/mm^3 of blood increases during gestation more rapidly than those of granulocytes and monocytes: at 17 weeks, the lymphocyte count reaches 50% of the value that will be observed at birth[4]. The high number of lymphocytes since early stages of embryo–fetal development might be related to the basic requirements needed for the immune system to function properly: first, synthesis and expression of an impressive number of distinct antigen-specific receptors on B and T lymphocytes and, secondly, induction of tolerance towards 'self' antigens[5,6].

Diversity of antigen-specific receptors

A fundamental immunological phenomenon that occurs at the fetal stage of development is the genetically determined and antigen-independent synthesis and expression of a very broad spectrum of diverse antigen-specific receptors on the membrane of B and T lymphocytes. This phenomenon requires a high rate of lymphocyte generation and, at single cell level, assembling of variable region genes (both for immunoglobulins and T-cell receptors) from germline gene segments by a common, site-specific DNA recombination system referred to as VDJ recombinase[7,8] (V = variability; D = diversity; J = joining). Immunoglobulin heavy chain V region gene rearrangement during early B-cell ontogeny develops in an ordered and restricted manner: at 130 days of gestation, the repertoire of Vh genes expressed by early B cells is restricted to only 9–39 genes[9]. After synthesis and expression of complete antigen-specific receptors and cessation of VDJ recombination, the virgin lymphoid cells migrate from the primary sites of generation to colonize the secondary or peripheral lymphoid organs. Primary B-cell follicles, that appear as nodular collections of small lymphocytes positive for surface IgM, can be observed in the human spleen at 23 weeks of gestation[10].

Induction of tolerance

During intrauterine life, the cells of the immune system progressively acquire antigen-specific receptors and other surface molecules; moreover, they develop the biochemical machinery needed to recognize foreign antigens and to react towards them after birth; but, on the other hand, when virgin cells bearing self-reactive receptors encounter the related autologous antigens, a tolerogenic signal must be delivered to the cell in order to avoid dangerous immune reactions towards autologous tissues. It can be hypothesized that during intrauterine life, some molecules on the membrane of lymphocytes and/or a peculiar milieu of cytokines or growth factors cause lymphocytes reacting with specific (mainly 'self') antigens to negative clonal selection by inducing apoptosis or functional anergy[5].

Lymphocyte differentiation antigens

Early in ontogeny, precursor lymphoid cells do not possess functional capabilities and express on their surface only few of the molecules (or differentiation antigens) that later on will be borne by mature and functionally active lymphocytes. In the last few years, rapid progress has been made in the identification, biochemical and functional analysis of many surface molecules synthesized and expressed by lymphocytes in a lineage and/or differentiation-restricted manner[11]. These surface molecules act as receptors, can transmit signals through the membrane and contribute in different ways to regulate cell activation beside the antigen-specific T- or B-cell receptors. Timing of appearance of several molecules on the membrane of lymphocytes during gestation reveals a sequence of expression that is common in several species. This finding strongly suggests that these surface molecules are indispensable for lymphoid differentiation and that their timely appearance is fundamental in deciding the fate of immature lymphocytes[12].

At early stages of development, immune reactivity of virgin cells is mainly committed towards tolerance induction, while at birth and later in life, reaction with foreign antigens induces clonal expansion, development of effector cells and generation of memory cells. We hypothesize that phenotypic and functional analysis of lymphoid cells at different stages of development might provide some clues to recognizing surface molecules relevant for transmission of tolerogenic signals in virgin cells reactive with self antigens.

The role of cytokines and growth factors

Specific cytokines and growth factors play a role in lymphocyte proliferation and development of specialized functions in effector cells. However, to date, little information is available on the capacity of fetal lymphocytes to produce different lymphokines and, the reverse, their responsiveness to cytokines. Knowing this, it might be anticipated that some cytokines can regulate tolerance induction during fetal life.

These hypotheses might be verified by phenotypic and functional studies of lymphoid cells obtained from human fetuses: the comparison between surface phenotypes and functions in human fetuses during gestation and the correlations with similar results in neonates and adults can allow a deeper understanding of the normal development of the immune system and the progressive acquisition of immune functions.

MATERIALS AND METHODS

Availability of fetal material

In humans, ethical issues, difficulties in obtaining fetal material and lack of availability of precisely timed samples during gestation are all limiting factors in studying ontogeny of the immune system during gestation. Nevertheless, several studies have been performed on this topic by using blood samples drawn by chordocentesis from fetuses undergoing prenatal diagnosis at 16–22 weeks of gestation, umbilical cord blood samples collected from neonates (after Cesarean section or spontaneous delivery), and blood or tissues (mainly liver, spleen, thymus, lymph nodes) obtained from spontaneously aborted fetuses.

Written informed consent from the pregnant women and approval of experimental research projects by ethical committees must be obtained by the researchers for complete respect of human rights.

Phenotypic analysis

Analysis of surface molecule expression on lymphocyte suspensions from blood samples or cell suspensions from tissues have been performed by immunofluorescence techniques. In the literature some discrepancies exist both in the percentages and in the absolute numbers of the three major lymphocyte populations (T, B and natural killer lymphocytes) and in their subsets. Changes in sample preparation, staining procedures (direct or indirect immunofluorescence techniques, staining of whole blood or separated lymphocytes) and instruments for analysis and counting of stained cells (fluorescence microscope or flow cytometer) account for most of the differences within the published results of phenotypic analysis of fetal or neonatal lymphocyte subsets. First of all, the interval of time between blood sampling, staining and analysis should be limited to a few hours. Direct immunofluorescence (by using mouse monoclonal antibodies conjugated to fluorochromes) reduces non-specific binding to lymphocytes and furthermore allows simultaneous analysis of two or three surface molecules on a single cell, by combined staining with distinct monoclonal antibodies conjugated to fluorescein isothiocyanate, phycoerythrin or peridinin chlorophyll and multidimensional 3-color analysis. In analyzing cord blood lymphocytes, the percentages of positive cells for several surface molecules can differ significantly, whether staining by fluorochrome-conjugated monoclonal antibodies is performed on leukocytes from lysed whole blood or on Ficoll–Hypaque separated mononuclear cells. Several factors justify these discrepancies. With the lysed whole blood technique, 'lymphoid' cells might be contaminated by erythroblasts, by immature red cells resistant to lysis (as shown by detection of glycophorin A-positive cells) and by monocytes, as indicated by the percentage of CD14+ cells[13]. However, mononuclear cell separation over a density gradient can lead to selective loss of lymphocyte subsets and does not avoid contamination of lymphoid cells with monocytes. Caution is needed in interpreting or comparing results obtained with different techniques and the potential pitfalls of each method must always be kept in mind. Flow cytometry analysis is now widely used to evaluate cell suspensions after staining with fluorochrome-conjugated monoclonal antibodies; indeed the time-consuming and tedious counting of fluorescent cells with a fluorescence microscope is just a memory of older immunologists. However, even with the most advanced instruments, correct calibration of flow cytometers and proper negative/positive controls are needed in order to obtain reproducible results.

Immunohistochemistry can be performed on 4-μm sections prepared from tissue blocks of frozen fetal tissue using enzyme-conjugated reagents[14].

Functional studies

Fetal or neonatal human lymphocytes have been analyzed in a variety of *in vitro* experimental systems in order to obtain data on immune functions such as the synthesis and secretion of immunoglobulins, ability to exert helper and/or suppressor activity, cytotoxicity and lymphokine production.

Methods in our studies

Phenotypic analysis by flow cytometry We have analyzed the phenotypes of circulating lymphoid cells on blood samples drawn by chordocentesis from fetuses at 18–22 weeks of gestation and from the umbilical cords on the placental side after spontaneous delivery of normal neonates and cutting of funis. In both cases, blood samples were obtained from the pregnant women after written informed consent. Fetal blood samples were drawn from fetuses undergoing prenatal diagnosis of Cooley's disease, by a two-needle, ultrasound and biopsy-guided procedure[15]. The results presented in this review refer to blood samples from fetuses not affected by Cooley's disease.

The determination of lymphoid cell immunophenotypes in fetal and neonatal blood samples has been performed by direct immunofluorescence staining with fluorescein isothiocyanate (FITC)- or phycoerythrin-conjugated murine monoclonal antibodies specific for human leukocyte antigens and by flow cytometry analysis. The monoclonal antibodies specific for CD1, CD2, CD3, CD4, CD5, CD10, CD16, CD19, CD20, CD23, CD28, CD38, CD56, CD57, T-cell receptors α/β, T-cell receptors γ/Δ, CD45RA, CD45RO and HLA-DR surface molecules were purchased from Becton Dickinson (Mountain View, CA, USA). The FITC-conjugated and affinity-purified goat antisera specific for human μ or δ heavy immunoglobulin chains were from Southern Biotechnology Associates Inc., Birmingham, AL, USA. Briefly, 40 μl aliquots of whole fetal blood or 100 μl aliquots of neonatal blood were incubated at room temperature for 20 min with 10 or 20 μl, respectively, of FITC- or phycoerythrin-conjugated monoclonal antibodies specific for two distinct leukocyte surface antigens. FITC- or phycoerythrin-conjugated murine monoclonal antibodies specific for molecules unrelated to human leukocyte antigens were used as negative controls.

To detect surface μ or δ immunoglobulin heavy chains, aliquots of fetal or neonatal blood were washed twice in phosphate-buffered saline (PBS) before incubation with 10 μl of goat anti-human IgM or IgD antisera, diluted 1:50 in PBS with 0.1% sodium azide.

After incubation, the red blood cells were lysed by adding 2 ml of FACScan lysing solution (from Becton Dickinson, Milan, Italy). The leukocytes were then washed twice in PBS, resuspended in 1 ml of filtered PBS and analyzed by a FACScan (Becton Dickinson) flow cytometer equipped with an argon-ion laser at 488 nm. The percentages of cells positive for the examined surface markers were calculated on the lymphoid cell population, 'gated' by forward scatter and side-scatter parameters. The intensity of antigen expression on lymphoid cells was determined by evaluating the mean channel number of fluorescence in the positive cell population. To detect the simultaneous expression of two different surface antigens on single cells, aliquots of blood were incubated as previously indicated with two monoclonal antibodies specific for distinct surface molecules and conjugated, respectively to FITC or phycoerythrin. The biparametric flow cytometry analysis of lymphoid cells was performed after compensation adjustment to minimize the spectral overlap of the FITC and phycoerythrin detector channels.

In vitro culture of neonatal lymphocytes

Lymphocyte cultures were carried out after purification of mononuclear cells from neonatal blood diluted 1:4 in PBS on a Ficoll–Hypaque density gradient. Mononuclear cells were resuspended in RPMI-1640 medium supplemented with 10% fetal calf serum, 2 mM L-glutamine, 100 units/ml of penicillin and 100 μg/ml of streptomycin at the concentration of 1×10^6 cells/ml. The lymphocyte cultures were established in flat-bottom wells of 24-well tissue culture plates (from Falcon, Cat. No.76.008.05) at the concentration of 2×10^6 cells/well and stimulated with 50 μl of phytohemagglutinin (from Difco Laboratories, Detroit, MI, USA). At intervals of 2–6 days, cultured cells were examined to evaluate the expression of activation molecules such as HLA-DR antigens, CD71 or receptor for transferrin and of different isoforms of the CD45 leukocyte molecule by CD3+ lymphocytes.

RESULTS

Phenotypic changes of lymphocytes during intrauterine life

T-cell lineage

As shown in Tables 1 and 2, more than 60% of lymphocytes in fetal (18–22 weeks of gestation) blood samples express the CD7 and CD2 membrane antigens. More than 95% of CD7+ cells bear the CD5 and CD3 molecules. A low proportion of fetal CD7+ lymphocytes does not express CD3; these cells are likely to co-express the CD1 antigen. A mean of 43% of lymphoid cells are CD4+, while the CD8 molecule is expressed by 20% of cells. Approximately 4% of lymphocytes bear simultaneously the CD4 and CD8 antigens. Indirect evidence suggests that these cells are CD1+. In the fetus, the great majority of CD7+ and CD3+ lymphocytes expresses, respectively, the CD38 and the CD28 molecules. The analysis of T-cell receptor expression has shown that 90% of CD3+ cells bear the α/β and 4% the γ/δ T-cell receptor. This observation implies that 5% of circulating CD3+ cells are still lacking the T-cell receptor at 18–22 weeks of gestation. Seven percent of CD3+ lymphocytes express the CD25 antigen or 55 kDa chain of the interleukin-2 receptor. A low percentage (< 2%) of T lymphocytes express the HLA-DR antigens.

Table 1 *Percentages of lymphoid cells in fetal or newborn blood samples expressing surface molecules related to leukocytes and lymphoid cells*

Surface molecules*	% Positive cells (mean ± SD)	
	Fetal blood	Newborn blood
CD7	63 ± 7	61 ± 8
CD2	60 ± 9	62 ± 6
CD3	59 ± 8	57 ± 5
CD5†	57 ± 7	56 ± 7
CD1	5 ± 3	3 ± 2
CD4	43 ± 8	47 ± 6
CD8	20 ± 6	19 ± 5
CD4 + CD8	4 ± 2	3 ± 1

*The CD designation refers to the classification of leukocyte surface antigens elaborated at the IVth International Workshop on Human Leukocyte Differentiation Antigens, Vienna, February 21–25, 1989; **the results refer to the values obtained in 20 fetal and 18 newborn blood samples; †the percentages refer to CD5+CD19− cells

Table 2 *Simultaneous expression of two surface molecules by CD7+ or CD3+ lymphoid cells in fetal or newborn blood samples*

Surface molecules*	Percentages of CD7+ or CD3+ cells expressing a second molecule (mean ± SD)**	
	Fetal blood	Newborn blood
CD7 + CD38	92 ± 6	90 ± 4
CD3 + CD28	95 ± 4	75 ± 18
CD3 + TCR (α/β)	92 ± 5	90 ± 3
CD3 + TCR (γ/δ)	4 ± 2	4 ± 2
CD3 + CD45RA	73 ± 9	81 ± 12
CD3 + CD45RO	11 ± 6	4 ± 2
CD3 + CD25	7 ± 3	5 ± 2
CD3 + HLA-DR	< 2	< 2

*The CD designation refers to the classification of leukocyte surface antigens elaborated at the IVth International Workshop on Human Leukocyte Differentiation Antigens, Vienna, February 21–25, 1989; **the results refer to the values obtained in 20 fetal and 18 newborn blood samples. TCR, T cell receptor

Finally 70% and 11% of fetal CD3+ cells bear, respectively, the RA and RO isoforms of the CD45 leukocyte antigens.

When similar analyses were performed on lymphocytes from umbilical cord blood, we observed a decrease in the percentages of CD1+ cells and a slight increase in the percentages of CD2+ and CD4+ lymphocytes. In cord blood, the CD38 molecule is still expressed by the majority of CD3+ cells, while only 75% of T cells bear the CD28 antigen. A decrease was observed in the percentages and fluorescence intensity (evaluated as mean fluorescence channel number for positive cells) of lymphocytes positive for CD25 and HLA-DR antigens. No significant changes were observed in the percentages of CD3+ T cells bearing the α/β or γ/δ receptors; compared to the fetal lymphocytes, 80% of neonatal CD3 T cells expressed the CD45RA isoform, while only 4% bore the CD45RO.

B-cell lineage

In fetal blood, approximately one out of four lymphoid cells is a B lymphocyte bearing the CD19 surface molecule (Tables 3 and 4). At this stage of development most CD19+ B cells co-express surface IgM and CD20; surface IgD is detectable on 65% of total B cells. It is noteworthy that 50% of CD20+ B cells express the CD10 antigen at low fluorescence intensity (Figure 1).

Table 3 *Percentages of lymphoid cells in fetal or newborn blood samples expressing B-cell-related surface molecules*

Surface molecules*	% Positive cells (mean ± SD)**	
	Fetal blood	Newborn blood
CD19	23 ± 8	13 ± 3
CD20	19 ± 5	12 ± 4
IgM	21 ± 9	12 ± 3
IgD	15 ± 7	11 ± 4
C5	17 ± 11	9 ± 3
CD10	10 ± 4	3 ± 2

*The CD designation refers to the classification of leukocyte surface antigens elaborated at the IVth International Workshop on Human Leukocyte Differentiation Antigens, Vienna, February 21–25, 1989; **the results refer to the values obtained in 20 fetal an 18 newborn blood samples

Table 4 *Simultaneous expression of two surface markers by CD19+ B lymphoid cells in fetal and newborn blood samples*

Surface molecules*	Percentages of CD19+ cells expressing a second molecule (mean ± SD)**	
	Fetal blood	Newborn blood
CD19 + CD5	74 ± 18	69 ± 13
CD19 + CD10	45 ± 16	13 ± 8
CD19 + IgM	91 ± 10	85 ± 15
CD19 + IgD	65 ± 15	82 ± 12
CD19 + CD20	85 ± 10	90 ± 8
CD19 + CD21	35 ± 11	75 ± 4
CD19 + CD23	31 ± 10	51 ± 21
CD19 + CD28	52 ± 13	45 ± 16
CD19 + CD38	91 ± 9	80 ± 11

*The CD designation refers to the classification of leukocyte surface antigens elaborated at the IVth International Workshop on Human Leukocyte Differentiation Antigens, Vienna, February 21–25, 1989; **the results refer to the values obtained in 20 fetal and 18 newborn blood samples

Table 5 *Percentages of lymphoid cells in fetal or newborn blood samples expressing surface molecules related to natural killer cells and progenitor/proliferating cells*

Surface molecules*	% Positive cells (mean ± SD)**	
	Fetal blood	Newborn blood
CD56	12 ± 7	14 ± 6
CD16	6 ± 3	9 ± 4
CD57	0	< 1
CD34	5 ± 3	4 ± 2
CD71	5 ± 3	4 ± 3
HLA-DR†	3 ± 1	3 ± 2

*The CD designation refers to the classification of leukocyte surface antigens elaborated at the IVth International Workshop on Human Leukocyte Differentiation Antigens, Vienna, February 21–25, 1989; **the results refer to the values obtained in 20 fetal and 18 newborn blood samples; †the percentages refer to HLA/DR+ CD19– cells

More than 75% of B cells bear the CD5 antigen while the CD21 and CD23 molecules are expressed by only one out of three B cells. More than 90% of B cells express the CD38, and only 50% of CD19+ lymphocytes bear the CD28 antigens.

The percentages of CB CD19+ cells are lower than those observed in fetal blood. The expression of surface IgM, CD20 and CD5 by CD19 B cells does not change significantly during intrauterine life. A marked reduction (down to 3%) is observed in the percentages of B cells co-expressing the CD10 molecule; on the contrary, up to 75% and 50% of neonatal B cells express the CD21 and CD23 surface molecules. The expression of CD28 and CD38 antigens by B lymphocytes tends to decline from 18 weeks of gestation until birth.

Natural killer cells

Twelve percent of fetal lymphoid cells bear the CD56 molecule (Table 5); approximately 50% of these cells co-express the CD16 surface antigen, while the CD57 is undetectable. This observation implies that 50% of fetal natural killer cells are CD56+ CD16– CD57–. In the neonate the CD57 molecule is still undetectable, while a slight increase in the percentages of CD16+ cells can be observed.

Precursor and proliferating cells

Three to eight percent of fetal mononuclear cells bear the CD34 antigen. Double marker experiments have shown that the majority of CD34+ cells are also positive for the CD71 or transferrin receptor and HLA-DR antigens. Similar observations have been made in the neonate.

Expression of activation antigens by cord blood lymphocytes

After 48 h of phytohemagglutinin activation more than 90% of cord blood CD3+ T lymphocytes synthesize and express on the membrane the CD25 and CD71 molecules, while 80% of T cells are positive for the HLA-DR antigens. At the 4th day of culture more than 95% of CD3+ T cells bear simultaneously the CD25, CD71 and HLA-DR antigens; on the 6th day, depending upon culture conditions, a decline in the percentages of T cells expressing CD25 and CD71 molecules is usually observed. Before stimula-

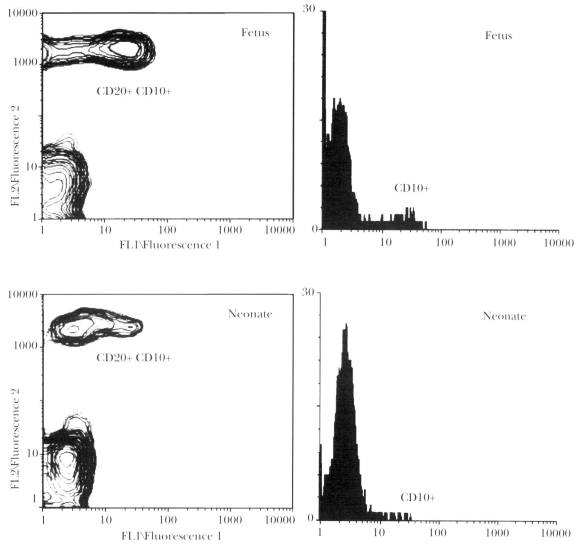

Figure 1 *The contour plots and the related histograms demonstrate the higher percentages of CD20+ B cells that co-express the CD10 molecule in fetal blood compared to the values observed in newborn's blood*

tion 80% of cord blood lymphocytes bear the RA isoform of the CD45 leukocyte surface antigen, while only 5% of cells express the CD45RO. After phytohemagglutinin stimulation, cells undergo a progressive and complete switch from synthesis of RA towards RO isoform (Figures 2 and 3).

DISCUSSION

These results confirm that at 18 weeks of gestation, lymphocytes of the three main lineages (T, B and natural killer cells) can be clearly distinguished in peripheral blood on the basis of their membrane phenotypes. These studies indicate also that during the intrauterine development of the immune system, T and B cells undergo several phenotypic changes. During fetal life, early precursors of T lymphocytes are generated in the liver and later in the bone marrow[16]. These cells migrate to the thymus, where they acquire the capacity to synthesize and mount on the membrane lineage-specific molecules and develop into functionally mature T lympho-

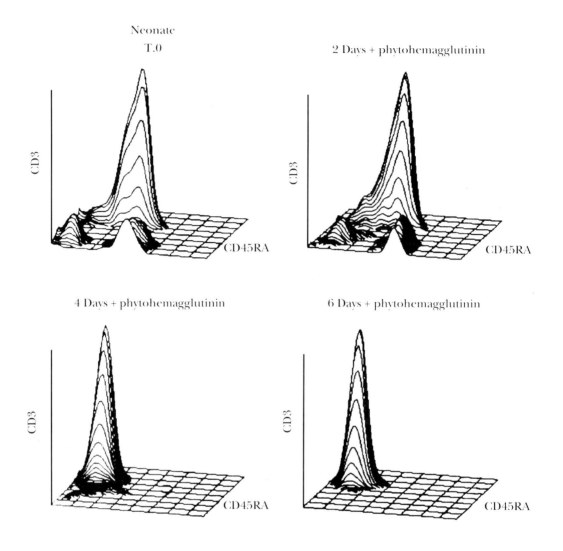

Figure 2 *The 3-D plots show that phytohemagglutinin-stimulated, CD3+ lymphocytes from newborn's blood lose progressively the ability to synthesize and express on the membrane the RA isoform of the CD45 leukocyte antigen, after 2, 4 and 6 days of in vitro culture*

cytes[17]. We have observed that in fetal life, T cells identified by the pan-T-cell markers CD7 and CD2 account for 60% of circulating lymphocytes. Most of the CD7+ lymphocytes express the CD5 antigen and the CD3 protein complex; furthermore, the majority of T cells express the CD4 (43%) and CD8 (20%) antigens in an almost mutually exclusive pattern. Compared to the fetal distribution, a slight increase in the percentage of CD4+ cells has been observed at birth. Several reports have provided inconsistent values of CD4+ and CD8+ cells; these discrepancies are probably due to technical differences[18]. Nevertheless, we can state that during intrauterine life circulating CD4+ T cells outnumber CD8+ cells by a ratio of 2 or more. Correlating with the lymphocytosis that develops during fetal life, the numbers of CD2, CD3 and CD4 cells increase exponentially during normal pregnancy to a plateau at 34 weeks, while CD8 cells increased in a linear fashion[19].

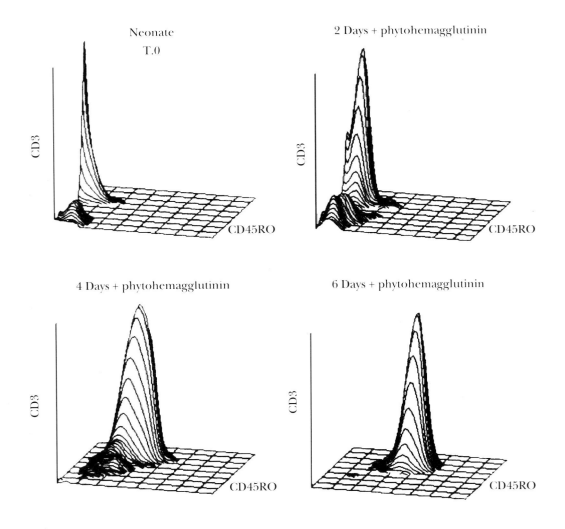

Figure 3 *The 3-D plots show that phytohemagglutinin-stimulated, CD3+ lymphocytes from newborn's blood acquire progressively the ability to synthesize and express on the membrane the RO isoform of the CD45 leukocyte antigen, after 2, 4 and 6 days of in vitro culture*

Both direct (demonstration by double marker staining) and indirect evidence prove that in fetal blood some lymphoid cells express phenotypic features of common or immature thymocytes: approximately 5% of T cells express the CD1 molecule and bear the CD4 and CD8 antigens simultaneously; few cells (3–4%) are positive for CD7 but negative for CD3[20]. These T cells with immature phenotypes might be thymocytes that have escaped the thymic environment before complete phenotypic maturation; they are still detectable in cord blood of normal neonates and their presence in the peripheral blood might reflect the high rate of lymphocyte generation in the thymus during intrauterine life. The majority of T cells in the fetus express the CD3 complex; 90% of them present the CD3 protein complex associated with the classical α/β T-cell receptor[21], 4% express the alternative γ/δ T-cell receptor[22] while 6% of CD3+ cells lack the antigen-specific receptors on the surface. In agreement with other published data[23] we have observed that the distribution of CD3+ cells expressing the α/β or γ/Δ T-cell receptor does not change through intrauterine life until birth.

We have shown that 70% and 10% of fetal CD3+ lymphocytes bear, respectively, the RA and RO isoforms of the CD45 leukocyte antigen. At birth, higher percentages (80%) of T cells express CD45RA while a decrease is observed in the percentage of CD45RO+ cells. This observation is in agreement with the data reported by Thilaganathan and colleagues[19] that the number of CD4+CD45RA+ cells increases exponentially during the pregnancy, while the CD8+CD45RA+ cells increase linearly. The selective expression of the RA and RO isoforms of the CD45 leukocyte antigen has been considered a marker of naive or unprimed T cells vs memory or activation-dependent differentiated cells[24–26]. The CD45 molecule contains a tyrosine phosphatase in its cytoplasmic region and probably acts in signal transduction; therefore, it has been proposed that CD45RA and CD45RO expression might correlate with different phases of the cell cycle[27]. It has been observed that the CD45RO isoform is also expressed by cortical thymocytes and that the CD45RO–T-cell receptor complex renders T cells more sensitive to antigenic stimulation. We suggest that the fetal CD3+ CD45RO+ cells might represent T lymphocytes activated *in vivo* by specific and mainly 'self' antigens. At this stage of development, activated T cells can express the receptor for interleukin-2 (CD25), but are deficient in expression of HLA-DR antigens, as suggested by the low (< 2%) values of CD3+HLA-DR+ cells, compared to higher percentages of CD3+CD25+ cells. This observation might imply that fetal T lymphocytes can undergo a short-term activation, with limited clonal expansion and meager generation of memory cells. We hypothesize that *in vivo* activation of fetal lymphocytes through antigen-specific receptors induces tolerance by means of apoptosis or clonal anergy. It has been demonstrated that CD4+ T cells can be separated into functionally distinct subsets depending upon expression of different isoforms of CD45 and/or CDw29. It has been proposed that the CD4+CD45R+ and CD4+CDw29+ subsets are mutually exclusive and correspond to virgin and memory T cells, respectively. Cord blood lymphocytes are deficient in CD4+CDw29+ T cells[28]; since CD4+CDw29+ cells mediate antigen-specific proliferation and helper activity[29], their absence in cord blood would explain the failure of neonatal lymphocytes to mediate helper functions[30] and to secrete γ-interferon[31]. The prevalence of 'naive' or unprimed CD4+CD45R+ T cells in cord blood might account for the suppressor activity that neonatal lymphocytes exert in several *in vitro* systems[32,33].

We have observed that after mitogen (phytohemagglutinin) activation cord blood lymphocytes undergo a switch from the synthesis and surface expression of the RA towards the RO isoform of the CD45 molecule. This phenomenon is complete within 6 days of *in vitro* culture of activated cord blood lymphocytes. These findings confirm previous data suggesting that the CD45RA+ and CD45RO+ T-cell subpopulations represent post-thymic, activation-induced differentiation stages in extrauterine life[34]. Therefore, we can state that neonatal T lymphocytes present surface phenotypes of cells committed to exert suppressor activity; however, these cells already possess the biochemical machinery to respond to activation, to proliferate and to undergo phenotypic and functional changes.

In our studies we have observed that most fetal T lymphocytes bear the CD28 and CD38 antigens; the CD28 molecule is a member of a heterophilic cell adhesion complex that serves as a surface component of a signal transduction pathway that stabilizes the mRNA and enhances lymphokine production[35]. The B7/BB-1 molecule, an activation antigen expressed on B cells, is supposed to be the natural ligand of the CD28 antigen; therefore it is likely that CD28 can play a role in B-cell antigen presentation to T cells and in T–B lymphocyte co-operation. The CD38 molecule, previously known as T10 antigen[36] acts as a transducer of activation signals; it is expressed by bone marrow precursors, activated T and B cells and plasma cells and is involved in a pathway of cell activation and proliferation that differs from those mediated by the T-cell receptor–CD3 complex or by CD2 and CD28[37]. We hypothesize that the expression of CD28 and CD38 molecules might render fetal T lymphocytes more sensitive to activation signals and to induction of tolerance towards antigens encountered at early stages of development.

In the second trimester of pregnancy, the CD19+ B lymphocytes represent 25% of circulating lymphoid cells. The CD19 antigen is the earliest differentiation antigen expressed by cells of the B lineage[38]. It has been recently demonstrated that this molecule lowers the threshold for antigen receptor stimulation of B lymphocytes[39]. This finding might, in some way, be correlated with the easy induction of tolerance during fetal and neonatal life. Surface IgM and CD20 antigen are expressed by more than 95% of CD19+ cells, while surface IgD is detectable on less than 70% of them. These findings suggest that in fetuses at 18–20 weeks of gestation, a few (5%) circulating CD19+sIgM-negative B cells can be detected; these cells might be defined more accurately as pre-B cells. Furthermore, 20–25% of fetal B cells are sIgM-positive but sIgD-negative. At birth, all newborns' B cells have been shown to express surface IgD[40]. The phenotypic immaturity of fetal B cells is confirmed by the observation that 50% of them express at low density the CD10 antigen, a membrane neutral endopeptidase, previously known as the common acute lymphoblastic leukemia antigen[41]. During intrauterine life, a decrease in the percentages of CD10+ cells occurs; indeed at birth less than 5% of B cells express this molecule at low density.

Seventy percent of fetal CD19+ cells bear the CD5 antigen. This finding is in good agreement with previous data[42,43]. The CD5+CD19+sIgM+ B cells synthesize and secrete 'natural' antibodies with low affinity and cross-reactivity with autologous antigens[44]. The CD23 antigen is a molecule that acts as a receptor for Fc-IgE, has some homology with lectins and, at least in adults, is expressed by activated B cells[45,46]. This molecule is expressed by 30% of fetal B lymphocytes and 50% of newborns' B cells. Similarly, 35% and 75% of B cells bear the CD21 antigen during fetal life and at birth, respectively; this molecule is the receptor for complement and Epstein–Barr virus and acts synergistically with CD19 as a signal transduction complex of B lymphocytes[47,48]. We have also observed that the great majority of fetal B cells bear the CD38 molecule, while only 65% of them are positive for the CD28 antigen; a reduction in the expression of these surface molecules is observed at birth.

These phenotypic findings represent the basis, at cell membrane level, to understand the functional characteristics of fetal or newborns' B lymphocytes. It is known that newborns' B cells differentiate poorly into immunoglobulin-producing plasma cells and are able to synthesize IgM but not IgG or IgA[49]. Indeed, these observations correlate with the phenotypic finding of high percentages of CD5+ cells in cord blood. We can speculate that the reduction of CD5 expression and, on the contrary, the progressive synthesis of CD21 by B cells might correlate with transition from a state of immune tolerance or poor response to antigenic stimulation during fetal life to immune competence and ability to mount a humoral immune response after birth.

Recently, the natural ligand of CD5 has been identified as CD72, a further surface protein of B cells[50]. This finding suggests that the CD5/CD72 interaction has some role in the T–B co-operation during the development of immune responses towards antigens. In this regard, the expression of CD5 by B cells might hamper the 'cognate' activation of B cells. However, we have also to consider that CD5+ CD10+ fetal human B cells can be induced *in vitro* to undergo isotype switching and immunoglobulin production[51].

Cells expressing the CD56 antigen, an isoform of the neural-cell adhesion molecule, represent 12–15% of lymphoid cells both in fetal and neonatal blood[52]. Approximately 50% of fetal CD56+ cells bear the CD16 antigen or Fc-IgG receptors, a molecule that is expressed on all functional natural killer cells in the peripheral blood and on neutrophils[53]. The CD57 antigen is not expressed by fetal lymphoid cells and less than 2% of cells bear this molecule at birth[54–56]. The ability to express the CD57 molecule develops late in the ontogeny of lymphoid cells of the natural killer and T lineages. In adults very low percentages of CD57+ cells can be detected in the bone marrow and in lymph nodes, while these cells can be easily observed in peripheral blood and spleen[55].

Finally, we have confirmed the presence in fetal blood of cells expressing the CD34 antigen and positive for HLA-DR antigens and CD71 molecule or transferrin receptor[57]; these findings suggest that these cells are in a proliferative state. We have previously demonstrated that nearly 5% of mononuclear cells in cord blood are in the S + G2m phases of the cell cycle[58]. These cells are likely to be precursor cells with broad hematopoietic potentials[59]. It has been suggested that the progenitor cells in cord blood might be a source of hematopoietic stem/progenitor cells that could be used for transplantation[60]. Indeed it has been demonstrated that umbilical cord blood can reconstitute bone-marrow in a patient with Fanconi's anemia[61]. Neonatal or *in utero* transplantation of fetal stem cells is an additional therapeutic approach that might be useful for treatment of several human genetic diseases[62,63].

In summary, the results we have presented and discussed delineate the phenotypes of human circulating lymphoid cells at the second trimester of pregnancy and at birth. They contribute to the knowledge of the development of the immune system during intrauterine life and provide reference values that could be used for prenatal diagnoses in fetuses supposed to be affected by congenital or acquired pathologic conditions. Finally, the phenotypic and functional data regarding lymphoid cells from umbilical cord blood might prove to be useful both for early diagnosis and for new therapeutical approaches in immunological and hematological genetic disorders.

ACKNOWLEDGEMENTS

This work has been partly supported by Grants from Regione Puglia, Italy (grant N. 3604-16.06.90), MURST (40% Funds to the Research Project 'Immunopathology') and C.N.R. (P.F. ACRO).

References

1. Keleman, E., Calvo, W., and Fliedner, T. M. (1979). *Atlas of Human Hemopoietic Development*. (Berlin: Springer-Verlag).
2. Gilmour, J. R. (1942). Normal hemopoiesis in intrauterine and neonatal life. *J. Pathol.*, **52**, 25–32
3. Gupta, S., Pahwa, R., O'Reilly, R., Good, R. A. and Siegal, F. P. (1976). Ontogeny of lymphocyte subpopulation in human fetal liver. *Proc. Natl. Acad. Sci. USA*, **73**, 919–22
4. Davies, N. P., Buggins, A. G. S., Snijders, R. J. M., Jenkins, E., Layton, D. M. and Nicolaides, K. H. (1992). Blood leukocyte count in the human fetus. *Arch. Dis. Child.*, **67**, 245–53
5. Nossal, G. J. V. (1989). Immunological tolerance. In Paul, W. E. (ed.) *Fundamental Immunology*, 2nd edn., pp. 571–86. (New York: Raven Press)
6. Vetro, S. W. and Bellanti, J. A. (1989) Fetal and neonatal immunocompetence. *Fetal Diagnosis Therapy*, **4**, 82–91
7. Hayward, A. R. (1981). Development of lymphocyte response and interaction in the human fetus and newborn. *Immunol. Rev.*, **57**, 39–62
8. Oettinger, M. A., Schatz, D. G., Gorka, C. and Baltimore D. (1990). RAG-1 and RAG-2 adjacent genes that synergistically activate V (D) J recombination. *Science*, **248**, 1517–23
9. Schroeder, H. W. Jr., Hillson, J. L. and Perlmutter, R. M. (1987). Early restriction of the human antibody repertoire. *Science (Wash. DC)*, **238**, 791–5
10. Alt, F. W., Blackwell, T. K. and Yancopoulos, G. D. (1987). Development of the primary antibody repertoire. *Science*, **238**, 1079–87
11. Knapp, W., Rieber, P., Dorken, B., Schmidt, R. E., Stein, H. and von der Borne, A. E. G. (1989). Towards a better definition of human leukocyte surface molecules. *Immunol. Today*, **10**, 253–8

12. Aspinall, R., Kampinga, J. and van der Bogaerde, J. (1991). T-cell development and the invariant series hypothesis. *Immunol. Today*, **12**, 7–10
13. Radacot, E. (1993). Cord-blood lymphocyte populations. *Immunol. Today*, **14**, 189–90
14. Robbins, B. A. (1987). Diagnostic immunohistochemistry of lymphoma and related disorders: practical aspects of frozen section technique and interpretation. *J. Clin. Lab. Anal.* **1**, 104–12
15. Bovicelli, L., Orsini, L. M., Grannun, P. A., Pittalis, M. C., Toffoli, C. and Dolcini, B. (1989). A new funipuncture technique: two needle ultrasound and needle biopsy-guided procedure. *Obstet. Gynecol.*, **73**, 428–31
16. Basch, R. S. and Kadish, J. L. (1977), Hematopoietic thymocyte precursors II: properties of precursors. *J. Exp. Med.* **145**, 405–19
17. Lepault, F. and Weissman, I. L. (1981). An *in vivo* assay for thymus-homing bone marrow cells. *Nature (London)*, **293**, 151–4
18. Ho, A. D. and Stehle, B. (1985). Characterization of immature T cell subpopulations in neonatal blood. *Blood*, **65**, 507–8
19. Thilaganathan, B., Mansur, C. A., Morgan, G. and Nicolaides, K. H. (1992). Fetal T-lymphocyte subpopulations in normal pregnancies. *Fetal Diagnosis Therapy*, **7**, 53–61
20. Reinherz, E. L., Kung, P. C., Goldstein, G., Levey, R. H. and Schlossman, S. F. (1980). Discrete stages of human intrathymic differentiation: analysis of normal thymocytes and leukemic lymphoblasts of T-cell lineage. *Proc. Natl. Acad. Sci. USA*, **77**, 1588–92
21. Marrack, P. and Kappler, J. (1987). The T-cell receptor. *Science*, **238**, 1073–9
22. Brenner, M. B., McLean, J., Dialynas, D. P., Strominger, J. L., Smith, J. A., Owen, F. L., Seidman, J. G., Ip, S., Rosen, F. and Krangel, M. S. (1986). Identification of a putative second T-cell receptor. *Nature (London)*, **322**, 145–9
23. Van Dongen, J. J. M., Comans-Bitter, W. M., Wolvers-Tettero, I. L. M. and Borst, J. (1990). Development of human T lymphocytes and their thymus-dependency. *Thymus*, **16**, 207–34
24. Serra, H. M., Krowka, J. F., Ledbetter, J. A. and Pilarski, L. M. (1988). Loss of CD45R (Lp220) represents a post-thymic T-cell differentiation event. *J. Immunol.*, **140**, 1435–41
25. Akbar, A. N., Terry, L., Timms, A., Beverley, P. C. L. and Janossy, G. (1988). Loss of the CD45R and gain of UCHL1 reactivity is a feature of primed T cells. *J. Immunol.*, **140**, 2171–8
26. Akbar, A. N., Salmon, M. and Janossy, G. (1991). The synergy between naive and memory T cells during activation. *Immunol. Today*, **12**, 184–8
27. MacKay, C. R. (1991). T-cell memory: the connection between function, phenotype and migration pathways. *Immunol. Today*, **12**, 189–92
28. Bradley, L. M., Bradley, J. S., Ching, D. L. and Shiigi, S. M. (1989). Predominance of T cells that express CD45R in the CD4+ helper/inducer lymphocyte subset in neonates. *Clin. Immunol. Immunopathol.*, **51**, 426–35
29. Morimoto, C., Letvin, N. L., Boyd, A. W., Hagan, M., Brown, H. M., Kornacki, M. M. and Schlossman, S. F. (1985). The isolation and characterization of the human helper inducer T cell subsets. *J. Immunol.*, **134**, 3762–9
30. Anderson, U., Bird, A. G., Britton, S. and Polacios, R. (1981). Humoral and cellular immunity in human studies at the cell level from birth to two years of age. *Immunol. Rev.*, **57**, 6–38
31. Lewis, D. B., Larsen, A. and Wilson, C. B. (1986). Reduced interferon-gamma mRNA levels in human neonates: evidence for an intrinsic T-cell deficiency independent of other genes involved in T cell activation. *J. Exp. Med.*, **163**, 1018–23
32. Hayward, A. R. and Kunick, J. (1981). Newborn T cell suppression: early appearance, maintenance in culture and lack of growth factor suppression. *J. Immunol.* **129**, 50–3
33. Rodriguez, M., Bankhurst, A. D., Ceuppens, J. L. and Williams, R. C. (1981). Characterization of the suppressor cell activity in human cord blood lymphocytes. *J. Clin. Invest.*, **68**, 1577–88
34. Clement, L. T., Yamashita, N. and Martin, A. M. (1988). The functionally distinct subpopulations of human CD4+ helper/inducer T lymphocytes defined by anti-CD45R antibodies derive sequentially from a differentiation pathway that is regulated by activation-dependent post-thymic differentiation. *J. Immunol.*, **141**, 1464–70
35. June, C. H., Ledbetter, J. A., Linsley, P. S. and Thompson, C. B. (1990). Role of the CD28 receptor in T-cell activation. *Immunol. Today*, **11**, 211–16
36. Reinherz, E. L., Kung, P. C., Goldstein, G., Levey, R. H. and Schlossman, S. F. (1980). Discrete stages of human intrathymic differentiation: analysis of normal thymocytes and leukemic lymphoblasts of T-cell lineage. *Proc. Natl. Acad. Sci. USA*, **77**, 1588–93
37. Funaro, A., Spagnoli, G. C., Ausiello, C. M., Alenio, M., Roggero, S., Delia, D., Zaccob, M. and Molovasi, F. (1990). Involvement of the multilineage CD38 molecule in a unique pathway of cell activation and proliferation. *J. Immunol.*, **145**, 2390–6
38. Nadler, L. M., Anderson, K. C., Marti, G., Bates, M. P., Park, E., Daley, J. F. and Schlossman, S. F. (1983). B4, a human B lymphocyte-associated antigen expressed on normal, mitogen activated, and malignant B lymphocytes. *J. Immunol.*, **131**, 244–50

39. Carter, R. H. and Fearon, D. T. (1992). CD19: lowering the threshold for antigen receptor stimulation of B lymphocytes. *Science*, **256**, 105–7
40. Durandy, A., Thuillier, L., Forveille, M. and Fisher, A. (1990). Phenotypic and functional characteristics of human newborns' B lymphocytes. *J. Immunol.*, **144**, 60–65
41. Greaves, M. F., Brown, G., Rapson, N. T. and Lister, T. A. (1975). Antisera to acute lymphoblastic leukemia cells. *Clin. Immunol. Immunopathol.*, **4**, 67–84
42. Antin, J. H., Emerson, S. G., Martin, P., Gadol, N. and Ault K. A. (1986). Leu-1+ (CD5+) B cells. A major lymphoid subpopulation in human fetal spleen: phenotypic and functional studies. *J. Immunol.*, **136**, 505–10
43. Bofil, M., Janossy, G., Janossa, M., Burford, G. D., Seymour, G. J., Wernet, P. and Keleman, E. (1985). Human B lymphocyte development. II. Subpopulation in the human fetus. *J. Immunol.*, **134**, 1531–8
44. Casali, P. and Notkins, A. L. (1989). CD5+ B lymphocytes, polyreactive antibodies and the human B-cell repertoire. *Immunol. Today*, **10**, 364–8
45. Bonnefoy, J. Y., Aubry, J. P., Peronne, C., Widjenes, J. and Banchereau, J. (1987). Production and characterization of a monoclonal antibody specific for the human lymphocyte low affinity receptor for IgE: CD23 is a low affinity receptor for IgE. *J. Immunol.*, **123**, 2970–5
46. Gordon, J., Flores-Romo, L., Cairns, J. A., Millsum, M. J., Lorne, P. J., Johnson, G. D. and MacLennan, I. C. M. (1989). CD23: a multifunctional receptor/lymphokine? *Immunol. Today*, **10**, 153–7
47. Weis, J. J., Toothaker, L. E., Smith, J. A., Weis, J. H. and Fearon, D. T. (1988). Structure of the human B lymphocyte receptor for C3d and the Epstein–Barr virus and relatedness to other members of the family of C3/C4 binding proteins. *J. Exp. Med.*, **167**, 1047–66
48. Matsumoto, A. K., Kopicky-Burd, J., Carter, R. H., Tuveson, D. A., Tedder, T. F. and Fearon, D. T. (1991). Intersection of the complement and immune systems: a signal transduction complex of the B-lymphocyte-containing complement receptor type 2 and CD19. *J. Exp. Med.*, **173**, 55–64
49. Hayward, A. R. and Lawton, A. R. (1977). Induction of plasma cell differentiation of human fetal lymphocytes: evidence for functional immaturity of T and B cell. *J. Immunol.*, **119**, 1213–8
50. Van-De-Velde, H., Von-Hoegen, I., Luo, W., Parnes, J. R. and Thielemans, K. (1991). The B-cell surface protein CD72/Lyb-2 is the ligand for CD5. *Nature (London)*, **251**, 662–5
51. Punnonen, J., Aversa, G. G., Vanderkerckhove, B., Roncarolo, M. G. and De Vries, J. E. (1992). Induction of isotype switching and Ig production by CD5+ and CD10+ human fetal B cells. *J. Immunol.*, **148**, 3398–404
52. Hercend, T., Griffin, J. D., Bensussan, A., Schmidt, R. E., Edson, M. A., Brennan, A., Murray, C., Daley, J. F., Schlossman, S. F. and Ritz, J. (1985). Generation of monoclonal antibodies to a human natural killer clone: characterization of two natural killer-associated antigens, NKH1 and NKH2, expressed on subsets of large granular lymphocytes. *J. Clin. Invest.*, **75**, 932–43
53. Lanier, L. L., Le, A. M., Phillips, J. H., Warner, N. L. and Babcock, G. F. (1983). Subpopulations of human natural killer cells defined by expression of the Leu-7 (HNK-1) and Leu-11 (NK-15) antigens. *J. Immunol.*, **131**, 1789–96
54. Abo, T. and Balch, C. M. (1981). A differentiation antigen of human NK and K cells identified by a monoclonal antibody (HNK-1). *J. Immunol.*, **127**, 1024–9
55. Abo, T., Miller, C. A. and Balch, C. M. (1984). Characterization of human granular lymphocyte subpopulations expressing HNK-1 (Leu-7) and Leu-11 antigens in the blood and lymphoid tissues from fetuses, neonate and adults. *Eur. J. Immunol.*, **14**, 616–23
56. Panaro, A., Amati, A., DiLoreto, M., Felle, R., Ferrante, M., Papadia, A. M., Porfido, N., Gambatesa, V., Dell'Osso, A. and Lucivero, G. (1990). Lymphocyte subpopulations in pediatric age. Definition of reference values by flow cytometry. *Immunol. Clin.*, **9**, 35–43
57. Goding, J. W. and Burns, G. F. (1981). Monoclonal antibody OKT-9 recognizes the receptor for transferrin on human acute lymphocytic leukemia cells. *J. Immunol.*, **127**, 1256–8
58. Lucivero, G., Surico, G., Mazzini, G., Dell-Osso, A. and Bonomo, L. (1988). Age-related changes in the proliferative kinetics of PHA-stimulated lymphocytes. Analysis by uptake of tritiated precursors of DNA, RNA and proteins, and by flow cytometry. *Mech. Ageing Dev.*, **43**, 259–67
59. Linch, D. C., Knott, L. J., Rodeck, C. H. and Huehns, E. R. (1982). Studies of circulating hematopoietic progenitor cells in human fetal blood. *Blood*, **59**, 976–9
60. Broxmeyer, H. E., Douglas, G. W., Hangoc, G., Cooper, S., Bard, J., English, D., Arny, M., Thomas, L. and Boyse, E. A. (1989). Human umbilical cord as a potential source of transplantable hematopoietic stem/progenitor cells. *Proc. Natl. Acad. Sci. USA*, **86**, 3828–32
61. Gluckman, E., Broxmeyer, H. E., Auerbach, A. D., Friedman, H. S., Douglas, G. W., Devergie, A., Esperou, H., Thierry, D., Soci, G.,

Lehn, P., Cooper, S., English, D., Kurtzberg, J., Bard, J. and Boyse, E. A. (1989). Hematopoietic reconstitution in a patient with Fanconi's anemia by means of umbilical cord blood from an HLA-identical sibling. *N. Engl. J. Med.*, **321**, 1174–8

62. Parkman, R. (1986). The application of bone marrow transplantation to the treatment of genetic diseases. *Science*, **232**, 1373–6
63. Touraine, J. L., Raudrant, D., Royo, C., Rebaud, A., Roncarolo, M. G. and Betuel, H. (1989). *In utero* transplantation of stem cells in bare lymphocyte syndrome. *Lancet*, **1**, 1382

Prenatal and perinatal development of the human cerebral cortex

I. Kostović and M. Judaš

INTRODUCTION

From the very dawn of modern neurobiological research, the development of the human central nervous system has strongly attracted the enquiring minds of neuroscientists, at the same time posing perhaps the greatest challenges to both their research facilities and their imagination. Understandably, these difficulties arose from ethical and methodological constraints related to research on human subjects, as well as from the limitations of the theoretical concepts prevailing in the period of classical developmental neuroanatomy. Not the least obstacle was the lack of an appropriate experimental animal model, since a number of crucial histogenetic events in the human and primate brain (contrary to the situation in, for example, the rodent brain) unfold and even complete themselves before birth.

As exemplified by the magnificent early monographs of His[1] and Hochstetter[2], the systematic study of early brain morphogenesis and the basic histological composition of embryonic cellular zones was a relatively easy task to accomplish. However, the subsequent research continued in the shadow of theoretical views derived from comparative neuroanatomy and the recapitulationist's drive to find parallels between ontogeny and phylogeny. This led to the firmly established 'progressivist' view regarding the development of the brain as a complex, intricately patterned and protracted process of ever increasing structural and functional complexity and perfection[3-7].

With the introduction of modern research methods, a wealth of new data rapidly accumulated, leading to profound changes in our views concerning the structural and functional development of the nervous system.

So, for example, the application of autoradiography provided detailed insight into the kinetics of neuronal proliferation and the systematic relationship between the time of neuronal generation and the acquisition of the final positions of neurons, as exemplified in the 'inside-out' pattern of corticogenesis[8]. The results of systematic studies of the mode of neuronal migration[9,10] and sequential growth of cortical afferents[11-15] in the developing telencephalon of the monkey and human were recently united in a coherent and testable 'radial unit hypothesis' of cerebral cortical development[16,17].

Finally, a number of recent studies points to the crucial role of so-called 'regressive events' in the normal histogenesis of the central nervous system: naturally occurring neuronal death, selective elimination of axonal collaterals, 'exuberant' initial production of connection fibers, and transient overproduction of dendritic spines and synapses[18-21]. The extent of these 'regressive' events, their relationship with 'progressive' histogenetic events (proliferation, migration and neuronal differentiation) and the continuity with the adult cortical organization are still poorly understood. However, it is obvious that both 'progressive' and 'regressive' events lead to a more advanced level of cortical organization. Therefore, it seems appropriate to replace the term 'regressive events' by the term 'reorganization'.

Our own views concerning the structural development and transient and reorganizational phenomena of the human prenatal and postnatal brain are based on two decades of continuous and systematic research, during which we applied different techniques for demonstrating the cytoarchitectonics (Nissl staining), neuronal morphology (Golgi impregnation), synaptogenesis (electron-microscopic analysis), growing pathways (acetylcholinesterase (AChE) histochemistry) and transmitter-related properties of developing neuronal populations (immunocytochemistry and AChE histochemistry) on a number of human brains of the Zagreb Neuroembryological Collection[22–25].

This research has led to the discovery of an early synaptogenesis within the human cortical anlage[26,27] as well as to the delineation of the hitherto undescribed and essential compartment of the telencephalic wall and cortical anlage – the subplate zone[15,27,28].

Furthermore, we have documented that during the development of the human cerebral cortex transient patterns of organization of cortical afferents, synapses and neurons are present from the 3rd intrauterine month to the 6th postnatal month[22,23,29–33]. In addition, postnatal overgrowth (i.e. the overproduction of synapses and spines) begins to slow down after only the 2nd year of life[34,35]. All this indicates that transient patterns of cortical organization and reorganization may extend for the impressively long period of more than 3 years.

We have proposed that the human cerebral cortex passes through two broad periods of the developmental reorganization characterized by different levels of rearrangement of cortical elements[23–25], as follows:

(1) The perinatal period of the 'first reorganization' involves disappearance of the fetal subplate zone and laminar relocation of afferent pathways. The exact timing and duration of these processes and the size of the transient subplate zone are proportional to the complexity of the cortico-cortical pathways in a given cortical area.

(2) The period of the 'second, fine reorganization' covers infancy and early childhood; it is characterized by dendritic and synaptic rearrangements.

In this review, after a concise account of general histogenetic processes, we summarize our current views on the prenatal and perinatal development and reorganization of the human cerebral cortex.

The readers interested in morphogenesis of the human fetal brain should consult classical[1,2] as well as recent accounts[22,36,37]. Those interested in the development of the human spinal cord, brain stem, cerebellum, diencephalon and basal ganglia, as well as the development of meninges and brain vascularization, should consult one of the comprehensive modern reviews of the development of the human brain[22,38,39].

GENERAL ACCOUNT OF HISTOGENETIC EVENTS

The histogenetic and cellular processes that contribute to the shaping and structural development of the brain are: proliferation, migration, differentiation (development of dendrites, axons and cytological maturation), development of connections with synaptogenesis and cell death. The development of glia (gliogenesis) begins somewhat later than the main neurogenesis, but significantly overlaps it in time.

All histogenetic processes can be determined by spatial and temporal parameters. The most important spatial parameters are embryonic zones and we shall describe them first, relying on the terminology of the Boulder Committee[40] as revised by Rakic[8] to incorporate the recently discovered subplate zone.

The neural tube initially consists of pseudostratified columnar neuroepithelium, which forms a single cytoarchitectonic lamina – the ventricular zone. This early proliferative zone occupies the full thickness of the neural tube. During the 5th postovulatory week, a cell-sparse marginal zone appears external to the ventricular zone. The early marginal zone is composed of elongated, growing processes of neuroepithelial cells, which reach an immature basal membrane already present around the central nervous system anlage. The basal membrane together with marginal end processes of neuroepithelial cells forms the earliest 'outer limiting membrane' of the central nervous system. Thus, this initial histogenetic period is characterized by neuronal proliferation and the presence of only two zones (ventricular and marginal). Starting from this early stage, the ventricular zone is the main proliferative zone in the whole central nervous system.

The next zone to develop between ventricular and marginal zone is the intermediate zone, which is the main site of neuronal migration. The intermediate zone has considerably lower cell-packing density than has the ventricular zone, but it contains significantly more cells than the marginal zone.

As is well known, all neurons are generated at places different from those which they attain in the adult brain and therefore must migrate for some distance in order to acquire their final positions. The mechanism of migration during the earliest stages of development is still unknown; however, there is very little doubt that during the later stages, when the intermediate zone is thicker, active migration of neurons represents one of the key histogenetic processes. The migration pathway in the large human brain may be very long (more than 1 cm!) and the length of the migrating neurons represents only a fraction of this total pathway length. According to the evidence obtained in the developing nervous system of the monkey[8-10], neurons follow radial glial guides, and cell-to-cell contact between neurons and radial glia is essential for the process of migration. Migratory neurons are bipolar and have two main cytoplasmic processes. One process is 'leading', i.e. directed towards the final site of the migrating neuron. The opposite is a 'trailing' process.

The next fundamental embryonic zone appearing between the ventricular and intermediate zone, is the subventricular zone. It contains proliferating cells and mitotic figures and may be included together with the ventricular zone in germinative zones of the brain. The subventricular zone is well developed in cerebral vesicles, where it may serve as a place of origin for neurons of the basal ganglia and cortex. Accordingly, it contains precursors of both neurons and glia.

These four zones (ventricular, subventricular, intermediate and marginal zone) are transient developmental elements and they do not have adult counterparts. The neurons born in the ventricular or subventricular zone migrate through the intermediate zone, eventually reach their final position and begin to differentiate into various types of neuron.

Although processes may grow out even during the migration, the main differentiation of dendrites and axons begins after the neurons have attained their final positions. The development of the main shape of dendrites is intrinsic to neurons, since this process continues even *in vitro*. The appearance of dendritic spines is a relatively late developmental event, occurring in the second half of gestation. In general, the principal efferent neurons mature and differentiate their dendritic trees earlier than do neurons of the local circuitry (interneurons). Furthermore, large neurons are generally produced and differentiate earlier than small neurons.

The most specific process in the brain is the development of neuronal connections. During this process several events can be distinguished: (a) growth of presynaptic axons, (b) development of postsynaptic elements, and (c) synaptogenesis.

The vast majority of presynaptic axons in the fetal brain are afferent axons from remote sites, not belonging to the local circuitry elements. In general, brainstem neurons mature very early and send their axons to the 'higher' brain regions. Similarly, axons from the basal forebrain and thalamus form early afferent systems for the cerebral cortex. During the outgrowth, axons tend to be arranged in bundles running through the intermediate zone (fetal 'white' matter) as well as through the marginal zone. Growing tips of axons are called growth cones. The membrane of growth cones contains macromolecules that probably enable 'recognition' of postsynaptic membranes of other neurons (so-called neuronal chemoaffinity molecules). During growth, axons may show transmitter properties, even before the establishment of synaptic contacts.

The main postsynaptic sites in the early fetal brain are dendrites (axodendritic synapses). The synapses (characterized by the presence of membrane-associated densities and synaptic vesicles) appear very early in the cortical development, at the beginning of the 3rd month of gestation. This early and rather surprising maturation of synaptic contacts between fetal neurons indicates a possible early functional development. Immature synapses have fewer synaptic vesicles than in the adult brain and their synaptic membranes are shorter (Figure 1). It is obvious that some, presumably older, neurons make synaptic contacts in a nucleus while other neurons still migrate through the intermediate zone or are produced in the ventricular or subventricular zone. This significant overlap in timing of neurogenetic events is characteristic for the development of the brain of the large primate, particularly the human. The overlap in cell production, cell migration, axonal ingrowth and synaptogenesis in the cortical anlage may last for 5–6 months.

In general, there are two types of cell death, both being normal developmental events: (1) morphogenetic cell death and (2) naturally occurring cell death. Morphogenetic cell death occurs where neural tube derivatives bend, fold or decrease in thickness. Thus, morphogenetic cell death participates in a morphological shaping of the brain and occurs during the earliest, embryonic phases of development. Naturally occurring cell death is related to the development of neuronal connections (the failure to establish synaptic contacts, competition for postsynaptic targets, or the lack of trophic influence from the target). This type of cell death occurs during the later developmental stages, but it is poorly studied in the brain of the human and monkey.

Other 'regressive' developmental changes are probably more significant than the actual cell death. The most interesting is the phenomenon of the establishment of transient synapses[21,35]. Another interesting phenomenon is the presence of transient neuronal projections[19,20], which later disappear, probably by a mechanism of axon retraction or pruning of axon collaterals[20].

Developmental studies performed on experimental animals have suggested that the development of glia (gliogenesis) is a relatively late event occurring after neurogenesis. However, studies on the brains of primates[8] and humans[41] have shown that gliogenesis starts at the beginning of fetal life and occurs parallel to neurogenesis. This correlates well with the very long prenatal development of the brain in humans. The earliest glial cells to differentiate are radially oriented, but already during the midfetal period, various types of astroglia may be observed. Although very little is known about the development of oligodendroglia, it probably occurs *in utero*, since the onset of myelinization occurs at the end of gestation.

HISTOGENESIS OF THE HUMAN CEREBRAL CORTEX

General pattern of cortical development

In addition to the embryonic zones common to the whole central nervous system, the developing cerebral (telencephalic) wall contains a number of special zones characteristic of the development of the cerebral cortex. Since all cellular events (proliferation, migration, differentiation, growth of fiber pathways, synaptogenesis, cell death as well as initial overproduction and subsequent elimination of axonal collaterals, dendritic spines and synapses) take place in one or more of these zones, it is logical to divide the whole prenatal histogenesis into a series of subsequent stages on the basis of complex cytoarchitectonic transformations of embryonic zones.

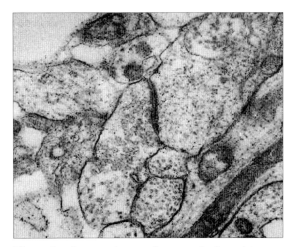

Figure 1 *Asymmetric synaptic contact in the early neocortical anlage of the human fetus. Note synaptic vesicles and thickened parts of the cellular membrane*

Therefore, before the detailed description of each period and cortical region, we shall briefly describe our staging system (see also Tables 2, 3 and 4, below). In a way, this staging system may be regarded as an updated and elaborated system of Poliakov[6] and Sidman and Rakic[38,39]. However, the main advantage and originality of our system lies in the fact that it fully recognizes the importance of two major developmental phenomena which were not taken into consideration in previous classifications: (a) the developmental history of the subplate zone, and (b) transient and reorganizational processes in the developing human brain.

On the basis of multiple structural features as well as the relative intensity of different histogenetic events (Table 1), we have divided the whole prenatal cortical development into six developmental phases containing 11 distinct stages (Table 2). However, to enhance the correlation with physiological and clinical data, these stages and phases can be easily brought

Table 1 *Relative intensity and timing of major histogenetic processes leading to the formation of the human neocortex (WG, weeks of gestation)*

Histogenetic processes	Embryonic period (4–7 WG)	Early fetal period (8–12 WG)	Mid-fetal period (13–24 WG)	Late fetus and premature infant (25–38 WG)	Newborn
Proliferation	+	+++	+	+–	–
Migration	+	+++	+++	+	–
Differentiation	–	+	+++	+++	+++
Growth of afferents	–	+	+++	+++	+
Growth of efferents	–	–+	+	+	+
Synaptogenesis	–	+	+	+++	+++
Cell death	–	+–	+–	?	?
Plasticity	–	?	?	?	?

Table 2 *Developmental phases and stages of human neocortical histogenesis during prenatal and perinatal life (WG, weeks of gestation; VZ, ventricular zone; SV, subventricular zone; IZ, intermediate zone; CP, cortical plate; SP, subplate zone; MZ, marginal zone; WM, white matter)*

Period	Age (WG)	Phase No.	Phase Description	Stage No.	Stage Description	Lamination pattern
Embryonic	4–7	I	universal embryonic zones	S1	2 embryonic zones	VZ, MZ
				S2	3 embryonic zones	VZ, IZ, MZ
				S3	4 embryonic zones	VZ, SV, IZ, MZ
Early fetal	8–9	II	formation of CP	S4	formation of CP	VZ, SV, IZ, CP, MZ
	10–12			S5	primary consolidation of CP	VZ, SV, IZ, CP, MZ
Mid-fetal	13–15	III	formation of typical fetal transitory compartments	S6	subplate formation	VZ, SV, IZ, SP, CP, MZ
	16–18			S7	secondary consolidation of CP	VZ, SV, IZ, SP, CP, MZ
	19–24	IV	typical fetal lamination pattern	S8	developmental peak of SP	VZ, SV, IZ, SP, CP, MZ
Late fetal	25–34	V	transformation of fetal lamination pattern	S9	initial lamination of CP, local resolution of SP	VZ, SV, IZ, SP, CP (layers II–VI), MZ
	35–38			S10	general resolution of SP, six-layered 'Grundtypus'	VZ, WM, SP, layers I–VI
Newborn		VI	immature adult-like lamination	S11	immature six-layered cortex	

Table 3 Basic features of the histogenesis of the pallium and cerebral cortex during prenatal and perinatal life (WG, weeks of gestation)

Period	Age (WG)	Phase	Main features
Embryonic	4–7	I	universal embryonic zones
Early fetal	8–12	II	formation of the cortical plate
Mid-fetal	13–15	III	formation of typical fetal transitory compartments
	16–24	IV	typical fetal lamination pattern, developmental peak of the subplate zone
Late fetus and premature infant	25–38	V	transformation of fetal lamination pattern (initial lamination within the cortical plate, resolution of the subplate zone)
Newborn		VI	immature adult-like six-layered cortex

Table 4 Four major periods of human cortical histogenesis

Developmental phase	Major histogenetic feature
Early fetal	progressive histogenetic events (proliferation, migration and differentiation)
Late fetal	transient patterns of cortical organization
Early postnatal and infancy	reorganization and overproduction of cortical circuitry elements
Late postnatal (childhood, puberty and adolescence)	prolonged structural and chemical maturation

into correspondence with five more plausible periods of human prenatal development: embryonic (first 2 months), early fetal (8–12 weeks of gestation), mid-fetal (13–24 weeks of gestation), late fetal and preterm (25–38 weeks of gestation) and newborn period (Table 3). Furthermore, they are easily fitted within the framework of four broadly defined periods covering the whole cortical histogenesis from the early embryonic to the fully mature adult brain (Table 4). Naturally, the exponential accumulation of new data within the rapidly expanding field of developmental neuroscience will inevitably lead to refinements or revisions of this staging system.

During the embryonic period (first 2 months of gestation) the wall of cerebral vesicles (telencephalic wall) is very thin (less than 1 mm) and consists of the same zones as in other parts of the neural-tube derivatives: the ventricular–subventricular, intermediate and marginal zones. This period of cytoarchitectonic development (4–7 weeks of gestation) can be described as a phase of universal embryonic zones (phase I, stages 1 to 3). The cortical plate (fetal zone specific for the cerebral cortex anlage) develops at the end of this period and during the subsequent early fetal period (phase II, stages 4 and 5). Another zone characteristic for the development of the cerebral cortex, the subplate zone, appears next (phase III, stages 6 and 7).

Thus, after the formation of these cortex-specific zones, the fetal cerebral pallium displays a typical fetal pattern of lamination (phase IV, stage 8) consisting of the following zones (starting from pia to ventricle): marginal zone (MZ), cortical plate (CP), subplate zone (SP), intermediate (IZ), subventricular (SV) and ventricular zone (VZ). Three of these fetal zones (MZ, CP and SP) represent the anlage of the future adult cerebral cortex. It is essential to emphasize that these cortical fetal zones are specific fetal elements: their neuronal content is permanently changing; they contain transient elements and have no direct relationships with layers of the adult cortex. Therefore, in order to describe a series of rather complex histogenetic events occurring from the early to the late fetal period, the whole fetal period should be divided into at least four broadly defined developmental phases:

(1) The period of formation and primary consolidation of the cortical plate and the pre-subplate stage (phase II, stages 4 and 5; 8–12 weeks of gestation);

(2) The period of the formation of characteristic fetal lamination in the neocortex: subplate formation stage and secondary consolidation of the cortical plate (phase III, stages 6 and 7; 13–18 weeks of gestation);

(3) The period of the developmental maximum of the characteristic fetal pattern of lamination in the neocortex: the developmental peak of the transient subplate zone accompanied by the initial, transitory lamination within the cortical plate (phase IV, stage 8; 19–24 weeks of gestation); and

(4) The period of transformation of the fetal pattern of lamination characterized by the gradual resolution of the subplate zone, the onset of areal differentiation, the appearance of the definitive adult-like six-layered pattern of lamination within the cortical plate, transient expression of neurotransmitter properties and laminar shifts and relocation of cortical afferents (phase V, stages 9 and 10; 25–38 weeks of gestation – the period of low-birth-weight premature infants). This period, critical for the structural shaping of the cerebral cortex, is characterized by the transformation of the typical fetal lamination into the adult-like six-layered '*Grundtypus*' within the neocortical anlage.

Accordingly, the definitive pattern of cortical lamination is already outlined in the newborn infant (phase VI, stage 11). However, the immaturity of the newborn cortex clearly indicates that histogenetic processes continue during the early postnatal period. Therefore, the newborn stage can be appropriately described as the stage of immature and transient neocortical organization.

In order to stress the continuity of development and both the differential timing and the significant temporal overlap of various histogenetic and reorganizational processes, as well as to enhance the understanding of their significance for the development of brain functions, the following sections are organized according to major developmental events. However, the correspondence with different stages and phases is always indicated in the text.

The neocortex and allocortex have a common developmental history in the early embryo (4–7 weeks of gestation)

During the third and fourth weeks of gestation, the thin wall of telencephalic vesicles consists solely of the ventricular zone, composed of immature, elongated neuroepithelial (ventricular) cells arranged into the pseudostratified epithelium. One end of these elongated cells is attached to the ventricular (ectodermal or inner) surface while the other stretches towards the superficial, mesodermal surface covered by the basal lamina. These cells proliferate intensively and undergo a characteristic mitotic cycle: during DNA synthesis (S phase) the cell nucleus moves away from the ventricular surface, later (post-synthetic gap phase – G_2) the nucleus moves towards the ventricular surface where mitosis (M phase) occurs. After the mitosis is completed, the nucleus once again moves away from the ventricular surface ('to-and-fro' movement).

During the 5th week of gestation, the superficial process of ventricular cells together with processes of the first post-mitotic neurons form a new pale layer – the marginal zone – so that the wall of the telencephalic vesicle now consists of two embryonic zones, marginal and ventricular (our stage 1 of cortical development). The major histogenetic event of this period is proliferation within the ventricular zone, which leads to the increase in number of neuroepithelial cells and gradual growth of the telencephalon. During the same period, morphogenetic cell death occurs along the midline, within the thin wall of the telencephalon medium (impar), thus contributing to its morphogenetic shaping.

During the 6th week of gestation, postmitotic cells generated within the ventricular zone detach from the ventricular surface and migrate away from it, thus forming a new intermediate zone at the interface between the marginal and ventricular zones. The telencephalic wall now consists of three embryonic zones characteristic for the development of all parts of the central nervous system: the marginal, intermediate and ventricular zones. Therefore, we designated the whole embryonic period as the phase of universal embryonic zones (phase I) and this particular stage as stage 2 of cortical development.

As a reflection of general histogenetic gradients, all three zones are significantly thicker in the basal mid-lateral than in the more dorsal, rostral, caudal or medial portions of the telencephalic wall. Furthermore, a special lamination pattern occurs in the most medial part of the telencephalic vesicle (the anlage of the limbic allocortex); the telencephalic wall is here slightly curved and the marginal zone is significantly enlarged. This is the site of the future formation of the hippocampus. From this hemispheric edge ('limbus') the cerebral wall continues as a thin epithelial lamina (area epithelialis, lamina tectoria) stretching from one hemispheric vesicle to the other.

By the end of the 6th week of gestation, another, subventricular, zone develops at the interface between the ventricular and intermediate zones. This zone, characteristic for the developing telencephalon, is a site of intensive proliferation and generates a substantial number of neurons destined for the future neocortex. Thus, in this stage (stage 3), the lateral cerebral wall consists of the following four zones: the ventricular, subventricular, intermediate and marginal zones. The subventricular zone becomes very thick within the basolateral part of the telencephalic wall, thus leading to the formation of the ganglionic eminence. Although the ganglionic eminence generates primarily the future neurons of the basal ganglia, it may contribute to the population of cortical neurons as well.

During the 7th week of gestation, characterized by a significant increase in the size of cerebral vesicles, an intensive proliferation continues within the ventricular zone and a number of cells migrate towards the subventricular and intermediate zones. The development of the subventricular zone and the establishment of regional differences in the thickness of the pallium indicate the end of the phase of universal embryonic zones and foreshadow the incipient development of specific fetal cortical zones.

The cortical histogenesis during the embryonic period may be summarized as follows: proliferation is the dominant event during early histogenesis and the first migratory wave of young (post-mitotic) neurons destined to form the cortical plate appears at the very end of the embryonic period.

The cortical plate and the first cytoarchitectonic differences between the neo-, archi- and paleocortex appear at the transition from the embryonic to the early fetal period (8–9 weeks of gestation)

The most important event for the delineation of a new developmental period is the appearance of the cortical plate within the basolateral pallium towards the end of the 8th week of gestation (Figure 2). After being generated within the ventricular–subventricular zone, young post-mitotic neurons migrate through the intermediate zone and finally form a cortical plate – a characteristic layer of tightly packed and vertically aligned immature neurons situated at the interface of the intermediate and marginal zones.

With the formation of the cortical plate, a true laminar cortical anlage is established. However, it is important to stress that some neurons are generated and arrive in the marginal zone even before the initial formation of the cortical plate. These special fetal neurons, called Cajal–Retzius cells, represent the major cellular component of the marginal zone throughout the prenatal development.

DEVELOPMENT OF THE HUMAN CEREBRAL CORTEX

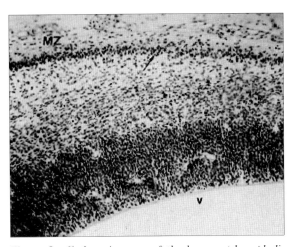

Figure 2 *Embryonic zones of the human telencephalic wall at the transition from the embryonic to early fetal period (8th week of gestation, Nissl staining). The first post-migratory neurons begin to form the cortical plate (arrow) below the marginal zone (MZ). Below the incipient cortical plate there is a pale intermediate zone, while dark ventricular and subventricular zones are situated alongside the embryonic ventricle (v)*

In order to reach the cortical plate, young neurons have to migrate a considerable distance. This process requires precise guidance, which is provided by a special type of radial glia. By means of membrane-to-membrane contact, through special adhesion macromolecules, neurons interact with radial glia and climb towards the cortical plate. By this mechanism, neurons find their path during late fetal development even when the cerebral wall becomes thicker than 1 cm. As a result of the proliferation and migration during the 8th and 9th weeks of gestation, new neurons are continuously added to the cortical plate of the lateral pallium. The cortical plate gradually spreads throughout the dorsomedial and rostrocaudal regions of the cerebral vesicle. With this process, the formation of the cortical plate is finished. After the formation of the cortical plate throughout the largest part of the cerebral pallium, clear differences appear between the lateral (neocortical), limbic (archicortical) and mediobasal (paleocortical) parts of the telencephalic pallium.

Although basic histogenetic processes are essentially the same in all these three major types of cortex, they occur with different time schedules, spatial relationships and laminar patterns. Thus, the lateral neocortex develops a prominent cortical plate and (later) the subplate zone; the limbic archicortex develops an exceptionally wide marginal zone and thin, convoluted cortical plate, while the mediobasal paleocortex never develops a true cortical plate.

First synapses develop above and below the cortical plate at 10–12 weeks of gestation

Formation of the cortical plate in the neopallial anlage is completed by 9 weeks of gestation. During the 10th, 11th and 12th weeks of gestation (stage 5), the cortical plate increases in thickness and becomes densely packed with post-migratory cells. The cortical plate is thickest in the mid-lateral part of the neocortical anlage, above the level of the ganglionic eminence (Figure 3). Below the cortical plate, there is a thin plexiform zone containing fibers and some post-migratory cells. This zone can be regarded as a part of the cortical anlage and as a forerunner of the subplate zone, thus a term presubplate zone is appropriate. In this developmental phase, the cortical anlage consists of three layers (from the pia to the ventricle): the marginal zone, cortical plate and presubplate zone. The cortical plate is the thickest part of the cortical anlage. Events related to the development of neuronal connections (ingrowth of axons, synaptogenesis and development of post-synaptic dendrites) begin during this early fetal period. The earliest afferent axons (of unknown origin) approach the cortical anlage through the marginal and pre-subplate zones.

The development of synapses in the human cerebral cortex begins after the formation of the cortical plate at the end of the 8th week of gestation. There are very few synapses in the cortical anlage during this period and they are distributed in bilaminar fashion: a superficial synaptic lamina is within the boundaries of the marginal zone, whereas the deep synaptic lamina is situated below the cortical plate and corresponds to the pre-subplate zone[15,26,27]

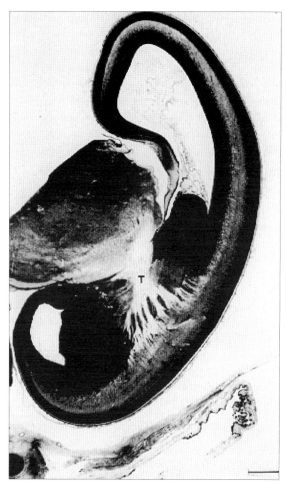

Figure 3 *Nissl-stained coronal section through the right telencephalic vesicle of the early human fetus (10th week of gestation, crown–rump length 55 mm). Well-developed cortical plate is in the stage of its primary consolidation. Note the dark proliferative (ventricular and subventricular) zone along the ventricular cavity and two pale zones: the narrow marginal zone (above the cortical plate) and the wide intermediate zone (the middle part of the telencephalic wall). Initial thalamocortical fibers (T) penetrate from the diencephalon into the telencephalic wall. Bar = 1 mm*

The earliest post-synaptic elements, dendrites, are also distributed within the marginal zone and belong to apical dendritic arborization of neurons from the cortical plate. In addition, some dendrites of the marginal zone belong to the fetal Cajal–Retzius cells. Deep dendrites are distributed within the pre-subplate zone and belong to the basal dendritic arborization of the neurons in the cortical plate. In addition, some of these dendrites belong to

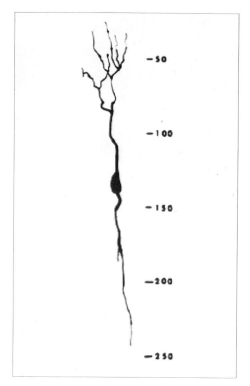

Figure 4 *Camera lucida drawing of the young bipolar neuron neuron situated within the cortical plate of the early human fetus. Note the initial terminal branching of the apical dendrite. Golgi impregnation; numbers indicate the subpial depth in micrometers*

early maturing neurons of the pre-subplate zone. Within the cortical plate, there are very few dendrites and one can see only cell bodies of bipolar, radially oriented neurons (Figure 4). Summarizing the early fetal development of the neural connections in the neocortical anlage, one can say that connectivity elements (axons, dendrites, synapses) develop in bilaminar fashion, above and below the cortical plate.

The subplate zone develops between the 13th and 15th weeks of gestation

During a relatively short period, between the 12th and 13th postovulatory weeks, in the deep part of the cortical plate, the cell-packing density decreases and the border between the cortical plate and the pre-subplate zone becomes obscured. The whole cortical plate shows bilaminar organization: its superficial part is cell-dense, while its deep part is characterized by low cell-packing density. Simultaneously there is an enlargement of the pale, cell-poor zone below the cortical plate.

Instead of the thin pre-subplate zone of the earlier stage, there now appears the permanently enlarging new layer, the subplate zone. This stage was called in classical literature the 'stage of the biliaminate cortical plate'[38]. The major histogenetic events contributing to this enlargement of the deep cortical anlage are: ingrowth of axons, loss of radial cell orientation in the deep part of the cortical plate and the growth of dendrites with intensive synaptogenesis. The number of synapses increases significantly within the newly formed subplate zone between the 13th and 15th weeks of gestation[15]. Since the enlargement of the deep, fibrous cortical anlage leads to the formation of the subplate zone, this developmental phase can be designated as a subplate formation stage.

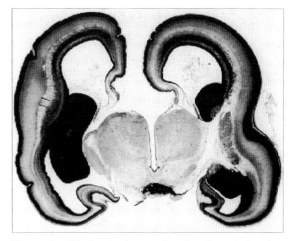

Figure 5 *Nissl-stained coronal section through the telencephalon of a 15-week-old human fetus (crown–rump length = 110 mm). The neocortical anlage displays a typical fetal pattern, consisting of three zones: the marginal zone, clearly delineated cortical plate ('second consolidation of the cortical plate') and prominent subplate zone below the cortical plate (arrows indicate the lower border of the subplate zone)*

Transient cortical organization during the mid-fetal period (16–24 weeks of gestation)

During the period between the 16th and 24th weeks of gestation (phase IV, stages 7 and 8), there is a developmental maximum of the fetal lamination pattern. This period, characteristic for the development of the human cortex, is also prominent in other primates.

At the beginning of this phase (stage 7, 16–18 weeks of gestation), the lower border of the cortical plate again becomes clearly delineated – in the classical literature it was designated as the 'secondary consolidation of the cortical plate'[38].

The main features of the lamination pattern are: a thick cortical plate which undergoes 'secondary' consolidation and a very large, prominent, fibrous, synapse-rich subplate zone (Figure 5) which is the thickest zone of the cortical anlage during this period (four times thicker than the cortical plate). The neocortical anlage consists of the following layers: the marginal zone, cortical plate and subplate zone. Below the subplate zone, there are other transient pallial compartments: the intermediate, subventricular and ventricular zones.

The proliferative activity within the ventricular zone continues and both glia and neurons are produced during this period. Autoradiographic data obtained for the corresponding period in the monkey indicate that neurons destined for superficial layers are produced in this period. These neurons destined for superficial cortical layers migrate through the intermediate zone towards the cortical plate, where they take positions superficial (external) to bodies of 'older' neurons, born during the earlier stages of cortical development. This is the so-called second wave of migration (the first wave occurred during the first consolidation of the cortical plate).

The most prominent histogenetic event in this period is ingrowth of afferent axons through the subplate zone. Afferent axons from the basal forebrain and thalamus grow through the subplate zone during a prolonged period (waiting period) between the 15th and 24th weeks of gestation. Basal forebrain afferents originate in the cholinergic nucleus basalis of Meynert while thalamic fibers originate in thalamic nuclei corresponding to a given thalamocortical projection. Many axons terminate within the subplate zone and this zone becomes the most significant site of synaptogenesis in the cortical anlage. The other zone with intensive synaptogenesis is the marginal zone. Dendritic development occurs concomitantly with synaptogenesis. The most differentiated dendrites belong to the polymorphic cells of the subplate zone and to neurons destined for the deepest cortical layers (layers VI and V). Finally, in the second half of this period the initial lamination of the cortical plate occurs, and only in the oldest fetuses from this developmental period do synapses develop within the cortical plate (from 19 weeks of gestation onwards)[15,26]. Furthermore, at the end of this period, the first cortical neurons develop peptidergic activity.

Summarizing this period, we emphasize that the major event is an ingrowth of afferent fibers through the special fetal subplate zone. The other important feature is the simultaneous occurrence of intensive proliferation, migration, neuronal differentiation, axonal ingrowth and intracortical synaptogenesis. In contrast to this, earlier developmental periods are dominated by proliferative, migratory processes while later, perinatal periods are dominated by neuronal differentiation and synaptogenesis. In general, there is a deep-to-superficial gradient of maturation in the cortex. Therefore, deep cortical layers are 'older' than superficial layers (II–IV). The marginal zone (layer I) is an exception, because it matures concomitantly with the deepest cortical zone (subplate zone).

Developmental reorganization and initial areal differentiation in the cortex of the late fetus and premature infants (25 weeks of gestation to term)

Histogenetic processes continue during late gestation with various intensities. Processes leading to an increase in the number of neurons, i.e. proliferation and migration, gradually decline in intensity and at birth all neocortical neurons are expected to be within the cortical layers. However, the production of glial cells, namely astroglia and oligodendroglia, continues with great intensity. Since some astroglia are formed from radial glial cells, one can observe numerous transitional forms[10]. As a morphological consequence of diminished proliferative activity, the ventricular and subventricular zones gradually become thinner. The exception is the ventricular zone of the mid-lateral neopallium, where it is in continuation with the still well-developed ganglionic eminence. In infants with low birth weight, this enlarged, vulnerable ventricular zone may be a site of periventricular bleeding.

In contrast to the decreasing intensity of 'productive' processes (proliferation and migration), the processes of neuronal differentiation, axonal ingrowth and synaptogenesis are of ever increasing intensity. In the process of neuronal differentiation, the most prominent developmental change occurs in the differentiation of pyramidal neurons of layer V, which develop rich basal and apical dendritic arborization. After 32–34 weeks of gestation, pyramidal neurons of layer III begin to differentiate dendritic trees[32,33], and their characteristic shape appears in some parts of the cortex. Simultaneously, there is an elaboration of terminal fields of thalamocortical axons within the prospective layer IV of the cortical plate; in some parts of the cortical anlage one can see the initial vertical segregation of the thalamocortical fibers[13]. This differentiation of dendrites within layers V and III, together with the laminar distribution of thalamocortical axons, leads to the new appearance of the cortical anlage with clear outlines of six-layered lamination throughout the neocortex after 32 weeks of gestation (Figure 6).

A transient deep concentration of presynaptic axons, synapses and postsynaptic elements within the subplate zone changes dramatically between the 24th and 28th weeks of gestation, when thalamocortical fibers penetrate the cortical plate[13–15] and intensive synaptogenesis occurs within the cortical plate[15,26,27]. During this phase of development, thalamocortical fibers display a transient intensive AChE reactivity and columnar distribution[13,23,29]. It should also be noted that the appearance of thalamocortical

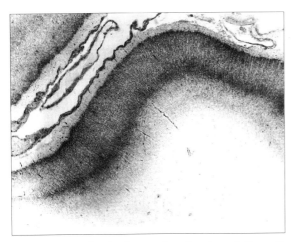

Figure 6 *Nissl-stained coronal section through the auditory cortex of the 34-week-old human fetus. Note the six immature adult-like layers within the cortical plate (six-layered 'Grundtypus of Brodmann')*

afferents in the prestriate visual[14,15], auditory[42,13] and somatosensory[15] cortices correlates well with the development of synapses in the cortical plate after the 23rd week of gestation[15,22,26,27].

This period of development is also characterized by intensive development of various transmitters and modulators, predominantly within the deep part of the cortical anlage, i.e. the subplate zone. Rapidly differentiating peptidergic neurons have been found within the subplate zone as well as deep parts of the cortical plate[31,44,45]. It is very likely that many peptidergic neurons coexist with GABAergic neurons, as was demonstrated in comparative stages of the fetal rhesus monkey[46].

The most important cytoarchitectonic event during the late fetal period is areal differentiation. Depending on the region, it begins between the 25th and 34th week of gestation (stage 9) and continues as a protracted process well into the postnatal period. In the frontal lobe, a primary cortical motor area can be recognized, due to the presence of differentiating Betz cells. Other areas of the frontal lobe begin to differentiate, too, but their landmarks are not yet definitive and clear. In the parietal lobe, a somatosensory area develops as a wide cytoarchitectonic belt with prominent granularity of layer IV. In the occipital lobe, one can clearly delineate the primary visual cortex (area 17). This area can be clearly delineated even before the 25th week of gestation on the basis of its histochemical reactivity. In the temporal lobe, the primary auditory cortex can be delineated on the basis of the vertical arrangement of its cells. There are many descriptions of areal differentiation in the literature[5], but this dynamic process is relatively poorly understood and requires future study. In particular, areal differentiation should be related to ingrowth of afferents, transmitter maturation and neuronal differentiation.

It should be emphasized that the cerebral cortex is still very immature, despite the appearance of an adult-like lamination pattern and initial areal differentiation. There are profound differences in both laminar and fibrillar organization between the late fetal (premature) and postnatal cortex, as follows:

(1) The first major difference is the presence of fetal zones or layers in the premature cortex. The fetal subplate zone is still prominent in most parts of the cortex. It first becomes resolved in the depth of the cortical sulci (formed throughout the late fetal period). The presence of the fetal subplate zone below six cortical layers is an important parameter of immaturity, since this zone contains growing afferent fibers, transient classes of fetal neurons and probably some transient synapses. The marginal zone still contains a transient fetal subpial granular layer, which gradually disappears during this period.

(2) The second major feature that distinguishes the premature cortex from the postnatal cortex is the high cell-packing density and relative paucity of the neuropil. An especially high cell-packing density is present in layer II, i.e. the youngest layer of the cortical anlage. The prospective layer IV also shows high cell-packing density and is present throughout the entire fetal neocortex.

(3) The third major difference is the permanent growth of afferents. On the basis of

a comparative analysis between the development of human and monkey cortex[13-15], one can expect growth of callosal afferents. That possibility is in accordance with the intensive differentiation of pyramidal neurons of layer III, known as the source of callosal projections.

(4) The fourth difference lies in the transient histochemical properties of certain classes of afferent fibers. For example, thalamocortical fibers destined for layer IV of the cortex show an intensive, transient AChE reactivity which disappears during later development (Figure 7). On the other hand, during this late fetal period, major cortical transmitter systems such as the cholinergic system develop intensive intracortical maturation and synaptogenesis[12].

The period of late gestation and prematurity is characterized by an intensive synaptogenesis. After the 24th week of gestation, synaptogenesis gradually occupies the cortical plate, in a deep-to-superficial fashion.

CORRELATION OF STRUCTURAL AND FUNCTIONAL DEVELOPMENT

Motor development

Up to the 7th week (crown–rump length about 18 mm), the fetus seems to remain immobile. The first spontaneous movements of the fetal trunk and limbs appear at 7.5 to 8 weeks of gestation[47]. Several days later, these movements are replaced by general movements and startles, involving the trunk, head and limbs; again later, small isolated limb movements are observed and the motor repertoire expands rapidly from the 10th week of gestation onward[48]. An exhaustive list of types of fetal movement during the first half of pregnancy can be found in the study of De Vries and colleagues[49].

Cortical areas important for goal-directed behavior as well as their connections with functionally important subcortical areas are not yet developed. It is therefore obvious that the dynamic pattern of neuronal production and migration during the early fetal period, together with the immaturity of cerebral circuits, are too immature for cerebral involvement in motor behavior. The appearance of the first quantifiable numbers of synapses within the cortical anlage towards the end of this period may form a substrate for the first cortical activity observed at 19 weeks of gestation.

During the second half of pregnancy, motor behavior becomes increasingly frequent and variable. In short, a rich variety of fetal and premature movements has been described[47,48,50] and it has been shown that the repertoire of fetal movements consists exclusively of motor patterns, which can also be observed postnatally, and that there is a high degree of continuity of neural functions before and after birth[47-52]. However, the newborn's behavioral repertoire rapidly expands with patterns never observed in the fetus, such as the Moro response[47,48,50]. Furthermore, there is apparently a strong organizing influence of supraspinal structures on normal fetal activity, as indicated by a study of the anencephalic fetus[53]. Finally, there are significant developmental changes in specific patterns of movement, such as eye movements, during the last trimester of pregnancy; isolated eye movements have been observed since the 16th week of gestation and rapid eye movements since the 19th week[54]. In fetuses between 32 weeks' menstrual age and term, both nystagmoid rapid eye movements (REMs) and slow rolling eye movements (SEMs) were detected; REMs occurred frequently and tended to be present in groups, whereas SEMs were isolated and less frequent[55].

One can conclude that in the late fetus and preterm infant one can see the fragments of future motor patterns underlying goal-directed behavior[47,48,50].

Electrophysiological development

Rapid structural and functional development of the central nervous system during the last weeks of gestation and in the neonatal period is reflected in the rapidly changing bioelectrical activity of the infant's brain as well as in its behavior. A characteristic pattern of a very early

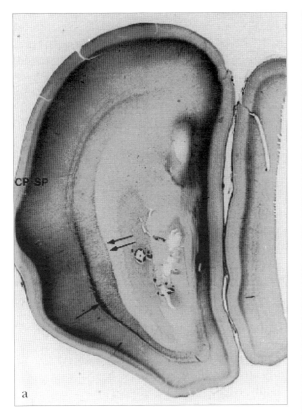
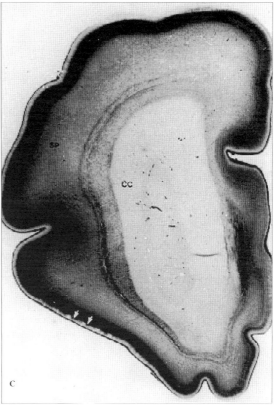
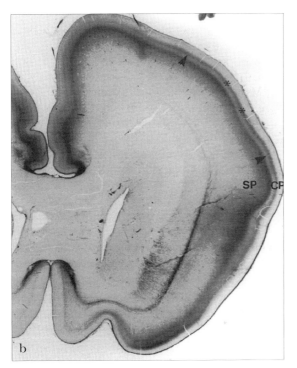

Figure 7 Laminar shifts and regional differences in AChE-reactive staining in the human prefrontal cortex at different fetal stages. In a 22-week-old fetus (a), AChE-reactive fibers originating in the basal forebrain (external capsule, arrow) and thalamus (internal capsule, double arrow) accumulate transiently in the superficial part (asterisk) of the subplate zone (SP), displaying the earliest cortical regional differences. In the 24-week-old fetus (b), AChE-reactive fibers gradually penetrate into the cortical plate (small asterisks) with a parallel decrease in staining of the subplate zone. At 28 weeks of gestation (c), strong AChE reactivity is evident in the cortical plate throughout the basolateral prefrontal cortex (arrowheads). Note laminar preference of AChE with heavy staining of layer IV, columnar pattern in the lateral and especially the basal portion of the frontal pallium (arrowheads), and regional differences related to the staining pattern of the cortical plate. Furthermore, at this stage the thickness of the subplate zone is 4–5 times that of the heavily stained cortical plate (developmental peak of subplate, between arrows). CC, corpus callosum; CP, cortical plate; SP, subplate zone

stage of bioelectrical development (24–27 weeks) is discontinuous bioelectrical activity with burst discharges[56].

In early premature babies (27–33 weeks' gestational age), the occipital areas tend to show higher voltage and lower frequencies than other scalp areas; delta brushes tend to increase in number between 27 and 32 weeks' gestational age[57] and attain the greatest abundance between 31 and 34 weeks of conceptional age[58]. Except for frontal sharp transients ('encoches frontales'), the spikes and sharp waves are only sporadic in early premature infants[57]. Anderson and co-workers[57] suggested that the sawtooth pattern, which tended to increase and then to decline between 27 and 32 weeks of conceptional age, may be characteristic for early premature infants. Furthermore, in these infants, they described an isolated slow delta wave ('delta crest') that was seen only in the frontopolar areas, was frequently symmetric and was synchronous on both hemispheres. Interhemispheric relationships on electroencephalogram (EEG) are weak in premature infants, have increased by the age of 40 weeks and increase even more later[59].

The main features of EEG maturation in preterm infants (29–38 weeks) are a progressive spatiotemporal differentiation, a decrease in discontinuous activity with burst discharges and an increase in various rhythmic activities[60]. Lombroso[58] found a progressively increasing interhemispheric synchrony with advancing conceptional age, as well as a dramatic decrease of delta brushes after 34 weeks' conceptional age, especially during REM sleep[58]. One of the maturational changes that occurs with increasing gestational age in premature infants is the evolution of the quiescent periods during the discontinuous portion of the EEG recording, known as interburst intervals[57].

As already stated, another major feature of premature infants is the presence of a number of transient EEG phenomena[61]. Two EEG patterns of non-rapid eye movements (NREM) sleep, 'slow wave' and 'trace alternant' stages, have a transient nature in premature infants[58]. Delta brushes represent one of the more characteristic signatures of prematurity in EEG[58]; these rhythms decrease with increasing postconceptional age and practically disappear after term[61]. According to Cioni and associates[61], specific waveforms typical of a given postmenstrual age are temporal theta at 29–31 weeks of postmenstrual age and delta brush after 31 weeks. It is important to stress that behavioral states are consistently present only after 36 weeks of gestational age[47,48,50].

Structural basis of physiological development in the late fetus and premature infant

Until recently, developmental neurologists considered the fetus and premature infant as having only subcortical functions. Now it is clear that the cortex of the fetus and premature infant is capable of receiving inputs through synaptic junctions and of responding to stimuli and exhibiting some kind of efferent motor activity.

After 15 weeks of gestation and in particular around 24 weeks of gestation, when thalamocortical and basal forebrain cholinergic input is established in the cortex, functional activity of synapses is very likely, because of their morphological maturity and the presence of transmitter machinery. The predominance of deep synaptogenesis together with the accumulation of thalamic and basal forebrain afferents in the deep 'waiting' compartment, just before the penetration of the cortical plate[15,22,23], correlates well with the first intermittent high-amplitude electroencephalographic bursts in the cerebral hemisphere found between 20 and 24 weeks of gestation[62]. The predominance of deep circuitry elements must have an influence on the prospective dipole of cortical electrical activity. The early electrical cortical response is surface-positive due to the predominance of deep synaptogenesis. Later, near birth, the cortical potential becomes surface-negative and changes again into surface-positive during postnatal life. Weitzman and Graziani[63] elicited widespread monophasic surface-negative cortical auditory evoked potential in preterm infants at 28 weeks of gestation; according to our data, thalamocortical axons are present in the middle third of the auditory cortical anlage at that period[42,43]. Geniculocortical axon terminals are also limited to layer IV throughout the early period of evoked potential ontogenesis[14,15]. Furthermore, studies of the somatosensory cortex of fetal sheep[64] and the auditory cortex of the neonatal kitten[65,66] have shown the ontogenetically earliest responses to be generated in the deep part of the cortical anlage. Both the visual and the auditory evoked potential become predominantly surface-positive over their respective primary sensory cortices between 36 and 40 weeks post-conceptional age in humans[67]. For example, the cortical auditory evoked potential displays a characteristic maturational sequence: a predominantly negative cortical waveform becomes positive in polarity near term, first over the frontocentral regions, and then over the temporal region at 1–2 months of age[63,68,69].

Such maturational change from a predominantly surface-negative sensory evoked potential to a predominantly surface-positive one, together with the abovementioned anatomical data, suggest that the developmental changes observed in human infant evoked potentials may result from an early preponderance of activation within the thalamo-recipient laminae rather than in the superficial cortex; the later developing surface-positive response may then reflect activation of the pyramidal cells within lamina III[69].

The establishment of thalamocortical connections seems to be the necessary prerequisite for the cortical analysis of sensory inputs, the perception of pain in the human fetus[70]. The basal forebrain afferent system may also participate in the establishment of transient behavioral patterns between 30 and 34 weeks of gestation[12], characterized by the irregularity of sleep organization, with an earlier appearance of active REM sleep[62,71].

Developmental state at birth

In contrast to the relative maturity of the external configuration of the cortex at birth, some histogenetic processes are not yet finished. There is no production of cortical neurons at birth and almost all neurons of the newborn cortex have attained their final positions.

Cytoarchitectonically, at birth all primary (motor, somatosensory, visual and auditory) cortical areas can be delineated on the basis of their characteristic lamination pattern or the presence of characteristic cells (e.g. Betz pyramids in the primary motor cortex). The delineation of secondary and tertiary (associated) cortical areas is rather uncertain. One of the reasons is that in the newborn the granular layer (prospective layer IV) is present in all neocortical areas regardless of their future differentiation into the agranular (e.g. motor) or granular cortex. As a further sign of the immaturity of the newborn cortex, one can find, below layer VI, a vestige of the fetal subplate zone and numerous neurons in the white matter. Although white matter 'interstitial' neurons are present in the adult brain, too, they are much more numerous in the newborn cortex[28].

Furthermore, the process of dendritic maturation is ongoing. In addition to the process of elaboration of the dendritic tree of the pyramidal cells, a major event is the dendritic differentiation of stellate (Golgi type II) local circuitry neurons[33]; many of these local circuitry neurons synthesize the transmitter GABA and are very likely inhibitory in action. The process of axonal ingrowth is finished for basal cholinergic and thalamocortical afferents[12–15]. However, synaptogenesis involving these axons continues. Our data support the premise that changes in the distribution and chemical properties of the subcortico-cortical pathways play a significant role in the perinatal reorganization of the prefrontal cortex in humans[23,25,29,30]. Whether cortico-cortical pathways are involved in structural rearrangements of the human infant cerebral cortex is not known.

In the human cortex, 'waiting' associative and commissural pathways are major constituents of the subplate zone after 28 weeks of gestation[15]. Considering the fact that most thalamocortical axons enter the cortical plate before birth[13–15,29,42,43], cortico-cortical fibers are the most likely constituents of the postnatal subplate zone. The prolonged persistence of the subplate zone in the frontal cortex may then be explained by the prolonged postnatal growth of the cortico-cortical pathways.

Accordingly, a significant redistribution of cortico-cortical axons during subsequent development can be expected[19,20,72,73]. Moreover, cortico-cortical axons are produced in excess during perinatal life. The final number is achieved by the process of competitive elimination during postnatal life[72,73]. That implies a considerable rearrangement (retraction or pruning of axonal collaterals?) in callosal and other cortico-cortical connections after birth. Unfortunately, virtually nothing is known about the status of the maturity of associative connections.

A special situation seems to occur with respect to the callosal connections. Recent experimental studies in the monkey have shown that commissural cortico-cortical fibers reside in the transient 'subplate' zone between embryonic days E100 and E123[74,75]. Ipsilateral cortico-cortical fibers also 'wait' in the subplate zone for several weeks before entering the cortical plate[75]. In addition, some subplate neurons transiently send their axons through the corpus callosum[75]. In the monkey, callosal axons at birth are three times more numerous than in the adult[72]. In the human newborn one can expect a similar situation, but somewhat later, since most newborn mammals are more mature at birth than is the human baby.

In summary, at birth all neurons destined for the cerebral cortex are extant and have attained their final position. Other histogenetic processes, e.g. synaptogenesis, neuronal differentiation and growth of association and commissural fibers, are very intensive. Since the newborn cortex sends and receives some supernumerary axons and contains the vestige of fetal elements, one can expect considerable rearrangements in organization during early postnatal ontogenesis.

CONCLUSIONS

During prenatal and postnatal ontogenesis, the human cerebrum undergoes prolonged maturation and substantial structural and chemical reorganization. These structural–chemical developmental changes correlate to some extent with electrophysiological maturational shifts as revealed by different electrophysiological methods applied to human fetuses, preterm infants and children. The correlation between electrophysiological maturation and structural changes (laminar development, synaptogenesis, dendritic maturation, axonal ingrowth, modular development, transmitter maturation, etc.) seems to be closer in the early and late fetus than during postnatal development. For example, shifts of synaptogenesis and transmitter distribution and growing axons within the deep cortical anlage (subplate zone) have an impact on the changing cortical dipole. Both structural and electrophysiological maturation of cortical neurons, layers and areas as well as their connections underlie the neurobiological basis of the ontogenesis of general behavioral patterns, goal-directed behavior and cognitive development.

During the early fetal period, early neurons make initial synapses, which form the basis for the earliest electrical activity of the human brain. The overall immaturity of neuronal connections, particularly in cortical areas, correlates with the absence of any behavioral pattern or goal-directed movements.

In the late fetus and preterm infant, transient accumulation of major afferent pathways, the presence of transient layers (subplate zone), and the transient pattern of transmitter-related organization form the neurological basis of cortical electric responses as well as changes of transient behavioral states, and transient sleep patterns, as described by numerous investigators[48,50]. Fragments resembling goal-directed movements may be the result of an initial neuronal connection established at both cortical and subcortical levels. In the neonatal period, transient fetal elements persist and correspond to transient behavioral patterns. Parallel to the profound structural and chemical reorganization during the first 6–8 months, there is the disappearance of transient motor and behavioral patterns. The structural and chemical reorganization includes the disappearance of the deep subplate zone, the final ingrowth of afferent pathways and changes in transmitter distribution and modular arrangement of neuronal elements. The appearance of fragments of skilled movements correlates with the parallel maturation of both associative, and motor and sensory cortical areas. The previously close spatiotemporal correlation between these events becomes progressively looser.

ACKNOWLEDGEMENTS

This work has been supported by scientific funds of the Ministry of Science of the Republic of Croatia.

References

1. His, W. (1904). *Die Entwicklung des menschlichen Gehirns während der esten Monate*, 176 pp. (Leipzig: Hirzel)
2. Hochstetter, F. (1919). *Beiträge zur Entwicklungsgeschichte des menschlichen Gehirns. I.*, 170 pp. (Vienna: Deuticke)
3. Filimonoff, I. N. (1929). Zur embryonalen und postembryonalen Entwicklung der Grosshirnrinde des Menschen. *J. Psychol. Neurol.*, **39**, 323–89
4. Filimonoff, I. N. (1947). A rational subdivision of the cerebral cortex. *Arch. Neurol. Psychiat. (Chicago)*, **58**, 296–311
5. Kahle, W. (1969). *Die Entwicklung der menschlichen Grosshirnhemisphäre*, Neurology Series Vol. 1, 116 pp. (Berlin: Springer)
6. Poliakov, G. I. (1979). *Entwicklung der Neuronen der menschlichen Grosshirnrinde*, 320 pp. (Leipzig: VEB Georg Thieme)
7. Yakovlev, P. I. (1969). The development of the nuclei of the dorsal thalamus and of the cerebral cortex, morphogenetic and tectogenetic correlation. In Locke, S. (ed.) *Modern Neurology. Papers in Tribute to Professor Derek Denny-Brown*, pp. 15–53. (Boston: Little, Brown)
8. Rakic, P. (1982). Early developmental events: cell lineages, acquisition of neuronal positions, and areal and laminar development. *Neurosci. Res. Prog. Bull.*, **20**, 439–51
9. Rakic, P. (1972). Mode of cell migration to the superficial layers of fetal monkey neocortex. *J. Comp. Neurol.*, **145**, 61–84
10. Schmechel, D. E. and Rakic, P. (1979). A Golgi study of radial glial cells in developing monkey telencephalon: morphogenesis and transformation into astrocytes. *Anat. Embryol.*, **156**, 115–52
11. Rakic, P. (1977). Prenatal development of the visual system in the rhesus monkey. *Phil. Trans. R. Soc. Lond. (Biol.)*, **278**, 245–60
12. Kostović, I. (1986). Prenatal development of nucleus basalis complex and related fibre systems in man: a histochemical study. *Neuroscience*, **17**, 1047–77
13. Kostović, I. and Goldman-Rakic, P. S. (1983). Transient cholinesterase staining in the mediodorsal nucleus of the thalamus and its connections in the developing human and monkey brain. *J. Comp. Neurol.*, **219**, 431–47
14. Kostović, I. and Rakic, P. (1984). Development of prestriate visual projections in the monkey and human fetal cerebrum revealed by transient cholinesterase staining. *J. Neurosci.*, **4**, 25–42
15. Kostović, I. and Rakic, P. (1990). Developmental history of the transient subplate zone in the visual and somatosensory cortex of the macaque monkey and human brain. *J. Comp. Neurol.*, **297**, 441–70
16. Rakic, P. (1988). Specification of cerebral cortical areas. *Science*, **241**, 170–6
17. Rakic, P. (1988). Defects of neuronal migration and pathogenesis of cortical malformations. *Prog. Brain Res.*, **73**, 15–37
18. Cowan, W. M., Fawcett, J. W., O'Leary, D. D. M. and Stanfield, B. B. (1984). Regressive events in neurogenesis. *Science*, **225**, 1258–65
19. Innocenti, G. M. (1982). Development of interhemispheric cortical connections. *Neurosci. Res. Prog. Bull.*, **20**, 532–40
20. O'Leary, D. D. M. (1992). Development of connectional diversity and specificity in the mammalian brain by the pruning of collateral projections. *Curr. Opinion Neurobiol.*, **2**, 70–7
21. Rakic, P., Bourgeois, J.-P., Zečević, N., Eckenhoff, M. F. and Goldman-Rakic, P. S. (1986). Concurrent overproduction of synapses in diverse regions of the primate cerebral cortex. *Science*, **232**, 232–5
22. Kostović, I. (1990). Zentralnervensystem. In Hinrichsen, K. V. (ed.) *Humanembryologie*, pp. 381–448. (Berlin–Heidelberg–New York: Springer-Verlag)
23. Kostović, I. (1990). Structural and histochemical reorganization of the human prefrontal cortex during perinatal and postnatal life. In Uylings, H. B. M., Van Eden, C. G., De Bruin, J. P. C., Corner, M. A. and Feenstra, M. G. P. (eds.) *The*

Prefrontal Cortex, Progress in Brain Research, Vol. 85, pp. 223–40. (Amsterdam: Elsevier)

24. Kostović, I., Judaš, M., Kostović-Knežević, Lj., Šimić, G., Delalle, I., Chudy, D., Šajin, B. and Petanjek, A. (1991). Zagreb Research Collection of human brains for developmental neurobiologists and clinical neuroscientists. *Int. J. Dev. Biol.*, **35**, 215–30

25. Kostović, I., Petanješk, Z., Delalle, I. and Judas, M. (1992). Developmental reorganization of the human association cortex during the perinatal and postnatal life. In Kostović, I., Knežević, S., Wisniewski, H. M. and Spillich, G. J. (eds.) *Neurodevelopment, Aging and Cognition*, pp. 3–17. (Boston–Basel–Berlin: Birkhäuser)

26. Molliver, M. E., Kostović, I. and Van der Loos, H. (1973). The development of synapses in cerebral cortex of the human fetus. *Brain Res.*, **50**, 403–7

27. Kostović, I. and Molliver, M. E. (1974). A new interpretation of the laminar development of cerebral cortex: synaptogenesis in different layers of neopallium in the human fetus. *Anat. Rec.* **178**, 395

28. Kostović, I. and Rakic, P. (1980). Cytology and time of origin of interstitial neurons in the white matter in infant and adult human and monkey telencephalon. *J. Neurocytol.*, **9**, 219–42

29. Kostović, I., Škavić, J. and Strinović, D. (1988). Acetylcholinesterase in the human frontal associative cortex during the period of cognitive development: early laminar shifts and late innervation of pyramidal neurons. *Neurosci. Lett.*, **90**, 107–12

30. Kostović, I., Lukinović, N., Judaš, M., Bogdanović, N., Mrzljak, L., Zečević, N. and Kubat, M. (1989). Structural basis of the developmental plasticity in the human cerebral cortex: the role of the transient subplate zone. *Metab. Brain Dis.*, **4**, 17–23

31. Kostović, I., Štefulj-Fučić, A., Mrzljak, L., Jukić, S. and Delalle, I. (1991). Prenatal and perinatal development of the somatostatin-immunoreactive neurons in the human prefrontal cortex. *Neurosci. Lett.*, **124**, 153–6

32. Mrzljak, L., Uylings, H. B. M., Kostović, I. and Van Eden, C. G. (1988). Prenatal development of neurons in the human prefrontal cortex. I. A qualitative Golgi study. *J. Comp. Neurol.*, **271**, 355–86

33. Mrzljak, L., Uylings, H. B. M., Van Eden, C. G. and Judaš, M. (1990). Neuronal development in human prefrontal cortex in prenatal and postnatal stages. In: Uylings, H. B. M., Van Eden, C. G., De Bruin, J. P. C., Corner, M. A. and Feenstra, M. G. P. (eds.) *The Prefrontal Cortex*, Progress in Brain Research, Vol. 85, pp. 185–222. (Amsterdam: Elsevier)

34. Huttenlocher, P. R. (1979). Synaptic density in human frontal cortex. Developmental changes and effects of aging. *Brain Res.*, **163**, 195–205

35. Huttenlocher, P. R., De Courten, C., Garey, L. J. and Van der Loos, H. (1982). Synaptogenesis in human visual cortex – evidence for synapse elimination during normal development. *Neurosci. Lett.*, **33**, 247–52

36. Chi, J. G., Dooling, E. C. and Gilles, F. H. (1977). Gyral development of the human brain. *Ann. Neurol.* **1**, 86–93

37. Fees-Higgins, A. and Larroche, J-C. (1987). *Le développement du cerveau foetal humain. Atlas Anatomique.* (Paris: Masson)

38. Sidman, R. L. and Rakic, P. (1973). Neuronal migration, with special reference to developing human brain: a review. *Brain Res.*, **62**, 1–35

39. Sidman, R. L. and Rakic, P. (1982). Development of the human central nervous system. In Haymaker, W. and Adams, R. D. (eds.) *Histology and Histopathology of the Nervous System*, pp. 3–138. (Springfield, Illinois: C. C. Thomas)

40. Boulder Committee Report (1970). Embryonic vertebrate central nervous system: revised terminology. *Anat. Rec.*, **166**, 257–62

41. Choi, B. H. and Lapham, L. W. (1978). Radial glia in the human fetal cerebrum: a combined Golgi, immunofluorescent and electron microscopic study. *Brain Res.*, **148**, 295–311

42. Krmpotić-Nemanić, J., Kostović, I., Kelović, Z. and Nemanić, D. (1980) Development of acetylcholinesterase (AChE) staining in human fetal auditory cortex. *Acta Otolaryngol. (Stockh.)*, **89**, 388–92

43. Krmpotić-Nemanić, J., Kostović, I., Kelović, Z., Nemanić, D. and Mrzljak, L. (1983). Development of the human fetal auditory cortex: growth of afferent fibres. *Acta Anat.*, **116**, 69–73

44. Kostović, I., and Štefulj-Fučić, A. (1985). Distribution of somatostatin immunoreactive neurons in frontal neocortex and underlying 'white' matter of the human fetus and preterm infant. *Soc. Neurosci. Abst.*, **11**, 352

45. Delalle, I. and Kostović, I. (1991). Laminar distribution of NPY-immunoreactive neurons in human prefrontal cortex during prenatal and postnatal development. *XIV Annual European Neuroscience Association Meeting*, Cambridge, UK, September 1991. (Abstr.) p.132

46. Meinecke, D. L. and Rakic, P. (1989). The temporal relationship between GABA and GABA-A/benzodiazepine receptor expression in neurons of the visual cortex of the developing rhesus monkey. *Soc. Neurosci. Abstr.*, **15**, 1335

47. Prechtl, H. F. R. (1985). Ultrasound studies of human fetal behaviour. *Early Human Dev.*, **12**, 91–8

48. Prechtl, H. F. R. (1989). Fetal behavior. In Hill, A. and Volpe, J. J. (eds.) *Fetal Neurology*, pp. 1–16. (New York: Raven Press)

49. DeVries, J. I. P., Visser, G. H. A. and Prechtl, H. F. R. (1985). The emergence of fetal behaviour. II. Quantitative aspects. *Early Hum. Dev.*, **12**, 99–120
50. Prechtl, H. F. R. (ed.) (1984). Continuity of neural functions from prenatal to postnatal life. *Clin. Dev. Med.*, **94**, 255
51. DeVries, J. I. P., Visser, G. H. A. and Prechtl, H. F. R. (1982). The emergence of fetal behaviour. I. Qualitative aspects. *Early Hum. Dev.*, **7**, 301–22
52. DeVries, J. I. P., Visser, G. H. A. and Prechtl, H. F. R. (1982). The emergence of fetal behaviour. III. Individual differences and consistencies. *Early Hum. Dev.*, **16**, 85–103
53. Visser, G. H. A., Laurini, R. N., DeVries, J. I. P., Bekedam, D. J. and Prechtl, H. F. R. (1985). Abnormal motor behaviour in anencephalic fetuses. *Early Hum. Dev.*, **12**, 173–82
54. Awoust, J. and Levi, S. (1983). Neurological maturation of the human fetus. In Levski, R. A. and Morley, P. (eds.) *Ultrasound '82*, pp. 583–7. (Oxford–New York: Pergamon Press)
55. Bots, R. S. G. M., Nijhuis, J. G., Martin, C. B. Jr and Prechtl, H. F. R. (1981). Human fetal eye movements: detection *in utero* by ultrasonography. *Early Human Dev.*, **5**, 87–94
56. Dreyfus-Brisac, C. (1968). Sleep ontogenesis in early human prematurity from 24 to 27 weeks of conceptional age. *Dev. Psychobiol.*, **1**, 162–9
57. Anderson, C. M., Torres, F. and Faoro, A. (1985). The EEG of the early premature. *Electroencephalogr. Clin. Neurophysiol.*, **60**, 95–105
58. Lombroso, C. T. (1979). Quantified electrographic scales on 10 preterm healthy newborns followed up to 40–43 weeks of conceptional age by serial polygraphic recordings. *Electroencephalogr. Clin. Neurophysiol.*, **46**, 460–74
59. Kuks, J. B. M., Vos, J. E. and O'Brien, M. J. (1988). EEG coherence functions for normal newborns in relation to their sleep state. *Electroencephalogr. Clin. Neurophysiol.*, **69**, 295–302
60. Nolte, R. and Haas, G. (1978). A polygraphic study of the bioelectrical brain maturation in preterm infants. *Dev. Med. Child Neurol.*, **20**, 167–82
61. Cioni, G., Biagioni, E. and Cipolloni, C. (1992). Brain before cognition: EEG maturation in preterm infants. In Kostović, I., Knežević, S., Wisniewski, W. H. and Spillich, G. J. (eds.), *Neurodevelopment, Aging and Cognition*, pp. 75–98. (Boston–Basel–Berlin: Birhäuser)
62. Dreyfus-Brisac, C. (1979). Ontogenesis of brain bioelectrical activity and sleep organization in neonates and infants. In Falkner, F. and Tanner, J. M. (eds.) *Neurobiology and Nutrition*, Human Growth Vol. 3, pp. 157–82. (London: Baillière Tindall)
63. Weitzman, E. D. and Graziani, L. J. (1968). Maturation and topography of the auditory evoked response of the prematurely born infant. *Dev. Psychobiol.*, **1**, 79–89
64. Persson, H. E. (1973). Development of somatosensory cortical functions – an electrophysiological study in prenatal sheep. *Acta Physiol. Scand.* (Suppl.), **395**, 1–64
65. König, N., Pujol, R. and Marty, R. (1972). A laminar study of evoked potentials and unit responses in the auditory cortex of the postnatal cat. *Brain Res.*, **36**, 469–73
66. Miyata, H., Kawaguchi, S., Samejima, A. and Yamamoto, T. (1982). Postnatal development of evoked responses in the auditory cortex of the cat. *Jpn. J. Physiol.*, **32**, 421–9
67. Vaughan, H. G. Jr and Kurtzberg, D. (1989). Electrophysiological indices of normal and aberrant cortical maturation. In Kellaway, P. and Noebels, J. L. (eds.) *Developmental Neurophysiology*. (Baltimore: Johns Hopkins University Press)
68. Kurtzberg, D., Hilpert, P. L., Kreuzer, J. A. and Vaughan, H. G. Jr (1984). Differential maturation of cortical auditory evoked potentials to speech sounds in normal full term and very low-birthweight infants. *Dev. Med. Child. Neurol.*, **26**, 466–75
69. Novak, G. P., Kurtzberg, D., Kreuzer, J. A. and Vaughan, H. G. Jr (1989). Cortical responses to speech sounds and their formants in normal infants: maturational sequence and spatiotemporal analysis. *Electroencephalogr. Clin. Neurophysiol.*, **73**, 295–305
70. Anand, K. J. S. and Hickey, P. R. (1987). Pain and its effects in the human neonate and fetus. *N. Engl. J. Med.*, **317**, 1321–9
71. Wolff, P. H. and Ferber, R. (1979). The development of behavior in human infants, premature and newborn. *Ann. Rev. Neurosci.*, **2**, 291–307
72. LaMantia, A. S. and Rakic, P. (1990). Axon overproduction and elimination in the corpus callosum of the developing rhesus monkey. *J. Neurosci.*, **10**, 2156–75
73. Chalupa, L. M. and Killackey, H. P. (1989). Process elimination underlies ontogenetic change in the distribution of callosal projection neurons in the postcentral gyrus of the fetal rhesus monkey. *Proc. Natl. Acad. Sci. USA*, **86**, 1076–9
74. Goldman-Rakic, P. S. (1982). Neuronal development and plasticity of association cortex in primates. *Neurosci. Res. Prog. Bull.*, **20**, 520–32
75. Schwartz, M. L., Rakic, P. and Goldman-Rakic, P. S. (1991). Early phenotype expression of cortical neurons: evidence that a subclass of migratory neurons have callosal axons. *Proc. Natl. Acad. Sci. USA*, **88**, 1354–8

Screening with ultrasound in obstetrics

G. P. Mandruzzato, G. D'Ottavio and M. A. Rustico

The diagnostic capabilities of ultrasound in obstetrics have been assessed in numerous papers in the literature, mainly in relation to high-risk pregnancies or specific clinical situations. The usefulness of ultrasonography is well established when it comes to resolving specific diagnostic problems. However, there is still considerable disagreement concerning the extension of this type of examination to all pregnant women, even where no risk factors are present.

Moreover, the ways in which ultrasound screening should be carried out have yet to be codified. In the early 1980s, it was recommended in the German Federal Republic that all pregnant women should undergo at least two ultrasound examinations. A subsequent 'consensus conference' in the United States in 1984 recommended, on the other hand, that ultrasound should only be carried out in specific cases, while in the same year in Norway and the United Kingdom it was suggested that ultrasound examinations should be carried out on all pregnant women. In Italy and France two scans – the first at 20 weeks and the second at 32 weeks – have been recommended. Attempts to resolve this problem by means of random clinical trials to assess reductions in perinatal mortality and morbidity resulting from routine ultrasound in all pregnant women have produced contrasting results.

In one study group, about 50% of major abnormalities were identified, with the consequent interruption of the pregnancy[1]. Perinatal mortality was reduced as compared with the controls. In a more recent trial carried out by the group RADIUS, no statistically significant differences, in terms of perinatal outcome, were found between the group of patients undergoing routine ultrasonographic screening and that in which ultrasound was used in a selective manner on a clinical basis[2].

None of the studies recorded examined more than 15 000 subjects, while Lilford and Chard[3] calculated that the number of examinations necessary to produce a reduction in the perinatal mortality rate from 10/1000 to 8/1000 would involve the study of 46 820 mothers. Consequently, the trials carried out so far have been based on an insufficient number of subjects. Moreover, perinatal outcome is a poor indicator unless uniform management is provided, considering that ultrasound offers only diagnostic information.

A different approach to the problem is that of defining specific objectives in prenatal screening. Recent surveys carried out among both European and American gynecologists reveal that obstetric ultrasound is fundamental in three specific fields: the early diagnosis of fetal malformations, the improved detection of intrauterine growth retardation (IUGR) and the precise dating of pregnancy.

As far as malformations and IUGR are concerned, the reason for extending this examination to all pregnant women is that more than 80% of fetal abnormalities and almost 50% of cases of IUGR are found in pregnancies in which there are no specific risk factors. The question, therefore, is whether diagnostic ultrasound has the necessary characteristics to be used as a screening test.

Screening is a tool which detects a predisposition for a particular disease or its treatable stages in people who are generally considered to be free of disease. A screening test is not always in itself diagnostic, but is should detect a subgroup of those tested who are at greater risk of having the disease or disorder than the original population screened. This group then needs to be investigated further using a diagnostic test, which is more time consuming, expensive and possibly invasive than the screening test. The requirements of a screening test are as follows:

(1) It must have enough sensitivity to avoid false-negatives;

(2) It must have high specificity to avoid taking unnecessary action in false-positive cases;

(3) Patients should find it comfortable and quickly performed;

(4) It should not cause adverse effects;

(5) Effective management should be available for any problems detected; and

(6) The benefit of its application should justify its cost.

As far as malformations are concerned, relatively few data are available with regard to the accuracy of a prenatal screening program for congenital defects. The assessment criteria, the number of examinations and gestational period in which they are carried out, the abnormalities considered and the level of preparation of the operators is also far from homogeneous. Table 1 contains the results that emerged from a review of the literature of the last few years.

Campbell and Smith[4] reported the results of five years' screening at King's College Hospital, London, where all the patients systematically underwent an ultrasound examination between the 16th and 18th week of pregnancy. Out of 16 670 women examined, 54 fetal malformations and just one false-positive result (hydrocephalus) were observed, for a sensitivity and specificity of 84% and 99.9%, respectively.

The results of a screening program performed at the hospital of Luton and Dunstable in 1988–89 are recorded by Chitty and colleagues[5]. Out of 8432 fetuses screened predominantly in the second trimester, 130 had some sort of abnormality (1.5%). In 93 cases these malformations were identified prior to the 24th week (74% sensitivity), and the presence of two false positives resulted in a specificity of 99.9%. By considering only the most serious malformations, the sensitivity increased to 82.8%.

Out of 8523 pregnant women screened at 19 weeks, Luck[6] recorded 166 malformations present at birth or during the first week of life (1.9% of a non-selected population), 140 of which were diagnosed at 19 weeks with a sensitivity of 85% and a specificity of 99.9%.

The data recorded by Levi and associates[7] in relation to a multicenter study involving four hospitals in Belgium between 1984 and 1989 revealed that 45% of fetal malformations could be diagnosed by a routine screening of the non-selected population, but only 21% of these were identified prior to the 22nd week.

The reduced accuracy which emerges from the study of Levy and colleagues is to a considerable extent due to the decision to include minor malformations as defined by Smith[8] and in the Eurocat register, a parameter which was not noted in any other study. It also reflects the reliability of ultrasound in peripheral hospitals, where the equipment and training of the operators is relatively heterogeneous, and provides a far more reliable picture of the real possibilities of applying a screening test on the entire population than do the results obtained in highly specialized centers, which undoubtedly have greater resources, but which would not be able, given their number, to handle the massive amount of work involved.

An attempt was made in our institute to answer this problem of the accuracy of an echographic screening program for fetal malformations in a non-selected population of pregnant

Table 1 Review of the literature concerning ultrasound screening programs

Reference	Number of subjects	Sensitivity (%)	Specificity (%)	Positive predictive value	Negative predictive value
Campbell and Smith[4]	16 670	84	99.9		
Levi et al.[7]	16 616	45.3	99.9	96	98.6
Chitty et al.[5]	8 432	74.4	99.9	97.9	99.6
Luck et al.[6]	8 523	85	99.9		

Table 2 *Methods used by the authors in ultrasound screening for fetal malformations*

	Requirements
Examinations	two, at 20–22 weeks and 30–32 weeks (at least one for checking fetal anatomy)
Follow-up	at birth and at 2 months of life (at least 2 years for malformed babies)
Confirmation	postnatal ultrasound examination or treatment surgery autopsy
Equipment	
1982	ATL MK300, 3.0 MHz M-sector probe
1986	AU 920, 3.5–5.0 MHz convex probes
1988	Acuson 128, 3.5 MHz E-sector probe
Operators	four gynecologists (with 2–4 years' experience) two gynecologists (with > 5 years' experience)

Table 3 *Sensitivity and specificity of ultrasound screening shown for individual organ systems*

	True positives (n)	False negatives (n)	Sensitivity (%)	Specificity (%)	Positive predictive value (%)	Negative predictive value (%)
Urinary	31	33	93.9	99.9	96.9	99.9
CNS	18	21	85.7	100	100	99.9
Skeletal	12	16	75.0	100	100	99.8
Lymphatic	11	11	100	100	100	100
Gastrointestinal tract	10	10	100	100	100	100
Miscellaneous	7	8	87.5	99.9	87.5	99.9
Total	89	99	89.9	99.9	97.8	99.9

women. A retrospective study was carried out on 8850 unselected pregnancies in which at least two sonographic examinations (at 20–22 and 30–32 weeks) were performed, from January 1982 to December 1990, for a total of 8910 fetuses (60 sets of twins). The positive features of this study were the homogeneity in the training of the operators, the use of instruments that were suitable for examining fetal anatomy at well-defined gestational ages and on the basis of a strict protocol (Table 2). Choroid plexus cysts, slight dilations of the renal pelvis and brain ventricles, in addition to abnormalities of the fingers and toes when isolated, were not defined as malformations. The clinical follow-up of all newborns was continued until the 2nd month after birth.

Data are available for all babies on which further examinations and/or surgery were performed. Autopsy findings are also available in all cases of termination of pregnancy or perinatal death. In this period 89 malformations (true-positive) were correctly identified before birth, and ten were missed (false-negative). Two cases defined as abnormal did not display any malformations at birth (false-positive). These were represented by a case of renal cystic dysplasia and one cystic adenomatoid malformation; these diagnoses did not in any case result in over-treatment, other than receiving more frequent ultrasound controls. Table 3 shows the accuracy of the test for any group of malformations, while Table 4 indicates the reliability of the test when carried out at 20–22 weeks' gestation.

As regards the number of false-negatives in the ultrasonographic examination during the second trimester (42), most of these (32) were detected at the subsequent examination. It can be observed that some abnormalities were not detected at the first examination, possibly as a result of their late appearance or the evolving nature of the lesion (microcephalia, intestinal obstructions, less severe cases of hydronephrosis). We therefore consider that only six cases (two cases of single kidney, two renal ectopia, one multicystic kidney and one umbilical hernia) were truly missed diagnoses during the second trimester. The first four were of little clinical relevance, while the other two could be treated surgically.

As regards the false-negatives at birth (not diagnosed at either the examination at 22 weeks or that at 32 weeks), generally speaking the considerations made above (progressive nature of some malformations or their low clinical relevance) hold true. The potentially disabling abnormalities which were not recognized (small lesions of the neural canal and the case of osteogenesis imperfecta type IV) proved not to be of serious clinical importance (Table 5). In our study, therefore we obtained for non-cardiac malformations a sensitivity of 89.9%, a specificity of 99.9%, a positive predictive value of 97.8% and a negative predictive value of 99.9% (Table 3). We believe that these results are good, given the type of population studied. It is not possible to compare these results with those of other studies, owing to the fact that heart

Table 4 *Sensitivity and specificity of ultrasound screening at 22 weeks of gestation, shown for individual organ systems*

	True positives (n)	False negatives (n)	Sensitivity (%)	Specificity (%)	Positive predictive value (%)
Urinary	17	16	51.5	100	100
CNS	17	4	80.9	100	100
Skeletal	12	4	75.0	100	100
Lymphatic	11	0	100	100	100
Gastrointestinal tract	2	8	20.0	100	100
Miscellaneous	3	5	38.5	100	100
Total	62	37	62.6	100	100

Table 5 *False-negatives in ultrasound screening for fetal malformations, shown for individual organ systems*

	At 20–22 weeks		At birth	
	n	Condition	n	Condition
CNS	1	microcephaly	1	communicating external hydrocephaly
			1	small occipital meningocele
			1	small lumbar lipomenigocele
Urinary	6	number/position abnormality	1	hydronephrosis
	1	ARPK	1	cystic dysplasia
	1	multicystic kidney		
	2	isolated cyst		
	4	hydronephrosis		
Gastrointestinal tract	2	small diaphragmatic hernia	0	
	1	duodenal stenosis		
	4	jejunal atresia		
Miscellaneous	1	omphalocele	1	Pierre Robin syndrome
	9	ovarian cysts		
	4	CCAM		
Skeletal	0		2	lubfoot
			1	OI (type IV)
			1	cleft lip
Lymphatic	0		0	
Total	33		10	

ARPK, autosomal recessive polycystic kidney; CCAM, congenital adenomatoid malformation (of the lung); OI, osteogenesis imperfecta malformations were not taken into consideration (these will be the subject of a later, separate study) and because the long follow-up period enabled us to detect later appearing abnormal cases.

ULTRASOUND SCREENING OF CONGENITAL CARDIOPATHIES

One aspect of prenatal diagnosis that has recently been introduced is the echographic screening of congenital cardiopathies. The fetal heart was in fact one of the last organs to be studied. This delay was due partly to the technical limitations of the echographic equipment which have now mainly been overcome, and partly to cultural factors: obstetricians for a long time considered the fetal heart a complex structure that was very difficult to explore. There has been, and to a certain extent still is, a tendency to leave any evaluation in pregnancies with a specific risk to cardiologists.

Recent epidemiological studies have indicated congenital heart malformations as the abnormalities most frequently encountered in postnatal life, and it has been shown that carrying out the examination in only high-risk cases makes it possible to diagnose only a small percentage of the cases that exist.

Accordingly, since the mid 1980s, the systematic inclusion of the four-chamber view in screening programs for fetal heart malformations has been advised. This scanning plane has certain important features: it is easy to teach and easy to learn, it can be carried out in a high percentage of cases (more than 95% in the second trimester), and, above all, it is on its own capable of detecting some of the most serious heart malformations[9].

The results found in the literature on this point are somewhat contradictory and difficult to compare as a result of the different methods of study used, the characteristics of the studied population, and the period of pregnancy. The rates of sensitivity range from 92%, obtained using a specific risk population, in which this high sensitivity reflected the high rate of the disease rather than the accuracy of the four chambers, to much lower sensitivities, as is shown by the most recently published studies on the general population.

Eik-Nes[10] has described the results of the Norwegian screening programme for heart malformations using the four-chamber view at 18 weeks. During the first stage of the research (3938 pregnancies studied), characterized by an approximate evaluation of the four-chamber section, the sensitivity was 14%. During the second stage (7182 pregnancies screened), thanks to the introduction of intensive teaching programs, the sensitivity increased to 36.3%, with the test capable of diagnosing 30% of serious heart defects. A third stage of this study is also planned, involving an assessment of arterial blood flow.

In Levi's perspective study carried out to check the accuracy of echography in the diagnosis of malformations (16 370 pregnant women studied in the second trimester), the sensitivity for the cardiovascular system was 23.5%; most of the diagnoses were made after 24 weeks[7].

In another perspective study[11], an initial period, in which the visualization of the four chamber view was left up to the operator (5336 pregnant women studied at 18–20 weeks), was compared with the next period (3680 patients observed at the same gestational period), characterized by an intense effort of the operators to obtain the section of the four chamber view in every examination. The sensitivity of echography in recognizing heart malformations increased from 43% to 81% without there being any significant increase in the length of the examination. Stoll and colleagues, in their prospective study[12], record a mean sensitivity for the four chambers of 9.2%, even though for certain serious abnormalities (such as the hypoplastic left-ventricle syndrome) the accuracy was much higher. They attributed the low sensitivity of the screening to the inadequate training of the operators and the insufficient time for the examination. They believed that a teaching program involving a complete evaluation of the fetal heart was feasible, however. Luck arrived at the same conclusion in her study involving 8523 pregnancies, in which a sensitivity of 36%[6] is described.

The prospective observational study, involving ten obstetric ultrasound units in England, UK, and more than 30 000 pregnant women in the second trimester, reveals that it is possible to diagnose with the four-chamber view almost 69% of the abnormalities that can be potentially recognized using this plane of screening, with an overall sensitivity of 77%[13].

Achiron and associates[14] compared the accuracy of the four chamber view echocardiography extended to the study of the ventricular–arterial connections in 5400 fetuses studied consecutively between 18 and 24 weeks. They concluded that a complete examination was feasible and increased sensitivity from 48% to 86%.

Our center for prenatal diagnosis carried out a study on a low-risk population of pregnant women in order to check the accuracy of ultrasound in the diagnosis of heart malformations[15]. From February 1986 to January 1992, fetal ultrasound examinations were carried out on 6557 patients at an average gestational age of 22 weeks. The examination included, in addition to a detailed observation of the entire fetal anatomy, a complete evaluation of the fetal heart: atrioventricular and ventricular-arterial connections and venous returns in accordance with the criteria codified in the literature. The operators involved and the instruments used were those described elsewhere. In one third of the cases the echocardiography has to be repeated during a more advanced gestational period (28–30 weeks) in order to arrive at a final decision on the normality of the fetal heart.

All the women delivered their babies in our institute. More than 95% of the babies were examined at birth and between the second and third month of life by the pediatrician, who informed the cardiologist of any pathologies which had not emerged previously. A complete cardiological examination was carried out immediately after birth on babies with an abnormal prenatal echocardiographic report. All autopsies were performed by the same anatomist–pathologist in our institute. During this period, 24 heart malformations were correctly diagnosed (0.36%) (Table 6).

Thanks to the accurate postnatal checking system, even after several months, 36 false-negatives (0.54%) were detected (Table 7).

Table 6 *True-positives in ultrasound screening for fetal cardiac malformations*

	n	Condition
Conotruncal anomalies	3	TOF
	2	TGA
	1	DORV
Atrioventricular defects	5	
Hypoplastic left heart	4	
VSD (large)	3	
ASD (secondary type)	3	
Others		
	1	EFE
	1	TV insufficiency
	1	PV stenosis + TV insufficiency
Total	24	

TGA, transposition of great arteries; TOF, tetralogy of Fallot; DORV, double outlet right ventricle; VSD, ventricular septal defect; ASD, atrial septal defect; EFE, endocardial fibroelastosis; TV, tricuspid valve; PV, pulmonary valve

Table 7 *False-negatives in ultrasound screening for fetal cardiac malformations*

	n	Condition
Conotruncal anomalies	2	TGA (1 dead)
	1	TOF (mild)
Coarctation	1	surgery (dead)
	1	surgery (alive and well)
Atrioventricular defects (incomplete)	1	dead
VSD	2	major surgery
	17	not critical
ASD (secondary type)	7	follow-up
PV stenosis	3	follow-up (not critical)
AV stenosis	1	follow-up (not critical)
Total	36	

Table 8 *False-positives in ultrasound screening for fetal cardiac malformations*

Condition	n
VSD	7
ASD (secondary type)	1
Aortic stenosis	1
Total	9

Among them, we consider as important false negatives the two cases of transposition of the great vessels, the aortic coarctation with hypoplasia of the arch, the incomplete atrioventricular canal and the two large defects of the interventricular septum. There were nine false-positives (0.13%) (Table 8). As the suspected abnormalities were in all cases of minor clinical relevance, the management of those pregnancies has not been influenced.

The relatively high number of diagnostic errors can be explained: (1) by the technical limitations of the echocardiography carried out in the second trimester (this explains the numerous failures to diagnose ventricular septal defect and atrial septal defect); (2) by the natural history of certain cardiopathies (such as aortic coarction, cases of mild valvular stenosis), which evolve during intrauterine life and cannot be clearly assessed on the basis of a single examination carried out during the second trimester; and (3) by the possibility of errors (two cases of transposition of the great vessels in our study), that could be avoided if the examiner always adhered strictly to the standard method of observation.

The accuracy of fetal echocardiography in our study, if calculated on the basis of what it is realistically possible to diagnose during the second trimester, is as follows: sensitivity 80% (important false-negatives 6/36), specificity 99%, positive predictive value 72.7%, negative predictive value 99%. It is possible to deduce the following from these experiences:

(1) The accuracy of the four-chamber view amongst the low-risk population is closely correlated with the gestational period in which the examination is carried out, which must not be less than 18 weeks;

(2) Objective limits, such as maternal obesity, unfavorable fetal positions, instruments with poor resolution and insufficient time for the examination, are factors which prevent an adequate evaluation of the fetal heart, and this must be kept in mind during a screening programme;

(3) In all the studies examined, the element around which the possibility of carrying out screening for heart malformations revolves (either four-chambers or a complete evaluation extended to the ventricular–arterial connections) is the level of training of the operators.

It is the opinion of most of the authors mentioned, and ours too, that the experience of operators in this particular field of prenatal diagnosis can be improved with a teaching program that actively involves the operator. The operator will be able, once correctly stimulated, first to carry out a correct four-chamber scanning and then, if constantly being taught, a complete evaluation of the fetal heart.

TRANSVAGINAL SONOGRAPHY

The rapid extension of transvaginal sonography (the enormous potential of which is well known, but which still presents technical and interpretative problems) is a good reason to analyze its present and future possibilities and its ability to replace or merely support transabdominal sonography as a screening test to be carried out for fetal malformations.

Our contribution in this area has been a prospective study, the purpose of which was to assess the efficacy of routine prenatal ultrasonography in detecting fetal structural abnormalities, comparing the results obtained using transvaginal sonography at 14 weeks' gestational age with those obtained using transabdominal scanning at 21 weeks.

From March 1991 to December 1992, 1229 pregnant women, bearing a total of 1239 fetuses, were recruited at their booking visit and were offered a vaginal scan in addition to the routine examination.

The scans were performed by seven operators using 5.0-MHz and 7.5-MHz vaginal transducers (Acuson 128, Diasonics CV 400). A maximum of 20 min of scanning time was allowed per patient (mean 15 min) in which the entire fetal anatomy was examined. A computerized form was filled in, indicating for each structure whether it was visualized and whether any abnormal findings were recorded. Gestational age was confirmed by measuring biparietal diameter and femur length.

Table 9 *True-positives in transvaginal ultrasound screening for fetal malformations*

Condition	n
Osteogenesis imperfecta (type III)	1
Multiple vertebral and rib anomalies	1
Absence of left arm	1
Clubfoot	1
Cleft lip and palate	1
Cystic hygroma	3
Megacystis and horseshoe kidney	1
Renal duplication and upper pole UPJ	1
Dandy–Walker malformation	1
Tetralogy of Fallot	1
Total	12

UPJ, uretero–pelvic junction

Table 10 *False-negatives in transvaginal ultrasound screening for fetal malformations*

Condition	n
Hypoplastic left heart	1
Atrioventricular septal defect	1
VSD and aortic coarction	1
Tetralogy of Fallot	1
Holoprosencephaly	1
Unilateral hypoplasia of the radius	1
Unilateral clubfoot	1
Bilateral cleft lip	2
Pelvic kidney	1
Unilateral hydronephrosis	1
Right diaphragmatic hernia	1
Agenesis of cerebellar vermis	1
Total	13

Table 11 *False-negatives in transabdominal ultrasound screening for fetal malformations*

Condition	n
Bladder exstrophy	1
Pierre Robin syndrome	1
Clubfoot	1
Heterozygous achondroplasia	1
Esophageal atresia and fistula	1
Intracranial neoplasm	1
Cerebral atrophy	1
Anorectal atresia	1
Total	8

All patients had a routine scan at 20–22 weeks (according to the previously mentioned protocol) and postnatal follow-up was obtained for all babies, including post-mortem examinations for fetuses which underwent termination of pregnancy. During the study period, 12 cases of fetal abnormality, including five skeletal malformations, three cystic hygromata, two urinary tract obstructions, one case of Dandy–Walker anomaly and a tetralogy of Fallot, were correctly diagnosed using the transvaginal approach (Table 9).

Thirteen malformations were missed at the first scan and only later identified: 12 at midgestation rescreening, and one at the autopsy following a termination of pregnancy for other reasons (Table 10). If we correct the rate of false-negatives for gestational age, excluding those pathologies that could not have been diagnosed because of their progressive nature, it is possible to say we failed to detect ten diagnosable abnormalities. Using the same criteria we can conclude that, as far as 21-week screening is concerned, we missed three malformations that could have been detected at that time (Table 11). In other words, this means that we obtained a 'realistic' (correct for gestational age) sensitivity of 54% for early transvaginal sonography versus an approximate rate of 80% related to transabdominal sonography.

If we examine in detail the false-negative results, it appears clear that congenital heart defects account for about one-third of missed diagnoses at transvaginal screening. Furthermore, they represent the most severe abnormalities. In our experience the visualization rate for each organ explored during 14-week screening ranges, for extracardiac structures, from 99.3% (for limbs) to 86% (for face), while a satisfactory four-chamber view was achieved in 84.7% of cases and the outlet flows of great vessels were sought in only 33.7% of cases.

In the literature, higher rates of visualization for cardiac structures are reported, involving small series of selected cases. The only paper dealing with a screening program involving a low-risk population concluded that for a complete evaluation of these structures more time should be made available early in pregnancy, using the transvaginal approach which is subject to well-known technical limitations (e.g. poor probe mobility)[16]. However, in a mass screening policy, we cannot spend too much time waiting for the fetus to move or bring the mother back for a second appointment.

We, too, think, therefore, that it is unlikely, at present, that transvaginal sonography will replace abdominal scanning for the screening of low-risk pregnancies. It could, however, represent an additional early examination for the high-risk population.

ULTRASONIC MARKERS OF FETAL CHROMOSOMAL DEFECTS

The identifying of fetuses that are potentially carriers of chromosomal defects in an inexpensive, non-invasive way is one of the most interesting challenges that has faced diagnostic ultrasound in recent years. Normally, owing to the inherent risks in the technique used to take samples and the costs of analysis, fetal karyotype evaluations (chorion villus sampling or amniocentesis) are limited to women at risk because of age. Other less frequent indications are a previous child or abortion with a chromosomal defect and the presence of balanced translocation in one of the parents.

Although aneuploidy – like Down's syndrome – is most frequent among older patients, no more than 20% of fetuses with trisomy 21 are born to these women. The screening of this disease using the level of α-fetoprotein in the maternal serum (α-fetoprotein ≤ 0.5 multiples of median) identifies only 20–25% of the fetuses affected. The use of three biochemical markers (α-fetoprotein, non-conjugated estriol, β-human chorionic gonadotropin) seems much more promising in terms of accuracy, but has not yet become a widespread routine practice. In the last few years, the need has also been felt in ultrasound for a more reliable method for selecting those patients (who do not belong to the classic risk categories) on whom invasive prenatal diagnosis should be carried out. Numerous ultrasound markers have been put forward – and the list is growing all the time – as an indication of the presence of chromosomal defects.

Nuchal fold

Benacerraf and colleagues was one of the first group of investigators to record an association between a thickening of the nuchal fold (≥ 6 mm between 15 and 20 weeks) and Down's syndrome. This was present in 9 of the 21 trisomic fetuses (42.8%) and in only 0.1% of normal fetuses[17]. Other authors[18] have observed this feature in only 21% of the fetuses affected, with a rate of false-positives of 9%. In Ginsberg's study (carried out between 14 and 20 weeks), in 41% of the fetuses with trisomy 21 (5/12), and in 50% of the fetuses with trisomy 18 (2/4), a nuchal fold ≥ 6 mm was noted; in the 212 control patients the fold was always below this value[19]. The gestational period (different in the various studies), the method of measuring (in some of the studies the thickness of the fold included the thickness of the cranium), the type of study (perspective/retrospective) are all factors which help to explain the different levels of accuracy achieved.

Clinodactyly and hypoplasia of the middle phalanx of the fifth finger/toe

Benacerraf and colleagues noted a hypoplasia of the ossification center of the middle phalanx together with clinodactyly of the fifth finger/toe in three of the four fetuses with trisomy 21 studied between 17 and 20 weeks. In a later study, she observed that a ratio between the ossification center of the middle phalanx of the fifth finger/toe and that of the fourth finger/toe, ≤ 0.7, characterized six of the eight fetuses with trisomy 21, with a rate of false-positives of 18%. There is no question that the clinical usefulness of these findings is reduced by the objective difficulty in measuring such small structures and the fact that these findings are also typical of other syndromes as well as the normal population[20].

Short femur – short humerus

Benacerraf has calculated the length of the femur as a function of biparietal diameter. She has recorded a sensitivity of 68% and a specificity of 98% in the diagnosis of trisomy 21 between 15 and 21 weeks, when the ratio of measured femur/anticipated femur is ≤ 0.91[21]. Perrella and colleagues[18], on the other hand, noted a much lower sensitivity (26%) with a rate of false-positives of 5% and a positive predictive value amongst the general population of 1%. Studying the length of the long bones of aborted fetuses, Fitzsimmon and colleagues[22] confirmed the presence of significant differences between the length of the femur of fetuses with Down's syndrome and normal fetuses, but stressed that the use of a measured femur/anticipated femur ratio of ≤ 0.91 only identified 18% of the fetuses affected. In the same work, they also recorded that the length of the humerus was far more affected than was that of the femur in fetuses with trisomy 21. This was confirmed by Benacerraf and colleagues, who noted that 50% of the fetuses with Down's syndrome (12/24) had a shorter humerus (measured humerus/anticipated humerus ratio of ≤ 0.90) compared with 6.25% among the control subject. Nyberg noted that 24.4% of trisomic fetuses (11/45) had a short humerus (measured humerus/anticipated humerus ratio of ≤ 0.89), compared with 4.5% of the control subjects. He also added that when both these long bones were shorter, the risk of Down's syndrome increased 11-fold.

In the study of Rotmensch and associates[23], they noted a measured humerus/anticipated humerus ratio of ≤ 0.90 with a sensitivity of 28%. The differences in terms of sensitivity may be due to the use of different instruments and transducers in the various studies and different levels of experience among individual operators, which implies that each laboratory should test its own accuracy in the field of biometric screening.

Pyelectasis

Benacerraf recorded an incidence of pyelectasis (renal pelvis ≥ 4 mm) in 18% of a series of 43 fetuses with Down's syndrome observed between 14 and 20 weeks. Having put more effort than anybody into the research into these echographic markers, she suggested introducing a score with a view to improving the accuracy of echography in the diagnosis of chromosomal defects. She considered the ultrasonographic finding of nuchal fold ≥ 6 mm a serious abnormality; this was given a score of 2. Short femur, short humerus and pyelectasis were given a score of 1. The use of a score of 2 in her study identified 81% of the fetuses with Down's syndrome and 100% of the fetuses with trisomy 13 and 18, with a rate of false-positives of 4.4%[21].

Choroid plexus cysts

The association between choroid plexus cysts and chromosomal defects, mainly trisomy 18, has been widely documented. In the majority of cases, however, the choroid plexus cysts were associated with important abnormalities that are easily identified using echography. Some authors have reported that in a few sporadic cases the choroid plexus cysts were the only abnormality in fetuses which turned out to be bearers of trisomy 18. For this reason, the decision on whether or not to carry out an amniocentesis in the presence of apparently isolated choroid plexus cysts is still a matter of controversy[24].

First-trimester translucency

Recent study has shown a possible association between nuchal translucency and chromosomal defects. A perspective study carried out on 827 pregnant women in the first trimester revealed that the presence of nuchal fluid of ≥ 3 mm increased the risk of chromosomal defects tenfold (recorded in 35% of these fetuses, compared with 1% in those with a fluid collection of < 3 mm). As yet none of the ultrasonographic markers proposed is capable of distinguishing with great accuracy and at an early enough stage a healthy fetus from one with a chromosomal defect. The latest marker proposed – nuchal translucency – calls for perspective studies to be carried out on a wider population[25].

There is an overlapping of individual markers with the population of normal fetuses which increases with the gestational period. It is difficult to detect them, as they have to be actively looked for, and the literature shows that only an operator who is expert in ultrasonographic prenatal diagnosis obtains satisfactory, reproducible results. Ultrasound does not yet have a leading role in the screening for chromosomal defects, even though its contribution in this field is undoubtedly going to increase.

Nuchal thickness and the other markers proposed can, however, be used – if the operator has sufficient time and the right equipment – together with other parameters (maternal age, biochemical tests) in the attempt to identify an increasing number of fetuses at risk because of chromosomal defects.

SCREENING FOR INTRAUTERINE GROWTH RETARDATION

IUGR should be defined as a reduction of fetal growth that can lead to a birth weight below the tenth centile for the gestational age. Consequently, two categories of IUGR can be defined: one is represented by fetuses undergoing a reduction of their growth in the last part of pregnancy as shown by biometry, but reaching a birthweight over the tenth percentile – appropriate-for-gestational-age IUGR (AGA IUGR); the other group is represented by fetuses showing a reduced fetal growth and showing also a birthweight below the tenth percentile – small-for-gestational age IUGR (SGA IUGR). In fact, reduction of fetal growth in the last period of pregnancy, as observed by ultrasonic biometry, can be registered even when the birthweight is over the tenth centile, considered as normal from a statistical point of view. Taking this fact into consideration, the prevalence of the condition is more than 10% in the general population.

IUGR is frequently associated with maternal diseases and abnormalities of the fetus or of the fetal adnexa. Moreover, IUGR can be complicated by hypoxemia and/or acidemia, which occurs in about 35% of the fetuses with IUGR, with little difference between AGA and SGA/IUGR. As a consequence, perinatal morbidity and mortality are increased.

Currently, as there is little possibility of effective management *in utero*, the crucial problem is the timing of the delivery and a careful assessment of the fetal condition, in order to avoid fetal demise or neonatal mortality, neonatal morbidity and late sequelae. As for any other disease, the first step in management is the diagnosis. In this condition, this represents the recognition of reduced growth. Little doubt exists that ultrasonic biometry is the most accurate method, which in many studies has shown a high specificity.

However, the sensitivity is not always satisfactory. This low sensitivity is mainly related to the gestational age at which the examination has been carried out, and to the time interval from ultrasound examination until the birth. The efficacy of the ultrasound diagnosis has usually been calculated from the birthweight. As fetal growth is a dynamic process, the number of false-negatives will be very high if the time between the last examination and the delivery is too long. A better sensitivity together with an excellent specificity has been reported in one study[26]. It has been shown that, when using serial biometry, the appearance of the first abnormal parameter indicating reduced growth is widely distributed during gestation[27].

It is more difficult, when discussing the possibility of using ultrasonic biometry as a screening method for detecting IUGR, to analyze cost/benefit considerations for any suggested screening program.

One end-point for assessing the efficacy of the screening procedure is of course represented by the perinatal outcome, which is influenced by many factors. It is important to consider that the recognition of the impairment of fetal growth (IUGR) is only the first step to a more complete assessment of the fetal condition.

Considering that maternal risk conditions for IUGR are recognizable in 35% of cases, it is logical to believe that, in order to improve the detection rate and consequently the perinatal outcome, a policy of mass screening, by using serial biometry, might be advisable. Currently however, it is very difficult to propose any kind of screening policy.

CONCLUSIONS

Diagnostic obstetric ultrasound has been proved to be very accurate in assessing many abnormal fetal conditions and often it represents the best available screening method. Fetal malformations and ultrasound markers of possible karyotype abnormalities are only observable by using this technology. As far as intrauterine growth retardation is concerned, it is necessary to remember that only in 35% of cases this condition will be detected on the basis of clinical judgement.

The opportunity to use this powerful technology as a routine procedure in pregnancy is currently debated and opinions are largely divergent. Some evidence has been given in the medical literature that a routine ultrasound examination, if properly used, can be useful. On the other hand, no study has produced convincing evidence that routine ultrasound examinations are without value.

When considering studies concerning screening ultrasound, the following critical points must be taken into consideration:

(1) The numerical size of the population must be large enough to draw valid statistical conclusions.

(2) A clear definition of the protocol of the ultrasound examination is necessary.

(3) It is essential that the expertise of the operator should be good enough to get the best possible results from the technology.

(4) An exact identification of the end-points and the availability of a uniform protocol of management is also crucial, especially if perinatal outcome is one of the chosen end-points.

Looking at this last point we consider that an ethical issue is evident. In one study, improvement in perinatal outcome was mainly related to the reduction of malformation at birth, subsequent to the termination of pregnancies carried out in positive cases[1]. However, termination of pregnancy can be considered as a kind of 'management', that reduces perinatal mortality and morbidity in the perinatal period even though it is not a form of fetal therapy[28].

In summary, the authors conclude that routine ultrasound examination in pregnancy is likely to offer improvement in obstetric care. Further clinical investigations with well-designed studies are necessary.

References

1. Saari-Kemppainen, A., Karjalainen, O., Ylostalo, P. and Heinonen, O. P. (1990). Ultrasound screening and perinatal mortality: controlled trial of systematic one-stage screening in pregnancy. *Lancet*, **336**, 387–91
2. Ewingman, B. G., Crane, J. P., Frigoletto, F. D., LeFevre, M. L., Bain, R. P., McNellis, D. and the RADIUS Study Group (1993). Effect of prenatal ultrasound screening on perinatal outcome. *N. Engl. J. Med.*, **329**, 821–7
3. Lilford, R. J. and Chard, T. (1982). The routine use of ultrasound. *Br. J. Obstet. Gynaecol.*, **89**, 338–41
4. Campbell, S. and Smith, P. (1984). Routine screening for congenital anomalies by ultrasound. In Nicolaides, R. Ch. (eds.) *Prenatal Diagnosis*, pp.325–30. (London: RCOG)
5. Chitty, L. S., Hunt, G. H., Moore, J. and Loob, M. O. (1991). Effectiveness of routine ultrasonography in detecting fetal structural abnormalities in a low risk population. *Br. Med. J.*, **303**, 1165–9
6. Luck, C. A. (1992). Value of routine ultrasound scanning at 19 weeks: a four year study of 8849 deliveries. *Br. Med. J.*, **304**, 1474–8
7. Levi, S., Hyjazi, Y., Schaaps, J. P., Defoort, P., Coulon, P. and Beukens, P. (1991). Sensitivity and specificity of routine antenatal screening for congenital anomalies by ultrasound: the

Belgium multicentric study. *Ultrasound Obstet. Gynecol.*, **1**, 102–10
8. Smith, D. W. (1982). *Recognizable Patterns of Human Malformation*, 3rd edn. (Philadelphia: WB Saunders)
9. Copel, J. A., Pilu, G., Green, J., Hobbins, J. C. and Kleinman, C. S. (1987). Fetal echocardiographic screening for congenital heart disease: the importance of the four chamber view. *Am. J. Obstet. Gynecol.*, **157**, 648–55
10. Eik-Nes, S. H. (1991). Four chamber view of the fetal heart. Part of the routine scan? In *Fetal Cardiology Perinatal Cardiac Management*, postgraduate course (Malmo, Sweden: International Perinatal Doppler Society)
11. Vergani, P., Mariani, S., Ghidini, A., Schiavina, R., Cavallone, M., Locatelli, A., Strobelt, N. and Cerruti, P. (1992). Screening for congenital heart disease with the four-chamber view of the fetal heart. *Am. J. Obstet. Gynecol.*, **167**, 1000–3
12. Stoll, C., Alembik, Y., Dott, B., Roth, P. M. and De Geeter, B. (1993). Evaluation of prenatal diagnosis of congenital heart disease. *Prenat. Diagn.*, **13**, 453–61
13. Sharland, G. K. and Allan, L. D. (1992). Screening for congenital heart disease prenatally. Results of a 2.5 year study in the South East Thames Region. *Fetal Neonat. Med.*, **99**, 220–5
14. Achiron, R., Glaser, J., Gelernter, I., Hegesh, J. and Yagel, S. (1992). Extended fetal echocardiographic examination for detecting cardiac malformations in low risk pregnancies. *Br. Med. J.*, **304**, 671–4
15. Rustico, M. A., Benettoni, A., D'Ottavio, G., Bogatti, P., Fontana, A., Pecile, V. and Mandruzzato, G. P. (1990). Fetal echocardiography: the role of the screening procedure. *Eur. J. Obstet. Gynecol. Reprod. Biol.*, **36**, 19–25
16. Johnson, P., Sharland, G., Maxwell, D. and Allan, L. (1992). The role of transvaginal sonography in the early detection of congenital heart disease. *Ultrasound Obstet. Gynecol.*, **2**, 248–51
17. Benacerraf, B. R., Gelman, R. and Frigoletto, F. D. (1987). Sonographic identification of second-trimester fetuses with Down's syndrome. *N. Engl. J. Med.*, **317**, 1371–5
18. Perrella, R., Duerinckx, A. J., Grant, E. G., Tessler, F., Tabsh, K. and Crandall, B. F. (1988). Second-trimester sonographic diagnosis of Down syndrome: role of femur-length shortening and nuchal-fold thickening. *Am. J. Radiol.*, **151**, 981–5
19. Ginsberg, N., Cadkin, A., Pergament, E. and Verlinsky, Y. (1990). Ultrasonographic detection of the second-trimester fetus with trisomy 18 and trisomy 21. *Am. J. Obstet. Gynecol.*, **163**, 1186–90
20. Benacerraf, B. R., Frigoletto, F. D. and Cramer, D. W. (1987). Down syndrome: sonographic sign for diagnosis in the second-trimester fetus. *Radiology*, **163**, 811–3
21. Benacerraf, B. R., Neuberg, D., Bromley, B. and Frigoletto, F. D. (1992). Sonographic scoring index for prenatal detection of chromosomal abnormalities. *J. Ultrasound Med.*, **11**, 449–58
22. FitzSimmons, J., Droste, S., Shepard, T. H., Pascoe-Mason, J., Chinn, A. and Mack, L. A. (1989). Long bone growth in fetuses with Down syndrome. *Am. J. Obstet. Gynecol.*, **161**, 1174–7
23. Rotmensch, S., Luo, J. S., Liberati, M., Belanger, K., Mahoney, M. J. and Hobbins, J. C. (1992). Fetal humeral length to detect Down syndrome. *Am. J. Obstet. Gynecol.*, **166**, 1330–4
24. Porto, M., Murata, Y., Warneke, L. A. and Keegan, K. A. (1993). Fetal choroid plexus cysts: an independent risk factor for chromosomal anomalies. *J. Clin. Ultrasound*, **21**, 103–8
25. Nicolaides, K., Shawwa, L., Brizot, M. and Snijders, R. (1993). Ultrasonographically detectable markers of fetal chromosomal defects. *Ultrasound Obstet. Gynecol.*, **3**, 56–9
26. Laurin, J. and Persson, P.-H. (1987). Ultrasound screening for detection of intra-uterine growth-retardation. *Acta Obstet. Gynecol.*, **66**, 493–500
27. Mandruzzato, G. P., D'Ottavio, G., Rustico, M. A., Alberico, S., Bogatti, P. and Nesladek, N. (1986). Management of intrauterine growth retardation: diagnostic and clinical aspects. *Fetal Ther.*, **1**, 126–8

Non-directive prenatal genetic counseling

Z. Papp, E. Tóth-Pál and Cs. Papp

Classical genetic counseling has aimed to help families by giving emotional support and by disclosing and discussing the causes of certain 'genetic' problems, the risks of recurrence, and the possibilities for prevention or other options. In many situations, no reliable figures for the risk of recurrence are available.

A number of diagnostic techniques, applicable in pregnancy, have now become available, together with a much better understanding of genetically determined disease at many levels. The classical options in many cases have included contraception, sterilization, adoption, or heterologous insemination by donor (AID)[1-7]. Now, in many disorders, one can suggest undertaking further pregnancies, with the offer of prenatal genetic counseling. The fetal phenotype may be examined (by ultrasound, for malformations or growth retardation; by cell biochemistry, for metabolic disorders), or the fetal genotype may be examined (by cytogenetic analysis, for chromosome disorders; by DNA testing, for direct or indirect identification of mutant genes)[8-10]. There remain disorders for which no diagnosis is available, or for which one can offer no more than 'classical genetics', but it is likely that many disorders at present of unknown cause will soon be understood at the biochemical or gene level, and that many presently 'unmapped' genes will be mapped within the next decade.

The increased availability of prenatal diagnosis (available in more centers, for more patients, for more disorders) has stimulated the development of screening for genetic disease. Subpopulations at particular risk may be easily identified (e.g. older mothers), or identified only after specific testing (e.g. for thalassemia, hemoglobinopathies, Tay–Sachs disease). The screening process may take place before or during an actual pregnancy; some screening methods, e.g. maternal serum α-fetoprotein (MSAFP), ultrasound, can only be applied during pregnancy[11,12].

The option of further pregnancies includes the option of prenatal diagnosis, which, in turn, includes the option of pregnancy termination. Many couples, even in high-risk situations, will be lucky, and have a healthy child. Only a few will go through the trauma of one or several terminations. Couples identified by screening as 'high risk' may be at very high risk (25%), in the cases of monogenic traits, at a lower risk (approximately 10%), if identified through raised MSAFP, or at relatively low risk (approximately 1%), if identified by maternal age or low MSAFP.

Decisions on pregnancy testing and termination must be the couple's own; it is the duty of the counselor to support and to inform, but not to persuade. Some couples refuse the option of interrupting pregnancy e.g. for religious reasons[13].

Unlike some infectious diseases, which may be controlled by immunization, compulsory screening and therapy, genetic diseases do not endanger society directly. It is families that are affected by them. Nevertheless, the indirect effect of genetic disease on society cannot be ignored. Unlike infectious diseases, genetic diseases do not threaten the health of other people, but they do burden society (e.g. the cost of institutional care for handicapped children). The question arises as to whether anybody has the right to insist on the birth of a child who will suffer from an undoubtedly incurable disease and also severely burden public finances. Some people do insist on continuing such pregnancies, and there is no doubt that the right to make individual decisions must be respected.

Often couples coming for genetic counseling are full of fears and anxiety, oppressed by the memory of one or more ill or dead children. Couples appreciate the opportunity for a counseling session and discussion, and the offer of prenatal diagnosis will be accepted by most of them[14].

Counseling sessions may often be strongly psychological in nature[15]. It is essential to present a clear and full description of the relevant disorder and to answer all questions honestly and promptly. A good and harmonious relationship should develop or be developed between the counselor and the couple. The physician–patient relationship, always important in medicine, is here replaced by a physician/counselor–family relationship, which deepens in the course of counseling. This sort of relationship is necessary for the proper help and management of high-risk couples in this situation. A great deal depends on the character of the individual physician[16–19].

Four questions should be addressed by the genetic counselor:

(1) What is the disease in question (clinical and laboratory diagnosis)?

(2) How severe is it (prognosis and therapeutic possibilities)?

(3) How is it caused/inherited (risk of recurrence)?

(4) What can be done to avoid or prevent the disease (prenatal diagnosis and therapy)?

DIAGNOSIS

Knowledge of the disease in question is a prerequisite of genetic counseling. Confirmation of an exact diagnosis, which is of basic importance, may be difficult. Obtaining old or recent medical records, pedigree analysis, careful history-taking, clinical examination of relatives, special laboratory tests and other investigations (perhaps involving referral to other specialist departments), can all be relevant or necessary procedures.

Disease, whether genetic or non-genetic, may be due to a variety of factors. Genetic disease is particularly likely to be heterogeneous in this respect. For example, a muscular dystrophy may result from a number of mutant genes. Among the common types of muscular dystrophy, there is the facioscapulohumeral form, which is characteristically autosomal dominant, and myotonic dystrophy, also autosomal dominant. 'Limb-girdle' muscular dystrophy, a diagnosis that probably includes a number of disorders, is autosomal recessive. Duchenne, Becker and Emery–Dreifuss muscular dystrophies are all X-linked recessive, with fairly distinct, but overlapping, phenotypes; under some conditions they can manifest, usually in mild degree, in females also (e.g. symptomatic carriers). Sometimes, investigation of a family with 'muscular dystrophy' reveals that the primary disease was not in the muscles at all, but, for example, a spinal muscular atrophy originating in the anterior horn cells, or a more generalized disorder, for example a glycogenosis.

A practically identical clinical picture is characteristic of some of the commoner types of mucopolysaccharidoses. However, Hurler, Scheie and Sanfilippo diseases are of autosomal recessive inheritance, whereas Hunter disease is X-linked recessive.

It should be noted that there are diseases which do not usually manifest until adulthood (e.g. Huntington disease, facioscapulohumeral muscular dystrophy), and that in connection with certain diseases of recessive inheritance, heterozygotes may also show clinical symptoms. For example, axillary and pubic hair may be sparse in heterozygotes for testicular feminization, cutaneous symptoms may be seen by gene carriers for Fabry disease, and nephrolithiasis occurs in heterozygotes for cystinuria.

In some cases, medical documents may be incomplete or unobtainable; certain tests that are now considered essential for the diagnosis may not have been carried out or available at that time. There may be no histological information, no post-mortem report, no roentgenograms, no photographs, no biochemical results. Genetic counseling cannot be based on a diagnosis such as 'mental retardation', 'growth disorder', or 'degenerative disease'. Sometimes an exact diagnosis, such as 'achondroplasia', may be clearly misleading. To make a correct diagnosis, with few exceptions, requires detailed and correct information.

PROGNOSIS AND THERAPY

Without a correct diagnosis, the genetic counselor cannot tell the parents whether there is a high or low risk of recurrence within the family, whether tests can be carried out to detect those persons/couples at high risk of having an affected child, whether prenatal diagnosis is possible (and if so, how, where and when), whether the disease is in any way treatable, whether the severity is highly variable within a family, whether there are other (as yet undiscussed) serious implications, or whether other 'reproductive options' are available.

Although much genetic disease remains untreatable, the counselor must know the possibilities for the disease in question. He must be up-to-date and informed about postnatal procedures and appliances (e.g. neonatal or prenatal surgery, transplantation, artificial limbs), about medical treatment (e.g. physiotherapy and antibiotic therapy for cystic fibrosis, use of restricted/special diets – for phenylketonuria/galactosemia, use of specific vitamins – pyridoxine for certain epilepsies, hydroxocobalamin for B_{12} transport disorders), and about what is available within the community (e.g. help from social services, financial help for parents with handicapped children, institutional care). He must be able to discuss more remote possibilities, such as 'gene therapy', within a realistic perspective. He must be able to talk to the parents in a way, and at a level, that is appropriate to their pre-existing knowledge and education, and their degree of anxiety or depth of grief. He must be prepared to educate them further. He/she must be understood and be supportive.

GENETIC RISK

This term covers two concepts: the general population risk of a disorder/disease and the

Table 1 *General population risks of some common conditions*

	Risk
Fetal loss	
in the first trimester	1/6
in the second and third trimesters	1/30–1/100
Neonatal death	1/100
Malformation detectable at birth	1/33
Mental retardation	1/50
Chronic disease in adulthood	1/5

risk, or recurrence risk, of a disorder/disease in a specific family/situation.

Many couples have no idea at all of general population risks. They may imagine that it is extremely unusual to abort spontaneously, bear a baby with a malformation, or have a child with mental retardation. They cannot understand how such things can happen, if they are not in the family already. They do not understand why a particular disaster has happened to them, as they have done nothing to deserve or provoke it.

The general population risks for a few commonplace situations are given in Table 1. All genetic counseling has to be given, and understood, against this general background risk. For example, a couple may be horrified to be told there is a 1% recurrence risk for a certain malformation; they may perceive this as a very high-risk situation (although 100 to 1 odds in a gambling situation are usually perceived as far from certainty!). It may help couples realize that an additional risk of 1% for a malformation is not so enormous when compared with the starting risk of 3–5%; they have only a 33% increase above the general risk level.

In some counseling situations, couples may be at increased risk for one or a number of problems, as compared with general population risks, yet one is not talking of a 'recurrence risk'; the condition provoking anxiety and the request for counseling has not yet happened. In these situations, the *actual risk* may not be very high, though much above the general population level. For example, a woman of 40 has a risk of bearing a live-born with Down's syndrome that is 20-fold the risk she ran when she was only 20, yet the actual risk is only 1/100. Similar low levels of risk (yet high, compared to general population risks) may be associated, for example, with exposure to teratogens or radiation. Slightly higher levels or risk will be run in cousin marriages[20].

Very high levels of risk, for a problem that has not yet appeared within the family, will seldom be found, except in connection with specific screening programs, for example detection of Tay–Sachs heterozygotes in Ashkenazi Jews, or of thalassemia carriers in Mediterranean populations. In these situations, when both (prospective) parents are heterozygotes, the risk of an affected child is 25%. In virtually all of these very high-risk situations identified by screening, a prenatal test can be offered, but this would not be acceptable to all couples.

When a disorder has already appeared within a family, recurrence risks may be high (> 1/10), intermediate (1/10–1/100) or low (< 1/100). Use of these words ('high', 'intermediate', 'low') is extremely arbitrary. The counselor's use of such words may be at variance with the use, or perception, of the counseled couple. To the counselor, a risk estimate may appear intermediate or low, yet to the counseled couple it is high. Risk figures can be 'rewritten' by turning statements around: a 1/100 recurrence risk, for a serious malformation, may appear formidable to the threatened parents; it is more reassuring to be told there is a 99% chance that the baby will be unaffected. Risk figures should be compared with general population risks. The nature of the disorder/problem itself, and the impossibility/possibility of prenatal diagnosis, will affect the way it is perceived[21].

In some situations, recurrence risk is very low. If problems with a previous pregnancy were due to teratogen exposure, and the teratogen can be avoided in further pregnancies, risks may not be much above the general population risk.

Most malformations are multifactorially determined. After a couple has had a child with an isolated exomphalos, or tracheo-esophageal malformation, recurrence risks may be 1–2% only. Although this represents a 20–40-fold increase over the general population level, it is still not a very daunting risk. After the birth of a child with congenital heart disease, recurrence risks are usually 2–5% (depending on the malformation type). The background rate for congenital heart disease is nearly 1% (8/1000).

When dealing with a malformation problem, the counselor must be sure that it is really isolated, and not part of a syndrome (that may be monogenic). For example, an occipital encephalocele alone might suggest a recurrence risk, for all types of neural tube defects, of about 3%; if the encephalocele was accompanied by cystic kidneys or polydactyly, however, the Meckel syndrome would probably be diagnosed, with a recurrence risk of 25%[22,23].

In families with monogenic disorders, many relatives will run risks that are intermediate or low. For example, with a heterozygote frequency of 1/25 for cystic fibrosis, the risk to the child of a woman whose brother was affected is 1/150, and the risk to a child of a woman whose brother's child was affected is 1/200. In families with X-linked recessive disease, some females, with no affected close relatives (but with many unaffected brothers or maternal uncles), will be at very low risk for being carriers or having affected sons.

The background general population risk is not identical with the risk within a given family (*specific risk*), nor with the risk calculated for a given pregnancy (*actual risk*). For example, the background risk (in Europe) for a healthy subject, of being heterozygous for cystic fibrosis, is 1/25, and the risk of his/her child being affected by the disease is 1/2500. However, the situation will change completely if it is revealed that the couple already have a child suffering from cystic fibrosis. In this case, the specific risk that both members of the couple are heterozygotes is 1/1, and the risk for a further child being affected is 1/4. If the couple undertake a pregnancy, and the pregnancy tests give normal results, the actual risk for an affected child will fall to about 1/100, as the reliability of prenatal diagnosis of cystic fibrosis is 99% with up-to-date DNA methods.

To talk about 100% reliability of a biochemical or molecular prenatal diagnosis is, in practice, nonsense. The counselor should not use words like 'never' or 'always'. Instead, expressions like 'probably not', 'a very high chance', 'almost certainly', are preferable, and might also avoid legal complications!

To explain the concept of risk, we may use analogies, e.g. one coin (heads/tails) may be useful in explaining autosomal dominant inheritance, and two coins may explain recessive inheritance.

Discussion of risk situations demands tact. In particular, one should avoid laying 'blame' on one member of the couple; this might be difficult in the case of monogenic disorders or inherited chromosome rearrangements. It is better, if possible, to spread the 'responsibility' to both members of the couple: for example, with an X-linked recessive disorder and an affected male child, the mother gave the mutant gene, but without the paternal Y chromosome all would have been well.

In cases of multifactorial determination, it is important not to accuse anybody, e.g. the physician who prescribed a drug, or the factory in which the counselee was exposed to chemicals (and which guaranteed the safety of her work). An unfortunate combination of environmental factors and predisposing genes may be stressed. The counselor should intervene to prevent any further, possibly dangerous, exposure[24].

PRENATAL DIAGNOSIS

In very many counseling situations, the specific recurrence risk is so low that, apart from a general screening for malformations, further tests are superfluous. A simple reassurance may disappoint certain couples if they feel that their problem has been oversimplified.

For most couples running a higher than average risk/recurrence risk, one can offer prenatal diagnosis.

Cases require individual assessment. The reliability and the safety of the diagnostic procedures should be discussed with the parents. These should be carefully weighed, bearing in mind the nature and severity of the disease/disorder prompting the desire for diagnosis/termination. It should be explained that the test(s) will be for one problem only, or a limited range of disorders, and normal results will not guarantee a child normal in *every* way.

The final decision, to accept or reject the offer of prenatal diagnosis, is for the couple to make. Their decision will reflect their attitude to the disorder in question, and also their feelings regarding termination of pregnancy, should the test show an 'affected' fetus. They should *not* be required to give any consent in advance, regarding abortion if the anomaly is detected.

DECISION MAKING

The couple decide whether or not to undertake pregnancy, and they decide whether or not to accept an offer of prenatal diagnosis. However, prenatal testing is time-consuming, laborious and expensive; it uses human resources and materials that are, as a result, not available to others; it involves certain risks to mother and to fetus. If a couple are convinced that they would not terminate pregnancy in any event (an 'affected' fetus), they will probably also be convinced that the risks, to mother and pregnancy, are not worth taking[25].

In some situations prenatal diagnosis is, at present, impossible, even though the genetic risk is high. In autosomal recessive disorders after the birth of an affected child, the recurrence risk is 25%. In this difficult situation, some counseled couples will decide the 25% recurrence risk is too high, and will choose termination of an existing pregnancy, sterilization, conception by artificial insemination, or divorce and remarriage. Other couples regard the 75% chance of a healthy child as sufficient encouragement to make at least one more attempt to have a healthy child[26,27].

The physician/counselor gives information, and the parents, in the light of their own individual circumstances and attitudes, make the decision[28]. The parental decision will depend on a number of factors. Of importance may be their optimistic or pessimistic attitude of mind, their ethical and religious principles, their level of education, or their social circumstances. Their previous experiences with the disease in question may also be of decisive importance. Many couples declare that they do not want to undergo another tragedy. This is a most convincing argument[29-34].

The personality of the counselor, too, is of great importance: the way in which information is imparted, the content and clarity of such information, the manner in which the couples' own questions, fears and problems are discussed and dealt with[35,36]. Decision making is extremely difficult and painful for some couples, and decisions will often have lifelong consequences. The counselor should help the couple to the best of his/her ability[37].

Finally, our own experiences in Hungary suggest that couples at high-risk for genetic disorders undoubtedly prefer to have a healthy child, and they ask for prenatal diagnosis if it is possible[17,38]. We do not need to persuade them to undertake prenatal diagnosis, and termination of pregnancy in the case of prenatal diagnosis of an affected fetus. We call our practice non-directive prenatal genetic counseling. It may be different in different parts of the world.

References

1. Abramovsky, I., Godmilow, L., Hirschhorn, K. and Smith, H. (1980). Analysis of a follow-up study of genetic counseling. *Clin. Genet.*, **17**, 1–12
2. Fuhrmann, W. and Vogel, F. (1982). *Genetische Familienberatung.* (Berlin: Springer)
3. Harper, P. S. (1981). *Practical Genetic Counseling.* (Bristol: John Wright)
4. Herrmann, J. and Opitz, J. M. (1980). Genetic counseling. *Postgrad. Med.*, **67**, 233–43
5. Lewis, R. (1992). The evolution of genetic counseling. *Scientist*, **6**, 1–13
6. Passarge, T. and Vogel, F. (1980). The delivery of genetic counseling services in Europe. *Hum. Genet.*, **56**, 1–5
7. Pullen, I. and Emery, A. E. H. (1985). Genetic counseling. A contemporary approach. *Br. J. Hosp. Med.*, **34**, 358–60
8. Papp, Z. (1990). *Obstetric Genetics.* (Budapest: Akadémiai Kiadó)
9. Papp, Z., Tóth, Z., Szabó, M., Csécsei, K. and Török, O. (1985). Prenatal screening for neural tube defects and other malformations by both serum AFP and ultrasound. In Kurjak, A. (ed.) *The Fetus as a Patient*, (Amsterdam, New York, Oxford: Elsevier Science Publishers)
10. Simpson, J. L., Elias, S., Gatlin, M. and Martin, A. O. (1981). Genetic counseling and genetic services in obstetrics and gynecology: implications for educational goals and clinical practice. *Am. J. Obstet. Gynecol.*, **140**, 70–80
11. Graber, A. P. and Hixon, H. E. C. (1990). Prenatal genetic counseling. *Clin. Perinatol.*, **17**, 749–59
12. Lorenz, R. P., Willard, D. and Botti, J. J. (1986). Role of prenatal genetic counseling before amniocentesis. A survey of genetics centers. *J. Reprod. Med.*, **31**, 1–3
13. Hof, J. O. and Kopinsky, S. M. (1982). Communication in genetic counseling. *S. Afr. Med. J.*, **62**, 758–64
14. Chadwick, R. F. (1993). What counts as success in genetic counseling? *J. Med. Ethics*, **19**, 43–6
15. Fassler-Trost, A. (1990). Genetic counseling: values orientation of the counselor and his effect on the decision process of clients. *Psychother. Psychosom. Med. Psych.*, **40**, 27–32
16. Aylsworth, A. S. (1992). Genetic counseling for patients with birth defects. *Pediatr. Clin. N. Am.*, **39**, 229–53
17. Curtis, D., Johnson, M. and Blank, C. E. (1988). An evaluation of reinforcement of genetic counseling on the consultand. *Clin. Genet.*, **33**, 270–6
18. Czeizel, A. (1981). Genetic counseling clinics in Hungary. *Am. J. Med. Genet.*, **9**, 75–7
19. Czeizel, A., Métneki, J. and Osztovics, M. (1981). Evaluation of information-guidance genetic counselling. *J. Med. Genet.*, **18**, 91–8
20. Sato, K., Kato, Y., Kayama, F., Suzuki, A., Tsutsumi, O., Morita, Y., Jimbo, T., Mizuno, M. and Sakamoto, S. (1982). A follow-up study of genetic counseling for malformation. *Jpn. J. Hum. Genet.*, **27**, 193–4
21. Evans, M. I., Bottoms, S. F., Critchfield, G. C., Greb, A. and LaFerla, J. J. (1990). Parental perceptions of genetic risk. Correlation with choice of prenatal diagnostic procedures. *Int. J. Gynaecol. Obstet.*, **31**, 25–28
22. Papp, Z., Tóth, Z., Török, O. and Szabó, M. (1987). Prenatal diagnosis policy without routine amniocentesis in pregnancies with a positive family history for neural tube defects. *Am. J. Med. Genet.*, **26**, 103–10
23. Stoll, C., Roth, M. P., Dott, B. and Bigel, P. (1986). Usefulness of a registry of congenital

malformations for genetic counseling and prenatal diagnosis. *Clin. Genet.*, **29**, 204–10
24. Langer, M. and Ringler, M. (1990). Prospective counseling after diagnosis of fetal malformations: interventions and prenatal reactions. *Acta Obstet. Gynecol. Scand.*, **68**, 323–9
25. Shiloh, S., Avdor, O. and Goodman, R. M. (1990). Satisfaction with genetic counseling: dimensions and measurement. *Am. J. Med. Genet.*, **37**, 522–9
26. Sorenson, J. R., Scotch, N. A., Swazey, J. P., Wertz, D. C. and Heeren, T. C. (1987). Reproductive plans of genetic counseling clients not eligible for prenatal diagnosis. *Am. J. Med. Genet.*, **28**, 345–52
27. Sorenson, J. R. and Wertz, D. C. (1986). Couple agreement before and after genetic counseling. *Am. J. Med. Genet.*, **25**, 549–55
28. Elder, S. H. and Laurence, K. M. (1991). The impact of supportive intervention after 2nd trimester termination of pregnancy for fetal abnormality. *Prenat. Diagn.*, **11**, 47–54
29. Frets, P. G., Duivenvoorden, H. J., Verhage, F., Niermeijer, M. F., Van de Berge, S. M. and Galjaard, H. (1990). Factors influencing the reproductive decision after genetic counseling. *Am. J. Med. Genet.*, **35**, 496–502
30. Frets, P. G., Duivenvoorden, H. J., Verhage, F., Ketzer, E. and Niermeijer, M. F. (1991). Model identifying the reproductive decision after genetic counseling. *Am. J. Med. Genet.*, **35**, 503–9
31. Frets, P. G., Duivenvoorden, H. J., Verhage, F., Peterson, B. M. and Niermeijer, M. F. (1991). Analysis of problems in making the reproductive decision after genetic counseling. *J. Med. Genet.*, **28**, 194–200
32. Frets, P. G. and Niermeijer, M. F. (1990). Reproductive planning genetic counseling. A perspective from the last decade. *Clin. Genet.*, **38**, 295–306
33. Wertz, D. C. and Fletscher, J. C. (1988). Attitudes of genetic counselors. A multinational survey. *Am. J. Hum. Genet.*, **42**, 592–600
34. Wertz, D. C. and Sorensen, J. R. (1986). Client reactions to genetic counseling. Self-reports of influence. *Clin. Genet.*, **30**, 494–502
35. Kessler, S. (1980). Genetic associates/counselors in genetic services. *Am. J. Med. Genet.*, **7**, 323–34
36. Scott, J. A., Walker, A. P., Eunpu, D. L. and Djurdjinovic, L. (1988). Genetic counselor training. A review and considerations for the future. *Am. J. Hum. Genet.*, **42**, 191–9
37. Papp, Z. (1989). Genetic counseling and termination of pregnancy in Hungary. *J. Med. Philos.*, **14**, 323–33
38. Papp, Z. (1992). Efficiency of genetic counseling and prenatal diagnosis in the prevention of congenital anomalies. In Macek, M., Ferguson-Smith, M. A. and Spála, M. (eds.) *Early Fetal Diagnosis: Recent Progress and Public Health Implications*, pp. 590–5. (Prague: Karolinum-Charles University Press)

The routine fetal examination

K. Å. Salvesen and S. H. Eik-Nes

Ian Donald introduced ultrasound to obstetricians in 1958. Since then the use of the technique in pregnancy has spread over the whole world. In the mid 1970s the indications for doing an ultrasound scan of a pregnancy increased to large numbers, but at the same time, obstetricians often found themselves left with a problem in late pregnancy: the wish that a scan had been done earlier. Since that time there has been continuous debate about how and when to use ultrasound in pregnancy.

The use of ultrasound in pregnancy has never been questioned whenever a clinical examination or the patient's history gives reason to suspect a problem. But suggesting an ultrasound examination in an apparently healthy pregnant woman can make emotions range high in some individuals – even cause a new national debate in countries where such examinations have been part of the general practice for years.

Why is it like that?

BACKGROUND FOR THE ROUTINE FETAL EXAMINATION

In general practice, the obstetrician sees various conditions of a low incidence that may become clinically manifest only late in pregnancy or not until delivery. Such conditions can be related to gestational age, or to the unexpected presence of multiple fetuses, adverse location of the placenta, clinically silent fetal demise in the second trimester or various kinds of developmental disorders of the fetus.

Most fetal developmental disorders occur in mothers without any risk factors, and most are not detected clinically until late in the pregnancy or only after delivery. The detection of developmental disorders in the fetus may benefit both the mother and the fetus. Most mothers carrying a fetus with a lethal disorder want to be given the choice to determine the type of intervention appropriate for them at a time when it is possible to make a decision about continuation of the pregnancy. In some cases of fetal developmental disorders, direct intervention can cure the fetus or lessen its handicap. More and more, we learn that just the knowledge of a special fetal condition prior to delivery can make a difference. For example, when we know that the fetus is suffering from defects that require immediate intervention by a team of neonatologists or pediatric surgeons, the fetus will be better off when the mother is hospitalized where there is equipment and expertise that can take care of the condition[1].

RANDOMIZED CONTROLLED TRIALS

In the rapidly advancing field of obstetrics and neonatology, the true impact of a systematically performed fetal examination in every pregnancy can be assessed in randomized controlled trials. A randomized controlled trial is the best scientific method to evaluate the use of new technology. Over the last 15 years, several such studies have been done (see Table 1). A number of meta-analyses addressing this question have also been published[2–4]. Thus, it may sound astonishing to outside viewers that the question of efficacy and efficiency of routine screening with ultrasound in pregnancy remains unsolved. To explain this controversy, it is necessary to review some of the trials and meta-analyses more closely.

The London trial

This was the first of the randomized controlled trials to be published[5]. The study addressed the

Table 1 *Randomized controlled trials addressing the question of routine use of ultrasound in pregnancy*

Trial site	Number of women	Number of planned scans in the screened group	Medical journal	Year
London[5]	1 095	1	Br. J. Obstet. Gynaecol.	1982
Ålesund[6]	1 628	2	Lancet	1984
Trondheim[7]	1 009	2	Lancet	1984
Glasgow[9]	877	2	Br. Med. J.	1984
Stockholm[10]	4 997	1	Lancet	1988
Helsinki[11]	9 310	1	Lancet	1990
Missouri[17]	915	2	Obstet. Gynecol.	1990
Copenhagen[12]	965	7	Br. J. Obstet. Gynaecol.	1992
RADIUS[14]	15 530	2	N. Engl. J. Med.	1993

possible benefit of an early dating of the pregnancy by measuring the fetal biparietal diameter (BPD) in a population of 1095 pregnant women. The final analysis was based on 1062 patients; a random half had the results initially withheld from the obstetrician. For 30% of the women for whom the results were intended to be withheld, the code was broken because of a clinical concern.

There was no difference in the fetal outcome as measured by the birth weight centile, Apgar score at one minute, and perinatal death. Overall, there was no difference between the groups in the number of women requiring induction of delivery.

The main deficiency of this study, as acknowledged by the authors, is the fact that the codes of 30% of the control group had to be broken. The clinicians had already become accustomed to the powerful new technology and found it unethical to withhold information from the ultrasound examinations. The effect of such a protocol deviation will be discussed later.

The Norwegian trials

During 1979 and 1980, two randomized controlled trials were conducted in Norway[6,7]. The Ålesund trial[6] included nearly all the pregnant women in a region. Thus, the study comprised a normal population of 1628 pregnant women. The Trondheim trial[7] did not include women who were referred to the obstetric outpatient clinic at the Trondheim University Hospital. Thus, the Trondheim trial included mostly low-risk pregnancies and consisted of 1009 women. Women were randomly selected to be offered two ultrasound scans (screened) or to have ultrasound for a clinically suspected problem only (controls). Both studies had identical design and ultrasonic devices (ADR 2130); however, the ultrasound operators in Ålesund were experienced compared to the operators in Trondheim, who were introduced to the technology only three months prior to the start of the study. Both studies had the same hypotheses. The calculation of the sample size was based on an expected 50% reduction in the number of induced post-term pregnancies in the screened group.

The Ålesund trial was primarily published as a letter to the editor[6] and later more extensively as a chapter in a textbook[8]. It was found that the primary null hypothesis of the trial could be rejected; the proportion of women being treated for post-term pregnancy was statistically significantly reduced. It was also demonstrated that the number of patients who needed antenatal hospitalization was smaller in the screened group, but the overall use of hospitalization (in days) was equal between the groups. There was no statistically significant effect of routine screening on perinatal mortality or morbidity.

The mean number of scans per pregnant woman was 2.5 among screened and 0.4 among control women. In all, 29% of control women were scanned with ultrasound during pregnancy, because of a clinical indication.

In the Trondheim trial[7] there were no differences in the condition of the newborns based on Apgar score, the need for resuscitation, the need to transfer to a neonatal intensive care unit, and perinatal statistics. In all, 6.5% of screened and 7.9% of the control women had labor induced (no significant difference). However, for 2.8% of all screened women, labor was induced because the pregnancy was believed to be post-term, based on the last menstrual period, despite the fact that the gestational age had been corrected by ultrasound. Thus, this failure of utilizing information from the ultrasound scan may explain why there was no statistically significant reduction in the number of screened women who had induced labor.

The mean number of scans per pregnant woman was 1.9 among screened and 0.2 among control women. In all, 13% of the control women were scanned with ultrasound during pregnancy because of a clinical indication, and 11% of the women in the screened group were never scanned.

The Glasgow trial

The main purpose of the Glasgow trial[9] was to evaluate the possible effect of screening 877 low-risk pregnancies to find small-for-gestational-age fetuses. All the women in the study had an ultrasound scan before 24 weeks of pregnancy for an assessment of gestational age. They were then randomized and a second ultrasound scan was performed of all women at 34–36 weeks. In 433 patients, the results of the second scan were reported to the clinician. In 444 controls, the results of the second scan were not reported unless there were complications (e.g. breech presentation or placenta previa).

There were no differences in obstetric management and outcome between the patients in the two groups, nor was there any difference in outcome when the babies who were considered to be small for gestational age were examined separately. There was no difference between groups in the number of labor inductions. This was, however, not a question under study, since all pregnancies had the result of an early scan revealed to the clinician.

The Stockholm trial

During 1985 to 1987, 8768 Swedish women were recruited to a randomized controlled trial of a one-stage screening program with ultrasound during pregnancy[10]. For various reasons, 1414 women were excluded, and 2357 (32%) of the remaining women fulfilled the criteria for elective ultrasound scans. Thus, the study population of 4997 women represents a highly selected low-risk group. The investigators stated two hypotheses: screening would be valuable if:

(1) There was a reduction in the number of pregnancies requiring labor induction because they were post-term; and

(2) If twin pregnancies had increased birth weight or length of gestation.

Labor was induced because the pregnancy was believed to be post-term in 1.7% of the screened women and 3.7% of the controls ($p < 0.0001$). The rate of overall labor inductions was 5.9% among screened and 9.1% among control women ($p < 0.0001$). Thus, the first null hypothesis was rejected. There was no statistically significant difference between groups with regard to birth weight or length of gestation among twins. There was, furthermore, no statistically significant effect of routine screening on perinatal mortality or morbidity.

In the trial, the authors found the mean birth weight to be 42 g higher ($p = 0.008$) and there were fewer babies with a birth weight below 2500 g (2.5% vs. 4.0%, $p = 0.005$) among the screened newborns. Babies of screened women who smoked were on average 75 g heavier at birth than babies of control women who smoked ($p = 0.01$). In comparison, newborns of screened non-smokers were 26 g (not significant) heavier than babies of non-smoking controls. The authors speculated that the greater differences in birth weight among newborns born to smokers may reflect that screened women may have reduced their smoking during pregnancy to a grater extent in response to watching their fetus on the screen.

The average number of scans per pregnant woman was 1.3 among screened and 0.5 among control women. Despite the fact that all women who fulfilled one or more of fifteen indications for elective scanning had been excluded from the study, 32% of the control women had ultrasound during pregnancy.

The Helsinki trial

During 1986 to 1987, 95% of all pregnant women in the Helsinki area entered a study to compare one-stage ultrasound screening with selective ultrasound use in pregnancy[11]. Thus, the trial evaluated the routine use of one early ultrasound scan in a normal population of 9310 pregnant women.

There were no differences in the number of labor inductions or mean birth weights in the two groups. Perinatal mortality was significantly lower in the screened (0.5%) than in the control group (0.9%) ($p < 0.05$). This 49% reduction in perinatal mortality was mainly due to improved early detection of major anomalies that led to induced abortion.

In 1.6% of the screened group, no ultrasound examination at all was performed (the women did not attend), whereas 77% of the control women had an ultrasound scan during pregnancy based on a clinical indication. The average number of scans per pregnant woman was 2.1 among screened and 1.8 among control women. Remembering that this trial evaluated a one-stage screening program, it is easy to argue that ultrasound examinations had already become too prevalent in Finland to be properly evaluated in a randomized controlled trial. This was acknowledged by the authors, who stated[11]: 'In such circumstances, the possibilities of revealing an effect in a controlled trial are less likely than when there is a sharper contrast between screening and selective use of ultrasound'.

The Copenhagen trial

The purpose of the Copenhagen trial[12] was to assess the value of fetal weight estimation during routine third-trimester ultrasound examinations for the identification of fetuses that were small for gestational age, and thereby promote active pregnancy management and so reduce perinatal morbidity. During 1985 to 1987, 965 pregnant women considered at risk were randomized to either a revealed-results group or a withheld-results group. All women had an early ultrasound scan for estimation of gestational age, and additional ultrasound scans every three weeks from 28 weeks until delivery.

Revealing the results of ultrasound estimates of fetal weight for gestational age during the third trimester resulted in statistically significantly increased diagnoses of fetuses considered to be small for gestational age, of elective deliveries based on this diagnosis, and of healthy preterm babies admitted to the neonatal care unit. No detectable overall improvement in weight for gestational age at birth, or in neonatal morbidity or mortality could be demonstrated. There was no difference in the number of emergency interventions between the randomized groups. However, a subgroup analysis of the small-for-gestational-age fetuses revealed a statistically significantly reduced number of emergency interventions ($p = 0.04$) and acute interventions for fetal distress ($p = 0.02$) in the screened group.

The authors concluded that screening improved the diagnosis of fetuses that were small for gestational age, but this was not followed by improved fetal outcome. However, as was demonstrated in the subgroup analysis, knowing about small-for-gestational-age fetuses reduced acute interventions. From a practicing obstetrician's point of view, this is a clear benefit of ultrasound screening. A similar finding was demonstrated in a Swedish randomized controlled trial comparing Doppler ultrasound velocimetry of the umbilical artery with conventional antenatal cardiotocographic surveillance[13]. Doppler ultrasound velocimetry demonstrated a statistically significant reduction in antenatal monitoring occasions, antenatal hospital admissions, inductions of labor, emergency Cesarean sections for fetal distress, and admissions to a neonatal intensive care unit[13].

The RADIUS trial

The RADIUS (Routine Antenatal Diagnostic Imaging Ultrasound Study) was a randomized controlled trial conducted in the United Sates from 1987 to 1991[14,15]. In all, 55 744 pregnant women were registered, but 32 317 (58%) of the women were excluded because they had indications for ultrasound scanning during pregnancy. Only 15 530 (28%) women were randomly assigned to a two-stage screening program or to ultrasound examination for medical reasons that developed after randomization. This highly selected group of women had a low risk of adverse pregnancy outcome. To maximize the ability to detect any differences between the screened and control groups, the authors grouped perinatal mortality and 19 outcome measures of perinatal morbidity into one single primary outcome measure: adverse perinatal. No rationale was given for including conditions such as fracture of the clavicle or other bones, or documented neonatal sepsis, in a study to evaluate antenatal ultrasound screening.

The rate of adverse perinatal outcome was 5.0% among the infants of the women in the screened group and 4.9% among the infants in the control group (relative risk = 1.0, 95% confidence interval 0.9 to 1.2). There were no significant differences between the groups regarding perinatal outcome in the subgroups of women with post-date pregnancies, twins, or infants who were small for gestational age.

The ultrasonographic detection of congenital anomalies had no effect on perinatal outcome in the study. However, one major objection to the RADIUS trial has been the poor detection of anomalies. Only 17% of anomalies were detected before 24 gestational weeks, whereas the overall sensitivity of ultrasound in six European centers was 51%[16]. Thus, there is good reason to question the quality of the ultrasound examinations performed in the RADIUS trial. The results concerning the detection of fetal developmental disorders is so poor, that if it really is representative for the rural United States, the main conclusion of that study is that there is a great need for teaching basic scanning skills. That is, of course, a very important finding. There is reason to believe that the skill level is less than appropriate outside the university clinics in other countries, as well.

The average number of scans per pregnant woman was 2.2 among screened and 0.6 among control women. Despite the fact that all women who fulfilled indications for elective scanning had been excluded from the study, 45% of the control women still had ultrasound scans during pregnancy.

META-ANALYSIS, 1993

A meta-analysis performed by Bucher and Schmidt[4] included 15 935 pregnancies from four randomized controlled trials[7,10,11,17]. Four outcome measures were analyzed: live birth rate, perinatal mortality, proportion of babies with Apgar score < 7 at 1 min, and rate of induced labor. The authors argued that induced abortions carried out because of malformations detected by ultrasound may bias the perinatal mortality results, since induced abortions decrease the numerator but leave the denominator of perinatal mortality evaluations basically unchanged. Thus, the rate of live births – that is, the number of live births per pregnancy – may be a better measure of the outcome of pregnancy.

The live-birth rate was identical in the screened and control groups (odds ratio = 0.99, 95% confidence interval 0.88 to 1.12), although the perinatal mortality was significantly lower in the group who had routine ultrasound scanning (odds ratio = 0.64, 95% confidence interval 0.43 to 0.97). There were no statistically significant differences between the groups in the rate of induced labor or the proportion of babies with low Apgar scores.

The authors of this meta-analysis have been criticized for their choice of outcome measures[18], but there is no agreement on what the most meaningful outcome measures should be. Another criticism of the meta-analysis has been the relative importance of the Helsinki trial results[19]. Because the Helsinki trial comprised 57% of the women in the meta-analysis, the results were strongly influenced by the pros and cons of the Helsinki trial. Thus, the finding of no effect on induced labor in the meta-analysis may be due to the large proportion of ultrasound exposure in the control group in the Helsinki trial[19].

DISCUSSION

With the speed of development that is taking place in medical technology nowadays, a controlled study can only be done within a short period of time. The medical technology needs to be developed enough to a stage where one can expect an impact to occur, the medical personnel performing the procedure need to be able to interpret their findings, and, finally, the clinicians involved in patient care need to understand the knowledge presented to them and use that information correctly. On the other hand, the medical technology to be evaluated should not be in widespread use in the population. If it is, this will influence the possibility of conducting a randomized controlled trial and the interpretation of the results. If a study is done too early, the full benefit from the technology might not be utilized (as probably was the case with inexperienced doctors in the Trondheim trial). If it is done too late, clinicians may believe it is unethical to withhold information (London trial) or a large proportion of the control group will be exposed to the technology on clinical indications (Helsinki and RADIUS trials).

Nowadays, ultrasound technology has become widespread in all developed countries. There are two ways to deal with this when conducting a randomized controlled trial. One approach is to exclude from the trial all pregnant women who will get ultrasound examinations on a clinical indication anyway (Stockholm and RADIUS trials). This will examine the use of the technology in a low-risk population. The study will then suffer from a low incidence of adverse perinatal outcomes. Also, the generalizability of the study results will suffer. Even a negative conclusion in a study performed in a large low-risk population cannot rule out the possibility of an effect to be found in a non-selected population.

The alternative approach is to enrol all pregnancies in a study, and thus examine the use of the technology in a normal population (Helsinki trial). The price to pay from this strategy would be a large proportion of the controls exposed to ultrasound. Benefits of the new technology will be 'watered down' by the high use of the technology in the control group. In the Helsinki trial there was no difference between the groups regarding labor inductions. This could be a consequence of the fact that 77% of controls were examined with ultrasound during pregnancy (most pregnancies in the control group were dated with ultrasound).

There is no agreement on the question of what is the best way to conduct a randomized controlled trial today. We may be past the historical time-window where routine ultrasound can be properly scientifically evaluated in randomized trials in developed countries.

THE COST ISSUE

The report from the RADIUS trial made cost an important finding of their trial. They found the mean number of scans per pregnant woman to be 2.2 among screened and 0.6 among control women. They even calculated that the costs of a two-stage screening program in the United States would be $1 billion. The question is, however, not as simple as it may seem.

We have no doubt that a screening program will increase the average number of scans per pregnant woman in a low-risk population (Stockholm and RADIUS trials). It is important to remember that a large proportion of the pregnant population was excluded because they were going to be examined by ultrasound anyway. The Helsinki trial, which was performed in a non-selected population, demonstrated no increase in the average number of scans per pregnant woman in a normal population (2.1 vs. 1.8).

A historical comparative study from Norway sheds important light on this issue. A nationwide survey to map the extent of the use of ultrasound was carried out in Norway in 1986. A new survey was performed in 1988 after Norway had introduced one routine scan between 16 and 19 weeks as part of prenatal care[20]. The survey was representative of the whole of Norway. In 1986, 71% of the women were offered a routine scan;

this increased to 79% in 1988. An average of 2.46 scans were done per pregnant woman in 1986, before one scan was introduced as routine practice. This decreased to 2.24 in 1988, 2 years after the official introduction of a routine fetal examination ($p < 0.01$). The cost of ultrasound scanning in pregnancy in Norway dropped 8% following the introduction of an offer to scan every woman at 16 to 19 weeks of pregnancy.

Based on the Helsinki trial and the Norwegian experience, there is good evidence to assume that the number of scans for the total population will not increase in a setup that offers the routine scan rather than the scan on indication.

SAFETY ASPECTS

Because of the exposure of vast numbers of the general population to ultrasound, any possibility of harmful effects becomes very important. Although no adverse effects arising from ultrasound examinations during human pregnancy have been identified, clinical safety is and will always remain a concern.

Until recently, most of our information concerning ultrasound safety has been obtained from *in vitro* studies. Follow-up studies of ultrasound exposure *in utero* in humans have been reported[21–24], but these studies suffer from lack of proper control groups, since the ultrasound exposure was done because of some clinical indication suggesting a problem in the pregnancy. Ideally, a long-term follow-up should be done on individuals in non-selected populations who were exposed to ultrasound in a random fashion. Thus, a follow-up of children who took part in randomized controlled trials as fetuses was needed to clarify questions about the effect on human development[25]. A need for long-term follow-up in prospective epidemiological studies has also been recommended by the Safety Committee of the European Federation of Societies for Ultrasound in Medicine and Biology[26].

Recently, the results from a follow-up of the children who took part in the Ålesund and Trondheim trials have provided new information regarding possible long-term effects of routine ultrasound during pregnancy[27–30]. In 1979–81, 2637 pregnant women were included in the two trials combined. Nine years later, 2428 children were eligible for follow-up, and 2161 (89%) children were included in the study.

Data were collected from parents, from nurses and doctors at maternal and child health centers, and from school teachers. Parents responded to a questionnaire about their child's development. Included in the questionnaire were 21 questions about handedness; three about hearing; four about vision; and six about attention, motor control and perception. Height and weight data were collected from the records of centers of maternal and child health from visits at 3, 6 and 12 months, and at 2, 4 and 7 years. Distant visual-acuity tests and pure-tone audiometry had been done at the visits at 4 and 7 years. Results of a short version of the Denver Developmental Screening Test recorded during the first year of life were available for most of the children. In the second year of primary school, 2011 were evaluated by their teachers with regard to reading aptitude, spelling, arithmetic and overall performance. A subsample of 603 children was tested with specific tests for dyslexia in the third year of school.

It was demonstrated that routine ultrasound scanning *in utero* had no effect on higher neurological functions as measured by teacher assessments of school performance, specific tests for dyslexia, and the Denver Developmental Screening Test during the first year of life, and parental assessments of attention, motor control and perception in childhood[27,28]. Deficits in sensory functions in children, and childhood growth, were also unrelated to ultrasound exposure status *in utero*[29,30]. The data suggested a possible association between routine ultrasonography *in utero* and non-right handedness among children[28]. Since the association was weak, and the remaining five null hypotheses were not rejected, this result may be due to chance. None the less, the study suggests that the association between ultrasound and non-right handedness should be tested in future studies.

Conclusively, the results from the follow-up of the Norwegian studies did not support the possible association between ultrasound exposure in utero and dyslexia in childhood reported in a study from Denver in 1984[24]. It is important to emphasize that the design of a randomized controlled trial rules out many of the biases that might have led to the possible association between ultrasound exposure and dyslexia.

WHAT HAVE WE LEARNED FROM THE RANDOMIZED CONTROLLED TRIALS?

The early randomized trials (London, Ålesund and Trondheim) are important, because ultrasound examinations were not too prevalent at that time. However, the study samples were limited and many questions remained unsolved. The Ålesund study demonstrated the importance of a more precise assessment of the gestational age in the ultrasound-examined group which led to reduced frequency of induction for overdue pregnancy.

The Stockholm trial was indeed important, because it was fairly large, and only 32% of the control women had ultrasound examinations during pregnancy. The study verified the Ålesund trial results and demonstrated that labor inductions were reduced through a one-stage screening program even in a low-risk population.

The consequences of a more precise estimate of the gestational age is obvious. It is of importance for the mother to deliver the baby around the date she was prepared for and not 3–5 weeks later. With the new rules in Scandinavia that guarantee a pregnant woman leave of absence from her work following the 37–38th week, it is also important to have the expected day of delivery as exact as possible. For the obstetrician, more precise information on gestational age has an impact on the management of most of the information concerning growth and development.

The Helsinki trial was also an important study, because it was done in a non-selected population. It demonstrated that perinatal mortality could be reduced in a one-stage screening program mainly due to improved early detection of major anomalies which led to induced abortion. Thus, this study demonstrated in a randomized setup the ability of ultrasound used routinely to detect fetal developmental disorders to a significantly larger extent than in the control group. The study did not demonstrate any reduction in labor inductions, but this may be due to the fact that almost 80% of the control group had a scan on a clinical indication, thus 'watering down' the effect of the routine ultrasound examinations.

The meta-analysis from 1993 did not add much to our knowledge, since it relied heavily on the data from the Helsinki trial. However, the authors introduced the live-birth rate as an outcome measure instead of perinatal mortality in randomized controlled trials.

The RADIUS trial is the largest one published to date. Historically speaking, it was possibly conducted too late, because ultrasound examinations had become so common in the United States at the time of the trial. The results are difficult to interpret, because the trial was done with an extremely highly selected low-risk population (28% of the registered women), and also because a large proportion of the control women (45%) had ultrasound examinations during pregnancy.

Data on perinatal mortality per 1000 deliveries in some of the randomized controlled trials

Table 2 *Perinatal mortality per 1000 deliveries as reported in some randomized controlled trials*

Trial	Screened group		Control group		Odds ratio	95% confidence interval
	n	Mortality	n	Mortality		
Trondheim	510	10.0	499	10.5	0.95	0.27–3.31
Ålesund	809	3.7	819	9.8	0.41	0.12–1.33
Stockholm	2482	4.9	2511	4.9	1.00	0.45–2.24
Helsinki	4691	4.6	4619	9.0	0.51	0.29–0.87
RADIUS	7812	4.4	7718	3.0	1.46	0.86–2.46

are shown in Table 2. The RADIUS trial did not demonstrate any reduction in perinatal mortality. However, the quality of the ultrasound examinations was poor; only 17% of the fetal developmental disorders were detected before 24 gestational weeks, which is far below the international standard[16,31]. The Helsinki trial demonstrated, on the other hand, a 49% reduction in perinatal mortality, mainly due to improved early detection of major anomalies that led to induced abortion. We believe that the RADIUS trial may have concluded differently if the quality of the ultrasound examinations had been better.

CONCLUSION

We think that there is enough evidence present for offering an ultrasound examination of the fetus routinely in every pregnancy. In the developed world, where ultrasound is widely used in pregnancy, there is no reason to believe that such an offer will increase the number of scans in relation to a system where the scans are offered on indication only.

In our opinion, the offer of a routine fetal examination integrated into general antenatal care is the way to organize the surveillance for the mother and her fetus beyond the year 2000. Pregnancy care has traditionally been directed towards the mother, as an indirect way of getting information from the fetus. Maternal care will remain important, but the routinely performed fetal examination with ultrasound gives us a unique opportunity to get in contact with our object, the fetus. Obviously, it will take time before the fetal examination is considered just as natural a part of antenatal care as the maternal examination.

References

1. Eik-Nes, S. H. (1993). Editorial. The fetal examination. *Ultrasound Obstet. Gynecol.*, **3**, 83–5
2. Thacker, S. B. (1985). Quality of controlled clinical trials. The case of imaging ultrasound in obstetrics: a review. *Br. J. Obstet. Gynaecol.*, **92**, 437–44
3. Neilson, J. and Grant, A. (1989). Ultrasound in pregnancy. In Chalmers, I., Enkin, M. and Keirse, M. J. N. C. (eds.) *Effective Care in Pregnancy and Childbirth*, Chapter 27, pp. 419–39. (Oxford: Oxford University Press)
4. Bucher, H. C. and Schmidt, J. G. (1993). Does routine ultrasound scanning improve outcome in pregnancy? Meta-analysis of various outcome measures. *Br. Med. J.*, **307**, 13–17
5. Bennett, M. J., Little, G., Dewhurst, J. and Chamberlain, G. (1982). Predictive value of ultrasound measurement in early pregnancy: a randomized controlled trial. *Br. J. Obstet. Gynaecol.*, **89**, 338–41
6. Eik-Nes, S. H., Økland, O., Aure, J. C. and Ulstein, M. (1984). Ultrasound screening in pregnancy: a randomised controlled trial. *Lancet*, **2**, 1347
7. Bakketeig, L. S., Eik-Nes, S. H., Jacobsen, G., Ulstein, M. K., Brodtkorb, C. J., Balstad, P., Eriksen, B. C. and Jörgensen, N. P. (1984). Randomised controlled trial of ultrasonographic screening in pregnancy. *Lancet*, **2**, 207–11
8. Eik-Nes, S. H. (1993). An overview of routine versus selective use of ultrasound. In Chervenak, F., Isaacson, G. and Campbell, S. (eds.) *Ultrasound in Obstetrics and Gynecology*, vol. 1, Chapter 21, pp. 229–38 (Boston: Little Brown)
9. Neilson, J. P., Munjanja, S. P. and Whitfield, C. R. (1984). Screening for small for dates fetuses: a controlled trial. *Br. Med. J.*, **289**, 1179–82
10. Waldenström, U., Axelsson, O., Nilsson, S., Eklund, G., Fall, O., Lindeberg, S. and Sjödin, Y. (1988). Effects of routine one-stage ultrasound screening in pregnancy: a randomised controlled trial. *Lancet*, **2**, 585–8
11. Saari-Kemppainen, A., Karjalainen, O., Ylöstalo, P. and Heinonen, O. P. (1990). Ultrasound screening and perinatal mortality: controlled trial of systematic one-stage screening in pregnancy. *Lancet*, **336**, 387–91
12. Larsen, T., Falck Larsen, J., Petersen, S. and Greisen, G. (1992). Detection of small-for-gestational-age fetuses by ultrasound screening in a high risk population: a randomized controlled study. *Br. J. Obstet. Gynaecol.*, **99**, 469–74
13. Almström, H., Axelsson, O., Cnattingius, S., Ekman, G., Maesel, A., Ulmsten, U., Årström, K.

and Marsál, K. (1992). Comparison of umbilical-artery velocimetry and cardiotocography for surveillance of small-for-gestational-age fetuses. *Lancet*, **340**, 936–40
14. Ewigman, B. G., Crane, J. P., Frigoletto, F. D., LeFevre, M. L., Bain, R. P. and McNellis, D. (1993). Effect of prenatal ultrasound screening on perinatal outcome. *N. Engl. J. Med.*, **329**, 821–7
15. LeFevre, M. L., Bain, R. P., Ewigman, B. G., Frigoletto, F. D., Crane, J. P. and McNellis, D. (1993). A randomized trial of prenatal ultrasonographic screening: impact on maternal management and outcome. *Am. J. Obstet. Gynecol.*, **169**, 483–9
16. Romero, R. (1993). Editorial. Routine obstetric ultrasound. *Ultrasound Obstet. Gynecol.*, **3**, 303–7
17. Ewigman, B., LeFevre, M. and Hesser, J. (1990). A randomized trial of routine prenatal ultrasound. *Obstet. Gynecol.*, **76**, 189–94
18. Owen, P. (1993). Routine ultrasound scanning in pregnancy. Apgar scores are poor predictors of outcome. *Br. Med. J.*, **307**, 559–60
19. Salvesen, K. Å. (1993). Routine ultrasound scanning in pregnancy. *Br. Med. J.*, **307**, 1064
20. Backe, B., Nafstad, P. and Saetnan, A. R. (1990). Reduced use of diagnostic obstetric ultrasound in Norway. Result of consensus panel recommending routine screening in pregnancy? *Acta Obstet. Gynecol. Scand.*, **69**, 649–50
21. Lyons, E. A., Dyke, C., Toms, M. and Cheang, M. (1988). *In utero* exposure to diagnostic ultrasound: a 6-year follow-up. *Radiology*, **166**, 687–90
22. Kohorn, E. T., Pritchard, J. W. and Hobbins, J. C. (1967). The safety of clinical ultrasonic examination. *Obstet. Gynecol.*, **29**, 272–4
23. Scheidt, P. C., Stanley, F. and Bryla, D. A. (1978). One-year follow-up of infants exposed to ultrasound *in utero*. *Am. J. Obstet. Gynecol.*, **131**, 743–8
24. Stark, C. R., Orleans, M., Haverkamp, A. D. and Murphy, J. (1984). Short and long term risks after exposure to diagnostic ultrasound *in utero*. *Obstet. Gynecol.*, **63**, 194–200
25. US Department of Health and Human Services. (1984). *Diagnostic Ultrasound Imaging in Pregnancy*, NIH Publication No. 84-667. (Washington: Public Health Service, National Institutes of Health)
26. European Committee of Radiation Safety (1994). The watchdogs. EFSUMB safety statement and reviews of recent literature. *Eur. J. Ultrasound*, **1**, 95–7
27. Salvesen, K. Å., Bakketeig, L. S., Eik-Nes, S. H., Undheim, J. O. and Økland, O. (1992). Routine ultrasonography *in utero* and school performance at age 8–9 years. *Lancet*, **339**, 85–9
28. Salvesen, K. Å., Vatten, L. J., Eik-Nes, S. H., Hugdahl, K. and Bakketeig, L. S. (1993). Routine ultrasonography *in utero* and subsequent handedness and neurological development. *Br. Med. J.*, **307**, 159–64
29. Salvesen, K. Å., Vatten, L. J., Jacobsen, G., Eik-Nes, S. H., Økland, O., Molne, K. and Bakketeig, L. S. (1992). Routine ultrasonography *in utero* and subsequent vision and hearing at primary school age. *Ultrasound Obstet. Gynecol.*, **2**, 243–7
30. Salvesen, K. Å., Jacobsen, G., Vatten, L. J., Eik-Nes, S. H. and Bakketeig, L. S. (1993). Routine ultrasonography *in utero* and subsequent growth during childhood. *Ultrasound Obstet. Gynecol.*, **3**, 6–10
31. Levi, S., Hyjazi, Y., Schaaps, J. P., Defoort, P., Coulon, R. and Buekens, P. (1991). Sensitivity and specificity of routine antenatal screening for congenital anomalies by ultrasound: the Belgian multicentric study. *Ultrasound Obstet. Gynecol.*, **1**, 102–10

Fetal brain pathology

R. N. Laurini

INTRODUCTION

The events between conception and the first year of life represent a biological continuum, with birth as the separating landmark between intra- and extrauterine life. Moreover, fetomaternal surveillance has drawn attention to antepartum events that contribute to subsequent neurological handicap in children[1]. We need therefore to define the fetal condition before delivery and identify and understand the pathology of birth itself as well as the possible influence of prenatal events on the perinatal and post-neonatal periods[2].

Fetal asphyxia represents a major form of prenatal pathology, with its morphological expression in the form of hypoxic–ischemic changes in fetal tissues. This type of fetal pathology is significantly related to the pathology of the placenta and uteroplacental circulation. Morphological examination of material obtained from spontaneous or induced abortions indicates that hypoxic–ischemic damage may occur during the embryonic and early fetal period. Although different organs and systems are affected by fetal asphyxia, the relationship between brain damage and neurological handicap underlines the importance of this aspect of fetal pathology. Severe mental retardation affects 3–4 children per 1000, and mild mental retardation occurs in 20–30 per 1000[3]. There may also have been an actual increase in certain neurological disabilities such as cerebral palsy in birth cohorts over the last 20 years[4,5].

Postnatal neurological development therefore can be considered as a measure of antenatal events, since intrapartum hypoxia and birth asphyxia seem not to play a major role in the etiology of neurological developmental defects. There is a growing body of evidence to suggest that defects in neurological development may be the consequence of prenatal hypoxic–ischemic encephalopathy[2,6].

The aim of this chapter is to stress the importance of developmental neuropathology as an integral part of the assessment of fetal development and disease. This chapter will therefore be biased towards the changes occurring during intrauterine life. The approach is both pathophysiological and clinicopathological, to further advance the concept of the fetus as a patient.

METHODS IN DEVELOPMENTAL NEUROPATHOLOGY

Although it is not the aim of this section to deal specifically with methodological aspects, these are highlighted in the assessment of the fetal neonatal and post-neonatal condition. It must be emphasized that the morphological examination of the central nervous system (CNS) and muscle is an integral part of a complete developmental post-mortem. As for any other organ or system, the final interpretation of the neuropathological findings will depend on the available clinical data together with the findings in the rest of the post-mortem.

The final aim of a fetal and neonatal neuropathological examination is to assess the findings in the context of the degree of maturity of the individual case, and to attempt to differentiate between a primary maldevelopment, and brain damage secondary to an environmental cause (e.g. asphyxia)[2]. This can be achieved only if one follows a comprehensive standard protocol consisting of a detailed gross examination combined with the absolutely necessary histological evaluation: the latter is essential since significant changes (e.g. gliosis) are not seen on gross examination[7,8].

The introduction of prenatal neurosonology and postnatal neurosonography, computerized tomography (CT) and magnetic resonance imaging (MRI) for the assessment of brain development and damage has resulted in an increased interest in the morphological examination of the fetal, perinatal and neonatal brain. In view of this, we have modified the traditional method for brain cutting to follow the coronal and sagittal planes used with brain imaging.

Routine histological examination should be performed in all cases. Sampling for histology is carried out on standard blocks from selected areas that are helpful for estimation of development, and represent target areas associated with hypoxic–ischemic changes. Some recommended tissue samples are illustrated in Figures 1 and 2.

In addition to routine histological stains, it is recommended that a standard selection of blocks is processed for immunoreactivity to glial fibrillary acidic protein (GFAP)[2]. The main aim is to differentiate between 'myelination gliosis', normal glial maturation, and pathological (reactive) gliosis as an expression of brain injury. The latter is characterized by the presence of reactive astrocytes, hypertrophic glial cells containing an increased amount of GFAP and thick fibrillary processes[9]. Table 1 summarizes the main histological parameters used to evaluate perinatal brain damage.

Finally, it is of prime importance to underline that all central nervous systems are examined, regardless of their condition. Maceration does

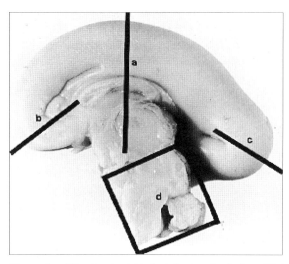

Figure 1 *The standard blocks taken routinely from fetal brains up to about 22 weeks' gestation: a, frontal; b, central; c, occipital; d, brain stem, fourth ventricle and cerebellum*

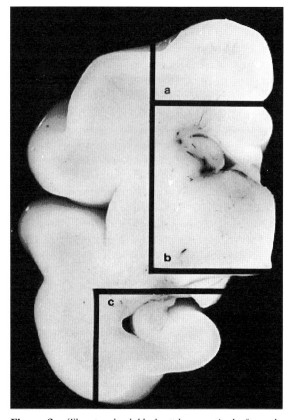

Figure 2 *The standard blocks taken routinely from the hemispheres of perinatal brains. Coronal section at the level of the mamillary bodies*

Table 1 *Perinatal brain damage: histology*

Karyorrhexis
Pyknosis
Neuronal eosinophilia
Pathological gliosis (hypertrophic astrocytes glial fibrillary acidic protein)

Table 2 *Perinatal brain gliosis*

Subpial
Centrum semiovale
Germinal matrix
Granular ependymitis
Cerebellum

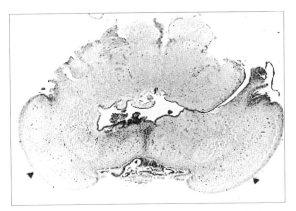

Figure 3 *Absence of external granular layer in both cerebellar hemispheres (arrowheads). Hematoxylin–eosin, × 4.4*

not represent a truly limiting factor for either gross or histological evaluation. Severely macerated cases can benefit from a gross examination *in situ* even if histology is technically impossible. In a recent review of 372 fetuses, we were able to carry out a complete neuropathological examination in 342 CNS; the remaining 30 were severely macerated and allowed only a gross examination *in situ*[10]. A recent review of 103 brains from macerated stillbirths confirms that this approach is meaningful[11]. In fact, Bridger and Wigglesworth[11] also concluded that perinatal anoxic–ischemic damage is more frequent than estimated by previous studies that have excluded macerated cases.

FUNCTIONAL MORPHOLOGY AND BRAIN PATHOLOGY

As a result of modern antenatal surveillance, the developmental pathologist can study embryos and fetuses at different stages of gestation accompanied by what can be considered a very detailed 'intrauterine clinical history'. This has resulted in a dramatic change in the approach to the pathology of early pregnancy, because the morphological findings encountered by the developmental pathologist can now be correlated with intrauterine structural and functional status. This dynamic rendering is defined as *functional morphology*[12].

We have previously discussed the role of the distinctive arterial anatomy in perinatal brains and its possible role in autoregulation. In this

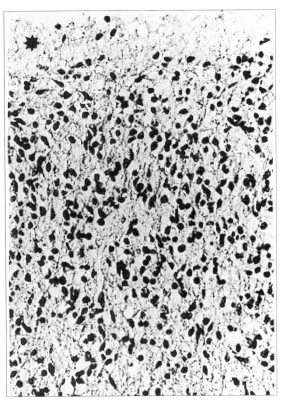

Figure 4 *Higher magnification of Figure 3 shows absence of external granular layer (✱) and an increased cellularity in the molecular layer compared with the control. Hematoxylin–eosin, × 280*

chapter I would like to highlight another aspect of correlation between morphological and functional findings.

Real-time ultrasound has resulted in the establishment of fetal monitoring which includes, among other variables, fetal body movements, fetal breathing movements and fetal tone as reflections of CNS function[13]. The quality and quantity of fetal movements and the development of behavioral states are probably the most sensitive parameters for the assessment of the function and integrity of the nervous system[14–16].

The following case illustrates the role of developmental neuropathology as an integral part of prenatal neurological examination. A healthy 22-year-old nulliparous woman attended for genetic counseling, since her mother had two brothers and two uncles with severe mental retardation. This expression of mental retardation in the family strongly suggested the likelihood of an X-linked disease. This possibility was reinforced by an amniocentesis that revealed a normal male karyotype. Therefore, a real-time ultrasound examination for fetal behavior was carried out, which showed a hyperactive fetus, with onset of abnormally abrupt and continuing movements[17]. The patterns of these movements showed a striking resemblance to the abnormal motility of anencephalic fetuses[18].

The post-mortem revealed a normal male fetus with development corresponding to 19 weeks' gestation. Gross examination of the CNS failed to show significant changes. Histology demonstrated a complete absence of the superficial granular layer in both cerebellar hemispheres (Figures 3 and 4). The cerebella from two normal male fetuses aborted for psychosocial reasons were used as controls (Figures 5 and 6). The morphological findings in this case correspond to those described as primary degeneration of the granular layer of the cerebellum[19]. In view of the gestational age, only the absence of the external granular layer could be observed, without the presence of Purkinje cells, as has been described at a later stage in gestation[20].

This correlation between prenatal neurological findings and developmental neuropathology is not limited to fetal anomalies[7,18], but has also been observed in Fanconi's anemia[17]. This correlation will gain importance when both prenatal neurological evaluations and neuropathological evaluations become a more established routine in antenatal care.

PRENATAL HYPOXIC–ISCHEMIC ENCEPHALOPATHY

In order to define the pathology of the previable fetus, we have recently reviewed 372 fetal post-mortems including 360 placentas and 342 central nervous systems[10]. Our findings regarding the pathology of spontaneous fetal intrauterine deaths are of particular importance in the context of prenatal brain injury. In this series, there were three main causes of death: infections (27 of 153), asphyxia (51 of 153) and

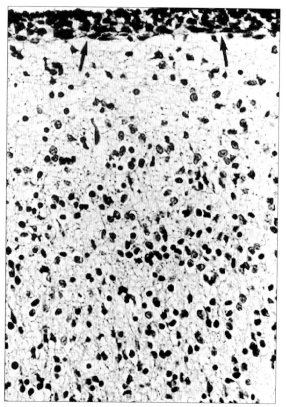

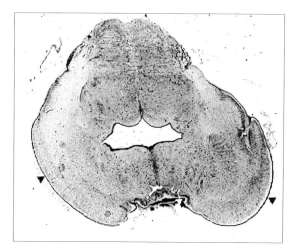

Figure 5 *Cerebellum from control case. Note presence of the external granular layer (arrowheads). Hematoxylin–eosin, × 5*

Figure 6 *Higher magnification of Figure 5 showing a well-developed external granular layer (arrows). Hematoxylin–eosin, × 280*

unknown (24 of 153). The group classified as death due to infections was overwhelmingly represented by the morphological expression of the infected amniotic fluid syndrome. The main cause was asphyxia: fetal lesions were frequently associated with ischemic and/or hemorrhagic pathology of the placenta. Finally, the third group was represented by cases classified as unknown cause of death[21].

The main placental pathology associated with these fetal deaths was not significantly different from that commonly seen in the perinatal period: chorioamnionitis, and hemorrhagic and ischemic pathology. The hemorrhagic lesions consisted of marginal and retroplacental hematomas. The most frequent morphological expression of fetal placental ischemia was 'accelerated maturation' and infarction. Furthermore, the decidual portion of spiral arteries sometimes showed insufficient trophoblast invasion and/or acute atherosis as a sign of pathology of the uteroplacental circulation. These results further underline the importance of the examination of the placenta and uteroplacental circulation. This examination plays a major role in the interpretation of the pathology at post-mortem as well as in liveborn infants[22].

A systematic examination of the CNS in the above mentioned groups of fetuses showed two main forms of brain pathology. One form was represented by acute hemorrhagic lesions seen in association with chorioamnionitis or with the use of prostaglandins to interrupt pregnancies. The other lesions of pathological gliosis, leukomalacia and abnormal cortication were frequently seen in association with ischemic pathology of the placenta. Sims and colleagues[23] have reported a similar relationship between brain and placental pathology in stillbirths.

The use of prostaglandins for termination of pregnancy represents a human model of fetoplacental hypoxic–ischemic pathology in normal pregnancies. A recent review of brain pathology in 116 consecutive fetuses from pregnancies interrupted for psychosocial reasons showed the presence of a germinal matrix hemorrhage in 21% and an intraventricular hemorrhage in 9%[24] (Figure 7). In 9% there

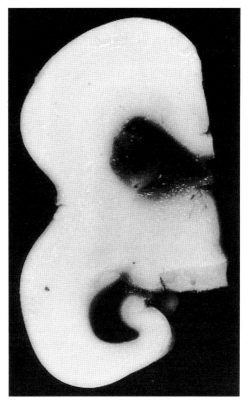

Figure 7 Germinal matrix and intraventricular hemorrhage in an interruption of pregnancy with the use of prostaglandins, at 20 weeks' gestation, for trisomy 21

were also periventricular radial hemorrhages. These lesions are identical to those observed in spontaneous fetal deaths following intrauterine asphyxia (Figures 8 and 9). Interestingly, a review of 158 placentas from pregnancies terminated with PGE_2 for psychosocial reasons demonstrated that it can also be considered as a human model of abruptio placenta in the fetal period[25].

Although the existence of different types of intrauterine brain damage is well established, the true incidence and etiology remain to be resolved. In this context, it is of interest to highlight the frequent association between fetal brain hemorrhage and chorioamnionitis[7,12]. A recent review of 140 post-mortems of fetuses between 12 and 24 weeks' gestation showed 34 brain hemorrhages; 18 were associated with chorioamnionitis while 16 were related to prostaglandin-induced termination of pregnancy[26]

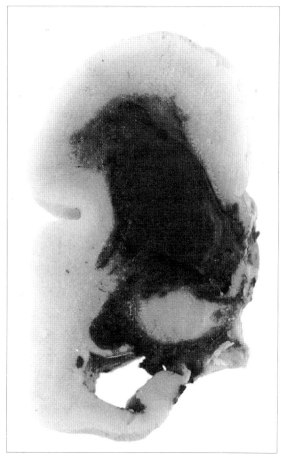

Figure 8 *Germinal matrix hemorrhage with intraventricular hemorrhage and extension into parenchyma. Intrauterine death of 2nd twin at 25 weeks' gestation, with intrauterine growth retardation and acute hydramnios*

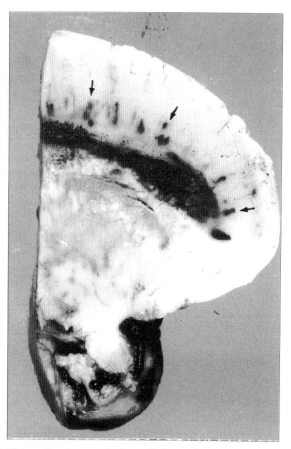

Figure 9 *Periventricular radial vascular congestion and hemorrhage (arrows) in a macerated fetus at 19 weeks' gestation. Retroplacental hematoma and infarction in the placenta*

(Figure 10). In this author's view, the frequent association between chorioamnionitis and fetal brain hemorrhage results from the biochemical cascade, including prostaglandins, released by the inflammatory process. The inflammatory infiltration of the fetal membranes results in a huge increase in prostaglandin E[27] and in interleukin-1[28].

Fetuses obtained following termination of normal pregnancy also allow the normal development and maturation of the glia to be defined by means of glial fibrillary acidic protein (GFAP) staining. This group of psychosocial interruptions of pregnancies corresponds to normal pregnancies in which a thorough post-mortem examination of these normal fetuses confirmed a development according to gestational age and the absence of any pathology. This allows the diagnosis of pathological gliosis, as observed in fetal deaths associated with ischemic and, occasionally, hemorrhagic pathology of the placenta. Careful histological examination of brains from fetuses dying *in utero* revealed the presence of hypertrophic astrocytes, foci of periventricular leukomalacia and areas of abnormal cortication[2]. GFAP staining in these cases confirmed the presence of reactive astrocytes both in areas of the germinal matrix and in the white matter. The mosaic appearance of the germinal matrix observed on staining with hematoxylin–eosin corresponded quite well with the distribution of the cellular

FETAL BRAIN PATHOLOGY

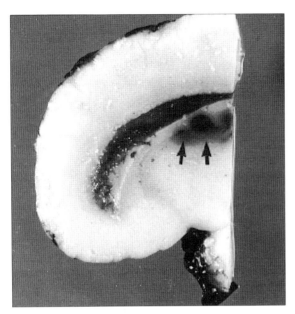

Figure 10 *Germinal matrix hemorrhage (arrows) in an intrauterine death at 22 weeks' gestation with acute asphyxia and congenital pneumonia. The placenta showed a chorioamnionitis*

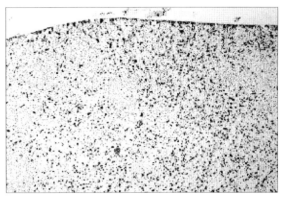

Figure 12 *Germinal matrix showing pathological gliosis and mosaic pattern. Intrauterine death at 27 weeks' gestation with signs of fetal distress and asphyxia. Placenta showed diffuse ischemia and centrocotyledon hemorrhages with infarction affecting 40% of placental volume. Glial fibrillary acidic protein, × 45*

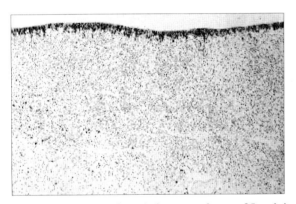

Figure 11 *Germinal matrix from control case at 28 weeks' gestation, with normal staining with glial fibrillary acidic protein, × 45*

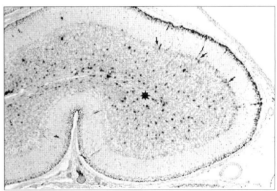

Figure 13 *Staining of cerebellum illustrating pathological gliosis of Purkinje layer (arrows) and white matter (✱) in a fetal brain at 20 weeks' gestation. Glial fibrillary acidic protein, × 90*

islands and GFAP-positive areas in these brains (Figures 11 and 12). Pathological gliosis in the cerebellum (Figure 13) was also frequently seen in these brains, commonly along the layer of Purkinje (Bergmann fibers) and/or in the white matter.

Periventricular leukomalacia represents another lesion of the white matter that can be associated with placental ischemia. In the fetal brain, it is unusual to find the characteristic small white spots restricted to the periventricular region, as is seen in the perinatal brain (Figure 14). Nevertheless, a detailed histological protocol can demonstrate occasional micro-foci of leukomalacia (Figure 15). These lesions are more commonly seen in brains showing a pathological gliosis.

Finally, a less frequent form of fetal brain damage is represented by focal abnormal cortication. At a time in gestation when the brain is normally lissencephalic, gross and histological examination demonstrates the presence of abnormal gyri (Figures 16 and 17). Preliminary results (Laurini, unpublished) suggest that

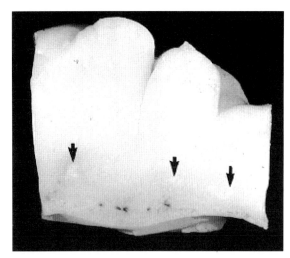

Figure 14 Section of brain hemisphere showing multiple white spots of periventricular leukomalacia (arrows). Early neonatal death (30 min) of second twin (28 weeks' gestation) with intrauterine growth retardation. Twin placenta with morphologically confirmed arteriovenous shunt

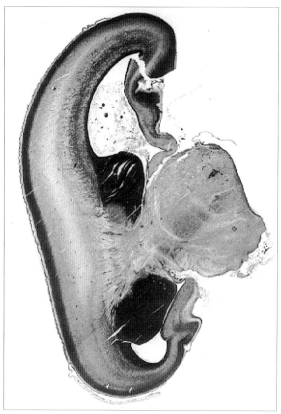

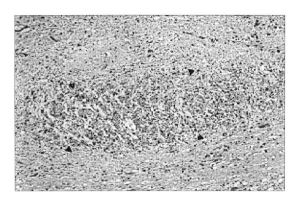

Figure 15 Histological presence of focal area of leukomalacia in a fetal brain (arrowheads). Hematoxylin–eosin, × 84

Figure 16 Central coronal section from brain hemisphere (see Figure 1a) from control case at 16 weeks' gestation. Note normal lissencephalia for gestational age. Hematoxylin–eosin, × 6

there is a relationship between gliosis of the centrum semiovale and abnormal cortication. A working hypothesis is that the pathological gliosis affects the radial glia and impairs the migration of neuroblasts from the germinal matrix to the cortex.

PERINATAL BRAIN PATHOLOGY

Brain pathology in prematurity

'Perinatal pathology' examines the pathology of the viable fetus, mainly in the context of the events in late fetal life, during delivery and in early neonatal life. For the purposes of this chapter I will concentrate on certain aspects of brain damage that are related to the two main forms of perinatal brain pathology: hemorrhagic and non-hemorrhagic.

First, we must highlight the role of the particular anatomy of the microcirculation of the perinatal brain in the pathogenesis of the different types of brain injury. Germinal matrix hemorrhage occurs predominantly at the time when there is a well-developed germinal matrix. The microcirculation of this structure is composed of capillary-like vessels, many of which are large in diameter but retain a thin, capillary-like wall (Figure 18). Regardless of the possible pathologic mechanism of germinal matrix hemorrhage, the vulnerability of the microcirculation, with its special morphology, remains one of the

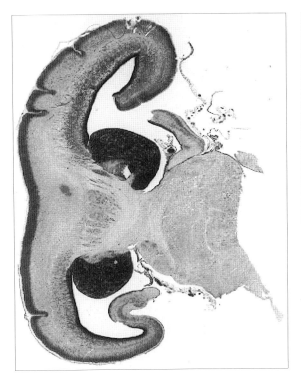

Figure 17 *Central coronal section from intrauterine death at 16 weeks' gestation. Note presence of multiple gyri and sulci. Hematoxylin–eosin, × 7.6*

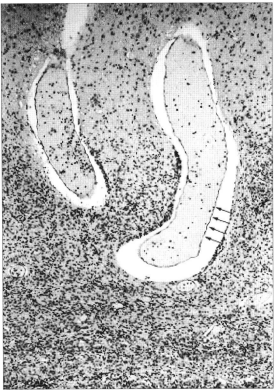

Figure 19 *Histological section from periventricular area illustrating marked vasodilatation of periventricular vessels with thin walls (arrows) in the absence of surrounding connective tissue. Early neonatal death (32 weeks' gestation) of a newborn with multiple malformations. In addition, lesions of acute asphyxia and germinal matrix haemorrhage. Hematoxylin–eosin, × 120*

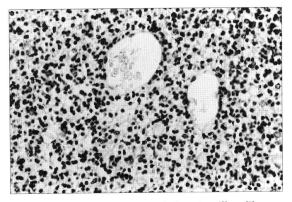

Figure 18 *Dilated microcirculation (capillary-like vessels) in the germinal matrix of a fetus following intrauterine death at 25 weeks' gestation. Note the delicate structure of the vessel wall that is one-cell thick, with absence of surrounding connective tissue. The fetus presented lesions of acute asphyxia and congenital pneumonia. The placenta showed a chorioamnionitis. Hematoxylin–eosin, × 178*

most important variables to consider. This singular vascular morphology is not limited to the germinal matrix, but is also present elsewhere in the brain parenchyma (Figure 19) and in most of the intracerebral veins forming the deep venous system. Furthermore, in the preterm infant, the deep venous system drains most of the area of the white matter into the Galenic system, without significant shunting between the deep and superficial venous systems.

These morphological aspects play a major role in the development of germinal matrix hemorrhage and periventricular venous infarction. Both arterial and venous hypotheses have been postulated to explain the pathogenesis of germinal matrix hemorrhage. A comprehensive routine histological examination of affected fetuses shows that, in early lesions, there is a dilation of the microcirculation associated with focal areas of hemorrhage around the capillary-like vessels. These changes are usually accompanied by a dilated terminal vein.

Germinal matrix hemorrhage can also be associated with periventricular vascular congestion, which ranges from simple dilatation of thin-walled vessels through progressive degrees of hemorrhage to the development of a periventricular venous infarction. These congested periventricular vessels adopt a radial disposition and correspond to the periventricular flares observed on ultrasound. The most common site is in the posterior half of the lateral ventricles (Figure 20).

The morphological changes associated with germinal matrix hemorrhage and periventricular venous pathology can be studied in detail in brains of normal fetuses obtained after termination of pregnancy by prostaglandins. In most cases, one is dealing with the early stages in the development of germinal matrix hemorrhages, that are usually very difficult to assess in neonatal deaths. These early changes are those of vasodilatation of the microcirculation of the germinal matrix and deep venous system, followed by endothelial damage and perivascular hemorrhage. Neither the germinal matrix nor the periventricular white substance shows changes suggesting the existence of an ischemic lesion (infarction) anteceding the perivascular hemorrhage. Although the prevailing hypothesis is that germinal matrix hemorrhage has an arterial origin[29], it is my contention that the pathology of the venous system also plays an important role in the development of both this condition and periventricular venous infarction. Recent work by Nakamura and associates[30] strongly supports this contention.

It is of great clinical importance to distinguish between periventricular venous infarction and hemorrhage into an area of periventricular leukomalacia. Periventricular leukomalacia is necrosis of the white matter with a hypoxic–ischemic character and is preferentially localized to the border zones of the main arterial territories, in the boundary between ventriculofugal and ventriculopetal cerebral arteries. The ischemic lesion underlying this condition is represented by a coagulative necrosis with

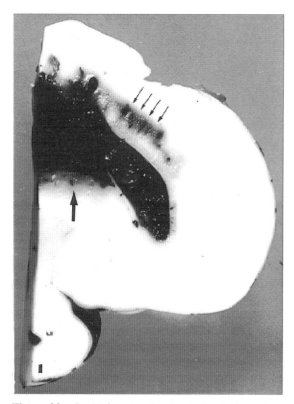

Figure 20 *Sagittal section from brain hemisphere showing a germinal matrix hemorrhage with intraventricular hemorrhage (large arrow) and periventricular radial congestion and hemorrhage (small arrows). Early neonatal death (26 weeks' gestation) with bronchopulmonary dysplasia, acute interstitial pulmonary emphysema and pulmonary hemorrhage. Placenta showed multiple foci of ischemic villitis*

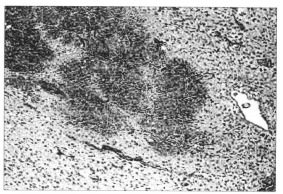

Figure 21 *Histological appearance of hemorrhagic periventricular leukomalacia showing diffuse hemorrhage associated with extensive coagulative necrosis. Neonatal death (31 weeks' gestation) with intrauterine growth retardation. Hematoxylin–eosin, × 45*

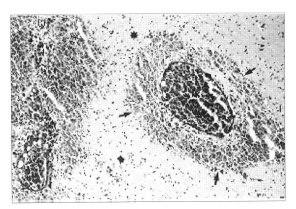

Figure 22 Histological pattern of periventricular venous congestion and hemorrhage. Note hemorrhagic necrosis limited to perivascular areas (arrows) and surrounded by normal brain parenchyma (✱). Early neonatal death (28 weeks' gestation) with hyaline membrane disease and acute pulmonary emphysema. Hematoxylin–eosin, × 45

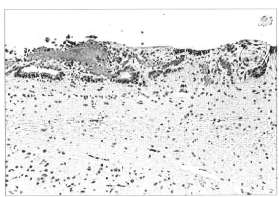

Figure 24 Histological section of granular ependymitis in a newborn suffering early neonatal death (36 weeks' gestation) with changes of asphyxia. Placenta with extensive infarction. Hematoxylin–eosin, × 81

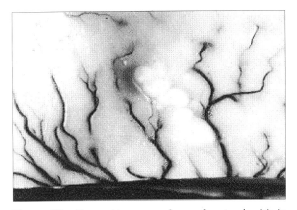

Figure 23 Gross appearance of granular ependymitis in a newborn suffering early neonatal death (34 weeks' gestation). Newborn with a neural tube defect and hydrocephalus, hyaline membrane disease and acute asphyxia

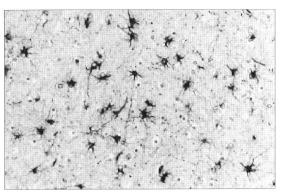

Figure 25 Pathological gliosis in centrum semiovale. Baby born at 37 weeks' gestation with severe hypoxic–ischemic encephalopathy. Placenta showed marked meconium deposition in membranes. Glial fibrillary acidic protein, × 90

granular cells (modified microglia) and gliosis (Figure 21). When hemorrhage develops in an area of periventricular leukomalacia, it is diffuse and not distinctly perivascular. Periventricular venous infarction, however, is characterized by the absence of underlying ischemic lesions and the presence of perivascular hemorrhage with white matter damage limited to the surrounding cerebral tissue, and absence of gliosis (Figure 22). The absence of pre-existing periventricular leukomalacia suggests a better prognosis for periventricular venous infarction than for hemorrhagic periventricular leukomalacia.

When assessing the main forms of perinatal brain pathology, more subtle associated lesions that can influence the prognosis of the main pathology should also be considered. A recent review of 29 perinatal brains stained with GFAP showed a significant association between the main types of perinatal brain damage and gliosis. It also stressed the relationship between granular ependymitis (Figures 23 and 24), pathological gliosis (Figure 25) and periventricular leukomalacia[2]. In addition, as was the case for the fetal brain, cerebellar gliosis was frequently seen in these brains. Table 2 summarizes the main localizations of pathological gliosis in the perinatal brain. There is no significant difference between the expression of pathological gliosis in the fetal or the neonatal brain.

In the view of the author there is a close relationship between the distinctive macro- and microcirculation of the perinatal brain and the development of diffuse gliosis. The hemodynamic and gas changes (O_2 and CO_2) referred to elsewhere can result in damage of endothelial cells with focal destruction of the blood–brain barrier and destruction of perivascular white matter (Figure 26), thus giving rise to pathological gliosis. Experimental work has demonstrated the development of reactive gliosis following disruption of the blood–brain barrier[32]. Reactive gliosis also develops around cortical vessels in rats exposed to alcohol, probably as a result of disruption of the developing blood–brain barrier[9]. These changes can only be demonstrated histologically (Figure 27), but might correspond to the diffuse transitory echodensities seen on ultrasound.

Pathological gliosis, periventricular leukomalacia and granular ependymitis are important tissue markers of hypoxic–ischemic events in the fetal, perinatal and postnatal brain. Their presence is a sign that one or several episodes of fetal stress were serious enough to cause brain damage.

The 'brain-sparing effect' is considered to be a physiological response of the fetus to stress, resulting in a redistribution of blood flow to sustain the brain, heart and adrenal glands. In my view, the existence of such redistribution indicates the presence of a pathological condition. Although it is agreed that this mechanism can reduce the deleterious effects of hypoxia, it is no guarantee that it will prevent tissue damage. Recent work suggests that the above mentioned markers of brain damage can develop despite the existence of the brain-sparing effect[32]. Birth asphyxia may therefore be better defined if end-organ damage is added to the other parameters such as Apgar score and pH. The presence of an organ lesion and dysfunction confirms the pathological character of the condition.

The increasing trend towards malpractice suits has stimulated pathologists to try and indicate the time of development of lesions observed at post-mortem. Although a number of brain lesions can be timed within a given range[22], one must be aware that certain injuries, such as gliosis, can be difficult to time. Pathologic gliosis is not necessarily associated with a chronic condition. It can also develop after an episode of asphyxia and/or hypoperfusion severe enough to give rise to brain damage. Our preliminary results with hypoxemia in fetal

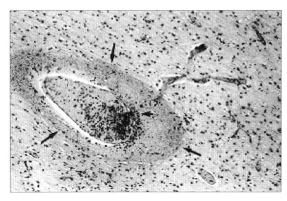

Figure 26 *Endothelial injury with focal thrombosis (short arrow) and destruction of the thin vessel wall, associated with perivascular white-matter damage (long arrows). Same case as in Figure 19. Hematoxylin–eosin, × 57*

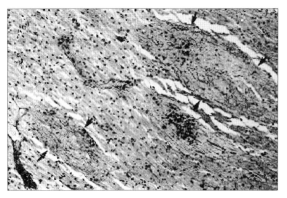

Figure 27 *Histological section of centrum semiovale showing multifocal congestion and rupture of the microcirculation. Note perivascular necrosis of the white matter (arrows). Intrauterine death at 26 weeks' gestation with intrauterine growth retardation, congenital pneumonia and acute asphyxia. The brain presented severe perivascular radial congestion and hemorrhage, bilateral small germinal matrix hemorrhages and a choroid plexus hemorrhage with intraventricular hemorrhage. Placenta showed chorioamnionitis. Periodic acid–Schiff, × 45*

sheep show that pathological gliosis detected by GFAP staining develops in about 3 days (Laurini, unpublished). This conclusion is in agreement with the findings that establish a minimum of 2 to 5 days for the development of hypertrophic astrocytes[33]. Nevertheless, after gliosis is established, it is difficult, though not impossible, to time the 'chronicity' of the brain damage. This is also applicable to other non-specific brain lesions once the injury is established (minimal response time). For example, the presence of macro-cavitation suggests a time span of about 14 days or more, without defining how much longer. Macro-cavitation present at birth therefore indicates an intrauterine event, but the same is not true when the lesion is first diagnosed at 4 weeks of postnatal life.

This concept is of cardinal importance in view of the frequent and undiscriminating use of the terms 'acute', 'subacute' and 'chronic'. A hemorrhage is not always a purely acute phenomenon (e.g. hemorrhagic periventricular leukomalacia) and gliosis is not a chronic lesion by definition (e.g. pathological gliosis 3 days after an episode of fetal asphyxia).

Brain pathology in the mature neonatal brain

A recent review of our perinatal post-mortems showed that approximately 12% of term infants had major brain pathology (germinal matrix hemorrhage, intraventricular hemorrhage and periventricular leukomalacia). Interestingly, this occurred in those weighing > 2500 g, clearly indicating that the mature brain is also at risk (Laurini, unpublished). In effect, although the incidence of cerebral palsy decreases with increasing gestational age and birth weight, the majority of disabilities occurs in appropriately grown infants[34].

Hypoxic injury in the mature neonatal brain is likely to affect the gray matter (Figure 28). Unfortunately, these lesions may coexist with other forms of brain pathology and are often overlooked.

Norman[33] established four different patterns of distribution of hypoxic–ischemic gray matter pathology: cortical, brainstem–thalamic, basal

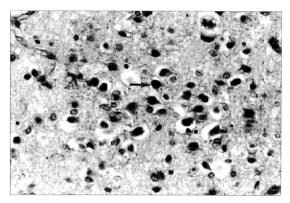

Figure 28 *Extensive acute neuronal necrosis of the pons. Note nuclear pyknosis (arrow). Neonatal death (term gestation) with severe asphyxia associated with placental ischemia. Hematoxylin–eosin, × 179*

ganglia and pontosubicular. Nevertheless, gray-matter necrosis in the early stages is difficult to recognize in the neonatal brain. There also exists a spectrum of mature brain lesions, ranging from cerebral edema through laminar necrosis, cortical necrosis, Purkinje cell loss, and Ammon's horn sclerosis, to cystic degeneration and ulegyria[8]. Extensive cortical damage is frequently associated with necrosis of the thalamus, striatum and hippocampus.

Intrauterine growth retardation and brain pathology

Intrauterine growth retardation (IUGR) is a recognized risk for increased perinatal morbidity, including neurodevelopmental defects, and mortality. However, it is uncertain how IUGR contributes to neurodevelopmental handicaps. It is incorrect to discuss brain damage in IUGR as a whole: several types of IUGR exist, and they differ significantly. Generally speaking, there are two major forms of IUGR. The symmetrical type develops early in pregnancy and is more frequently associated with infection, chromosomal aberrations, hereditary diseases, multifactorial malformations, toxins and malnutrition. In my experience, fetuses with this type of IUGR frequently show a combination of brain pathology associated with the primary cause, i.e. congenital anomaly, as well as lesions secondary to fetal hypoxia. Unfortunately, the latter may be misinterpreted as being part of the malformative syndrome rather than the result of a hypoxic–ischemic insult.

The asymmetrical type of IUGR develops late in pregnancy and is commonly associated with pathology of the uteroplacental circulation, with resulting placenta ischemia and fetal hypoxia. The main lesions are those of hypoxic–ischemic brain pathology: gliosis and periventricular leukomalacia. In this context, one must bear in mind that the early stages of these lesions are difficult to detect by means of sonography[35]. Periventricular leukomalacia can be diagnosed only after several days, when the lesion has evolved. Other lesions resulting from asphyxia and/or hypoperfusion, e.g. gliosis, can only be detected by means of a comprehensive histological examination.

The adverse neurodevelopmental outcome associated with IUGR, particularly the asymmetrical type, is the result of episodic or sustained fetal distress, which results in brain damage. However, not all cases of IUGR have an adverse neurodevelopmental outcome, and one must try to distinguish between IUGR with and without fetal hypoxia[36,37].

Recent work on intrauterine blood flow and postnatal neurological development has shown that small-for-gestational-age infants with abnormal fetal aortic blood-flow classes appear to have an increased risk of minor neurological handicap at 7 years of age, when compared to those with normal blood-flow classes[38]. A morphological evaluation of available placentas from this study showed a probable relationship between placental infarction and minor neurological deficiency[39].

In my experience, fetal distress is the important variable in the context of neurological developmental outcome, and pathological gliosis is its most important morphological marker. IUGR remains an indicator of a high risk for fetal distress and of an increased vulnerability of the fetal brain to develop significant tissue damage. Moreover, the pathology of the placenta and uteroplacental circulation represents a major factor in the development of intrauterine pathology, which can influence the postnatal condition.

POSTNATAL BRAIN PATHOLOGY

The aim of this chapter is to define intrauterine brain pathology and to highlight its influence on postnatal neurodevelopment. Therefore, I want to conclude by discussing briefly the neuropathology of sudden infant death syndrome (SIDS) and schizophrenia.

Neuropathology of SIDS

Today, SIDS represents the most common form of postnatal pathology in the industrialized world. There is evidence to suggest that, in a significant number of cases of SIDS, the uterine environment was less than optimal. SIDS shows a significant relationship with IUGR, prematurity and admission to neonatal intensive care units[40–42] (Laurini, unpublished): in fact, SIDS can be associated with the same obstetric factors previously mentioned when discussing the pathology of the perinatal brain.

We reviewed the brain pathology in a series of 235 cases of sudden infant death, 198 of which fell into the category of true SIDS[43]. In 34 cases, we found sequelae of hypoxic–ischemic lesions, as reported in the literature[44]. Preliminary evaluation using GFAP staining showed a pattern of gliosis similar to that previously described for the perinatal brains (Laurini and Janzer, unpublished). The localization of pathological gliosis was similar to that shown in Table 2. There was a strong correlation between the presence of granular ependymitis and diffuse pathological gliosis, demonstrated with the GFAP method. Kinney and colleagues[44] have also reported a mild telencephalic gliosis in SIDS.

Table 3 summarizes the neuropathology of SIDS. Interestingly, the occurrence of delayed

Table 3 *Neuropathological findings in sudden infant death syndrome*

Heavy brain
Brainstem gliosis
White matter abnormalities
  periventricular leukomalacia
  cerebral gliosis
  cerebellar gliosis
  ↑ lipid-laden macrophages
  retarded myelin formation

myelinization in SIDS can also be an epiphenomenon of pathological gliosis. The intrauterine development of reactive gliosis at a time of transformation of radial glia into multipolar astrocytes[45] can result in delayed or reduced myelinization.

In conclusion, SIDS remains a multifactorial phenomenon in which the intrauterine environment plays a major role in a significant number of cases. In particular, events leading to IUGR and prenatal hypoxic–ischemic encephalopathy define a subset of cases with subtle changes consistent with episodic or sustained intrauterine hypoxia–ischemia that increases the risk of SIDS. Gliosis and other brain lesions may, therefore, be the primary pathology in this subset of SIDS cases, and the neonatal disturbances in state (e.g. apnea) might be a result rather than a cause of gliosis[2].

Neuropathology of schizophrenia

Although it is accepted that schizophrenia has a genetic basis, there is also evidence to suggest that other factors are also involved. Studies using computed tomography have confirmed the presence of ventricular enlargement and abnormal cortication in schizophrenics. These changes, which are seen at an early stage and are non-progressive, are compatible with the sequelae of earlier (i.e. antenatal) events. Furthermore, they are more common in schizophrenics with a history of obstetric complications[46]. These obstetric complications are similar to those associated with perinatal brain pathology. Imaging studies in premature infants, may also show periventricular lesions that result in non-progressive enlargement of the lateral and third ventricles[47].

The presence of structural changes in brains of schizophrenics is now well documented. These changes are characterized by two main types of pathology: multifocal neural developmental defects, and periventricular damage, including gliosis of the periventricular, periaqueductal and forebrain areas[48,49]. These defects of neurological development are consistent with a single pathogenic event or genetic influence during the second trimester[49], while periventricular damage is compatible with the usual adverse perinatal factors described previously.

There are two main interpretations of these findings. One advances the hypothesis that a genetic factor causes a defect of neurological development that in turn increases the vulnerability to perinatal obstetric complications, resulting in periventricular damage[49]. One can also argue that a hypoxic–ischemic event in early pregnancy can produce patterns of brain injury similar to those reported in schizophrenics and give rise to a clinical, imaging and morphological presentation compatible with the schizophrenia spectrum disorder. Published evidence indicates that environmental factors (i.e. periventricular damage) are required for overt schizophrenia[49].

The existence of gliosis in schizophrenia is still a matter for debate, since there is no consensus among the available reports[48,50,51]. The main report which failed to find pathological gliosis in brains of schizophrenics found increased GFAP staining in 17 of 20 areas and admitted that a larger study is needed to examine the possibility that significant gliosis exists in a clinically defined subgroup of schizophrenics[50]. In this context one must bear in mind that remodelling of gliosis has been reported in experimental work: astrogliosis induced by alcohol exposure in rats can be transient[9].

Finally, we must explain the silent interval between the antenatal damage and postnatal expression of abnormality in the first year of life (SIDS) or in the second decade (schizophrenia). A latent period between obstetric complications and their sequelae has been noted in epilepsy and dyskinesias[52] and further confirmed by experimental work in primates[53]. A similar process may account for SIDS and schizophrenia: lesions may lie dormant until there is a functional need for the damaged structure. This hypothesis has been advanced for the onset of schizophrenic symptoms[54].

CONCLUSIONS

Correlation between findings obtained by antenatal surveillance and morphological examination of post-mortems, placentas and uteroplacental circulation strengthens the belief that postnatal neurological developmental deficits can be the consequence of prenatal hypoxic–ischemic encephalopathy. The incidence of antenatal brain damage may be greater than expected if all central nervous systems, including those from macerated fetuses, undergo a comprehensive examination. Further support for this line of thought will develop with the establishment of prenatal neurological examination as an integral part of antenatal diagnosis and surveillance. In this context, we have shown that developmental neuropathology can help explain findings of prenatal neurological examination.

Fetal brain damage can result from episodes of asphyxia and/or hypoperfusion or from more sustained fetal disress. The resulting brain pathology can find an immediate expression during the perinatal period or remain latent until the first year of life (sudden infant death syndrome) or even later, as suggested for schizophrenia.

A routine correlation between findings on antenatal surveillance and developmental pathology enhances our capacity to assess the fetal condition and identify cases at risk or with damage *in utero*, allowing optimal planning of perinatal care. In addition, it helps us to understand the etiology and pathogenesis of disease as an important step in prevention and therapy.

References

1. Visser, G. H. A. (1992). Antepartum events and subsequent handicap. In Fukuyama, Y., Suzuki, Y., Kamoshita, S. and Caesar, P. (eds.) *Fetal and Perinatal Neurology*, pp. 216–22. (Basel: Karger)
2. Laurini, R. N. (1994). Prenatal brain damage, placental pathology and SIDS. *J. Dev. Physiol.*, in press
3. Hagberg, B., Hagberg, G., Lewerth, A. and Lindberg, V. (1981). Mild mental retardation in Swedish schoolchildren. I. Prevalence. *Acta Pediatr. Scand.*, **64**, 193–200
4. Stanley, F. and Blair, E. (1991). Why have we failed to reduce the frequency of cerebral palsy? *Med. J. Aust*, **154**, 623–6
5. Hagberg, B., Hagberg, G., Olow, I. and von Wendt, L. (1989). The changing panorama of cerebral palsy in Sweden. V. The birth year period 1979–82. *Acta Pediatr. Scand.*, **78**, 283–90
6. Bejar, R., Wozniak, P., Allard, M., Bernischke, K., Vaucher, Y., Coen, R., Berry, C., Schragg, P., Villegas, I. and Resnik, R. (1988). Antenatal origin of neurologic damage in newborn infants. I. Preterm infants. *Am. J. Obstet. Gynecol.*, **159**, 357–63
7. Laurini, R. N. (1986). *Aspects in Developmental Pathology*, p. 11–33. (Groningen: Drukkerij van Denderen BV)
8. Laurini, R. N. (1987). Acquired disorders of the central nervous system. In Keeling, J. W. (eds.) *Fetal and Neonatal Pathology*, pp. 491–507. (Berlin, Heidelberg: Springer-Verlag)
9. Goodlett, C. R., Leo, T. J., O'Callaghan, P. O., Mahoney, J. C. and West, J. R. (1993). Transient cortical astrogliosis induced by alcohol exposure during neonatal brain growth spurts in rats. *Dev. Brain Res.*, **72**, 85–97
10. Laurini, R. N. and Hack, I. (1993). L'apport de la pathologie du développement a la génétique médicale. *Rev. Med. Suisse Romande*, **113**, 319–23
11. Bridger, J. E. and Wigglesworth, J. S. (1993). Prenatal anoxic-ischaemic brain damage. *J. Pathol.*, (Suppl.), **172**, A200
12. Laurini, R. N. (1990). Abortion from a morphological viewpoint. In Huisjes, H. J. and Lind, T. (eds.) *Early Pregnancy Failure*, pp. 79–113. (Edinburgh: Churchill Livingstone)
13. Maning, F. A. (1985). Assessment of fetal condition and risk: analysis and combined biophysical variable monitoring. *Sem. Perinatol.*, **9**, 168–83
14. de Vries, J. I. P., Visser, G. H. A. and Prechtl, H. F. R. (1982). The emergence of fetal behaviour. I. Qualitative aspects. *Early Hum. Dev.*, **7**, 301–22
15. de Vries, J. I. P., Visser, G. H. A. and Prechtl, H. F. R. (1982). The emergence of fetal behaviour. II. Quantitative aspects. *Early Hum. Dev.*, **12**, 99–120
16. Nijhuis, J. G. (1986). Behavioural states: concomitants. Clinical implications and the assessment of the condition of the nervous system. *Eur. J. Obstet. Gynecol. Reprod. Biol.*, **21**, 301–8
17. de Vries, J. I. P., Laurini, R. N. and Visser, G. H. A. (1989). Prenatal motor disorders in cases with abnormal cerebral development. In Versteegh, F. G., Ens-Dokkum, E. C. M., Kuypers, J. C., Peters, P. W. J. and van Velzen, D.

(eds.) *1st International Congress in Paediatric Pathology*, p. 30. (Pijnacker, The Netherlands: Dutch Efficiency Bureau)
18. Visser, G. H. A., Laurini, R. N., de Vries, J. I. P., Bekedam, D. J. and Prechtl, H. F. R. (1985). Abnormal motor behaviour in anencephalic fetuses. *Early Hum. Dev.*, **12**, 173–82
19. Norman, R. M. (1940). Primary degeneration of the granular layer of the cerebellum: an unusual form of familial cerebellar atrophy occurring in early life. *Brain*, **63**, 365–79
20. Friede, R. L. (1989). *Developmental Neuropathology*, pp. 361–71. (Springer-Verlag: Berlin)
21. Laurini, R. N. (1994). The role of developmental pathology in foetal medicine. In van Gejn, H. P. and Copray, F. J. A. (eds.) *A Critical Appraisal of Fetal Surveillance.* (Amsterdam: Elsevier Science Publishers), in press
22. Laurini, R. N. (1993). The perinatal postmortem. In Spencer, J. A. D. and Ward, R. H. T. (eds.) *Intrapartum Fetal Surveillance*, pp. 199–212. (London: RCOG Press)
23. Sims, M. E., Beckwith-Turkel, S., Halterman, G. and Paul, R. H. (1985). *Am. J. Obstet. Gynecol.*, **151**, 721–3
24. Laurini, R. N. and Akalin-Sel, T. (1993). Brain lesions and prostaglandins. *J. Maternal Fetal Invest.*, **3**, 176
25. Laurini, R. N. and Akalin-Sel, T. (1993). Placental changes and prostaglandins. *J. Maternal Fetal Invest.*, **3**, 177
26. Hack, I. and Laurini, R. N. (1990). Hémorragie cérébrale fetale et chorioamnionite. *Schweiz. Med. Wschr.*, **120**, 1064
27. Lopez-Bernal, A., Hansell, D. J., Khong, T. Y., Keeling, J. W. and Turnbull, A. C. (1989). Prostaglandin E production by the fetal membranes in unexplained preterm labour associated with chorioamnionitis. *Br. J. Obstet. Gynaecol.*, **96**, 1133–9
28. Taniguchi, T., Matsuzaki, N., Kameda, T., Shimoya, K., Jo, T., Saji, F. and Tanizawa, O. (1991). The enhanced production of placental interleukin-1 during labour and intrauterine infection. *Am. J. Obstet. Gynecol.*, **165**, 131–7
29. Wigglesworth, J. S. (1988). Pathological anatomy of intraventricular haemorrhage in the preterm baby. In Kubli, F., Patel, N., Schmidt, W. and Linderkamp, O. (eds.) *Perinatal Events and Brain Damage in Surviving Children*, pp. 205–10. (Berlin, Heidelberg, New York: Springer-Verlag)
30. Nakamura, Y., Okudera, T., Fukuda, S. and Hashimoto, T. (1990). Germinal matrix haemorrhage of venous origin in preterm neonates. *Hum. Pathol.*, **21**, 1059–62
31. Norton, W. T., Aquino, D. A., Hozumi, I., Chiu, F.-C. and Brosnan, C. F. (1992). Quantitative aspects of reactive gliosis: a review. *Neurochem. Res.*, **17**, 877–85
32. Akalin-Sel, T., Bewleys, S., van Geijn, H. P., Laurini, R. N. and Nicolaides, K. H. (1993). The significance of MCA Doppler assessment in preterminal decompensation of the severely growth retarded fetus. Presented at the *2nd World Congress of Perinatal Medicine*, Rome, September
33. Norman, M. G. (1978). Perinatal brain damage. In Rosenberg, H. S. and Bolande, R. P. (eds.) *Perspectives in Pediatric Pathology*, vol. 4, pp. 41–92. (Chicago, London: Year Book Medical Publishers)
34. Stanley, F. J. and Blair, E. (1991). Why have we failed to reduce the frequency of cerebral palsy? *Med. J. Aust*, **154**, 623–6
35. Hope, P. L., Gould, S. J., Howard, S., Hamilton, P. A., Costello, A. M. de L. and Reynolds, E. O. R. (1988). Precision of the ultrasound diagnosis of pathologically verified lesions in the brains of very preterm infants. *Dev. Med. Child Neurol.*, **30**, 457–71
36. Jouppila, P. and Kirkinen, P. (1989). Non invasive assessment of fetal aortic blood flow in normal and abnormal pregnancies. *Clin. Obstet. Gynecol.*, **32**, 703–9
37. Berg, A. T. (1989). Indices of fetal growth retardation, perinatal hypoxic related factors and childhood neurological morbidity. *Early Hum. Dev.*, **19**, 271–83
38. Marsal, K. and Ley, D. (1992). Intrauterine blood flow and postnatal neurological development in growth retarded fetuses. *Biol. Neonate*, **62**, 258–64
39. Laurini, R. N. (1993). Functional pathology of the placenta: role in perinatal medicine and the legal considerations. In Cosmi, E. V. and Di Renzo, G.-C. (eds.) Progress in Perinatal Medicine, pp. 433–8 (Carnforth, UK: Parthenon Publishing)
40. Buck, G. M., Cookfair, D. L., Michalek, A. M., Nasca, P. C., Standfast, S. J., Sever, I. E. and Kramer, A. A. (1989). Intrauterine growth retardation and risk of sudden infant death syndrome (SIDS). *Am. J. Epidemiol.*, **129**, 874–84
41. Gibson, A. A. M. (1992). Current epidemiology of SIDS. *J. Clin. Pathol. (Suppl.)*, **45**, 7–10
42. Allen, D. M.., Buehler, J. M., Samuels, B. N. and Brann, A. W. (1989). Mortality in infants discharged from neonatal intensive care units in Georgia. *J. Am. Med. Assoc.*, **261**, 1763–6
43. Vanney, A.-C. and Laurini, R. N. (1990). Syndrome de mort subite entre 1970 et 1988 a l'Institut de Pathologie de Lausanne. *Schweiz Med. Wschr.*, **120**, 1064

44. Kinney, H. C., Filiano, J. J. and Harper, R. M. (1992). The neuropathology of the sudden infant death syndrome. *J. Neuropathol. Exp. Neurol.*, **51**, 115–26
45. Pixley, S. R. and de Vellis, J. (1984). Transition between immature radial glia and mature astrocytes studied with a monoclonal antibody to vimentin. *Dev. Brain Res.*, **15**, 209–19
46. Murray, R. M. and Lewis, S. W. (1987). Is schizophrenia a neurodevelopmental disorder? *Br. Med. J.*, **295**, 681–2
47. DeVries, L. S., Dubowitz, V. and Leiser, A. (1985). Predictive value of cranial ultrasound in the newborn baby. *Lancet*, **2**, 137–40
48. Stevens, J. R. (1982). Neuropathology of schizophrenia. *Arch. Gen. Psychiatry*, **39**, 1131–9
49. Cannon, T. D., Mednick, S. A. and Parnas, J. (1989). Genetic and perinatal determinants of structural brain deficits in schizophrenia. *Arch. Gen. Psychiatry*, **46**, 883–9
50. Roberts, G. W., Colter, N., Lofthouse, B., Bogerts, B., Zech, M. and Crow, T. J. (1986). Gliosis in schizophrenia: a survey. *Biol. Psychiatry*, **21**, 1043–50
51. Roberts, G. W. and Crow, T. J. (1987). The neuropathology of schizophrenia – a progress report. *Br. Med. Bull.*, **43**, 599–615
52. Hadders-Algra, M., Touwen, B. C. L. and Huisjes, H. J. (1986). Neurologically deviant newborns: neurological and behavioural development at the age of six years. *Dev. Med. Child Neurol.*, **28**, 569–78
53. Goldman, P. S. and Galkin, T. W. (1978). Prenatal removal of frontal association cortex in the fetal rhesus monkey. *Brain Res.*, **152**, 451–85
54. Weinberger, D. R. (1986). The pathogenesis of schizophrenia: a neurodevelopmental theory. In Nasrallah, H. A. and Weinberger, D. R. (eds.) *The Neurology of Schizophrenia*, pp. 387–405. (Amsterdam: Elsevier)

Reproductive decisions after genetic counseling of couples at high risk for cystic fibrosis: a perspective from the last two decades

Z. Papp, M. Németi, Cs. Papp and E. Tóth-Pál

The aim of genetic counseling is to inform couples about the nature of a mental and/or physical handicap in the family and its risk of occurrence or recurrence. An important aspect of genetic counseling is to assist consultants in reaching a decision regarding the future reproductive behavior that is appropriate to their life situation[1].

In the last 10 years, the possibility of the diagnosis of monogenic disorders has increased. The scope of prenatal diagnosis has been widened with the introduction of chorionic villus sampling and the increased possibility of fetal diagnosis using DNA technology. The diagnosis of cystic fibrosis is the most prominent example of these changes[2-27].

Cystic fibrosis is, in Europe, the most common autosomal recessive disease. The association of pancreatic disease and lung disease was described in the 1930s, and the high sweat chloride in the early 1950s. Recent research suggests that the basic defect relates to opening of chloride channels across membranes. Although present treatment is not directed towards this defect, substantial improvements in life expectancy have been achieved; in some countries, half or more of affected infants live into adulthood[4,7].

Despite improving prospects, this is still a crippling disorder, and many parents of affected children seek prenatal diagnosis for subsequent pregnancies. Effective prenatal diagnosis has been available since the early 1980s, and by DNA technology, from 1986–7[2-27].

THE CLINICAL PICTURE

All mucus-producing tissues are affected, in particular the respiratory and gastrointestinal tracts and the epididymis. The glandular ducts are obstructed by tenacious mucus, and the gland parenchyma develops cystic degeneration. Dense mucus may form meconium plugs *in utero*, leading to intestinal obstruction (meconium ileus). The intestinal wall may perforate, and meconium entering the abdominal cavity produces a foreign-body type of fibrinous reaction and concomitant peritoneal calcification (meconium peritonitis, meconium pseudocyst). (Meconium peritonitis may also develop independently of cystic fibrosis!)

In cases without meconium obstruction, no signs, except perhaps unusually thick or viscid meconium, call attention, in the newborn infant, to presence of the disease. Symptoms develop gradually, as the exocrine glands are damaged. The major problems are those associated with pancreatic exocrine insufficiency (malabsorption, chronic offensive diarrhea, poor weight gain), and chronic respiratory-tract disease (pneumonia, empyema, otitis, sinusitis). Affected babies usually taste, on kissing, unduly salty; this is something that may be noticed by the parents.

Clinical diagnosis depends on recognition of the malabsorption and the pulmonary problems, with confirmation of high sweat concentrations of sodium and chloride.

Pathological confirmation of the diagnosis is easier in older children than in newborn infants or fetuses. Excess connective tissue, and cystic degeneration, are seen histologically in both pancreas and lungs in at least 80–85% of the cases[28–30]. Many affected children used to die during the first year of life. Because of improved symptomatic treatment, especially more vigorous treatment of infections with a much wider range of antibiotics, and also better prophylaxis, prospects have much improved in the last decades. Excluding infants who die in the first year of life, over half of patients may reach their 10th birthday, and many live into adulthood. Owing to diagnosis of increasing reliability, mild cases, which were not diagnosed earlier, are now included among the survivors, undoubtedly contributing to the improved statistics.

Neonatal screening programs have been organized to facilitate genetic counseling before any subsequent pregnancies, and in the hope of improving life expectancy by instituting early treatment. The sweat test, although diagnostic, is impracticable for screening, and a number of alternative (screening) tests have been devised. Proposed screening tests have included assays for albumin in meconium (elevated), and stool trypsin (depressed). Both of these tests have a 10–15% false-negative rate.

Despite the possibility of effective population screening (by radioimmunoassay), the advantages of early diagnosis are doubtful, because 20% of newborn infants have meconium ileus and another 60% of affected infants can be diagnosed clinically during the first year of life. Thus, if a heterozygous couple does not undertake another pregnancy within a year, genetic counseling can be offered to 80% of the unscreened families; at most, 20% may be exposed to a 25% recurrence risk in an unscreened pregnancy.

The improved survival expected from early diagnosis is questionable. There seems to be no difference between the survival of cases diagnosed at birth and that of cases diagnosed at 1 year of age. Meconium ileus is an exception, because prognosis in that condition is poor, not because of the underlying disease, but because of the ileus[4,31].

INHERITANCE

Mode of inheritance is autosomal recessive (McKusick catalogue number 219700). Males and females are at equal risk; there is no sex difference in severity. The heterozygote/carrier rate is 1/20 to 1/25 in most European populations, corresponding to a birth prevalence of 1/1600 to 1/2500. Aspects of genetic counseling and genetic risk are shown in Table 1.

Some affected females, surviving into adulthood, undertake pregnancy. With an unrelated husband, with a 1/25 risk that he is a carrier (heterozygote), there is a 1/50 (2%) risk of producing a child with cystic fibrosis. Pregnancy in women with cystic fibrosis is, in any case, fraught with risks for the woman; 10% may die of cardiovascular complications. Affected men are sterile, because of obstruction of the vas deferens.

PRENATAL MID-TRIMESTER DIAGNOSIS

Our first attempt at prenatal diagnosis of cystic fibrosis was the measurement of acid-soluble glycoproteins in amniotic fluid[32–34]. We offered this test to couples who already had one or more children with cystic fibrosis and who would not undertake further pregnancies without prenatal diagnosis. With the biochemical result of normal amniotic fluid, their chances of having a healthy child, theoretically 75%, rose to at least 90%.

Estimating the efficacy/accuracy depends not only on scrupulously thorough follow-up and testing of all live-born infants submitted to prenatal diagnosis, but also on careful post-mortem examination of all aborted fetuses. There is evidence that histological changes are already present in affected fetuses by 18 weeks' gestation, and are not found in similar-aged normal fetuses. We believe such changes are demonstrable, though they are not so striking as in affected infants dying after live birth[28,30].

In our laboratory between 1976 and 1982, 46 prenatal diagnoses were carried out using amniotic fluid for measurement of acid-soluble glyco-

Table 1 The risks for having a child with cystic fibrosis (CF), in various pedigree situations. The probability of heterozygosity (printed in italics) and the risk of passing the gene to the child are in parentheses. The risks in rows 1 to 7 apply to every autosomal recessive (AR) inherited disease. The values in rows 8 to 13 can be calculated for other AR inherited diseases by replacing the fraction 1/25 with the fraction representing the probability of heterozygosity for the disease in question; e.g. the probability of heterozygosity for Tay–Sachs disease is 1/30 for Ashkenazim and 1/300 for the general population

Pedigree situation	Risk of CF for the child
1. Both parents suffer from CF	1/1
2. One parent suffers from CF; the other is a proven heterozygote	1/2 (*1/1* × 1/2)
3. One parent, and a sibling of the other, suffer from CF	1/3 (*2/3* × 1/2)
4. The parents have already had a child suffering from CF	1/4 (*1/1* × 1/2 × *1/1* × 1/2)
5. The parents are first cousins, and one suffers from CF	1/8 (*1/4* × 1/2)
6. Both parents have a sibling suffering from CF	1/9 (*2/3* × 1/2 × *2/3* × 1/2)
7. The parents are first cousins, and one has a sibling suffering from CF	1/24 (*2/3* × 1/2 × *1/4* × 1/2)
8. One parent suffers from CF	1/50 (*1/25* × 1/2)
9. One parent has a child with CF by another partner	1/100 (*1/1* × 1/2 × *1/25* × 1/2)
10. One parent has a sibling suffering from CF	1/150 (*2/3* × 1/2 × *1/25* × 1/2)
11. One parent has a nephew/niece suffering from CF	1/200 (*1/2* × 1/2 × *1/25* × 1/2)
12. The parents are first cousins; no family history of CF	1/800 (*1/25* × 1/2 × *1/8* × 1/2)
13. The parents are not consanguineous; no family history of CF	1/2500 (*1/25* × 1/2 × *1/25* × 1/2)

Table 2 Prenatal diagnosis of cystic fibrosis between 1976 and 1993

	Acid-soluble glycoproteins in amniotic fluid (1976–82)	Trehalase activity in amniotic fluid (1983–89)	DNA analysis (RFLP, haplotypes, mutations) in chorionic villus cells (1987–93)
High-risk (25%) couples attending genetic counseling	73	126	77
Couples not undertaking pregnancy	10	13	5
Pregnancies with no requested prenatal diagnosis	17	19	7
Pregnancies with prenatal diagnosis	46/73 (65.7%)	94/126 (74.6%)	65/77 (84.4%)
	46/63 (73.0%)	94/113 (83.2%)	65/72 (90.3%)
normal result and unaffected child	34	68	51
normal result and affected child	7	3	0
abnormal results and affected child	4	23	14
abnormal results and unaffected child	1	0	0

proteins (Table 2). Following this and other unreliable attempts at prenatal diagnosis in the 1970s, attention turned to the microvillar enzymes that are secreted directly into the gut lumen. These enzymes, due to fetal intestinal movements, normally reach the amniotic fluid from 11–12 weeks onwards; a low activity in the amniotic fluid may be of value in the diagnosis of intestinal obstruction. It was shown that at 16–20 weeks of gestation the amniotic fluid activity of some isoenzymes of alkaline phosphatase and γ-glutamyltranspeptidase was low in some pregnancies involving a fetus with cystic fibrosis[35–44].

We have observed that at 18–20 weeks of gestation, the activity of a certain disaccharidase (trehalase) in the amniotic fluid of the fetus with cystic fibrosis may be strikingly low even without demonstrable intestinal obstruction[45–49]. These results were supported by other authors[50–52].

Table 3 Distribution of fetuses with prenatally diagnosable cystic fibrosis (CF) (within block outline) in consecutive pregnancies of 1024 couples, both heterozygous for CF (with no reliable CF heterozygote test) HE, healthy

[Tree diagram showing distribution across 1st through 5th pregnancies]

Starting from 1024:
- 1st pregnancy: 256CF, 768HE
- 256CF branches to: 64CF, 192HE (2nd pregnancy)
- 768HE branches to: 192CF, 576HE (2nd pregnancy)

3rd pregnancy:
- 64CF → 16CF, 48HE
- 192HE → 48CF, 144HE
- 192CF → 48CF, 144HE
- 576HE → 144CF, 432HE

4th pregnancy:
- 16CF → 4CF, 12HE
- 48HE → 12CF, 36HE
- 48CF → 12CF, 36HE
- 144HE → 36CF, 108HE
- 48CF → 12CF, 36HE
- 144HE → 36CF, 108HE
- 144CF → 36CF, 108HE
- 432HE → 108CF, 324HE

5th pregnancy:
- 4CF → 1CF, 3HE
- 12HE → 3CF, 9HE
- 12CF → 3CF, 9HE
- 36HE → 9CF, 27HE
- 12CF → 3CF, 9HE
- 36HE → 9CF, 27HE
- 36CF → 9CF, 27HE
- 108HE → 27CF, 81HE
- 12CF → 3CF, 9HE
- 36HE → 9CF, 27HE
- 36CF → 9CF, 27HE
- 108HE → 27CF, 81HE
- 36CF → 9CF, 27HE
- 108HE → 27CF, 81HE
- 108CF → 27CF, 81HE
- 324HE → 81CF, 243HE

	1st pregnancy	2nd pregnancy	3rd pregnancy	4th pregnancy	5th pregnancy
Number of offspring with CF	256	256	256	256	256
Prenatally diagnosable fetuses with CF					
number	0	64	112	148	175
percent	0	25	44	58	65
Reduction of the prevalence of CF at birth (%) (for all pregnancies)	0	12.5	22.9	31.6	38.9

Table 4 *The effect of reproductive compensation on prenatal diagnostic practice in cystic fibrosis (CF) with no reliable CF heterozygote test (see Table 5)*

	Without reproductive compensation	With reproductive compensation
Number of couples, both heterozygous for CF	1024	1024
Number of pregnancies undertaken per couple	2	8/3
Conceptions	2048	2731
Healthy offspring	1536	2048
CF-affected offspring	512	683
Demanded for prenatal diagnosis	256	939*
Diagnosable CF fetuses	64	235
Non-diagnosable CF fetuses	448	448
Ratio of diagnosable CF fetuses/all CF fetuses	12.5%	34.4%

* Calculable from the data of Table 5

Table 5 *Numbers of pregnancies and prenatal diagnoses necessary for the birth of two healthy children in marriages between two heterozygotes for cystic fibrosis (CF), in the absence of a reliable CF-heterozygote screening test*

Number of pregnancies	Number of couples*	Number of prenatal diagnoses
2	576	–
3	288	432†
4	108	288
5	36	135
6	11.25	54
7	3.38	20
8	0.98	7
9	0.28	2
10	0.08	
11	0.02	1
12	0.01	
Totals	1024	939

* This value is given by the formula, $\dfrac{576^{(n-1)}}{4^{(n-2)}}$,

where n = number of pregnancies (the values can also be computed from the data of Table 3). †In the case of three pregnancies, two sequences are possible: healthy, affected, healthy or affected, healthy, healthy. In the former case one, in the latter two prenatal diagnoses are necessary. If the distribution is the same, one prenatal diagnosis is necessary in half of the cases and two procedures in the other half of the cases. Further values in this column can be similarly calculated

In our laboratory between 1983 and 1989, 94 prenatal diagnoses were carried out using amniotic fluid for measurement of trehalase activity (Table 2).

PRENATAL FIRST-TRIMESTER DIAGNOSIS

The cystic fibrosis gene has been mapped to chromosome 7 (7q22.3–23.1), and a large number of closely-linked probes are now available. These permit prenatal diagnosis in almost all couples with a previous living child with cystic fibrosis, and in some situations in which the affected child has died and DNA is not available! Chorionic villus sampling is done at 8–12 weeks' gestation. (DNA can now sometimes be obtained, if critical for the analysis, from Guthrie blood-spots of dead babies – amplification with the polymerase chain reaction has been successful[2–27].)

Table 3 shows that during the second, third and fourth pregnancies of couples both heterozygous for cystic fibrosis, 25, 44 and 58%, respectively, of the fetuses with cystic fibrosis would be detectable, based on the suppositions that all cases would be diagnosed before the parents had another child, that prenatal diagnosis would always be offered, and that it would always be accepted. For couples having two pregnancies, not more, the prevalence of cystic fibrosis at birth would be reduced by 12.5% (64/512); if all couples undertook three or four pregnancies, the birth prevalence might be reduced by 23% or 32%, respectively. It should be noted that the number of heterozygotes would grow considerably in the population by following this method of prenatal screening.

REPRODUCTIVE BEHAVIOR

The magnitude of the genetic risk was earlier thought to be one of the decisive factors in reproductive planning after genetic counseling[53]. Our study shows that in non-directive prenatal genetic counseling the genetic risk has only a relative importance in reproductive planning. Between 1976 and 1993, 276 couples at high risk (25%) for cystic fibrosis attended our genetic counseling center (Table 2). During three 7-year periods (1976–82, 1983–89 and 1987–93), in parallel with the obvious improvement of prenatal diagnosis, the number of couples not undertaking pregnancy has decreased, and the number of pregnancies with requested prenatal diagnosis has increased.

While prenatal diagnosis was not available, the reproductive decision was strongly influenced by a genetic risk of 25% for cystic fibrosis in future offspring. A considerable proportion of parents of a child with cystic fibrosis changed their intended family size or abstained from further childbearing[54].

There is substantial evidence that the availability of prenatal diagnosis is especially valuable for couples with a genetic risk of 1/4[55-58]. Table 2 shows that after prenatal diagnosis became available, even in the period of 1976–82 when an unreliable method was used, 63 out of 73 couples (86.3%) decided to undertake pregnancy and 46/63 (73.0%) requested prenatal diagnosis. These ratios increased in the period of 1983–89 to 113/126 (89.6%) and 94/113 (83.2%), respectively, and in the period of DNA methods (1987–93) to 72/77 (93.5%) and 65/72 (90.3%), respectively.

The availability of prenatal diagnosis induced a change in reproductive planning in a majority of the parents of one or more children with cystic fibrosis[56]. Our results confirm that the availability and reliability of prenatal diagnosis are the most decisive factors in reproductive planning of couples at high risk for cystic fibrosis.

Many couples at high risk would like to have two healthy surviving children. Since the chance of producing a healthy child is 3/4 in each pregnancy, on average, 4/3 pregnancies are necessary to have one, and 8/3 to have two, healthy children. If reproductive compensation envisages the birth of two healthy children, then demands for prenatal diagnosis will increase considerably (Tables 4 and 5). In the absence of reproductive compensation, the number of heterozygotes contributing to the next generation would not increase. If reproductive compensation were widespread, then there would be a small increase in heterozygote frequency: 0.7% per generation.

The strength of the desire to have children can be inferred from the number of affected and healthy children the couples had during decision-making[58]. The desire to have children is also reflected in the position in the birth order of the affected child. Our experiences show that couples were more likely to plan a subsequent pregnancy when the affected child was the firstborn. Table 2 shows that we prefer the non-directive approach to genetic counseling. This approach is a logical consequence of the principle that consultands must be assisted in reaching an informed and autonomous decision that is appropriate to their life situation[58]. The option to undertake a pregnancy and to request prenatal diagnosis belongs to the parents. That is the principle of non-directive prenatal genetic counseling. Nevertheless, supportive counseling by social workers and clinical psychologists attached to prenatal genetic counseling centers can be essential in helping consultants in their decision-making process.

References

1. *Ad Hoc* Committee on Genetic Counseling of the American Society of Human Genetics (1975). *Am. J. Hum. Genet.*, **27**, 240–2
2. Beaudet, A. L. (1992). Genetic testing for cystic fibrosis. *Pediatr. Clin. N. Am.*, **39**, 213–28
3. Campbell, P. W., Phillips, J. A., Krishnam, M. R., Maness, K. J. and Hazinski, T. A. (1991). Cystic fibrosis. Relationship between clinical status and F 508 deletion. *J. Pediatr.*, **118**, 239–41
4. Christian, C. L. (1990). Prenatal diagnosis of cystic fibrosis. *Clin. Perinatol.*, **17**, 779–91
5. Cutting, G. R., Antonarakis, S. E., Buetow, K. H., Kasch, L. M., Rosenstein, B. J. and Kazazian, H. H. (1989). Analysis of DNA polymorphism haplotypes linked to the cystic fibrosis locus in North-American black and Caucasian families supports the existence of multiple mutations of the cystic fibrosis gene. *Am. J. Hum. Genet.*, **44**, 307–18
6. Dannecker, G., Rommens, J. M., Zengerling, S., Burns, J., Melmer, G., Kerem, B., Plavsic, N., Zsiga, M., Kennedy, D., Markiewicz, D. and Rozmahel, R. (1988). Identification and regional localization of DNA markers on chromosome-7 for cloning of the cystic fibrosis gene. *Am. J. Hum. Genet.*, **43**, 645–63.
7. Dodge, J. A. (1988). Cystic fibrosis in the United Kingdom 1977–85. An improving picture. *Br. Med. J.*, **297**, 1599–602
8. Editorial (1990). Worldwide survey of the delta F508 mutation. Report from the cystic fibrosis genetic analysis consortium. *Am. J. Hum. Genet.*, **47**, 354–9
9. Estivill, X., Chillon, M., Casals, T., Bosch, A., Morral, N., Nunes, V., Gasparin, P., Seia, A., Pignatti, P. F. and Novelli, G. (1989). Delta-F-508 gene deletion in cystic fibrosis in Southern Europe. *Lancet*, **2**, 1404
10. Farrall, M., Scambler, P., North, P. and Williamson, R. (1986). The analysis of multiple polymorphic loci on a single human chromosome to exclude linkage to inherited disease cystic fibrosis and chromosome 4. *Am. J. Hum. Genet.*, **38**, 75–83
11. Feldman, G. L., Williamson, R., Beaudet, A. L. and O'Brien, W. E. (1988). Prenatal diagnosis of cystic fibrosis by DNA amplification for detection of KM-19 polymorphism. *Lancet*, **2**, 102
12. Fujimura, F. K. (1991). Cystic fibrosis gene analysis. Recent diagnostic applications. *Clin. Biochem.*, **24**, 353–61
13. Gasparin, P., Novelli, G., Savoia, A., Dallapiccola, B. and Pignatti, P. F. (1989). 1st-trimester prenatal diagnosis of cystic fibrosis using the polymerase chain-reaction. Report of 8 cases. *Prenat. Diagn.*, **9**, 349–55
14. Halley, D. J. J., VanDamme, N. H., Deelen, W. H., Oostra, B. A., Jahoda, M. G. J., Sachs, E. S., Los, F. J. and Niermeijer, M. F. (1989). Prenatal detection of major cystic fibrosis mutation. *Lancet*, **2**, 972
15. Harris, A., Beards, F. and Mathew, C. (1990). Mutation analysis at the cystic fibrosis locus in the British population. *Hum. Genet.*, **85**, 408–9
16. Kerem, E., Corey, M., Kerem, B. S., Rommens, J., Markiewicz, D., Levison, H., Tsui, L. C. and Durie, P. (1990). The relation between genotype and phenotype in cystic fibrosis. Analysis of the most common mutation (delta-F 508). *N. Engl. J. Med.*, **323**, 1517–22
17. Miedzybrodzka, Z. H., Kelly, K. F., Davidson, M., Little, S., Shrimpton, A. E., Dean, J. C. S. and Haites, N. E. (1992). Prenatal diagnosis for the cystic fibrosis mutation 1717-1, G-A using arms. *Prenat. Diagn.*, **12**, 845–9
18. Németi, M., Johnson, J. P., Papp, Z. and Louie, E. (1992). The occurrence of various non-delta F508 CFTR gene mutations among Hungarian cystic fibrosis patients. *Hum. Genet.*, **89**, 245–6
19. Németi, M., Louie, E., Papp, Z. and Johnson, J. P. (1991). Molecular analysis of cystic fibrosis in the Hungarian population. *Hum. Genet.*, **87**, 511–12
20. Németi, M. and Papp, Z. (1990). First trimester diagnosis of cystic fibrosis with linked DNA probes. *Acta Univ. Carol. Med.*, **36**, 135–8
21. Riordan, J. R., Rommens, J. M., Kerem, B., Alon, N., Rozmahel, R., Grzelczak, Z., Zielenski, J., Lok, S., Plavsic, N., Chou, J.-L., Drumm, M. L. and Iannuzzi, M. C. (1989). Identification of the cystic fibrosis gene: cloning and characterization of complementary DNA. *Science*, **245**, 1066–73
22. Rommens, J. M., Zengerling, S., Burns, J., Melmer, G., Kerem, B., Plavsic, N., Zsiga, M., Kennedy, D., Markiewicz, D., Rozmahel, R., Riordan, J. R. and Buchwald, M. (1988). Identification and regional localization of DNA markers on chromosome 7 for the cloning of the cystic fibrosis gene. *Am. J. Hum. Genet.*, **43**, 645–63
23. Sullivan, M. J., Myles, T., Murphy, J., George, P. and Dawson, K. P. (1990). DNA analysis using polymerase chain reactions in the families of children with cystic fibrosis. *NZ Med. J.*, **103**, 216–17
24. Tsui, L. C. (1990). Population analysis of the major mutation in cystic fibrosis. *Hum. Genet.*, **85**, 391–2
25. Wainwright, B. J., Scambler, P. J., Schmidtke, J., Watson, W. A., Law, H. Y., Farrall, M., Cooke, H. J., Eidberg, H. and Williamson, R. (1985).

Localization of cystic fibrosis locus to human chromosome 7cen–q22. *Nature London*, **318**, 384–5

26. Watson, E., Williamson, B., Brueton, L. and Winter, R. (1990). Genetic counseling for cystic fibrosis based upon mutation haplotype analysis. *Lancet*, **336**, 190–1
27. Williamson, R. (1990). Gene mapping in cystic fibrosis and its clinical applications. *Acta Paediatr. Scand.*, **363**, 7–9
28. Damjanovich, L., Szeifert, G. T., Szabó, M. and Papp, Z. (1990). Pathological confirmation of foetal cystic fibrosis following prenatal diagnosis. *Acta Morph. Hung.*, **38**, 141–8
29. Ornoy, A., Arnon, J., Katznelson, D., Granat, M., Caspi, B. and Chemke, J. (1987). Pathological confirmation of cystic fibrosis in the fetus following prenatal diagnosis. *Am. J. Med. Genet.*, **28**, 935–47
30. Szeifert, G. T., Szabó, M. and Papp, Z. (1985). Morphology of cystic fibrosis at 17 weeks of gestation. *Clin. Genet.*, **28**, 561–5
31. Dankert-Roelse, J. E., Meerman, G. J. T., Knol, K. and Kate, L. P. T. (1987). Effect of screening for cystic fibrosis on the influence of genetic counseling. *Clin. Genet.*, **32**, 271–5
32. Alhadeff, J. A. (1978). Glycoproteins and cystic fibrosis: a review. *Clin. Genet.*, **14**, 189–201
33. Ember, I., Juhász, E., Tasnády, Z., Karsai, T. and Papp, Z. (1977). Acid soluble glycoproteins in amniotic fluid. In Szabó, G. and Papp, Z. (eds.) *Medical Genetics*. pp. 713–18. (Amsterdam–Oxford: Excerpta Medica)
34. Papp, Z., Ember, I., Juhász, E., Tasnády, Z., Karsai, T. and Elödi, P. (1977). Acid-soluble glycoproteins in amniotic fluid and cystic fibrosis of the foetus. *Clin. Genet.*, **11**, 431–2
35. Aitken, D. A., Beaudet, A. L., Boué, A., Brock, D. J. H., Carey, W. F., Kleijer, W. J., Papp, Z., Petersen, L., Potier, M., Schwartz, M. and Wauters, J. (1987). Current status of microvillar enzyme testing. In Vogel, F. and Sperling, K. (eds.) *Human Genetics*, pp. 631–2. (Berlin, Heidelberg, New York, London: Springer)
36. Aitken, D. A., Jaqoob, M. and Ferguson-Smith, M. A. (1985). Microvillar enzyme analysis in amniotic fluid and prenatal diagnosis of cystic fibrosis. *Prenat. Diagn.*, **5**, 119–27
37. Brock, D. J. H., Clarke, H. A. K. and Barron, L. (1988). Prenatal diagnosis of cystic fibrosis by microvillar enzyme assay on a sequence of 258 pregnancies. *Hum. Genet.* **78**, 271–5
38. Buffone, G. J., Spence, J. E., Fernbach, S. D., Curry, M. R., O'Brien, W. E. and Beaudet, A. L. (1988). Prenatal diagnosis of cystic fibrosis. Microvillar enzymes and DNA analysis compared. *Clin. Chem.*, **34**, 933–7
39. Carbarns, N. J., Gosden, C. and Brock, D. J. H. (1983). Microvillar peptidase activity in amniotic fluid possible use in the prenatal diagnosis of cystic fibrosis. *Lancet*, **1**, 329–31
40. Carey, W. F., Nelson, P. V., Raymond, S. and Morris, C. P. (1990). Cystic fibrosis prenatal diagnosis. Confirmation of an equivocal microvillar enzyme result by direct analysis of the common gene mutation. *Prenat. Diagn.*, **10**, 613–16
41. Dictus-Vermeulen, C., Ameryckx, J., Gueuning, C., Van Bogaert, E. and Graff, G. L. A. (1988). Alkaline-phosphatase isoenzyme pattern in human amniotic fluid is dependent on the level of total activity. Implications in cystic fibrosis diagnosis. *Clin. Chim. Acta*, **173**, 173–82
42. Mulivor, R. A., Cook, D., Muller, F., Boué, A., Gilbert, F., Mennuti, M. T., Pergament, E., Potier, M., Nadler, H. L., Punnett, H. and Harris, H. (1987). Analysis of fetal intestinal enzymes in amniotic fluid for the prenatal diagnosis of cystic fibrosis. *Am. J. Hum. Genet.*, **40**, 131–46
43. Muller, F., Berg, S., Frot, J. C., Boué, J. and Boué, A. (1985). Prenatal diagnosis of cystic fibrosis. I. Prospective study of 51 pregnancies. *Prenat. Diagn.*, **5**, 97–108
44. Stinson, R. A. and McPhee, J. (1987). Isoenzymes of alkaline phosphatase in amniotic fluid: implications in prenatal screening for cystic fibrosis. *Clin. Biochem.*, **20**, 241–4
45. Szabó, M., Münnich, A., Teichmann, F., Huszka, M., Veress, L. and Papp, Z. (1990). Discriminant analysis for assessing the value of amniotic fluid microvillar enzymes in the prenatal diagnosis of cystic fibrosis. *Prenat. Diagn.*, **10**, 761–9
46. Szabó, M., Teichmann, F. and Papp, Z. (1984). Low trehalase activity in amniotic fluid: a marker for cystic fibrosis? *Clin. Genet.*, **25**, 475–6
47. Szabó, M., Teichmann, F., Szeifert, G. T., Tóth, M., Tóth, Z., Török, O. and Papp, Z. (1985). Prenatal diagnosis of cystic fibrosis by trehalase enzyme assay in amniotic fluid. *Clin. Genet.*, **28**, 16–22
48. Szabó, M., Teichmann, F., Huszka, M., Münnich, A., Veress, L. and Papp, Z. (1990). Genetic counselling and prenatal diagnosis of cystic fibrosis in Debrecen (Hungary). Prenatal diagnosis by microvillar enzyme assay from amniotic fluid. *Acta Univ. Carol. Med.*, **36**, 132–4
49. Szabó, M., Teichmann, F., Huszka, M., Münnich, A., Veress, L. and Papp, Z. (1991). Prenatal diagnosis of cystic fibrosis by microvillar membrane enzyme analysis in amniotic fluid. *Acta Paediatr. Hung.*, **31**, 263–74
50. Kirschbaum, T. H. (1987). Prenatal diagnosis of cystic fibrosis by trehalase enzyme assay in amniotic fluid. In Mishell, D. R., Kirschbaum, T. H. and Morrow, C. P. (eds.) *Year Book of Obstetrics*

and Gynecology 1987, pp. 224–6. (Chicago: Year Book Medical Publishers)
51. Kleijer, W. J., Janse, H. C., Van Diggelen, O. and Niermeijer, M. F. (1985). Amniotic fluid disaccharidases in the prenatal detection of cystic fibrosis. *Prenat. Diagn.*, **5**, 135–43
52. Morin, P. R., Melancon, S. B., Dallaire, L. and Potier, M. (1987). Prenatal detection of intestinal obstructions, aneuploidy syndromes, and cystic fibrosis by microvillar enzyme assays (disaccharidases, alkaline phosphatase, and gamma-glutamyltransferase) in amniotic fluid. *Am. J. Med. Genet.*, **26**, 405–15
53. Carter, C. O., Fraser, R. J. A., Evans, K. A. and Buck, A. R. (1971). Genetic clinic: a follow up. *Lancet*, **1**, 281–5
54. Niermeijer, M. F., Halley, D. J. J., Kleijer, W. J., Neijens, H. J. and Sinaasappel, M. (1990). Prenatal diagnosis and genetic counselling of cystic fibrosis. *Acta Paediatr. Scand.*, **363**, 20–4
55. Borgo, G., Fabiano, T., Perobelli, S. and Mastella, G. (1992). Effect of introducing prenatal diagnosis on the reproductive behaviour of families at risk for cystic fibrosis. A cohort study. *Prenat. Diagn.*, **12**, 821–30
56. Evers-Kiebooms, G., Denayer, L., Cassiman, J. J. and Van den Berg, H. (1988). Family planning decisions after the birth of a cystic fibrosis child. The impact of prenatal diagnosis. *Scand. J. Gastroenterol.*, **23**, 38–46
57. Evers-Kiebooms, G., Denayer, L. and Van den Berg, H. (1990). A child with cystic fibrosis. 2. Subsequent family planning decisions, reproduction and use of prenatal diagnosis. *Clin. Genet.*, **37**, 207–15
58. Frets, P. G. and Niermeijer, M. F. (1990). Reproductive planning after genetic counselling: a perspective from the last decade. *Clin. Genet.*, **38**, 295–306

Computer applications in fetal medicine

I. E. Zador, V. Salari and R. J. Sokol

INTRODUCTION

Perhaps it is not entirely coincidental that the quantum leap in fetal medicine during the last three decades parallels the massive proliferation of computer technology. As fetal medicine evolved from its embryonic beginning in the mid-1960s, analog computers were on hand to aid in the early research concerning signal processing of uterine contractions and fetal heart rate. The introduction of the Digital Equipment Corporation's PDP 11 series of computers rapidly advanced the work in areas of computerized fetal monitoring. A decade later the first rudimentary perinatal databases started to appear. When the personal computer (PC) was introduced in the early 1980s, significant advancement took place. It was the digital scan converter and the resulting first clinically useful real-time ultrasound scanner (ADR 2130) that opened a window of opportunities into the mysterious world of fetal medicine. In this chapter, we briefly review the current trends in computer hardware and mention some new operating systems and application software that might be of interest and relevance to the perinatologist. We then focus on two of the major applications of computers in perinatology, namely fetal electronic monitoring and ultrasound fetal imaging. The chapter concludes with descriptions of some of the 'emerging' new computer technologies.

HARDWARE

As PCs are becoming increasingly 'user friendly', there are a few things that a perinatologist has to understand about the computer hardware functions. The most common utilization of a computer by a perinatologist is truly for 'personal use'. The decision in selecting a PC starts with a choice between the two dominant platforms on the market: Apple or the IBM and its compatibles. For the majority of common applications, either of these two computer systems will perform adequately. For a novice user, the Apple might be somewhat 'friendlier' but even this is becoming less of a difference between the two platforms. Since IBM and its compatibles share around 80% of the market, the available software seems to prefer the IBM base. In addition, the so-called OEM (original equipment manufacturers) products are available in a much larger variety and at a lower price for the IBM and its compatibles.

The next decision in the hardware selection process is to choose between a 'desktop' and a 'notebook' type of computer. The increasingly popular notebook computers, weighing 1.5 kg or less, are rivaling the power and storage capacity of their desktop counterpart. The difference might still be in the higher cost of the notebook, especially when equipped with an active-matrix color type of screen display – an increasingly popular feature. In the active matrix screens, each dot on the screen is controlled by its own transistor, unlike the alternative passive matrix, in which a transistor controls a whole row or column of dots. The advantage of active-matrix screens is that colors are much brighter than those in passive-matrix screens. The drawback is that active-matrix screens are expensive and power-hungry. A typical hardware configuration for years to come will require more than 16 MB of dynamic memory, hard disks exceeding 500 MB, and processors of a Pentium type or faster. Standard options will include a network interface card, a CD-ROM for multimedia applications and a modem/fax for telecommunication.

In hardware applications where massive computing power is needed, the move is from mainframes to client-server environments. Client-server systems split processing chores between powerful servers and desktop machines, enabling both desktop and servers to run more efficiently.

OPERATING SYSTEMS

The emerging new operating systems such as Microsoft's NT (for New Technology) are poised to be the key players in the developing market of client/server computing. Because modern medical management will require more work with limited resources, the ability to link small, inexpensive PCs on a network is very attractive, especially in the larger hospital/university-based perinatal units. These types of operating platforms will offer an open environment for more efficient integration of computing resources. They will work equally well with DOS, Windows, Unix, Macintosh, OS/2 and leading networks. They will enable better integration of the numerous stand-alone computer systems one can find in any hospital department. Such systems are now used to perform a variety of tasks, including billing, administrative and secretarial support, payrolls, laboratory data processing, and research applications, as well as numerous clusters of special purpose applications (residence database, fetal monitoring system, etc.).

APPLICATIONS SOFTWARE

In applications software for personal computers, the trend is for integrated software packages to include word processing, database, spreadsheet and telecommunication applications all in one package. This 'works' type of software package (e.g. LotusWorks, Microsoft Works, WordPerfect Office, etc.) suffered up till now from a reputation of being deficient in all but one or two areas. For example, a works-like package might serve reasonably well for word processing and spreadsheet tasks but too often its database, graphics, and telecommunications capabilities were substandard. At present, however, integrated software packages offer a remarkably consistent set of features that should fit the needs of almost anyone as evidenced by about 15 DOS, Windows and Macintosh packages available on the market.

In terms of integrated applications software available for larger medical centers, there are several systems in various stages of development. The one system commonly referred to is from the Medical College of Virginia (T. Peng, personal communication). The primary focus of this Hospital Information System (HIS) is to provide clinical data in an easily accessible format for the clinician. In addition, it was designed to provide data sets for quality assurance purposes, residence review statistics, and for *ad hoc* research. The key advantages of designing a clinical system on a HIS platform are multiple, directly accessible sites and the elimination of duplication of data entry. For example, once the patient's basic demographic and clinical information (name, birth date, last menstrual period, etc.) was entered, this would eliminate any further redundant entry of the same data by other providers. It is well known from the various forms that are utilized by the health care providers that there are many common data elements which are entered repetitively from form to form. Multiple terminal accessibility is of utmost importance, so that the clinician can access patient information from an office, a hospital floor, and from sites outside the hospital, e.g. other hospitals or offices. An additional advantage of the HIS-based system is that data of all users of the system such as pharmacy, laboratory, nursing and radiology are stored with the patient on the mainframe.

There are some disadvantages of the mainframe-based HIS systems. One drawback is that manipulating data on the mainframe is extremely tedious. For research, quality assurance and other *ad hoc* inquiries, it is generally easier to download the specific data set required and use PC-based database software. Redesign of formats for data entry, windows and screens are cumbersome and restricted in design. In that sense, a PC platform offers much broader versatility and flexibility but limited accessibility and storage. An additional disadvantage of the mainframe, HIS-based system which is especially critical for the obstetric patient is that data are not maintained on-line in perpetuity. In the Virginia system, for example, data are purged every three days and backed up onto magnetic tape. As such, the data entered when the patient was admitted for preterm labor is lost and would need to be re-entered when the patient returns in term labor.

SELECTED PERINATAL APPLICATIONS OF COMPUTERS

Fetal monitoring

From the early reports of successful intrapartum fetal monitoring done nearly 30 years ago, this modality has become an integral part of modern perinatal medicine. The relative maturity in the field of antepartum and intrapartum electronic fetal monitoring is perhaps best demonstrated by the small number of research papers available as measured by the Medline search of the last several years. For example, in 1992 the Medline search reveals only 15 articles on the subject, a relatively small number when compared to hundreds of articles appearing in the late 1970s and throughout the 1980s. Furthermore, at the 3rd World Symposium on Computers in Obstetrics and Gynecology held in Anchorage, Alaska, in 1992, there was not even a single session dedicated to the subject, while previous meetings in 1987 and 1990 each devoted a full day to the topic of computerization of electronic fetal monitoring.

Computerized fetal monitoring systems are currently marketed by several companies worldwide. In the United States, the most popular systems are made by Hewlett-Packard and Corometrics. In general, the computer system incorporated into the perinatal monitoring system is capable of sampling several channels of analog information at a rate of 1–1000 Hz. Calibrated digital values are displayed on the computer monitor and stored on the disk. The computer system performs algebraic computations and estimates derivatives. Pattern recognition algorithms are included for the detection and characterization of uterine contraction, fetal heart rate, fetal breathing movements and fetal behavioral states. Several different noise-rejection filters are usually available. Most of the systems support outputs of signals via a digital-to-analog converter.

Perinatal ultrasound imaging

Color Doppler, three-dimensional imaging, and digital beam forming are just a few examples of significant recent technological advancement in perinatal ultrasound imaging. It is well recognized that many of these innovations are in part due to dramatic changes in computer technology during the last decade. The challenge that computers will present in medical imaging in general and in perinatal ultrasound in particular are enormous. In perinatal ultrasound, the control over the parameters imposed by the manufacturer (i.e. image quality) will improve slightly, but there will be an explosion in applications related to 'ease of operation'. This will be determined by optimal use of computers and predominantly by availability of appropriate software that focuses on the development of a computer-controlled environment for a perinatal ultrasound laboratory. These components will include:

(1) Automatic capture of salient measurements;

(2) Simple rapid coding for common, normal and abnormal findings;

(3) Near real-time electronic and hard-copy report generation;

(4) Simple editing capability with automatic update of the database;

(5) Access to images and video record of the examination;

(6) Generation of a clinical and research database with a simple query scheme;

(7) Automated measurement of the fetal head, abdomen and femur;

(8) On-line availability of an image encyclopedia and clinical decision support; and

(9) Connectivity to other components of an integrated medical database.

Areas of active research involving computer applications in perinatal ultrasound imaging are described in greater detail in the next several paragraphs.

Automatic capture of fetal measurements

In fetal ultrasound, biparietal diameter (BPD), occiput–frontal diameter (OFD), head circumference (HC), abdominal circumference (AC) and femur length (FL) are the most commonly used fetal measurements. To minimize the limitations associated with manual measurements (e.g. inter- and intraobserver variability, examination time, etc.), several investigators studied the feasibility of computerized automation of these measurements. Thomas and colleagues[1] studied the feasibility of computer-determined measurement of fetal femur length. In their study, 49 images of fetal long bones were collected during routine fetal examinations and recorded on conventional multi-image films. Several different imaging algorithms were tried to obtain the straight measurement of the length of the femur without the occasionally visible curvature (side lobe artifact) of the medial aspect. The best results were obtained using the morphological operators that allow the processing of images based on shape characteristics. The correlation between the computed and measured values was very high ($r = 0.9985$) with a trend for the computed measurement to be slightly smaller than the measured values. The computation of each femur length was performed in about 10 min. Zador and associates[2] undertook an investigation with the focus on (a) the design of a PC-based system for automated measurements of BPD, OFD and HC, and (b) the integration of such a system into the routine obstetric ultrasound examination. In their study, data were obtained from 75 consecutive singleton ultrasound examinations free of any obvious structural anomalies. The computer obtained acceptable measurements of BPD, OFD and HC from 74 images and failed only on 1 image. There was a highly significant correlation between computer-determined measurements of BPD ($r = 0.986$), OFD ($r = 0.958$) and HC ($r = 0.972$) and those obtained by the operators. The mean measurement difference (computer minus operator) was 1.87 mm for BPD, 2.82 mm for OFD, and −0.36 mm for HC. These differences were independent of the operator's identity, the instrument used and gestational age.

The key finding from these studies was that, utilizing relatively inexpensive PC technology, it is possible to design and implement a system that can deliver fetal measurements with high correlations and in a fraction of the time, when compared to manual determination by a skilled operator. Operator-assisted image processing via interactive area-of-interest (AOI) specification have been shown to produce consistently accurate interactive measurements of BPD, OFD and the femur. The next level of technology would explore the possibility of free-form, full-screen automated search for the objects of interest. Using clinical ultrasound images, a methodology for the automatic location of the skull to perform BPD and OFD measurements has been developed (L. Chik, personal communication). However, the location of the femur might prove to be very difficult, since the femur is often presented as a somewhat 'inconspicuous' structure with disjointed segments. The sonographers appear to rely on the human ability to integrate the information from many frames to arrive at an acceptable visualization of the objects of interest. It is speculated that very elaborate image processing technology would be needed to emulate such human ability.

Ultrasound fetal tissue characterization

In contrast to the investigations involving adults and animals, there are few studies concerned with ultrasound fetal tissue characterization. The reason for this relates to an apparent lack of clinical feasibility, since most of the non-fetal studies focus on detection of tumors, which are rare in the fetus. Another limitation relates to the inability of direct application of ultrasound to the tissue of interest, increasing the complexity of the signal processing. Few of the existing fetal studies focused on assessment of organs in which maturational changes could be observed, most notably the placenta and lungs. The initial studies have been based on subjective assessment of fetal morphological differentiation and have been limited by interobserver variation and reproducibility. The major impetus for the more recent investigations came from the commercial availability of relatively inexpensive imaging workstations.

The basic components of a typical imaging/graphics workstation consists of a computer platform with a PC and the proper video interface for picture inputs and outputs. Generally, a variety of applications programs are needed for effective operation – these include contrast enhancement, histogram equalization, smoothing, sharpening and other filtering and convolution procedures. A pointing device, such as a digitizer pen or a 'mouse' are of great help if areas of interest are to be identified. A video printer or a laser printer with gray-scale video adapters are important assets. Video inputs might be derived from a video camera, a recorder, ultrasound equipment, or a still video camera. The images are usually stored within the video frame-grabber electronics, using high-speed random-access memory for faster display or interactive processing. A typical 512×512 image requires more than one-quarter million characters of display memory for black-and-white and up to three times more for red/green/blue or hue/saturation/intensity color coding. Many imaging packages and graphics packages are equipped to handle only image or graphic work and not both. The users have to make the choices according to their needs. As imaging input, display and printing equipment might have different aspect ratios or non-square pixels, mixed equipment might not match. Image compression trades storage requirements for computing time. Certain formats could be tedious to program if the 'uncompress' program is not available. While file compression schemes generally provide uncompressed files without the loss of data, many image-compression schemes are intended for file size economy with predetermined levels of filtering or quality degradation.

While investigating fetal tissue characterization, the composite video from the ultrasound hardware is input into a workstation. The ultrasound image can be either 'frozen' or captured during the real-time examination. Zador and associates[3], using such a setup, analyzed anterior placental images from 27 patients in the plane that included the long axis and the umbilical cord insertion. To control for external factors (gain, focusing, etc.), they calculated the ratio of the coefficient of variation of the placental echo amplitude to that of the tissue equivalent phantom. They reported good discrimination between grades 0/I vs. II/III but little distinction between grades 0 and I and grades II and III.

In the same investigation, they also examined the ultrasound tissue properties of the fetal lungs, liver and bowel. Since the lungs, liver and bowel are adjacent structures, their images were assessed relative to each other using longitudinal scans, including sections of both. The study on 10 fetuses showed a rise in lung echogenicity with gestational age, which coincided with pulmonary functional maturation and increasing alveolar surfactant excretion[3]. Similarly, increased bowel echogenicity corresponded to a previously described period of functional maturation. These preliminary results encouraged the suggestion that computerized ultrasound tissue characterization shows promise as a method of evaluating the anatomical counterparts of functional maturation in the fetus. Sohn and co-workers[4] analyzed fetal lung maturity by a computerized system in which frequency rather than amplitude was used to assess the changes along the fetal lung–liver interface. The A-scan envelope was digitized and entered into a computer for spectral analysis. From the resulting A-scan spectra of 222 patients, the mean, maximum and minimum frequencies were determined, and ratios of lung/liver were plotted against gestational age. The results showed a progressive change of the ratio with gestational age, with the largest change observed after 35 weeks.

Ultrasound 3-dimensional imaging

Amniography and fetoscopy are among the few tools available to view the fetus in three dimensions. Unfortunately, these are invasive techniques that cannot be safely repeated. Ultrasound three-dimensional (3-D) imaging is a non-invasive technique that can be used safely and repeatedly, and can provide even the most experienced sonographer with details not easily obtainable from serial tomographic images. The most common advantages of 3-D imaging include:

(1) The enhancement in visualization of small anatomical details, refining the diagnoses of subtle abnormalities (face, extremities, spine);

(2) An improved diagnosis related to better imaging of the fetal surface;

(3) Volumetric measurement (fetal weight, placental weight, amniotic fluid);

(4) Decrease in data acquisition time (increased patient throughput, bioeffect); and

(5) The integration of vessel dimension with velocity profiles to obtain true flow.

Up until now, the major research in perinatal 3-D ultrasound was performed only in a limited number of academic institutions, due mostly to the significant demand on financial resources needed for transducer design and computer processing[5–11]. Several prototype systems generated an 'approximation' of a 3-D scanner rather than a product for clinical applications. In general, a 3-D ultrasound scanner requires a computer system that can register the position and orientation of its images in a three-dimensional spatial coordinate system that is independent of the ultrasound transducer. The real-time images and spatial coordinates are transmitted to a computer that controls the system operation and provides a means for subsequent 3-D analysis of the acquired data. The current emphasis in perinatal 3-D imaging is on:

(1) The design of a transducer (weight, slice thickness and lateral resolution), which can be an integral part of the routine ultrasound scanners; and

(2) The development of a computer workstation for interactive rapid review of 3-D data.

Based on its theoretical potential and the experiences gained in 3-D image reconstruction in radiology, it appears that this modality will become an exciting area of perinatal imaging in the near future. Several ultrasound equipment manufacturers worldwide (Philips, Acoustic Imaging/Dornier, Kretztechnik, and Aloka) have introduced commercially available 3-D ultrasound units. However, clinical applications will have to await the outcomes of trials demonstrating the benefits and safety of this technology in fetal medicine.

Networked imaging system

Computer networking might offer the best opportunity to enhance the ultrasound laboratory through the sharing of high-performance resources. Even with low end equipment, an ultrasound image file can be transmitted to a host computer in less than 15 s without compression. This makes protocols for network file sharing (NFS) feasible for the support of clinical ultrasound machines or of teaching/research workstations equipped with 'bare-bone' imaging capabilities. A major problem in the ultrasound imaging laboratories remains the ability to interface ultrasound hardware from various manufacturers. At present, there is not an accepted standard for ultrasound image capture and storage. With the emerging 'digital imaging and communication' (DICOM) standard proposed by the National Electrical Manufacturers Association (NEMA) and endorsed by several major ultrasound manufacturers (Siemens, ATL, Acuson, Philips, and GE), it appears that major progress towards a standard for transferring images and other medical information between computers is forthcoming.

NEW TRENDS

In conclusion, we describe some emerging 'buzzwords' related to some new applications with potential for some exciting future applications in perinatal medicine.

Virtual reality

Just as flight simulators have long been used to train pilots before they climb into the actual airplanes, 'virtual reality' has a potential to provide a 'dry run' through risky and costly medical procedures. Virtual reality is an interactive technology that creates an illusion of being immersed in an artificial world. It involves the use of electronic sensors and computer-generated images to give the illusion of participating in simulated events. In a typical setup, a participant wears a helmet with a pair of miniature televisions aimed at the eyes to create a three-dimensional image. By using a combination of joystick, sensor-laden gloves or other hand-held devices, the person may mimic a surgical procedure. The only report related to application of virtual reality in ultrasound fetal imaging we could find includes work on 3-D imaging of the fetus superimposed on the pregnant woman's abdomen. Further research in virtual reality is expected to merge with robotics, producing telepresence, the ability of a person to observe and manipulate objects in distant locations. Applications of such technologies in fetal medicine is at best very speculative at present.

Digital convergence – multimedia

This application refers to the expected technological melding of computers, telecommunications, television and publishing. It is a rapidly growing area, with great potential for applications in perinatal medicine, mostly in the area of teaching and education.

Telemedicine

The September 1993 launch of the space shuttle Discovery deployed an Advanced Communication Technology Satellite which represents an entry into new frontiers of health care. Called 'telemedicine', this technology would bring high-quality health care to remote areas of the world by allowing scans to be examined, discussed and diagnosed by specialists in tertiary-level centers. Rather than transporting the patient to a specialist, images from ultrasound or other imaging modalities could be transmitted electronically to the specialist. The technology is expected to be in full use by the end of the decade.

Videoconferencing

Today, literally dozens of executives, managers, and project leaders can be rounded up in minutes and herded into a videoconference room to see, hear and speak to the 'big boss' on the 'big screen' – live and direct from New York or Amsterdam or Tokyo. The technology is still rather new and costly, but the ability to participate in a videoconference from an operating room, lecture room or private home is becoming an important competitive tool.

Internet

The International Network (Internet) is the successor of an experimental network built by the U.S. Defense Department in the 1960s. The Internet links at least 3 million computers, many of them related to universities and research, around the world. We encourage computer users, whether in the private office, university, hospital or at home, to explore the possibility of getting on Internet or some similar network (e.g. Bitnet) to gain an inexpensive and rapid link to the vast array of information of the outside world being disseminated through the modern electronic highways.

SUMMARY

In this chapter concerning computers in perinatal medicine, we have focused on applications we felt might be of relevance to the professionals involved in perinatal medicine. We have tried to provide some guidelines that might help in the personal computer selection process, a task which in today's rapidly changing technology is an extremely difficult one, even for the computer professional. We have also reviewed some selected applications of computers in perinatal medicine. Major emphasis was placed on ultrasound imaging, since this represents an area of extensive current and future computer applications. We have avoided detailed technical descriptions of various aspects of computer technology (central processor unit, hard disk, etc.). This is of little use to clinicians with today's increasing 'user friendly' computers. The real power of computers in perinatology can be discovered in the remaining chapters of this book. It is with some sense of wonder that we realize that most of these chapters exist only because of this marvelous invention called a computer, which was used to find applications in perinatal medicine nearly 30 years ago.

References

1. Thomas, G. T., Jeanty, P., Peters, R. A. and Parrish, E. A. (1991). Automatic measurements of fetal long bones: a feasibility study. *J. Ultrasound Med.*, **10**, 381
2. Zador, I. E., Salari, V., Chik, L. and Sokol, R. J. (1991). Ultrasound measurement of the fetal head: computer versus operator. *Ultrasound Obstet. Gynecol.*, **1**, 208
3. Zador, I. E., Bottoms, S. F., Chik, L., Salari, V., Evans, M. I. and Sokol, R. J. (1989). Development of ultrasound tissue characterization technique: computer differentiation of placenta, lung, liver and bowels. *Proceedings of the meeting of the Society for Gynecologic Investigation*, San Diego, March, p. 96
4. Sohn, C. H., Stolz, W. and Bastert, G. (1991). Diagnosis of fetal lung maturity by ultrasound: a new method and first results. *Ultrasound Obstet. Gynecol.*, **1**, 345
5. Sohn, C. H., Stolz, W., Nuber, B., Hesse, A. and Hornung, B. (1991). Three-dimensional ultrasonic diagnosis in gynecology and obstetrics (German). *Geburts. Frauenheilk.*, **51**, 335–40
6. Baba, K., Satoh, K., Sakamoto, S., Okai, T. and Ishii, S. (1987). Non-invasive three-dimensional imaging system for fetus *in utero*. In Maeda, K. (ed.) *The Fetus as a Patient*, pp. 111–16. (Excerpta Medica)
7. Baba, K., Satoh, K., Sakamoto, S., Okai, T. and Ishii, S. (1989). Development of an ultrasonic system for three-dimensional reconstruction of the fetus. *J. Perinat. Med.*, **17**, 19–24
8. Smith, S. W. and von Rann, O. T. (1988). High speed 3-D imaging with a two-dimensional array. *Ultrasonic Imaging and Tissue Characterization Symposium*
9. Brinkley, J. F., McCallum, W. D., Muramatsu, S. K. and Liu, D. Y. (1982). Fetal weight estimation from ultrasonic three-dimensional head and trunk reconstructions: evaluation *in vitro*. *Am. J. Obstet. Gynecol.*, **144**, 715–21
10. Pretorius, D. H. and Nelson, T. R. (1991). Three dimensional ultrasound imaging in patient diagnosis and management: the future. *Ultrasound Obstet. Gynecol.*, **1**, 381
11. Nelson, T. R. and Pretorius, D. H. (1992). Three-dimensional ultrasound of fetal surface. *Ultrasound Obstet. Gynecol.*, **2**, 166

Section 2

New dimensions in fetal and placental imaging

Early detection of congenital anomalies using transvaginal ultrasonography

M. M. van Zalen-Sprock, J. M. G. van Vugt and H. P. van Geijn

INTRODUCTION

Thanks to the advanced technology of ultrasonography, especially through the transvaginal approach, it is possible to investigate embryological development. Patients' acceptance of the transvaginal approach is good, not in the least since in early pregnancy transvaginal examination does not require a filled bladder. The distance between transducer and subject is considerably shorter in the transvaginal technique compared to abdominal scanning. High ultrasound frequencies can be used and accordingly better axial and lateral resolution is obtained. Clearer images are acquired and smaller structures are distinguished. Potential advantages are early diagnosis of fetal viability, assessment of correct dates and certainty about single or multiple gestation. Particularly early detection of structural anomalies is possible, which facilitates a correct prognosis and effective therapeutic action.

The number of malformations that can be detected in the first and early second trimester of pregnancy has extended in recent years. Rottem and co-workers[1] are among the first authors to describe the detection of anencephaly and cystic hygroma in the first trimester of pregnancy with transvaginal ultrasonography. Benacerraf and colleagues[2] have reported on first trimester ascertainment of fetal cephalocele, cystic hygroma followed by fetal hydrops and a case of thanatophoric dysplasia. One of the most commonly detected malformations between 10 and 14 weeks of pregnancy is cystic hygroma. Other anomalies that can be diagnosed early in pregnancy concern defects of the central nervous system, urinary tract anomalies, abdominal wall defects, cardiac anomalies and abnormalities of the skeletal system[3,4].

Thorough understanding of embryological and fetal development is required for correct interpretation in case of fetal abnormalities[5]. Furthermore, in applying transvaginal ultrasound scanning, knowledge of pitfalls is necessary to prevent inappropriate diagnoses. Caution and particular points of attention in regard to correct diagnosis are described in the separate subheadings of this chapter.

CYSTIC HYGROMA

The development of the lymph vascular system begins at the end of week 5 of gestation. Lymphatic vessels grow out of primary lymph sacs. The lymphatic ducts connect with the internal jugular veins[6]. In case of defective formation of the lymphatic vessels, the jugular sacs enlarge and lymph accumulates in tissues, resulting in nuchal cystic hygroma or jugular lymphatic obstruction sequence[7]. In the presence of this congenital malformation of the lymphatic system, originating in the soft tissue of the neck, the fetus has an intact skull and spinal column[8]. Cystic hygroma can already be diagnosed in the first trimester of pregnancy[9-12]. Hygromas can be single or multiloculated and are located lateral or posterior in the cervical region (Figures 1 and 2). Measurements of 3 mm are generally accepted as a cut-off level for abnormal development[9,11]. A hygroma may very well regress and resolve[11]. The outcome of 69 fetuses with a cystic hygroma detected between 10 and

THE FETUS AS A PATIENT

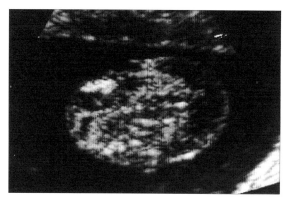

Figure 1 *Non-septated hygroma in a fetus of 10 weeks' gestation with trisomy 21*

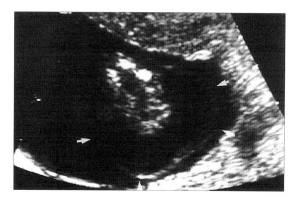

Figure 2 *Septated hygroma in a fetus with monosomy X*

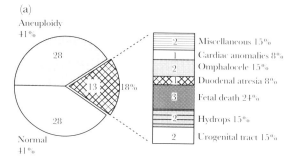

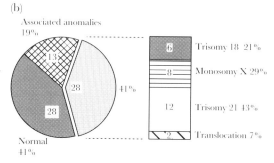

Figure 3 *Outcome of 69 fetuses with a cystic hygroma detected between 10 and 16 weeks of pregnancy in relation to (a) associated anomalies and (b) aneuploidy*

16 weeks of pregnancy is given in Figure 3. In about 40% of the euploid fetuses with a hygroma, regression of the abnormality occurs, always before 16 weeks of pregnancy. In about 40% of fetuses with cystic hygroma, an abnormal karyotype can be found, such as trisomy 21, trisomy 18, monosomy X or an unbalanced translocation[13]. Associated anatomic malformations with various etiology are found in 20–25% of the fetuses with a cystic hygroma, such as omphalocele, polycystic kidneys, urethral stenosis, cardiac anomalies or cystic adenomatoid malformation of the lung.

One of the pitfalls in the early diagnosis of cystic hygroma is amnion not yet merged with the chorion. A translucent area close to the head of the fetus can mistakenly be held for a uniloculated hygroma. This mainly occurs when the fetus is positioned close to the (posterior) gestational sac wall. Discrimination between amnion and hygroma is possible when the fetus changes position. Movements of the fetus may be provoked if the investigator taps the patient's abdomen with his free hand. If a hygroma is suspected, it has to be differentiated from occipital cephalocele[8]. Characteristics that can help this differentiation are the echogenic aspect of the cele, the presence or absence of a defect in the occipital skull, possible septation of the lesion and the presence of associated anomalies such as microcephaly or hydrops.

If the diagnosis of hygroma has been made, a structured and detailed ultrasonographic examination of the fetus is advised and fetal karyotyping is strongly recommended. In case of a resolving hygroma in a euploid fetus, follow-up ultrasound examinations are suggested to exclude malformations only detectable later in pregnancy[8].

CENTRAL NERVOUS SYSTEM

Development of the central nervous system (or neurulation process) starts at the beginning of week 5 of gestation with the formation of a plate of thickened ectoderm. The lateral edges of this neural plate elevate, thus forming the neural folds and finally forming the neural tube. The neuropores, cranial and caudal openings of this neural tube, are the last parts to close in this neurulation process, at the end of week 6 of gestation[14]. Abnormal central nervous system development is divided into neurulation and post-neurulation defects[15]. In neurulation defects, the caudal and/or cranial neuropores fail to close. In post-neurulation defects there is primarily an ossification defect of calvarium or the vertebrae, and secondly the meninges bulge through this bony opening, whether or not accompanied by neural tissue.

The most common malformation of the central nervous system is failure of the cranial part of the neural tube to close. This anomaly has an incidence of one in every 1000 births. It is characterized by acrania and there is no formation of parietal, occipital and frontal bones. The neuroepithelium at first develops normally. The abnormality is classified as exencephaly[16]. With continuing pregnancy, progressive hemorrhagic necrosis occurs and exencephaly changes to anencephaly[17]. Exencephaly is, in contrast to anencephaly, more often diagnosed in the first trimester of pregnancy. Failure of the caudal neuropore to close results in myeloschisis or myelocele. The spinal canal has an open connection with the amniotic fluid. Post-neurulation defects are characterized by bony defects, either in the cranial vault, or in the vertebrae. The meninges, with or without neural tissue, bulge through this opening. A cephalocele is formed when the defect is located in the calvarium (Figure 4). Depending on the content of the cele, a meningocele, meningoencephalocele, or meningohydroencephalocele develops. When one or more vertebrae are affected, a meningocele or meningomyelocele is formed. The term 'spina bifida' is often used for all different types of spinal defects and does not regard the specific etiology.

The ultrasonographic diagnosis in the first trimester of exencephaly can be made through the presence of free floating neural tissue in the head region and the absence of normal calvarium. Often the eyes have a bulging, frog-like appearance[18]. The spine is discernable with transvaginal ultrasonography from week 7 of gestation onwards as two parallel lines[1]. Early in pregnancy, abnormal closure of the caudal neuropore may be suspected if a widening of the parallel lines of the spine is observed. This may be obvious even before the ossification process of the vertebrae is completed. Calvarium and spine are completely ossified after week 12 of gestation resulting in the typical echogenic aspect of skull and vertebrae. Consequently, the detection with ultrasonography of a bony defect in either calvarium or vertebrae is only possible after week 12 of gestation[19].

Lateral ventricles in the normal first trimester fetus take a large part of the cranial vault contents and are almost completely filled with the prominent echogenic oval shaped choroid plexus. Hydrocephalus, often associated with spinal defects, can be diagnosed early in pregnancy through a changed aspect of the choroid plexus[20]. First trimester diagnosis of hydrocephalus is not so much based on the size and shape of the lateral ventricles, but relies more on a change in the aspect of the choroid plexus. In case of early development of hydrocephalus, the choroid plexus shrinks and dangles free in the posterior part of the lateral ventricles (Figure 5). Vibrations of an abnormal choroid plexus may be provoked when the patient's abdomen is tapped with the investigator's free hand.

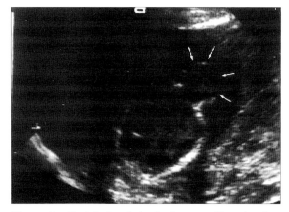

Figure 4 *Occipital cephalocele shown at 13 weeks of gestation*

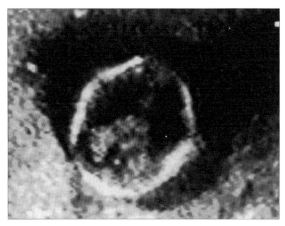

Figure 5 *Caput in the fourteenth week of pregnancy showing hydrocephalus and lemon sign*

ABDOMINAL WALL

The embryo folds in week 5 of gestation, forming head and tail folds. Through folding of the sides of the embryo towards the midline, the so-called 'lateral folds', a roughly cylindrical embryo is formed. In this process, part of the yolk sac is incorporated into the embryo as the midgut. The connection of midgut with yolk sac is reduced to a narrow yolk stalk and adjacent umbilical cord. At the beginning of week 8 of gestation the rapidly growing midgut herniates into the umbilical cord, because there is not enough room in the abdominal cavity. The relatively massive liver and kidneys are responsible mainly for this shortage of space. This normal migration of the midgut is called physiological umbilical herniation. During week 10 and 11 of gestation, the loops of the bowel return rapidly into the abdomen. As the intestines return in the fetal abdomen, they undergo a counter-clockwise rotation that gives the bowel its normal intra-abdominal orientation[6]. The embryologic process of physiological midgut herniation can be visualized with high frequency ultrasound[21,22] (Figure 6). After 12 weeks of gestation no physiologic umbilical herniation is seen in normal developing fetuses.

Omphalocele is a midline defect in the abdominal wall that results after failure of the lateral folds to fuse, or persistence of the body stalk, occurring once in every 5000 births[23]. The protruding mass, usually part of the liver and small bowel, is covered with peritoneum and amnion. In 75%, associated anomalies are present, and in approximately 40–50%, aneuploidy is detected[24]. Differentiation between omphalocele and physiologic umbilical hernia is not always possible, therefore it is suggested that abdominal wall defects should not be diagnosed with ultrasonography, prior to 12 weeks of gestation[21]. However, if the herniated sac contains fetal liver, besides the echogenic loops of the bowel, the diagnosis of omphalocele can be made earlier than 12 weeks of gestation[25,26]. Omphalocele is also likely if the diameter of the herniated mass is equal to or exceeds the abdominal circumference diameter[26] (Figure 7).

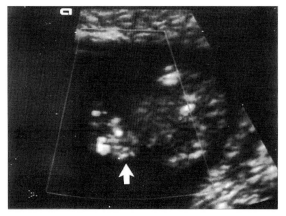

Figure 6 *Physiologic midgut herniation in the tenth week of pregnancy*

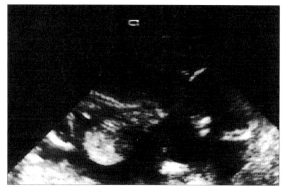

Figure 7 *Omphalocele in a euploid fetus of 14 weeks' gestation*

URINARY TRACT

Three overlapping kidney systems are formed in early prenatal life, the pronephros, the mesonephros and the metanephros or permanent kidney. The metanephric mesoderm provides the excretory units of the kidneys. The ureteric bud, an outgrowth of the mesonephric duct, gives rise to the collecting system[6]. Connection between the collecting and excretory tubule systems is essential for normal development. Failure to connect may cause congenital cystic disease and renal agenesis. The fetal urinary bladder is formed partially from a division of the cloaca, the primitive urogenital sinus, and secondly from the caudal portions of the mesonephric ducts. Production of fetal urine starts at the end of the first trimester.

The fetal kidneys have reached their adult shape and position by 10–12 weeks of gestation. With high frequency transvaginal probes, the fetal kidneys can be demonstrated in the first trimester as hyperechogenic masses on both sides of the fetal spine[27]. Fetal bladder filling can be observed from week 10 onwards[5]. Failure to demonstrate the fetal urinary bladder during an examination of 30 min or longer is highly suspect for urinary tract pathology[28]. In case of low urinary tract obstruction, the fetal bladder is identified as a large cystic mass occupying the whole fetal abdomen[29]. Oligohydramnios is a uniform finding with bladder outlet obstruction, renal agenesis and dysplastic renal non-functioning. Oligohydramnios, though, seldom develops early in pregnancy. Usually it is not present before 16 weeks of gestation. With early diagnosis of urethral stenosis or renal non-function syndrome, amniotic fluid volume can be normal and only decreases gradually after week 14 of pregnancy[29,30]. Abnormal kidney formation such as multicystic dysplastic kidneys can be demonstrated early in pregnancy. The mainly unilateral kidney appears as a cystic mass, with cysts of different size. Infantile polycystic kidneys can be diagnosed through the bilateral appearance of homogeneous echogenic kidneys[31]. The multiple cysts are small and may be difficult to distinguish. Fetal bladder filling cannot be visualized in case of non-functional poly-

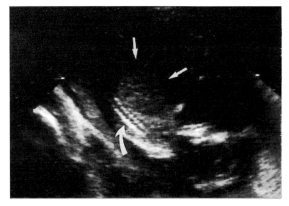

Figure 8 *Polycystic kidney in a fetus with Meckel–Gruber syndrome*

cystic kidneys. Polycystic kidneys may be part of the autosomal recessive Meckel–Gruber syndrome, which consists of the triad polycystic kidneys, polydactyly and occipital cephalocele (Figure 8).

Other malformations of the urinary system such as hydronephrosis or pyelectasis can also be diagnosed in the first trimester. Hydronephrosis is identified if the renal pelvis measures more than 3 mm in week 13 of pregnancy[13]. It can be present unilaterally or on both sides. Hydronephrosis may be a transient observation in normal developing fetuses, disappearing before week 16 of gestation, but it can also be a (transient) marker for chromosomal abnormalities especially trisomy 21[32,33].

CARDIOVASCULAR SYSTEM

The cardiovascular system originates from the mesodermal germ layer as two separate tubes. Initially, the cardiogenic area is located anterior to the neural plate. The central nervous system grows rapidly in the cephalic direction so that the cardiogenic plate is pulled forward and rotated 180°. The two lateral heart tubes come closer to each other and fuse. The heart tube continues to elongate and begins to bend. This bending creates the cardiac loop. With transvaginal ultrasonography it is possible to visualize the four chamber view from weeks 11 and 12, onwards[5,34,35]. The features of a normal four chamber view include the following[36]:

(1) The heart occupies about one-third of the fetal thorax;

(2) There are two atria of approximately equal size;

(3) There are two ventricles of approximately equal size and thickness; and

(4) The two atrioventricular valves meet the atrial and ventricular septa at the crux or center of the heart.

Approximately 80% of cardiac abnormalities can be detected through an abnormal four chamber view[36]. Evaluation of the outflow tract should also be a part of the detection of congenital heart defects[37,38]. Anomalies of the heart detected before the sixteenth week of gestation and described in the literature are ventricular septal defect in combination with tetralogy of Fallot[38-40], complete atroventricular canal defect[41], hypoplastic left ventricle, single ventricle and overriding aorta[37]. The incidence of cardiac anomalies is 3-9 per 1000 live births and almost 50% of these affected fetuses have associated anomalies or have an abnormal karyotype[36].

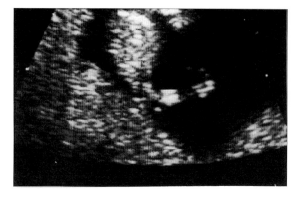

Figure 9 Hand as detected at 12 weeks of pregnancy

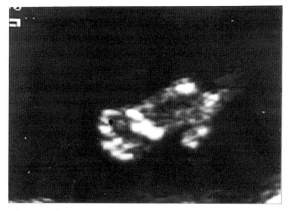

Figure 10 Foot as detected at 12 weeks of pregnancy

SKELETAL SYSTEM

The limb buds become visible as outpocketing of the ventrolateral body wall at the beginning of the seventh week of gestation. The hind limbs are 2 days behind in development in comparison with the fore limbs. At 8 weeks, the hand and foot plates become separated. Ossification centers in the long bones become visible at the end of the tenth week. With transvaginal ultrasonography, the limb buds can be seen in week 7 of pregnancy. Distinct digits are delineated at 11 weeks of gestation[1] (Figure 9 and 10). Normal growth of the fetal skeleton has been studied and measurements of the long bones are available from 12 weeks onwards[42]. It is possible to detect skeletal dysplasia early in pregnancy especially if a patient is at risk for a known skeletal dysplasia with a recurrence risk of 25% or 50% in case of autosomal recessive or dominant disorders, respectively[3,43-46]. Other abnormalities of upper and lower limbs i.e. polydactyly and club foot, detected before the sixteenth week of pregnancy, have also been described[4,5,47].

CONCLUSION

Transvaginal ultrasound scanning of the fetus in the first trimester of pregnancy should be considered in case of a family or obstetric history of fetal structural abnormalities with an elevated recurrence risk, in case of maternal use of medication early in pregnancy and in case of vaginal blood loss.

References

1. Rottem, S., Bronshtein, M., Thaler, J. and Brandes, J. M. (1989). First trimester transvaginal sonographic diagnosis of fetal anomalies. *Lancet* (letter), **1**, 444–5
2. Benacerraf, B. R., Lister, J. E. and DuPonte, B. L. (1988). First trimester diagnosis of fetal abnormalities. A report of three cases. *J. Reprod. Med.*, **33**, 777–80
3. Cullen, M. T., Green, J., Whetham, J., Salafia, C., Gabrielli, S. and Hobbins, J. (1990). Transvaginal ultrasonographic detection of congenital anomalies in the first trimester. *Am. J. Obstet. Gynecol.*, **163**, 466–76
4. Rottem, S. and Bronshtein, M. (1990). Transvaginal sonographic diagnosis of congenital anomalies between 9 weeks and 16 weeks, menstrual age. *J. Clin. Ultrasound*, **18**, 307–14
5. Timor-Tritsch, I. E., Farine, D. and Rosen, M. G. (1988). A close look at early embryonic development with the high-frequency transvaginal transducer. *Am. J. Obstet. Gynecol.*, **159**, 676–81
6. Moore, K. L. (1982). *The Developing Human*, pp. 339–41 (New York: WB Saunders)
7. Chervenak, F. A., Isaacson, G., Blakemore, K. J., Greg, R., Hobbins, J., Berkowitz, R. L., Tortoras, M., Mayden, K. and Mahoney, M. J. (1983). Fetal cystic hygroma. Cause and natural history. *N. Engl. J. Med.*, **309**, 822–5
8. Van Zalen-Sprock, M. M., van Vugt, J. M. G. and van Geijn, H. P. (1992). Cephalocele and cystic hygroma: diagnosis and differentiation in the first trimester of pregnancy with transvaginal sonography. Report of two cases. *Ultrasound Obstet. Gynecol.*, **2**, 289–92
9. Cullen, M. T., Gabrielli, S., Green, J., Rizzo, N., Mahoney, M. J., Salafia, C., Bovicelli, L. and Hobbins, J. C. (1990). Diagnosis and significance of cystic hygroma in the first trimester. *Prenatal Diagnosis*, **10**, 643–51
10. Exalto, N., van Zalen-Sprock, M. M. and van Brandenburg, W. J. A. (1985). Early prenatal diagnosis of cystic hygroma by real time ultrsound. *J. Clin. Ultrasound*, **13**, 655–8
11. Van Zalen-Sprock, M. M., van Vugt, J. M. G. and van Geijn, H. P. (1992). First trimester diagnosis of cystic hygroma, course and outcome. *Am. J. Obstet. Gynecol.*, **167**, 94–8
12. Nicolaides, K. H., Azar, G., Byrne, D., Mansur, C. and Marks, K. (1992). Fetal nuchal translucency: ultrasound screening for chromosomal defects in first trimester of pregnancy. *Br. Med. J.*, **304**, 867–9
13. Van Zalen-Sprock, M. M., van Vugt, J. M. G. and Van Geijn, H. P. (1992). Non-echogenic nuchal oedema as a marker in trisomy 21 screening. *Lancet* (letter), **339**, 1480–1
14. Sadler, T. W. (1990). Central nervous system. In *Langman's Medical Embryology*, pp. 352–89. (Baltimore: Williams & Wilkins)
15. Lemire, R. J. (1988). Neural tube defects. Review. *J. Am. Med. Assoc.*, **259**, 558–62
16. Kennedy, K. A., Flick, K. J. and Thurmond, A. S. (1990). First trimester diagnosis of exencephaly. *Am. J. Obstet. Gynecol.*, **162**, 461–3
17. Hendricks, S. K., Cyr, D. A., Nyberg, D. A., Raabe, R. and Mack, L. A. (1988). Exencephaly – clinical and ultrasonic correlation to anencephaly. *Obstet. Gynecol.*, **72**, 898–900
18. Achiron, R. and Achiron, A. (1991). Transvaginal ultrasonic assessment of the early fetal brain. *Ultrasound Obstet. Gynecol.*, **1**, 336–44
19. Goldstein, R. B., Filly, R. A. and Callen, P. W. (1989). Sonography of anencephaly: pitfalls in early diagnosis. *J. Clin. Ultrasound*, **17**, 397–402
20. Bronshtein, M. and Ben-Shlomo, I. B. (1991). Choroid plexus dysmorphism detected by transvaginal sonography: the earliest sign of fetal hydrocephalus. *J. Clin. Ultrasound*, **19**, 547–53
21. Cyr, D. R., Mack, L. A., Schoenecker, S. A., Patten, R. M., Shepard, T. H., Shuman, W. P. and Moss, A. A. (1986). Bowel migration in the normal fetus: US detection. *Radiology*, **161**, 119–21
22. Timor-Tritsch, I. E., Warren, W. B., Peisner, D. B. and Pirrone, E. (1989). First trimester midgut herniation: a high-frequency transvaginal study. *Am. J. Obstet. Gynecol.*, **161**, 831–3
23. De Vries, P. A. (1980). The pathogenesis of gastroschisis and omphalocele. *J. Ped. Surgery*, **15**, 245–51
24. Van de Geijn, E. J., van Vugt, J. M. G., Sollie, J. E. and van Geijn, H. P. (1991). Ultrasonographic diagnosis and perinatal management of fetal abdominal wall defects. *Fetal Diagn. Ther.*, **6**, 2–10
25. Brown, D. L. Emerson, D. S., Shulman, L. P. and Carson, S. A. (1989). Sonographic diagnosis of omphalocele during 10th week of gestation. *Am. J. Roentgenol.*, **153**, 825–6
26. Curtis, J. A. and Watson, L. (1988). Sonographic diagnosis of omphalocele in the first trimester of fetal gestation. *J. Ultrasound Med.*, **7**, 97–100
27. Bronshtein, M., Kushner, O., Ben-Rafael, Z., Shalev, E., Nebel, L., Mashiach, S. and Shalev, J. (1990). Transvaginal sonographic measurements of fetal kidneys in the first trimester of pregnancy. *J. Clin. Ultrasound*, **18**, 299–301
28. Bronshtein, M., Bar-Hava, I. and Blumenfeld, Z. (1993). Differential diagnosis of the non-visualized fetal urinary bladder by transvaginal sono-

graphy in the early second trimester. *Obstet. Gynecol.*, **82**, 490–3
29. Bronshtein, M., Yoffe, N., Brandes, J. M. and Blumenfeld, Z. (1990). First and early second-trimester diagnosis of fetal urinary tract anomalies using transvaginal sonography. *Prenatal Diagnosis*, **10**, 653–66
30. Stiller, R. J. (1989). Early ultrasonic appearance of fetal bladder outlet obstruction. *Am. J. Obstet. Gynecol.*, **160**, 584–5
31. Mahoney, B. S., Callen, P. W., Filly, R. A. and Golbus, M. S. (1984). Progression of infantile polycystic kidney disease in early pregnancy. *J. Ultrasound Med.*, **3**, 277–9
32. Bronshtein, M. and Blumenfeld, Z. (1992). Transvaginal sonography; detection of findings suggestive of fetal chromosomal anomalies in the first and early second trimesters. *Prenatal Diagnosis*, **12**, 587–93
33. Benacerraf, B. R., Mandell, J., Estroff, J. A., Harlow, B. L. and Frigoletto, F. D. (1990). Fetal pyelectasis: a possible association with Down syndrome. *Obstet. Gynecol.*, **76**, 58–60
34. Dolkart, L. A. and Reimers, F. T. (1991). Transvaginal fetal echocardiography in early pregnancy: normative data. *Am. J. Obstet. Gynecol.*, **165**, 688–91
35. Johnson, P., Sharland, G. and Allan, L. (1992). The role of transvaginal sonography in the early detection of congenital heart disease. *Ultrasound Obstet. Gynecol.*, **2**, 248–51
36. Allan, L. D., Crawford, D. C., Chita, S. K. and Tynan, M. J. (1986). Prenatal screening for congenital heart disease. *Br. Med. J.*, **292**, 1717–19
37. Bronshtein, M., Zimmer, E. Z., Milo, S., Ho, S. Y., Lorber, A. and Gerlis, L. M. (1991). Fetal cardiac abnormalities detected by transvaginal sonography at 12–16 weeks' gestation. *Obstet. Gynecol.*, **78**, 374–8
38. Bronshtein, M., Zimmer, E. Z., Berlis, L. M., Lorber, A. and Drugan, A. (1993). Early ultrasound diagnosis of fetal congenital heart defect in high-risk and low-risk pregnancies. *Obstet. Gynecol.*, **82**, 225–9
39. Bronshtein, M., Siegler, E., Yoffe, N. and Zimmer, E. Z. (1990). Prenatal diagnosis of ventricular septal defect and overriding aorta at 14 weeks' gestation, using transvaginal sonography. *Prenatal Diagnosis*, **10**, 697–702
40. DeVore, G. R., Steiger, R. M. and Larson, E. J. (1987). Fetal echocardiography: the prenatal diagnosis of a ventricular septal defect in a 14 week fetus with pulmonary artery hypoplasia. *Obstet. Gynecol.*, **69**, 494–8
41. Gembruch, U., Knöpfle, G., Chatterjee, M., Bald, R. and Hansmann, M. (1990). First trimester diagnosis of fetal congenital heart disease by transvaginal two-dimensional and Doppler echocardiography. *Obstet. Gynecol.*, **75**, 496–8
42. Brons, J. T. J., van der Harten, J. J., Wladimiroff, J. W., van Geijn, H. P., Dijkstra, P. F., Exalto, N., Reuss, A., Niermeijer, M. F., Meijer, C. J. L. M. and Arts, N. F. Th. (1988). Prenatal ultrasonographic diagnosis of osteogenesis imperfecta. *Am. J. Obstet. Gynecol.*, **159**, 176–81
43. Brons, J. T. J., van Geijn, H. P., Bezemer, P. D., Nauta, J. P. J. and Arts, N. F. Th. (1990). The fetal skeleton: ultrasonographic evaluation of the normal growth. *Eur. J. Obstet. Gynecol. Reprod. Biol.*, **34**, 21–36
44. Soothill, P. W., Vuthiwong, C. and Rees, H. (1993). Achondrogenesis type 2 diagnosed by transvaginal ultrasound at 12 weeks' gestation. *Prenatal Diagnosis*, **13**, 523–8
45. Bronshtein, M. and Weiner, Z. (1992). Anencephaly in a fetus with osteogenesis imperfecta: early diagnosis by transvaginal sonography. *Prenatal Diagnosis*, **12**, 831–4
46. Graham, D., Tracey, J., Winn, K., Corson, V. and Sanders, R. C. (1983). Early second trimester sonographic diagnosis of achondrogenesis. *J. Clin. Ultrasound*, **17**, 336–8
47. Bronshtein, M., Keret, D., Deutsch, M., Liberson, A. and Bar Chava, I. (1993). Transvaginal sonographic detection of skeletal anomalies in the first and early second trimester. *Prenatal Diagnosis*, **13**, 597–601

Three-dimensional ultrasound in obstetrics and gynecology

12

D. Jurković, E. Jauniaux and S. Campbell

Ultrasound imaging plays a dominant role in the modern management of many gynecological and obstetric problems. Continuous improvements in the quality of imaging and the introduction of new techniques such as transvaginal sonography and color Doppler have resulted in the further expansion of ultrasound diagnosis in recent years. Although some have predicted that ultrasound technology has already reached its theoretical limits[1], the recent introduction of three-dimensional ultrasonography may lead to the development of entirely new clinical applications.

TECHNIQUE OF THREE-DIMENSIONAL ULTRASONOGRAPHY

There are many ways of acquiring information necessary for three-dimensional imaging. At present, the most advanced systems use specially designed mechanical transducers that perform a co-ordinated sequence of parallel cross-sectional scans. This is achieved by a slow rotation of the scan head perpendicular to the scanning plane. A large number of two-dimensional images are thus stored as a volume in the machine's computer memory in an organized way, which permits three-dimensional reconstruction of an organ or area of interest. However, technical details of these calculations are beyond the scope of this chapter and those interested are advised to consult the specialized literature[2-4].

To obtain three-dimensional information, a conventional two-dimensional scan is first performed. This helps to identify an area of interest and an estimation of the size of the volume which needs to be analyzed. The volume size and shape depend on the design of the probe and may be modified depending on the size and position of the area of interest. Small organs such as the ovaries can be easily analyzed, while maximal volumes are usually required for successful analysis of larger structures such as the fetal head or limbs.

Although larger volumes provide more information, more time is necessary for their acquisition, which increases the number of artefacts caused by patients' movements and in particular by fetal body and breathing movements. This reduces the quality of stored information and may decrease the accuracy of reconstruction. It usually takes around 5 s to complete the storage of a volume of average size. During that time the operator holds the probe steadily while the rotation of the scanning head is automatically controlled.

The stored information can be analyzed in two ways. The analysis of planar reformatted sections is similar to the images produced by conventional two-dimensional scanning. However, scanning is performed by using the position controls on the key-board instead of the ultrasound probe. A typical display is shown in Figure 1. Three perpendicular planes are simultaneously displayed, thus enabling easier understanding of anatomical relations within the organ. The number and orientation of reformatted planes are not limited, thus providing additional information not seen during the initial two-dimensional scan.

Three-dimensional reconstruction of stored images (surface and volume rendering) is the other possible method of re-examining the stored ultrasound volumes. Additional computer work stations are usually required to complete this part of the examination. The

THE FETUS AS A PATIENT

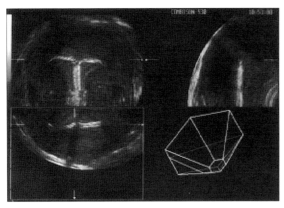

Figure 1 Three-dimensional display of the uterine anatomy. A Nova-T intrauterine contraceptive device is shown in great detail

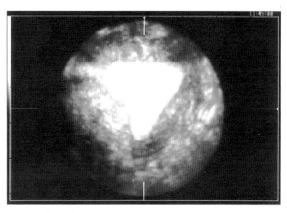

Figure 3 The internal structure of the uterus as seen on three-dimensional reconstruction using the transparency mode. (Courtesy of Kretztechnik, Austria)

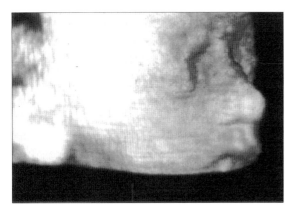

Figure 2 Fetal facial features at 20 weeks obtained by three-dimensional surface reconstruction. (Courtesy of Kretztechnik, Austria)

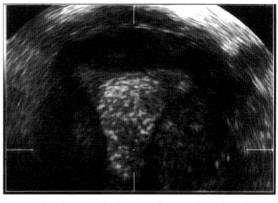

Figure 4 A coronal planar reformatted section through the uterus showing details of the uterine cavity that are not normally seen on a transvaginal scan

structure of interest is first identified and manually delineated, followed by an automatic process of echo extraction. In this way, the surface of the organ of interest is displayed in three dimensions (Figure 2). This enables a detailed morphological analysis of structures such as fetal face or tumor surface tissue. A transparency mode is another way of showing ultrasound images in three dimensions. In this mode, only the strongest and lowest signals are displayed, so that the internal structure of the organ of interest can be analyzed (Figure 3).

Once the examination is completed, all information can be permanently stored on computer disks and re-examined later. However, an average volume requires 4 to 8 MB of memory, which is available only on removable hard-disk cartridges such as SyQuest® 88 MB.

CLINICAL APPLICATIONS

Scanning using planar reformatted sections

Three-dimensional technology offers an entirely new approach to the analysis of ultrasound images which may improve diagnostic accuracy in the future. Ultrasound volumes stored in the machine's memory may be re-examined by using scan planes which are normally not obtainable by conventional scanning. This is particularly important when the transvaginal probe is used. Although the ultrasound resolution is superior when high-frequency transvaginal probes are used, the narrow vagina greatly reduces the number of available scanning planes. The major problem is an inability to obtain the transverse section through the pelvis that is accepted by many as particularly useful for the assessment of the uterus. Although this plane lies perpendicular to the ultrasound beam, it can be easily reconstructed from the stored volumes as shown in Figure 4. The uterine cavity can thus be analyzed in great detail, including the intramural parts of the Fallopian tubes. This should help the diagnosis of congenital uterine anomalies as well as the diagnosis of interstitial ectopic pregnancy[5], which is rare and dangerous.

Planar reformatted sections may be even more useful for the examination of fetal anatomy. Sagittal sections of the fetal head, which are usually particularly difficult to obtain, are easily obtained by using three-dimensional equipment (Figure 5). This should help the diagnosis of facial defects such as micrognathia or nasal hypoplasia, which are useful morphological markers of chromosomal anomalies[6].

Recently, Hong-Chang and colleagues[7] have described the value of planar reformatted sections for the examination of the fetal heart. In their experience, it was easy to perform a complete assessment of cardiac anatomy, including the four-chamber view as well as several long-axis views of the great vessels. This may simplify detection of fetal cardiac defects and reduce the time necessary for the diagnosis of complex congenital defects. However, cardiac movements may interfere with the quality of reconstruction and it remains to be seen to what extent this may affect diagnostic accuracy.

Volume measurements

Volume measurements are particularly useful in gynecology. Ovarian volume is routinely measured on a pelvic scan, facilitating the diagnosis of polycystic ovaries and early ovarian cancer. The volume of the pre-ovulatory follicle is also often calculated before follicular puncture for *in vitro* fertilization. This is usually done

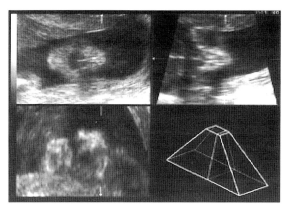

Figure 5 *A display of the fetal facial anatomy on three perpendicular sections. The fetal profile was obtained in the sagittal section (lower left image)*

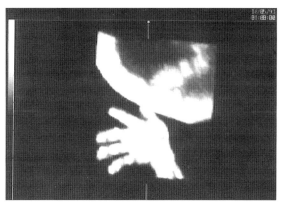

Figure 6 *A three-dimensional reconstruction showing the fetal hand at 20 weeks. (Courtesy of Kretztechnik, Austria)*

by measuring maximum diameters in three orthogonal planes. The volume is then calculated by using mathematical formulas for a sphere or ovoid[8]. Although this method is reasonably accurate when organs are of regular shape, it cannot be used in other circumstances.

By using planar reformatted sections, it is possible to obtain volume measurements regardless of the shape of the structure under investigation. The organ boundaries are marked on a number of consecutive parallel scans. Once the whole length of the organ of interest is included, the volume is calculated automatically. Lin and associates[9] have recently reported a good correlation between follicular volume estimated in this way and the actual amount of fluid aspirated at puncture.

The size of the primary tumor is an important prognostic parameter in patients with vulval or cervical cancer and this correlates well with the local and distant tumor spread. In cases of tumors involving deeper pelvic structures such as endometrial cancer, an accurate preoperative estimation of tumor size is not possible. However, three-dimensional equipment overcomes this problem and may help the decision about the extent of the surgical procedure.

The measurement of the abdominal circumference at the level of the fetal liver is used routinely for the assessment of fetal growth. An abnormally low circumference is usually caused by the depletion of liver glycogen stores in fetuses with hypoxic intrauterine growth retardation. The measurement of the liver volume itself, rather than the abdominal circumference, may enable earlier detection of the hypoxic fetus and help in differential diagnosis of other causes of abnormal growth. Measurement of the placental volume, which could not be accurately measured before, may also be useful in this group of patients.

The diagnostic value of three-dimensional reconstruction

A three-dimensional image of the fetal surface may improve the ultrasound diagnosis of various congenital malformations. Although many fetal anomalies can be reliably diagnosed by using conventional scanning, the diagnosis of minor defects and the assessment of a fetus with complex anomalies require particular expertise. By using three-dimensional imaging, the diagnosis of defects such as cleft lip or nasal abnormalities becomes obvious even to the least experienced operator. Positional limb defects, talipes, rocker-bottom feet or overlapping fingers can also be accurately demonstrated (Figure 6).

The ability to visualize fetal surfaces in three dimensions may help the diagnosis of a greater number of fetal anomalies in the first trimester of pregnancy. Because of the small size of the embryo and the complexity of developmental anatomy in early pregnancy, very few defects are diagnosed before 10 weeks' gestation. Clear three-dimensional reconstructions of embryos as early as 8 weeks, which can be magnified several times, enable the demonstration of anatomical details such as limbs or face, which cannot normally be seen with two-dimensional equipment (Figure 5).

Three-dimensional reconstruction could play a particularly important role in the diagnosis of cardiac defects. At present, suspected cardiac defects are examined by specially trained echocardiographers in tertiary centers. Using the transparency mode, intracardiac anatomy can be demonstrated and assessed by a pathologist or cardiologist with no particular scanning expertise. Although the heart is not a static organ, our initial experience shows that good-quality cardiac images can be obtained at 20 weeks' gestation.

Reconstructed images may play an important role in the assessment of early endometrial carcinoma. Three-dimensional reconstruction should demonstrate intramyometrial spread more accurately, and also help to demonstrate multiple foci of invasion. The assessment of patients with benign intrauterine pathology, such as submucous fibroids or intrauterine synechiae, could also be improved. In patients with intrauterine contraceptive devices, the type of device and its accurate location inside the uterus can be easily demonstrated. The potential advantages in cases of congenital uterine anomalies has already been discussed.

The impact on the organization of the scanning unit, training, quality control and referrals

The quality of ultrasound diagnosis depends primarily on the skill and experience of the operator. In most cases, the final diagnosis can only be reached by the person actually performing the scan. The examination of recorded findings on photographs and videotapes is rarely helpful. This considerably increases the responsibility of ultrasonographers, who have to achieve a very high standard of examination. In unusual cases, a long time is required to complete the examination and patients may be asked to return for an examination by other more experienced operators. Often the final diagnosis cannot be reached and the patients are referred to distant centers with particular expertise in diagnosis of fetal malformations. This can cause considerable inconvenience to the patients and aggravate the distress caused by abnormal ultrasound findings. Appointment schedules in a busy ultrasound unit are also often affected by the lengthy scans, and long delays are not uncommon. By using three-dimensional equipment, some of these problems can be solved for the first time.

Volume information stored on hard-disk cartridges contains all the important diagnostic information, which can be re-examined by independent observer. By using planar reformatted sections, a full examination of the organ of interest can be performed and the diagnosis checked without the patient being present in the scanning room. The benefits of this facility in terms of patient convenience and the more effective organization of work in the ultrasound unit are obvious. In the future, the examination of hard disks with stored volumes should enable an expert to reach a final diagnosis in most cases and offer appropriate advice without the need to see the patient. Furthermore, three-dimensional information can be transferred by telephone optic cables to obtain instant advice from centres of expertise.

The training of new ultrasonographers can start by the examination of stored volume scans rather than '*in vivo*' sessions on patients who require competent diagnosis. The principles of scanning by using planar reformatted sections are nearly the same as during routine two-dimensional scanning and basic skills can be developed without affecting the quality of patients' care. In those patients with abnormal or uncertain findings, the stored volumes can be examined later by the most experienced ultrasonographer in the unit. This will be of particular benefit to patients in whom the unusual appearances of normal anatomical features are cause for concern.

The ability of the examiner to store and examine an ultrasound volume later can significantly shorten a patient's examination time. A transvaginal scan can be completed and stored on the hard disk within 2–3 min. A scan for a fetal anomaly, which requires around 30 min of the ultrasonographer's time, can be completed in less than a few minutes with detailed analysis and measurement performed later. This can significantly increase the cost-effectiveness of the ultrasound equipment and increase the overall effectiveness of the ultrasound unit.

We have recently completed a study which has investigated the reproducibility and diagnostic accuracy of planar reformatted sections in comparison with the findings on two-dimensional scans. A very good correlation was found between uterine and ovarian size as well as a concordance in the final ultrasound diagnosis in all cases. We believe that the stored volumes are of sufficient quality to permit their use for diagnostic purposes in a clinical setting.

CONCLUSION

Three-dimensional ultrasound may significantly improve both the diagnostic accuracy and organization of ultrasound scanning in the future. We believe that this new technique will soon be accepted as a standard for routine ultrasound examination, as is real-time B-mode scanning today.

References

1. Kossoff, G. (1984). Prospects for ultrasound in tumour diagnosis. In Kossoff, G. and Fukuda, M. (eds.) *Ultrasonic Differential Diagnosis of Tumours*, pp. 283–93. (New York: Igaku-Shoin)
2. Baba, K., Satch, K., Sakamoto, S., Okai, Y. and Shiego, I. (1989). Development of an ultrasonic system for three dimensional reconstruction of the fetus. *J. Perinat. Med.*, 17, 19–24
3. Halliwell, M., Key, H., Jenkins, D., Jackson, P. C. and Wells, P. N. T. (1989). New scans from old: digital reformatting of ultrasound images. *Br. J. Radiol.*, 62, 824–9

4. King, D. L., King, D. L. and Shao, M. Y. (1990). Three-dimensional spatial registration and interactive display of position and orientation of real-time ultrasound images. *J. Ultrasound Med.*, **9**, 525–32
5. Feichtinger, W. (1993). Transvaginal three-dimensional imaging. *Ultrasound Obstet. Gynaecol.*, **3**, 375–8
6. Nicolaides, K., Shawwa, L., Brizot, M. and Snijders, R. (1993). Ultrasonographically detectable markers of fetal chromosomal defects. *Ultrasound Obstet. Gynaecol.*, **3**, 56–69
7. Kuo, H. C., Chang, F. M., Wu, C. H., Yao, B. L. and Liu, C. H. (1992). The primary application of three-dimensional ultrasonography in obstetrics. *Am. J. Obstet. Gynecol.*, **166**, 880–6
8. Sample, W. F., Lippe, B. M. and Gyepes, M. T. (1977). Grey scale ultrasonography of the normal female pelvis. *Radiology*, **125**, 477
9. Lin, M. T., Chen, G. D., Lin, L. Y. and Lee, M. S. (1991). Measurements of follicle size and the volume of follicular fluid by 3-dimensional ultrasound scanning compared with aspirated findings in IVF programs. *J. Obstet. Gynaecol. ROC*, **30**, 47–9

Sonoembryology in the central nervous system

H. Takeuchi

The explosive progress of transvaginal ultrasound has recently enabled us to obtain anatomical images of even the small embryo or fetus in the uterus of early pregnancy. As a result, the new clinical field, which was termed 'sonoembryology', was established. The feasibility of more detailed visualizing of the embryo in the process of development or the fetus which is about to develop is extremely useful for the general understanding of development, and the early detection of anomaly.

The central nervous system (CNS), mainly occupying the head, which is a comparatively simple anatomical structure, is the easiest part of the fetus for sonographic depiction. In terms of the embryo or fetus of early pregnancy, the ratio of the head to the whole body is as large as one-half to one-third. Accordingly, the central nervous system occupies the main part of the morphological observations of fetal development. In addition, anomalies in the CNS, due to their high incidence, should be recommended for antenatal diagnosis.

Brain anomalies, frequently occurring with cystic changes, can be clearly depicted by ultrasound and therefore early detection should be expected. For early detection of CNS anomalies, knowledge of the sonoembryology of the normal CNS is of paramount importance.

This paper describes the results of a study of the sonoembryology of the CNS using transvaginal ultrasound.

MATERIALS AND METHODS

Pregnant women who had no complications with regular menstrual cycles of 25 to 33 days, and with an uneventful course of pregnancy, who finally delivered an appropriate for date baby at term, were included in this study.

An assessment of gestational weeks was obtained from measurement of the crown–rump length (CRL) at the time of exploration, and compared with weeks of amenorrhea. If the difference was within 3 days, the latter was adopted. When the difference was more than 3 days, gestational weeks by CRL were applied.

Among over 300 cases in which transvaginal ultrasound was performed in the first trimester, 120 cases fulfilled the above prerequisites, with gestational ages of 6 weeks and 0 days to 12 weeks and 6 days, and were chosen for the study.

As diagnostic equipment, Mochida Sonovista CS and SLC with an exclusive transvaginal probe were used. The frequencies of 5, 6 and 7.5 MHz were available. The images obtained by 7.5 MHz were used in this study.

The head and spine of the embryo and fetus were depicted through three sectional views, namely the sagittal, transverse and coronal views, by conventional transvaginal methods. All the three sectional images could not always be successfully obtained. Only the good images were adopted.

RESULTS

In the observations, the following structures were investigated: the neural tube, brain vesicle, forebrain (prosencephalon), midbrain (mesencephalon), hindbrain (rhombencephalon), diencephalon, telencephalon, lateral ventricle, third ventricle, fourth ventricle, falx cerebri, choroid plexus, brainstem, thalamus, cerebellum, cysterna magna, spinal cord and skull. The results of the visualization and observation of the CNS of the embryo or fetus in each gestational week are as follows.

Six weeks of gestation (3–6 mm CRL)

In this gestational week, the heart beat was observed. Except for confirmation of the heart, no other anatomical structures of the embryonic organs were discernible. The shape of the embryo itself was, up to 6 mm of CRL, only like a 'stick' adjacent to the yolk sac. The cranial side and the caudal side were most difficult to differentiate. When the CRL attained 7 mm, the whole embryo in sagittal section was visualized as a triangular shape (Figure 1). Each side of the triangle was considered to be as follows: the outer line from the forehead to the back of the head; the line from the back of the head through the back region to the tail; and the line from the forehead through the abdomen to the tail.

Seven weeks of gestation (10–16 mm CRL)

When the CRL attained 10 mm, an echo-free space, which was though to be the brain vesicle, was initially detected in the intracranial area. As shown in Figure 2, in sagittal section, a small cystic part had appeared at the edge of the cranial area, and in transverse section, as shown in Figure 3, a cystic structure was similarly observed.

When this size of embryo was observed further in coronal section, two parallel linear echoes could be depicted in the back (Figure 4). Judging from the location and morphology of the echoes, this image was considered to be the neural tube. This could be confirmed by imaging these echoes, like 'double parentheses', when visualizing these parallel lines in transverse section (Figure 3).

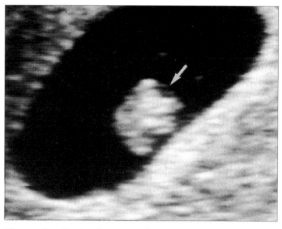

Figure 2 *Sagittal sectional view of an embryo with crown–rump length of 10 mm, at 7 weeks and 1 day of amenorrhea. A small cystic structure, which is considered to be the pontine flexure (arrow), is seen at the cephalic pole of the embryonic configuration*

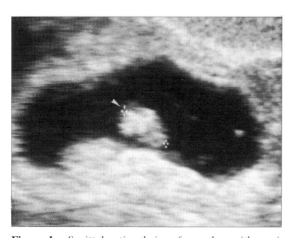

Figure 1 *Sagittal sectional view of an embryo with maximum length of 7 mm at 6 weeks and 4 days of amenorrhea. Rhomboid outline of the embryo is delineated, but no configuration of organs or anatomical structures is seen. Arrowhead indicates cephalic pole*

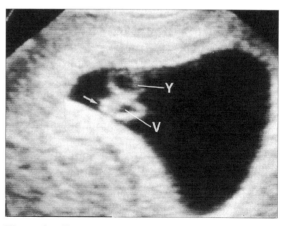

Figure 3 *Transverse sectional view at the cephalic pole of an embryo of 10 mm crown–rump length, at 7 weeks and 1 day of amenorrhea. A simple cystic structure (V), which is considered to be a part of the forebrain and midbrain, is visualized at the rostral portion. The echoes, like double parentheses (arrow), considered to be the neural tube, are seen at the dorsal portion. Y, yolk sac*

Eight weeks of gestation (17–24 mm CRL)

The head occupied one-third of the body length. The echo-free space within the head had become larger. In sagittal section or in parasagittal section, it represented a curved and twisted tubular structure, as shown in Figure 5. The morphology of the tubular structure was recognized as the developed brain vesicle itself. By using the well-depicted sagittal section image, it was possible to identify every part of what had already become the ventricle. Namely, when observing from the most rostral portion, as shown in Figure 5, a serial structure was discernible, comprising prosencephalon (lateral ventricle), third ventricle, mid-ventricle and fourth ventricle. Being a tubular structure, these could be delineated as almost one chamber in transverse section (Figure 6) or in coronal section (Figure 7).

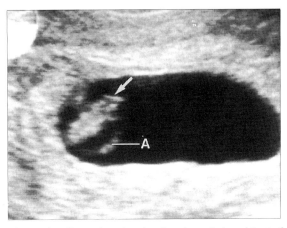

Figure 4 Coronal sectional view through dorsal part of an embryo with crown–rump length of 11 mm, at 7 weeks and 2 days of amenorrhea. Two parallel linear echoes from the neural tube are seen. Arrow indicates cephalic pole. A, amnion

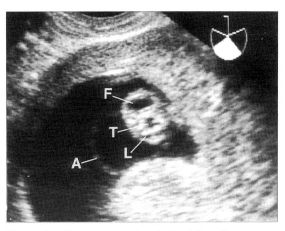

Figure 6 Transverse section obtained from the same embryo as shown in Figure 5. The curved tubular structure, when sectioned by one plane, produces two or three cystic parts. A, amnion; F, fourth ventricle, L, lateral ventricle; T, third ventricle

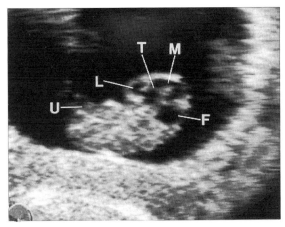

Figure 5 Sagittal sectional view of an embryo with crown–rump length of 20 mm, at 8 weeks and 3 days of amenorrhea. In the head space, a twisted and curved tubular structure is depicted. This structure shows, rostrally to caudally, the lateral ventricle (L), third ventricle (T), midbrain ventricle (M) and fourth ventricle (F) of the brain. U, umbilical cord

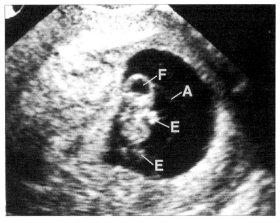

Figure 7 Coronal sectional view through dorsal part of an embryo of 21 mm crown–rump length, at 8 weeks and 3 days of amenorrhea. A cystic structure occupies almost the whole area of the head, and is considered to be the fourth ventricle. A, amnion; E, limb bud; F, fourth ventricle

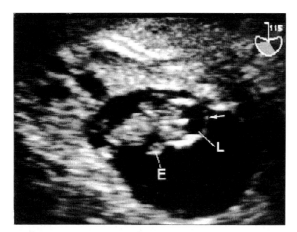

Figure 8 *Coronal sectional view of an embryo of 19 mm crown–rump length, at 8 weeks and 4 days of amenorrhea. The cystic part of the forebrain is divided into two by a thin membraneous echo (arrow) at the center, showing the development of the falx cerebri. E, limb bud; L, lateral ventricle*

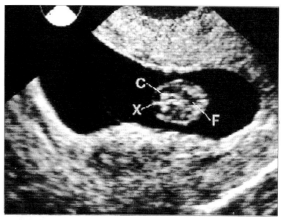

Figure 10 *Transverse sectional view of the same embryo as shown in Figure 9. In this transverse section of the head, the following are visualized: the lateral ventricles divided by the falx cerebri, the comma-shaped choroid plexuses within the lateral ventricles, a sonolucent space of the fourth ventricle and the skull echo. C, choroid plexus; F, fourth ventricle; X, flax cerebri*

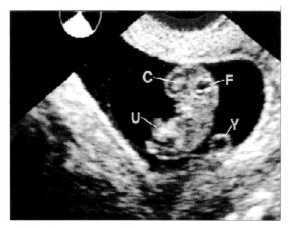

Figure 9 *Sagittal sectional view of an embryo with crown–rump length of 25 mm, at 9 weeks and 1 day of amenorrhea. At the most rostral portion of the head, an expanded lateral ventricle with choroid plexus is clearly shown. The third and midbrain ventricles cannot be delineated in this sectional view. The size of the fourth ventricle is about to diminish. C, choroid plexus; F, fourth ventricle; U, umbilical cord; Y, yolk sac*

At the end of 8 weeks of gestation, when the CRL had attained 20 mm, as shown in Figure 8, it could sometimes be seen that the middle of the forebrain, which had now grown large, was divided into two by a thin membranous structure, the development of the falx cerebri. Subsequently, the lateral ventricle could be specifically identified. The morphology of the brainstem was not discernible.

The fourth ventricle remained unclear. Two parallel lines which indicated the spine could be observed in coronal section, but the spinal cord could not be visualized within it.

9–10 weeks of gestation (25–30 mm CRL, 8–16 mm biparietal diameter)

When the CRL attained 25 mm, the first characteristic embryonic intracranial manifestation was the disappearance of a serial structure which had existed in the ventricle before. In consequence, the following were noted: the appearance of the falx cerebri, the separation and expansion of the lateral ventricle, the appearance of the choroid plexus within the lateral ventricle, the disappearance of the third ventricle and mid-brain ventricle, and the isolation of the fourth ventricle. Although the change within the lateral ventricle was already recognizable from the end of the 8th week of gestation, as described above, the change now became more definite. In the sagittal section of Figure 9, the choroid plexus in the lateral ventricle and the fourth ventricle at the occipital region could be distinctly depicted. In the same case, in transverse sectional view (Figure 10), the morphology of the falx cerebri, lateral ventricle, choroid plexus and fourth ventricle were perfectly delineated. Observation of a further transverse sectional view of the caudal portion revealed a structure which seemed to be the brainstem (Figure 11). In a transverse sectional view, a dotted echo from the cerebellum at both sides of the lateral ventricle wall could occasionally be visualized, as shown in Figure 12.

Another characteristic of the head image of 9 weeks of gestation was the feasibility of obtaining a skull echo. The correct recognition of the skull was possible, especially when observing in transverse section. Within the spine, the spinal cord initially became discernible.

Ten weeks of gestation was the period at which the intracranial structure became increasingly distinct. The mineralization of bone progressed especially and, as shown in Figure 13, the maxilla and mandible were also recognized.

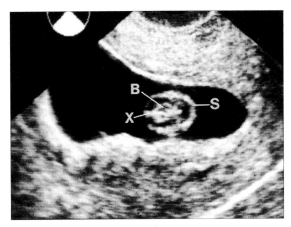

Figure 11 *Transverse sectional view at a plane slightly caudal to that of Figure 10. At the center of the intracranial space, the structure of the brainstem with falx cerebri can be visualized. B, brainstem; S, skull; X, falx cerebri*

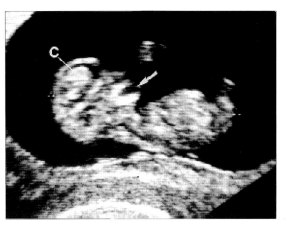

Figure 13 *Sagittal section of a fetus with crown–rump length of 35 mm, at 10 weeks and 1 day of gestation. In the head region, a clear profile of the face with maxilla and mandible can be recognized. Arrow indicates the mouth. C, choroid plexus*

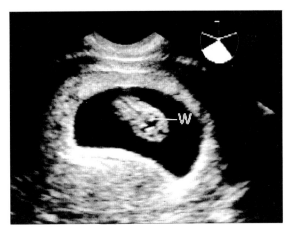

Figure 12 *Transverse section obliquely through fourth ventricle of an embryo of 24 mm crown–rump length at 9 weeks and 2 days of amenorrhea. This section was selected for delineation of the cerebellum (W). At both sides of the fourth ventricle wall, small dotted echoes, obtained from separate parts of the cerebellum, are seen*

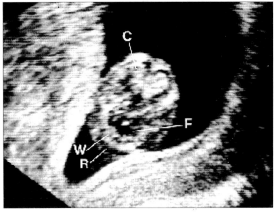

Figure 14 *Transverse section of the head of a fetus with crown–rump length of 40 mm, at 11 weeks and 3 days of gestation. Rostrally to caudally, the section shows the lateral ventricles filled with choroid plexuses (C), the space of the fourth ventricle (F), a 'dumb-bell'-shaped cerebellum (W) and the sonolucent space of the cisterna magna (R)*

11–12 weeks of gestation (40–56 mm CRL, 17–25 mm biparietal diameter)

The development and growth of each intracranial structure facilitated the clear recognition of their sonographic appearance. The initial depiction of the outline of the cerebellum was the first characteristic of this gestational week. Figure 14 shows the so-called 'dumb-bell'-shaped cerebellum delineated in transverse sectional view. An almost coronal section of the head in the same case enabled visualization from the morphologically completed brainstem through the spinal cord, as shown in Figure 15.

The nearly completed structures of the CNS were successfully delineated in a coronal section through the occipital region of the same case (Figure 16). It was not until this gestational week that most of the anatomical structures of the CNS, mainly of the intracranial region, could be discerned.

From 6 weeks of gestation, the initial depiction of anatomical structures of the CNS was possible. By 12 weeks of gestation, almost all of the CNS structures were completed. The time that each structure could be depicted was investigated. Every case did not show the same struc-

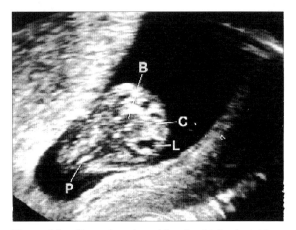

Figure 15 Coronal section obliquely obtained at plane slightly caudal to that of Figure 14. This section through the brainstem and spine shows the linear echo from the spinal cord. B, brainstem; C, choroid plexus; L, lateral ventricle; P, spinal cord

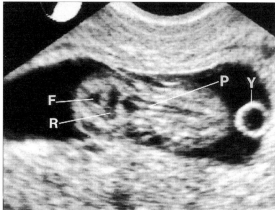

Figure 16 Coronal section view through dorsal portion of the same fetus as shown in Figures 14 and 15. Cranially to caudally, the sonolucent space of the fourth ventricle and cisterna magna, as well as the linear echo of the spinal cord are delineated. F, fourth ventricle; P, spinal cord; R, cisterna magna; Y, yolk sac

Table 1 Delineation of structures of the central nervous system in early gestation: sagittal section (125 cases). CRL, crown–rump length

	Week of gestation						
	6 (CRL 3–9 mm) (n = 20)	7 (CRL 10–16 mm) (n = 24)	8 (CRL 17–24 mm) (n = 24)	9 (CRL 25–31 mm) (n = 21)	10 (CRL 32–39 mm) (n = 16)	11 (CRL 40–47 mm) (n = 9)	12 (CRL 48–56 mm) (n = 11)
Brain vesicle (single space)	2	18	6				
Brain vesicle (bent)		6	18	6			
Fourth ventricle (isolated)			4	15	15		
Lateral ventricle			2	15	16	9	11
Thalamus					3	4	8
Spine				3	16	9	11
Spinal cord				5	8	8	8
Cranial calcification				10	16	9	11

Table 2 Delineation of structures of the central nervous system in early gestation: coronal and transverse sections (95 cases). CRL, crown–rump length

	Week of gestation						
	6 (CRL 3–9 mm) (n = 14)	7 (CRL 10–16 mm) (n = 15)	8 (CRL 17–24 mm) (n = 20)	9 (CRL 25–31 mm) (n = 18)	10 (CRL 32–39 mm) (n = 8)	11 (CRL 40–47 mm) (n = 9)	12 (CRL 48–56 mm) (n = 11)
Brain vesicle (single space)		13	10				
Fourth ventricle (isolated)			6	10	8	8	8
Lateral ventricle			6	14	8	9	11
Thalamus				4	2	3	8
Cerebellum ('dumb-bell' shape)						3	5
Neural tube	1	9	8				
Spine				10	6	9	11
Spinal cord				1	2	7	8
Cranial calcification				9	8	9	11

tures in every section. In terms of each anatomical structure, the time of visualization differed with the choice of section. Therefore, the sagittal section and the transverse or coronal sections were studied separately. The results are shown in Tables 1 and 2.

The possibility of visualization of the CNS depended on the location of the embryo or fetus. Therefore, the increase of the gestational week did not always facilitate better visualization. Table 3 shows the gestational week when each anatomical structure was almost definitely visualized.

CLASSIFICATION OF STAGES OF CENTRAL NERVOUS SYSTEM DEVELOPMENT

It was found that the time of sonographic appearance of anatomical structures differed according to development and growth of each. This indicates that sonographic features of anatomical structures differ with every gestational week. From 6 weeks to 12 weeks of gestation, it was considered that the sonographic findings of anatomical structures could be classified into five stages, as follows:

Stage 0 No visualized CNS structure (corresponded to 6 weeks of gestation, less than 9 mm CRL);

Table 3 Anatomical structures of the central nervous system and the week of gestation of their initial sonographic depiction

	Sectional view	
	Sagittal	Coronal/transverse
Brain vesicle (single space)	7	7
Brain vesicle (bent)	8	—
Fourth ventricle (isolated)	8–9	8–9
Lateral ventricle	9–10	9–10
Thalamus	11	9–12
Cerebellum ('dumb-bell' shape)	—	11–12
Neural tube	—	7–8
Spine	10	11
Spinal cord	10	10–11
Cranial calcification	9	9

Stage 1 Visualization of single brain vesicle and neural tube (corresponded to 7 weeks of gestation, 10–16 mm CRL);

Stage 2 Depiction and differentiation of prosencephalon, mesencephalon and rhombencephalon (corresponded to 8 weeks of gestation, 17–24 mm CRL);

Stage 3 Formation of brain hemispheres by falx cerebri and lateral ventricles with choroid plexus. Visualization of calvarium (corresponded to 9 weeks of gestation, 25–32 mm CRL);

Stage 4 Depiction of fused cerebellum and spinal cord; completion of intracranial structures (corresponded to 11 weeks of gestation, more than 40 mm CRL).

DISCUSSION

In terms of the young embryo, the CNS is relatively huge and occupies anatomically large spaces. Therefore, the use of high-frequency transvaginal ultrasound has enabled us to observe the process of early development of the brain.

The development of the CNS starts from 18 to 20 postconceptual days, when embryonic surface ectoderm differentiates into the neural plate[1–3]. Although this is the first visible indication of the human nervous system, even the whole configuration of the embryo, which is less than 3 mm in length, cannot be visualized echographically. Four to five days later, the folding of the neural plate forms the neural tube, which differentiates into the CNS, consisting of the brain and spinal cord[3]. Continuation of the fusion rostrally and caudally leaves both ends of the neural tube with a temporary opening, which is called the neuropore. The rostral neuropore closes in about 24 days (5 weeks and 3 days of gestation), and the caudal neuropore closes about two days later[2,3]. This closure of the rostral neuropore results in the formation of three primary brain vesicles, from which the brain develops.

During the fifth week of gestation, three primary brain vesicles form: the forebrain (prosencephalon), the midbrain (mesencephalon) and the hindbrain (rhombencephalon). During the sixth week of gestation, the forebrain partly divides into two vesicles – the telencephalon and the diencephalon – and the hindbrain partly divides into the metencephalon and the myelencephalon[2]. As a result, there are five secondary brain vesicles in the head of the embryo. However, these embryological structures are still undiscernible by ultrasound. From the viewpoint of sonoembryology of the CNS, 6 weeks of gestation is the period when the configuration of the embryo is discernible, whereas the anatomical morphology of the CNS, which has already developed, cannot be seen.

The brain grows rapidly and bends ventrally with the formation of the midbrain flexure in the mesencephalon region and the cervical flexure at the junction of the rhombencephalon and the spinal cord. Furthermore, between these flexures, unequal growth in the hindbrain produces the pontine flexure in the opposite direction in the middle of the 6th week of gestation[1]. This flexure results in thinning of the roof of the rhombencephalon, and produces the fluid content of the fourth ventricle. At the end of 6 weeks of gestation, on account of their enlargement, the sonographic features of the brain vesicles are first available.

Sagittal sections of the embryo at 9 to 10 mm CRL, from 6 weeks and 6 days to 7 weeks and 1 day of gestation, showed a small echo-free space at the top of the cephalic pole. This space is considered to be consistent with that of the pontine flexure. In a transverse section obtained from almost the same size of embryo, a simple hypoechoic vesicle, which was consistent with the mesencephalic and telencephalic vesicles, could be visualized at the rostral portion. These vesicles were the first images of the brain structures delineated by ultrasound. Achiron and Achiron[4] found that, between 7 and 8 menstrual weeks, the forebrain appeared as a hypoechoic vesicle below the calvarial roof, and they showed an image of the hypoechoic vesicle of an embryo with 7.3 mm biparietal diameter at 8 weeks and 1 day of gestation. Although no image was shown, Timor-Tritsch and colleagues[1] reported that the telencephalic vesicle and mesencephalic vesicle were seen during 7 weeks and 0–6 days of gestation. Our results show that by using high-frequency transvaginal ultrasound, the first anatomical structure of the brain can be depicted from an embryo of around 10 mm CRL at as early as 6 weeks and 6 days of gestation.

As the author[2] has already described, the neural tube could be successfully depicted as parallel lines in coronal section, and as double parentheses in transverse section, at as early as 6 weeks and 6 days of gestation. Timor-Tritsch and associates[1] also observed the neural tube in the coronal plane at 6 weeks of gestation. Seven weeks of gestation is the important period when in every section, sagittal, transverse and coronal, parts of the anatomical structures of the CNS are first visualized by the ultrasound image.

Rostrally, the neural tube becomes bent in three regions:

(1) At the mesencephalon, the mesencephalic flexure;

(2) At the junction of the brain and spinal cord, a slight curve, the cervical flexure; and

(3) Ventrally, the convex pontine flexure in the rhombencephalon.

By 8 weeks of gestation, these concavities of three brain vesicles result in the production of a W-shaped convoluted arrangement of the vesicular space in sagittal view. The most rostral portion of the vesicle divides into two parts, the telencephalon (lateral ventricle) and diencephalon (third ventricle). The very thin membrane-like falx cerebri, between both sides of the lateral ventricle, can be delineated in coronal section at the end of 8 weeks of gestation.

Another characteristic of the ultrasound image of the embryo at 8 weeks of gestation is the observation of the enlarged brain vesicle or ventricle as a considerably larger sonolucent space in coronal section. Its best example is the fourth ventricle, which entirely occupies the intracranial space visualized in coronal section through the occipital region. Eight weeks of gestation is the time that almost all the brain vesicles, which have developed with complicated bending, can be observed. It is the time that accurate confirmation of the development of the CNS is more available sonographically than at 7 weeks of gestation.

The cerebral hemispheres develop from the telencephalon at 6 to 7 weeks of gestation[1]. As the cerebral hemispheres expand, the lateral ventricles increase rapidly in size, and they cover successively the diencephalon, midbrain and hindbrain. The two hemispheres meet in the midline, forming the falx cerebri. Concurrently, choroid plexuses develop in the medial wall of the lateral ventricle at 8 weeks and 5 to 6 days of gestation[1]. Therefore, in the ultrasound image of 9 weeks of gestation, the lateral ventricles become distinct along with the depiction of the choroid plexus. Four choroid plexuses develop in each lateral ventricle, the third ventricle and the fourth ventricle, at the end of 8 weeks of gestation. Among them, those in the lateral ventricles are discernible for the first time in the echogram from the middle of the 9th week of gestation. They soon grow enough to fill the cavity of the lateral ventricles. The falx cerebri, lateral ventricles and choroid plexus are the structures that can definitely be depicted in the 9-week embryo. In particular, the choroid plexus within the lateral ventricle is considered to be the distinct sonographic marker of this age.

The thalamus develops in the superior portion of the diencephalon as early as 5 weeks and 1 to 2 days of gestation[1]. It is subdivided into a dorsal and a ventral part. As a main portion of the thalamus, the dorsal thalamus grows rapidly from each side of the third ventricle, and fuses in the midline during the 9th week of gestation[1]. In the transverse sectional image obtained at 9 weeks of gestation, the thalamus was occasionally seen, as described by the author[3] and Timor-Tritsch and co-workers[2]. The skull becomes definitely recognizable from this stage of the embryo, due to increasing mineralization. As a result, 9 weeks of gestation is the significant period when a part of the basic structures of the CNS, about to develop, can first be confirmed.

From 10 weeks of gestation, the fetal period begins. All the major organs of the body have already developed during the preceding embryonic period. Therefore, development during the fetal period is thought to be the growth of organs. Regarding ultrasound visualization of the CNS, completion of its basic structures can be confirmed at 11 weeks of gestation. The cerebellum and spinal cord are examples of the organs that are first confirmed in their typical morphology by ultrasound at 11 weeks of gestation.

The cerebellum develops bilaterally from thickening of the dorsal parts of the alar plates during 6 weeks of gestation[2,3]. Initially, the cerebellar swellings (rhombic lips) project partly into the fourth ventricle. These swellings at both sides of the fourth ventricle can be seen in the coronal section of the embryo at 9 weeks of gestation. The cerebellum then bulges externally. Rapid bulging of the rhombic lips and deepening of the pontine flexure result in fusion of the rhombic lips to the ventral portion of the alar plates. Eventually, fusion in the midline forms the dumb-bell-shaped cerebellum[2]. This could be successfully delineated for the first time in the transverse section of the 11-week fetus.

The neural tube, caudal to the fourth pair of somites, develops into the spinal cord[3]. From 7 weeks of gestation, the neural tube itself is discernible by ultrasound. Chondrification of the vertebral column begins at 6 weeks of gestation, and ossification of the vertebrae is detectable at about 11 weeks of gestation[3]. Meanwhile, leaving the central canal, the alar laminae become the dorsal horn, and the basal laminae become the ventral horn, and form the spinal cord. A fine linear echo which seems to be this central canal can be observed continuously from the brain stem to the spine first at 9 weeks of gestation. At 11 weeks, the linear echo is clearly apparent.

After 12 weeks of gestation, it is needless to mention that the depiction of each organ of the CNS becomes easier, because of its enlargement. As a result, when observing the development of the CNS by using high-frequency transvaginal ultrasound, it was found that the appearance of the basic structures was discernible from stage to stage during 6–11 weeks of gestation. Therefore, the confirmation of the normal development of the CNS and the detection of anomalies are now possible from very early in gestation. To perform sonographic examinations correctly, detailed knowledge of the CNS at each stage is required. The author would like to propose that the developmental process of the CNS discerned by ultrasound should be classified into five stages, from stage 0 to stage 4.

References

1. Timor-Tritsch, I. E., Monteagudo, A. and Warren, W. B. (1991). Transvaginal ultrasonographic definition of the central nervous system in the first and early second trimesters. *Am. J. Obstet. Gynecol.*, **164**, 497–503
2. Takeuchi, H. (1992). Sonoembryology. In Kurjak, A. (ed.) *An Atlas of Ultrasonography in Obstetrics and Gynecology*, pp. 17–26. (Carnforth, UK: Parthenon Publishing)
3. England, M. A. (1988). Normal development of the central nervous system. In Levene, M., Bennett, M. and Punt, J. (eds.) *Fetal and Neonatal Neurology and Neurosurgery*, pp. 3–27. (Edinburgh: Churchil Livingstone)
4. Achiron, R. and Achiron, A. (1991). Transvaginal ultrasonic assessment of the early fetal brain. *Ultrasound Obstet. Gyencol.*, **1**, 336–44
5. Moor, K. L. (1988). *The Developing Human*, 4th edn., pp. 379–90. (Philadelphia: W. B. Saunders)
6. O'Rahilly, R. and Müller, F. (1992). *Human Embryology and Teratology*, pp. 261–78. (New York: Willey–Liss)

The multifetal pregnancy: sonographic determination of chorionicity and amnionicity in the first and early-second trimesters

14

A. Monteagudo and I. E. Timor-Tritsch

INTRODUCTION

In the United States, approximately 1–1.5% of all live births are multiple[1,2]. Of all types of multiple births, twins are the most prevalent. There are two types of twins: fraternal or dizygotic twins, which result from multiple ovulation, and identical or monozygotic twins, which are the result of cleavage of a single fertilized ovum. The incidence of spontaneous twin pregnancies in the United States is about 1 : 80 pregnancies[1]. If zygosity is taken into consideration when assessing the incidence of twins, the prevalence of the two types of twins is different. The incidence of monozygotic twinning is constant throughout the world, with a frequency of 3.5–4.0/1000 conceptions, and this accounts for approximately 30% of all twins. In contrast, the incidence of dizygotic twinning ranges from 4–50/1000 conceptions, and is influenced by factors such as maternal age, parity, family history and ethnicity. Dizygotic twinning accounts for approximately 70% of all twins[1,3]. Spontaneously occurring pregnancies of high order are quite rare, but their incidence can be roughly calculated by using Hellin's hypothesis, which states that if the frequency of twins is n, then the frequency of triplets is n^2 and quadruplets n^3, etc. In the United States, the reported incidence of pregnancies of higher order are for triplets, 1/7925 pregnancies; for quadruplets, 1/5370 to 1/600 000 pregnancies; for quintuplets, 1/15–20 million deliveries[1].

With the increased use of ovulation-induction agents and assisted reproductive techniques over the past 30 years the number of multifetal pregnancies has risen dramatically. This has become especially true over the past decade. Between 1978 and 1988, the incidence of triplets and higher-order multiple pregnancies has increased by 101%[5]. In 1981, Schenker and associates[6] reviewed the data on multiple pregnancies induced by ovulation induction and found that, following the administration of human menopausal gonadotropins (hMG), the reported incidence ranged from 18 to 53.5%, and after clomiphene administration, the incidence ranged between 6 and 8%, with most multifetal pregnancies being twins. The incidence of multifetal pregnancies after *in vitro* fertilization and embryo transfer (IVF/ET) was dependent upon the number of embryos placed back in the uterine cavity; therefore, the greater the number of embryos transferred, the greater the chances of having a multifetal pregnancy. The overall incidence of multiple pregnancies was approximately 22%[7]. When three embryos were transferred, the reported incidence of multiple pregnancies was about 33%, with 25% being twins and 8.3% triplets[8].

The main objective of this chapter is to enhance and simplify the diagnostic process of the different types of twins by using transvaginal sonography (TVS) in the first and early second trimester. This information not only can be applied to twin pregnancies, but also can be extrapolated to pregnancies of higher order. Although the emphasis of this chapter is on the diagnosis of chorionicity and amnionicity using

TVS, an attempt has also been made to review some of the major problems encountered in multiple pregnancies.

TWINNING: REVIEW OF EMBRYOLOGY

There are two types of placentas encountered in twin pregnancies: the *dichorionic* and the *monochorionic*. Dizygotic twins have dichorionic placentas, but monozygotic twins can have either a dichorionic or a monochorionic placenta. All twins with dichorionic placentas are diamniotic, but the monochorionic twins can either be diamniotic or monoamniotic, depending upon when during development the zygote divided. In approximately 30% of monozygotic twins, division occurs within the first three days after fertilization. This pre-implantation division results in the formation of two blastocysts, the end result of which is a dichorionic–diamniotic placenta. In 70% of monozygotic twins, division of the zygote occurs post-implantation, usually between days 4 to 8 and before the development of the amniotic cavity. The end result of this division is a monochorionic–diamniotic placenta. If the zygote divides between days 8 to 13, after the amniotic cavity has developed, a monochorionic–monoamniotic placenta will result. If the zygote divides between days 13 and 16, this late division will result in conjoined twins (Figure 1)[1,9]. These events are summarized in Table 1.

SCANNING THE MULTIFETAL PREGNANCY

Mapping the pregnancy

When using TVS, multifetal pregnancies can be diagnosed as early as 5–6 weeks' gestation. Careful mapping of the multifetal pregnancy is necessary, especially in those cases in which more than three fetuses are present, or in those twin pregnancies in which chorionic villus sampling or amniocentesis will be performed. When more than three fetuses are present, the uterus should be carefully scanned in the sagittal and coronal planes. The location of each fetus within the uterus should be described in both planes. In the sagittal plane, as per obstetrical convention, the fetus closest to the cervix will be A, and the next closest B, etc. In addition, fetuses can be described as anterior or posterior, depending upon the wall of the uterus to which they are closest. In the coronal plane, they can be further assigned as right or left. Therefore, each particular fetus has a very specific set of coordinates that can consistently be used to locate it.

ASSESSING CHORIONICITY AND AMNIONICITY

Determining chorionicity and amnionicity of a multifetal pregnancy is very important, because multifetal pregnancies are associated with an

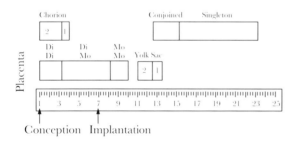

Figure 1 *Timing of the different types of cleavage that can occur in monozygotic twins. Adapted from reference 1. Di, dichorionic; Mo, monochorionic*

Table 1 *Summary of the embryology of monozygotic twinning. Note implantation occurs between days 6 and 7*

Timing of cleavage (days from ovulation)	Number of fetuses	Type of placenta	Number of amniotic sacs	Number of yolk sacs
1–3	2	dichorionic	2	2
4–8	2	monochorionic	2	2
8–10	2	monochorionic	1	2
13–16	conjoined	monochorionic	1	1

MULTIFETAL PREGNANCY: CHORIONICITY AND AMNIONICITY

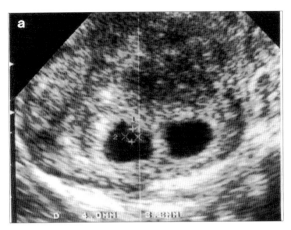 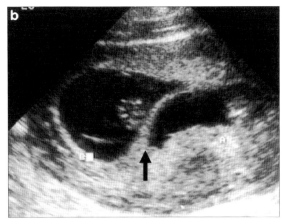

Figure 2 Dichorionic–diamniotic twin pregnancy. (a), Both chorionic sacs are seen at 6 weeks' gestation. In the left gestational sac, the yolk sac is seen and measured; (b), follow-up scan at 9 weeks' gestation demonstrates the 'thick' intertwin membrane. The arrow points to the 'lambda' or 'twin peak' sign

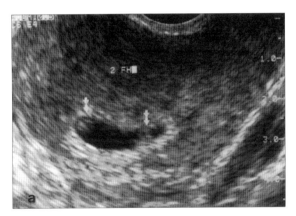 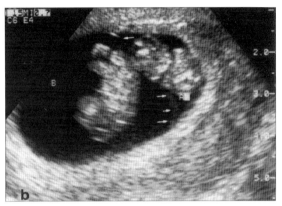

Figure 3 Monochorionic–diamniotic twin pregnancy. (a), Single chorionic sac containing both embryos (arrows point to the embryos). 2FH, two fetal hearts seen under real-time sonography; (b), follow-up scan at 9 weeks' gestation demonstrates both fetuses and the 'thin' intertwin membrane. Arrows point to the amniotic membranes

increased incidence of complications, such as preterm labor and delivery, placental complications, growth retardation, and malformations. In addition, monochorionic pregnancies are at increased risk of malformations and complications, including twin–twin transfusion syndrome, cord entanglement and conjoined twins.

The first trimester

By 5 weeks' gestation, the number of gestational sacs present can be accurately assessed using TVS[10]. The TVS appearance of the 5 weeks' multifetal pregnancy is rather simple. They are composed of round sonolucent structures (gestational sacs) surrounded by a bright echogenic rim of tissue, the chorion. Therefore, the chorionicity of the multifetal pregnancy is established as early as 5 weeks' gestation. Unfortunately, the determination of the number of fetuses has to wait until the 6th week of gestation, when the onset of the fetal cardiac activity first becomes apparent (Figures 2a, 3a). Although by 5.5 weeks' gestation the yolk sacs can be imaged and counted using the number of yolk sacs alone, it can be misleading to assess the number of fetuses at this time. This is because at times, the cleavage occurs late, just before the formation of conjoined twins; therefore only one yolk sac may be present in the presence of twins. If only one fetus is seen within each gestational sac, the pregnancy must be dichorionic (or trichorionic, etc. depending on the number of chorionic sacs present) (Figures 2, 4, 5). If two live fetuses are seen within the same chorionic sac, amnionicity cannot be reliably determined until 8 weeks (Figure 3a). However, using TVS, the earliest identification of the amnion is at 6–6.5 weeks' gestation. At this early gestational age, the amnion snugly surrounds the fetus and the amniotic cavity contains a small amount of amniotic fluid. Therefore, clear identification of it may be quite difficult until 7.5–8 weeks' gestation. At this time, the amnion separates from the fetal body and becomes quite easy to image (Figure 5)[11–13]. The sonographic appearance of a monochorionic–diamniotic pregnancy is a single sonolucent chorionic sac, which contains both amniotic sacs, within which the fetuses are found (Figures 3b, 6a). In a monochorionic–monoamniotic pregnancy, there is a single chorionic and amniotic sac

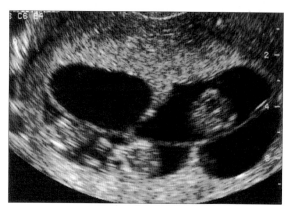

Figure 4 *Quadruplet pregnancy at 9.5 weeks' gestation demonstrating a quadrochorionic–quadroamniotic pregnancy*

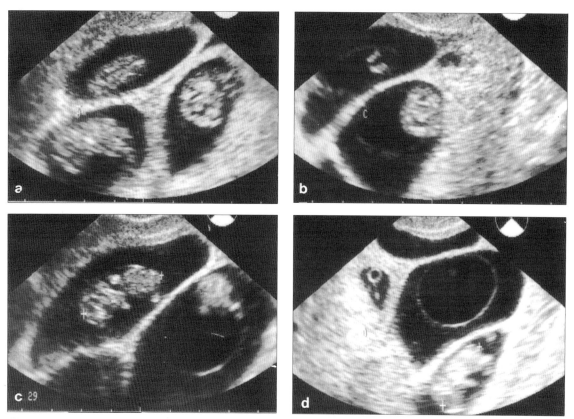

Figure 5 *Sextuplet pregnancy at 9 weeks 6 days of gestation. (a), Three of the six chorionic sacs each containing a single fetus; (b) and (c), amniotic sacs containing the fetuses clearly seen within the extraembryonic space; (d), round sonolucent amniotic sac contained within the extraembryonic space, which contains low-level echoes*

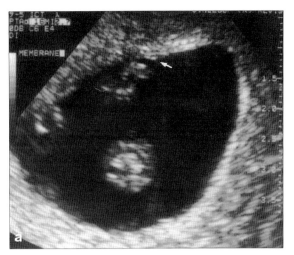 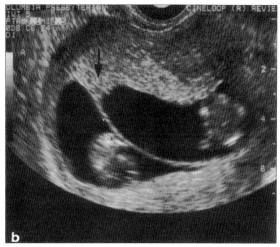

Figure 6 Two different twin gestations at 9 weeks. (a), Monochorionic–diamniotic twin pregnancy. The 'intertwin' membrane is thin and the junction between the fused amnions and the chorion is T-shaped (arrow); (b), dichorionic–diamniotic twin pregnancy. The 'intertwin' membrane is thick and the 'lambda' or 'twin peak' sign (arrow) is evident

containing both fetuses[10]. In multifetal pregnancies of high order, the sequential appearance of the embryonic structures holds true and their multichorionicity and amnionicity can be assessed (Figures 4, 5, 7).

The second trimester and beyond

Determining chorionicity and amnionicity beyond 14 weeks' gestation at times can be quite challenging, but by using the following guidelines a reasonable degree of accuracy can be achieved.

1. Counting the number of placentas

Careful evaluation of the uterus may show one or two placentas, but commonly two separate placentas may be fused, giving the false impression of only a single placenta[14].

2. Determining if each fetus is within its own amniotic sac

This is extremely important, because classically monochorionic–monoamniotic twins are associated with up to a 50% perinatal mortality for both twins. More recently, Tessen and colleagues[15] reported an overall survival rate of 70% and a survival rate for both twins of 65%.

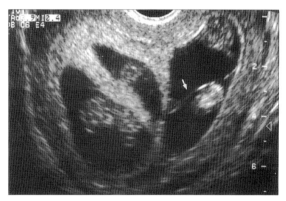

Figure 7 Quadruplet pregnancy at 9 weeks' gestation, demonstrating a trichorionic–quadramniotic pregnancy. Arrow points to the fused amniotic membranes of this monochorionic twin pair

3. Describing the appearance of the dividing membranes

The separating membranes can appear to be thick or thin. However, this is an extremely relative notion and depends upon comparisons at different gestational ages as well as the experience of the observer. In dizygotic twins, the opposing membranes are always thick, because each membrane is composed of four layers. These thick membranes are formed by each twin's chorion in addition to the amnion. Thick membranes measuring 2 mm or more are 95% predictive of dichorionic twins[16]. On the other hand, monozygotic twins may have both thick and thin dividing membranes, depending upon the type of placenta that is present (monochorionic vs. dichorionic). The thin dividing membranes are composed of two layers of amniotic membrane. These membranes are difficult to measure and are usually described as 'hair-like' or 'too thin to measure'[17–20]. In addition, the number of layers of the membranes can be counted. A two-layer intertwin membrane is consistent with monochorionic–diamniotic and a four layer intertwin membrane is suggestive of a dichorionic–diamniotic pregnancy[21].

4. *Looking for the presence of a triangular projection of placental tissue beyond the chorionic surface*

Bessis and Papiernik[22] called this projection (Figure 6b) the 'lambda sign' and they were able correctly to predict 20 out of 24 dichorionic pregnancies. Kurtz and colleagues[23] found the 'lambda sign' to be present only in six out of 85 dichorionic–diamniotic twin pregnancies. Finberg[24] made a similar observation and referred to it as the 'twin peak sign', and was able to predict the multichorionicity in 15 twins and five triplet pregnancies scanned between 14 and 35 weeks' gestation. The presence of the 'lambda' or 'twin peak sign' is a reliable indicator that the pregnancy is dichorionic, but its absence does not rule out the presence of dichorionicity[10].

5. *Determining the sex of the twins*

If the fetuses are of different sex, dizygotic twinning can be assured, but if the fetuses are of the same sex, zygosity may not be determined until after birth.

COMPLICATIONS OF MULTIFETAL PREGNANCIES

Vanishing twin syndrome

Vanishing twin syndrome refers to the phenomenon in which one member of the twin pair is lost. Usually the loss is very early and can only be detected if a timely sonogram is performed. Approximately 20% of twin pregnancies diagnosed by ultrasound are lost during the first trimester, resulting in a singleton pregnancy[25,26].

Growth discrepancy

Growth discrepancy complicates approximately 12–47% of twin pregnancies[27]. A 15–25% weight difference between twins raises the suspicion of growth discrepancy. A weight discrepancy of 25% or more is considered significant. An abdominal circumference difference of ≥ 20 mm between the twins is suggestive of growth discrepancy. Discrepancy of the biparietal diameter (BPD) is not a reliable indicator of growth retardation. Growth discordance can occur as early as 23–24 weeks' gestation[28].

Malformations and aneuploidies

In general, twins have a higher incidence of structural anomalies when compared to singletons[2,29]. This is the result of an increased incidence of structural anomalies seen in monozygotic twins[30]. The incidence of malformations is reported to be about 2.12%[31], with a higher rate found in monozygotic twins compared to dizygotic twins. The types of malformations that occur can be divided into two general groups: those that are unique to twins, especially monochorionic twins (see below), and those anomalies not unique to twin gestations (such as hydrocephalus, congenital heart disease, single umbilical artery and neural tube defects).

In addition, twins have an increased incidence of aneuploidies. This is because each fetus has an *a priori* risk, therefore the chance that at least one of the two fetuses is affected is greater than for singletons[32]. In monozygotic twins, both fetuses will be affected, although, rarely, an exception can occur and they will be of different karyotypes, usually as a result of a postzygotic non-disjunction. Therefore, when performing amniocentesis for genetic studies, both sacs should be tapped, even in the presence of a monochorionic placenta.

Placental 'problems'

In gestations of high order, there is a 6–9-fold increase in the incidence of velamentous insertion of the cord[33]. The incidence of vasa previa is also increased.

COMPLICATIONS UNIQUE TO MONOCHORIONIC PREGNANCIES

Resulting from vascular connections

Monochorionic twins have a higher frequency of vascular anastomosis in the placenta. These vascular connections between the twins can result in the twin–twin transfusion syndrome, brain or visceral lesions and in acardiac twin.

Twin-to-twin transfusion

The reported incidence of twin-to-twin transfusion (TTS) ranges from 5.5 to 38%[33,34]. The 'donor' twin is on the arterial side and shunts blood to the 'recipient' twin[35]. Sonography of the donor twin reveals severe oligohydramnios, microcardia and intrauterine growth retardation. Because of the severe oligohydramnios present, this twin appears to be 'stuck' to the wall of the uterus[36]. The 'stuck' twin does not move, because the constricting amnion fits like a glove and compresses this fetus against the uterine wall. In contrast, the 'recipient' twin shows severe polyhydramnios, macrosomia, cardiomegaly and even hydrops. The perinatal morbidity is 10% for all twin pairs with TTS. The perinatal mortality is 88% for the recipient twin and 96% for the donor twin[37].

Twin embolization syndrome

This syndrome is usually associated with the intrauterine death of one twin. Brain lesions in the recipient twin may result from embolization of thromboplastic material from the dead co-twin or from episodes of hypotension[38]. Bejar and co-workers[39] found that the incidence of antenatal necrosis of the cerebral white matter (periventricular leukomalacia) occurred in 30% of monochorionic twins vs. 3.3% in dichorionic twins.

Twin reversed arterial perfusion syndrome or acardiac twin

The incidence of twin reversed arterial perfusion syndrome (TRAP) has been reported to be one in 30 000 deliveries or 1/100 monozygotic twins[1]. This syndrome is characterized by vascular anastomoses (artery–artery and vein–vein) between the fetuses. The 'perfused' twin has multiple abnormalities, including absence of the heart, abdominal organs, fetal head and upper extremities. The 'pump' twin is morphologically normal. The reported perinatal mortality for the 'pump' twin is 55%. Approximately 50% of the twins have a chromosomal abnormality. The mortality rate for the normal twin is 50%[40].

Cord entanglement

Entanglement of the umbilical cords can only occur in monochorionic–monoamniotic twins. Monochorionic–monoamniotic twin pregnancies are uncommon and account for approximately 1% of all monochorionic twins. Mortality in monoamniotic twins has been reported as high as 50%[1]. This high mortality results from cord entanglement between the twins.

Conjoined twins

Conjoined twins occur rarely. The incidence of conjoined twins is reported to be one in 33 000 to one in 165 000 births[2]. Thirty-nine per cent of the conjoined twins are stillborn and another 34% die shortly after birth[41]. Survival of the twins depends upon the type of union and other associated anomalies. The most common types of conjoined twins are thoraco-omphalopagus (28%), thoracopagus (18%), omphalopagus (10%), incomplete duplication (10%) and craniopagus (6%)[41].

References

1. Benirschke, K. and Kim, C. K. (1973). Multiple pregnancy (first of two parts). *N. Engl. J. Med.*, **288**, 1276–84
2. Benirschke, K. and Kim, C. K. (1973). Multiple pregnancy (second of two parts). *N. Engl. J. Med.*, **288**, 1329–36
3. Westrom, K. D. and Gall, S. A. (1988). Incidence, morbidity, mortality and diagnosis of twin gestations. *Clin. Perinatol.*, **15**, 1
4. Petrikovsky, B. M. and Vintzielos, A. M. (1989). Management and outcome of multifetal pregnancy of high fetal order: literature review. *Obstet. Gynecol. Surv.*, **44**, 578–84
5. Luke, B. and Keith, L. G. (1992). The contribution of singleton, twins and triplets to low birth weight infant mortality and handicap in the United States. *J. Reprod. Med.*, **37**, 661
6. Schenker, J. G., Yarkoni, S. and Granat, M. (1981). Multiple pregnancies following induction of ovulation. *Fertil. Steril.*, **35**, 105–23
7. Ezra, Y. and Schenker, J. G. (1993). Appraisal of *in vitro* fertilization. *Eur. J. Obstet. Gynecol. Reprod. Biol.*, **48**, 127–33
8. Bollen, N., Camus, M., Staessen, C., Tournaye, H., Devroey, P. and van Steirteghen, A. C. (1991). The incidence of multiple pregnancies after *in vitro* fertilization and embryo transfer, gamete, or zygote intrafallopian transfer. *Fertil. Steril.*, **55**, 314–18
9. Moore, K. L. (1988). *The Developing Human. Clinically Oriented Embryology*, pp.122–5. (Philadelphia: W.B. Saunders)
10. Monteagudo, A. and Timor-Tritsch, I. E. (1994). Early and simple determination of chorionic and amniotic type in multifetal gestations in the first fourteen weeks by high-frequency transvaginal sonography. *Am. J. Obstet. Gynecol.*, **170**, in press
11. Goldstein, S. R. (1988). Early pregnancy scanning with the endovaginal probe. *Contemp. Obstet. Gynecol.*, **31**, 54–64
12. Goldstein, S. R., Snyder, J. R., Watson, C. and Dannon, M. (1988). Very early pregnancy detection with endovaginal ultrasound. *Obstet. Gynecol.*, **72**, 200–4
13. Warren, W. B., Timor-Tritsch, I. E., Peisner, D. B., Rajv, S. and Rosen, M. G. (1989). Dating the pregnancy by sequential appearance of embryonic structures. *Am. J. Obstet. Gynecol.*, **161**, 747–53
14. Mahoney, B., Filly, R. and Callen, P. (1985). Amnionicity and chorionicity in twin pregnancies; prediction using ultrasound. *Radiology*, **155**, 205
15. Tessen, J. A. and Zlatnik, F. J. (1991). Monoamniotic twins: a retrospective controlled study. *Obstet. Gynecol.*, **77**, 832–4
16. Winn, H. N., Gabrielli, S., Reece, E. A., Roberts, J. A., Salafia, C. and Hobbins, J. C. (1989). Ultrasonographic criteria for the prenatal diagnosis of placental chorionicity in twin gestations. *Am. J. Obstet. Gynecol.*, **161**, 1540
17. Townsend, R. R., Simpson, G. F. and Filly, R. A. (1988). Membrane thickness in ultrasound prediction of chorionicity of twin gestations. *J. Ultrasound Med.*, **7**, 326
18. Hertzberg, B. S., Kurtz, A., Choi, H. Y., Kaczmarczyk, J. M., Warren, W., Wapner, R. J., Needleman, L., Baltarowich, O. H., Pasto, M. E., Rifkin, M. D., Pennel, R. G. and Goldberg, B. B. (1987). Significance of membrane thickness in the sonographic evaluation of twin gestations. *Am. J. Roentgenol.*, **148**, 151–3
19. Barss, V. A., Benacerraf, B. R. and Frigoletto, F. D. (1985). Ultrasonic determination of chorion type in twin gestation. *Obstet. Gynecol.*, **66**, 779
20. Lavery, J. P. (1992). Ultrasound in the multifetal pregnancy. *Female Patient*, **17**, 116–23
21. D'Alton, M. E. and Dudley, D. K. (1989). The ultrasound prediction of chorionicity in twin gestation. *Am. J. Obstet. Gynecol.*, **160**, 557
22. Bessis, V. A. and Papiernik, E. (1981). Echographic imagery of amniotic membranes in twin pregnancies. In Gedda, L. and Parisi, P. (eds.) *Twin Research, Vol. 3: Twin Biology and Multiple Pregnancy*, pp. 183–7. (New York: Alan R. Liss)
23. Kurtz, A., Mata, J., Wapner, R., Mata, J., Johnson, A. and Morgan, P. (1992). Twin pregnancies: accuracy of first trimester abdominal US in predicting chorionicity and amnionicity. *Radiology*, **185**, 759–62
24. Finberg, H. J. (1992). The 'twin peak' sign. Reliable evidence of dichorionic twinning. *J. Ultrasound Med.*, **11**, 571
25. Landy, H. J., Weiner, S., Corson, S. L., Batzer, F. R. and Bolognese, R. J. (1986). The 'vanishing twin': ultrasonographic assessment of fetal disappearance in the first trimester. *Am. J. Obstet. Gynecol.*, **155**, 14
26. Jauniaux, E., Elkazen, N., Leroy, F., Wilkin, P., Rodesch, F. and Hustin, J. (1988). Clinical and morphologic aspects of the vanishing twin phenomenon. *Obstet. Gynecol.*, **72**, 577
27. Chitkara, U., Berkowitz, G. S., Levine, R., Riden, D. J., Fagerstrom, R. M., Chevernak, F. A. and Berkowitz. (1985). Twin pregnancy: routine use of ultrasound examinations in the prenatal diag-

nosis of intrauterine growth retardation and discordant growth. *Am. J. Perinatol.*, **2**, 49–54
28. Finberg, H. J. (1994). Ultrasound evaluation in multiple gestation. In Callen, P. W. (ed.) *Ultrasonography in Obstetrics and Gynecology*, 3rd edn. (Philadelphia: W.B. Saunders)
29. Little, J. and Bryan, E. (1986). Congenital anomalies in twins. *Semin. Perinatol.*, **10**, 50–64
30. Schinzel, A. A. G. L., Smith, D. W. and Miller, J. R. (1979). Monozygotic twinning and structural defects. *J. Pediatr.*, **96**, 921–30
31. Kohl, S. G. and Casey, G. (1975). Twin gestation. *Mt Sinai J. Med.*, **42**, 523
32. Rodis, J. F., Egan, J. F. X., Craffey, A., Ciarleglio, L., Greenstein, R. M. and Scorza, W. E. (1990). Calculated risk of chromosomal abnormalities in twin gestations. *Obstet. Gynecol.*, **76**, 1037–41
33. Dudley, D. K. and D'Alton, M. E. (1986). Single fetal death in twin gestation. *Semin. Perinatol.*, **10**, 65–72
34. Giles, W. B., Trudinger, B. J., Cook, C. M. and Connelly, A. J. (1990). Doppler umbilical artery studies in the twin–twin transfusion syndrome. *Obstet. Gynecol.*, **76**, 1097–9
35. Blickstein, I. (1990). The twin–twin transfusion syndromes. *Obstet. Gynecol.*, **76**, 714–22
36. Mahoney, B. S., Petty, C. N., Nyberg, D. A., Luthy, D. A., Hickok, D. E. and Hirsch, J. H. (1990). The 'stuck twin' phenomenon: ultrasonographic findings, pregnancy outcome, and management with serial amniocentesis. *Am. J. Obstet. Gynecol.*, **163**, 1513–22
37. Patten, R. M., Mack, L. A., Harvey, D., Cyr, D. R. and Pretorius, D. H. (1989). Disparity of amniotic fluid volume and fetal size: problem of the stuck twin: US studies. *Radiology*, **172**, 153
38. Larroche, J. C. L., Droulle, P., Delezoide, A. L. and Nessmann, F. N. (1990). Brain damage in monozygous twins. *Biol. Neonate.*, **57**, 261–78
39. Bejar, R., Vigliocco, G., Gramajo, H., Solana, C., Benirschke, K., Berry, C., Coen, R. and Resnik, R. (1990). Antenatal origin of neurologic damage in newborn infants. II Multiple gestations. *Am. J. Obstet. Gynecol.*, **162**, 1230–6
40. Moore, T. R., Gale, S. and Bernirschke, K. (1990). Perinatal outcome of forty-nine pregnancies complicated by acardiac twining. *Am. J. Obstet. Gynecol.*, **163**, 907
41. Romero, R., Pilu, G., Jeanty, P., Ghidini, A. and Hobbins, J. C. (1988). *Prenatal diagnosis of congenital anomalies*. (Norwalk, CT: Appleton & Lange)

The first 3 weeks of gestation assessed by transvaginal color Doppler

15

S. Kupešić and A. Kurjak

INTRODUCTION

Remarkable advances in the understanding of early human development have been achieved with the introduction of transvaginal color Doppler technology. This new technique has provided the unique ability to study both morphology and physiology virtually from conception to implantation.

The fundamental unit of the ovary is the follicle, which consists of the female germ cell (oocyte) surrounded by a series of specialized cell layers, the granulosa and the theca cells. Every month during a woman's reproductive life, one oocyte is released from the single mature follicle that has completed development. After ovulation, the follicle cells undergo luteinization. A number of biochemical, morphological and vascular changes occurs during this process, a significant proportion of which can be studied by transvaginal color Doppler. If the oocyte is fertilized, the embryo is transported into the uterus where, under the proper hormonal and environmental conditions, it will implant and develop into a new individual. Transvaginal ultrasonography with color flow imaging and blood flow analysis allows detailed examination of small arteries supplying the pre-ovulatory follicle, corpus luteum and endometrium. We will review and illustrate these in detail.

OVARY

Transvaginal sonography allows the production of increasingly detailed images of ovarian morphology[1]. The addition of color flow imaging has facilitated the measurement of sequential changes in ovarian arteries during the ovarian cycle[2–5]. The highest resistance to flow is observed on day 1 of the menstrual cycle, while the lowest occurs on the day of the luteinizing hormone (LH) peak[2,3].

Pre-ovulatory follicle and follicular blood flow during ovulation

Pre-ovulatory follicles have a more permeable capillary network than follicles destined to undergo atresia, allowing the accumulation of higher levels of circulating gonadotropins[6–8]. In response to the LH surge, there is an immediate increase in blood flow, as evidenced by hyperemia. Blood flows through the newly formed capillary network, producing edema in the theca layer of the follicle. There is an increase in follicular fluid volume, probably caused by osmotic uptake of plasma due to the action of hyaluronic acid synthesized by granulosa cells. Rupture is preceded by thinning of part of the follicle wall and overlying surface epithelium, producing a transparent area or stigma which is characterized by a loss of capillaries. This reduction in blood flow at the follicle apex is followed by epithelial cell death. Disintegration of the apex of the follicle, final maturation of the oocyte and liberation of the highly viscous cumulus–oocyte mass are required for successful ovulation. The very thin stalk of cells which connects the oocyte to the mass of granulosa cells breaks easily, allowing the oocyte to be extruded in the flow of follicular fluid. This ovulation process takes place over a period of one or more minutes. The ovum is the follicle's most valuable cargo, surrounded by thousands of cells that provide nourishment and protection for the journey.

The evaluation of follicular development by ultrasound is now well established in routine clinical work (Figure 1). Transvaginal color Doppler reveals areas of vascularity on the follicular rim[2,3] (Figure 2): follicular flow velocity waveforms are usually detected when the dominant follicle reaches 10 mm in diameter. The resistance index (RI) is around 0.54 when ovulation approaches[9] (Table 1, Figure 3), declining from 2 days prior to ovulation (Figure 4) and reaching its nadir of 0.44 ± 0.04 at ovulation (Figure 5). The marked increase in the peak systolic blood flow velocity within the follicle in the presence of a relatively constant resistance index is an important finding which might herald impending ovulation[2]. This may represent dilatation of new vessels that have developed between the vascular theca cell layer and the hypoxic granulosa cell layer of the follicle[10]. Changes in oxygen tension within the follicle and their effect on cellular function have been described: these are necessary for normal ovulation to occur. Transvaginal sonography with color flow imaging could become the method of choice for studying subtle vascular changes within the ovary in women with normal and abnormal ovarian function.

Corpus luteum – morphology, function and vascularization

The cells of the former follicular wall undergo structural and functional transformation as they make up the corpus luteum[11]. Capillaries and fibroblasts from the theca proliferate and penetrate the basement membrane. The mural granulosa cells undergo morphological changes, collectively referred to as luteinization. Cells, capillaries, and blood vessels intermingle to give rise to a corpus luteum[12]; this is colored by a golden pigment, from which it derives its name, which means 'yellow body'.

Microscopically, the corpus luteum undergoes four stages of development and demise: proliferation, vascularization, maturation and regression. During the proliferative stage the theca interna is invaginated, and its vascular channels are greatly dilated. Endothelial sprouts from the vessels penetrate the granulosa and the hemorrhagic cavity of the ruptured follicle (Figure 5). In the stage of vascularization, the blood-filled cavity of the ruptured follicle undergoes rapid organization (Figure 6). As maturation progresses, the theca cells and luteinized cells that have originated from the granulosa become vacuolated and physiologically active. The mature corpus luteum usually measures 1–3 cm in diameter, and shows low impedance signals (mean RI = 0.43) (Figure 7). Regressive changes occur in the corpus luteum as early as the 23rd day after menstruation. Decreased blood velocity and an increased resistance index (mean RI = 0.49) are the typical signs of these changes (Figure 8). If pregnancy occurs the corpus luteum, maintained by human chorionic gonadotrophin (hCG), a hormone secreted by the trophoblast, produces progesterone, to support the developing conceptus. The corpus luteum normally begins to regress after 10 weeks, when the placenta assumes production of the progesterone, and completely resolves by 16 weeks[13]. Doppler ul-

Table 1 *Follicular and corpus luteum blood flow*

	No	Resistance index[a]
Follicular blood flow (days before ovulation)		
−5	2	0.54 ± 0.04[a]
−4	2	0.54 ± 0.04
−3	18	0.53 ± 0.04
−2	26	0.51 ± 0.04
−1	38	0.49 ± 0.04*
Corpus luteum blood flow (days after ovulation)		
1	43	0.44 ± 0.04**
2	6	0.44 ± 0.06
3	7	0.45 ± 0.04
4	5	0.44 ± 0.04
5	1	0.43 ± 0.04
6	9	0.46 ± 0.07
7	17	0.47 ± 0.04
8	18	0.47 ± 0.04
9	8	0.48 ± 0.02
10	7	0.48 ± 0.02
11	7	0.47 ± 0.02
12	11	0.48 ± 0.04
13	7	0.49 ± 0.04
14	5	0.51 ± 0.01
15	6	0.50 ± 0.02

[a]Resistance index for follicular blood flow ± 1 SE
*Compared with day −5: $p < 0.001$
**Compared with pre-ovulatory level: $p < 0.001$

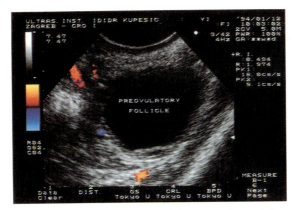

Figure 1 Transvaginal scan of the mature preovulatory follicle demonstrating the triangular echo of the cumulus oophorus

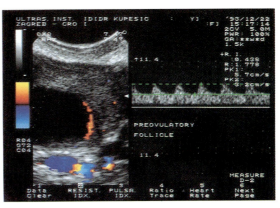

Figure 4 During the moment of presumed ovulation the velocity of the follicular blood flow tends to increase, while the resistance index (RI) decreases to 0.43

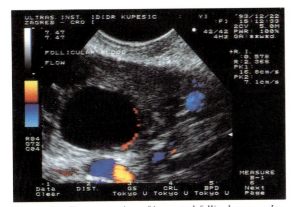

Figure 2 Demonstration of increased follicular vascularity at the time of luteinizing hormone peak

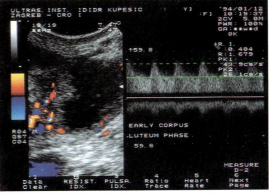

Figure 5 Demonstration of increased vascularity on the periphery of collapsed follicle (left). Note echogenic fluid (blood) within the cavity of a ruptured follicle, increased blood flow velocity, and decreased resistance index (RI = 0.40) (right)

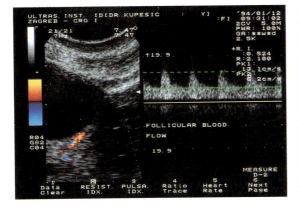

Figure 3 Transvaginal scan demonstrating a ring of angiogenesis in a growing follicle (left). Flow velocity waveforms show resistance index (RI) of 0.52

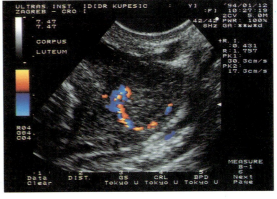

Figure 6 A mature corpus luteum, occupying the half of the entire ovary. Note color-coded area representing corpus luteum vascular network

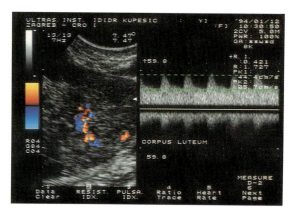

Figure 7 *Transvaginal color Doppler indicates increased ovarian vascularity in the luteal phase of the cycle. High blood flow velocity and low resistance index (RI = 0.42) represent the typical flow patterns of a mature corpus luteum (right)*

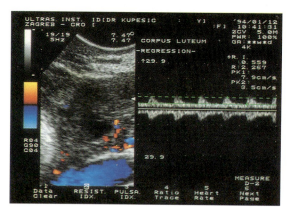

Figure 8 *Less prominent color-coded area demonstrates ovarian vascularization in late luteal phase (left). Pulsed Doppler shows high resistance index (RI = 0.56) blood flow during the regression of corpus luteum (right)*

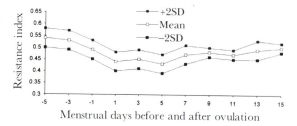

Figure 9 *Follicular and corpus luteum blood flow*

Table 2 Luteal blood flow in normal early pregnancy (resistance index ± SD)

Gestational age (weeks)	No. patients	Luteal flow	p
5	8	0.452 ± 0.04	NS
6	10	0.448 ± 0.05	NS
7	19	0.444 ± 0.04	NS
8	19	0.451 ± 0.04	NS
9	18	0.450 ± 0.03	NS
10	18	0.458 ± 0.05	NS
12	17	0.450 ± 0.02	NS
Total	127	0.452 ± 0.04	

trasound studies at this stage can yield important information[14,15]. This method permits non-invasive assessment of corpus luteum blood velocities, and therefore gives direct information concerning the active ovarian arterial circulation[16,17]. After ovulation, the resistance index is significantly different from pre-ovulatory values (Figure 9). Women with documented ovulation show an RI of 0.43 ± 0.04 shortly after ovulation (Figure 7), with a return to the earlier cycle level of 0.49 ± 0.02 ($p < 0.001$) (Figure 8). None of 127 pregnant women between the fifth and twelfth weeks of gestation had an RI > 0.50 (Table 2). The resistance and pulsatility indices between 6 and 12 weeks of gestation do not change significantly ($p > 0.05$). Beyond 12 weeks of gestation, it is thought that these luteal velocity waveforms disappear following regression of the corpus luteum.

Studies on intra-ovarian vascularity raise the interesting question of whether factors other than hCG play a role in maintaining the function of the corpus luteum[18–22]. Although in the non-pregnant state, in which hCG plays no role, the luteal flow appears during the whole second part of the ovarian cycle.

Kratzer and colleagues[23] found that corpus luteum function in early pregnancy is primarily determined by the rate of change of hCG levels. There is a significantly slower rate of change in hCG levels in patients with ectopic pregnancy and spontaneous abortion than in normal intrauterine pregnancy. The resistance and pulsatility indices in ectopic pregnancies are similar to those seen in the non-pregnant state during the late luteal phase[17]. We analyzed corpus luteum blood flow in normal and abnormal pregnancies (Table 3) and found no difference between ectopic and normal early pregnancy ($p > 0.05$). During the first trimester of

Table 3 *Corpus luteum blood flow in normal and abnormal pregnancy (resistance index ± SD)*

Group	No. patients	Luteal flow	p
Normal pregnancy	127	0.452 ± 0.04	
Missed abortion	11	0.536 ± 0.06	< 0.01
Anembryonic pregnancy	11	0.448 ± 0.04	NS
Molar pregnancy	9	0.449 ± 0.05	NS
Ectopic pregnancy	10	0.485 ± 0.07	NS
Threatened abortion	6	0.532 ± 0.08	< 0.01
Incomplete abortion	7	0.539 ± 0.05	< 0.01
Total	181		

NS = non significant (Anova and Tukey HSD type A, $p > 0.05$)

pregnancy luteal flow was similar to that in the early luteal phase of the non-pregnant state. In women with threatened, incomplete or missed abortions the resistance and pulsatility indices were significantly higher than those in normal pregnancy ($p < 0.001$). Zalud and Kurjak[5] studied luteal blood flow in the non-gravid ovary and in normotopic and ectopic pregnancy. The lowest resistance index of luteal flow (0.42 ± 0.12) was found in non-pregnant women and the highest (0.53 ± 0.09) occurred in women with early intrauterine pregnancy. Those with ectopic pregnancy had an RI of 0.48 ± 0.07, and ipsilateral luteal flow was detected in 86.4%. Measurement of luteal blood flow may, therefore have some prognostic value in patients with threatened abortion[24]. An increase in RI is indicative of less chance that the embryo will survive, especially after 8 weeks of gestational age, when the critical time for natural selection of survival has passed[25].

Luteal flow may be a useful indicator of corpus luteum regression, and can be correlated to factors that influence corpus luteum function, such as progesterone, relaxin, prostaglandin or angiogenic growth peptide factors[25]. Prostaglandin F2-α, known as luteolysin[25], is produced locally by the lutein cells near the time of regression. As prostaglandin F2-α is a powerful vasocontrictor it may increase the impendence to flow (measured as resistance or pulsatility indices) in blood vessels within the corpus luteum. Whether endothelium derived relaxation factor (EDRF) plays any important role here is yet to be determined. It is not yet clear whether inadequate vascularization plays a role in luteal phase defects. Transvaginal sonography coupled with pulsed wave Doppler seems to be sensitive enough to answer these questions and to be used as a clinical tool.

FERTILIZATION, EMBRYOGENESIS AND IMPLANTATION

Several hours before ovulation the Fallopian tube has probably received signals as to the site on the ovary's surface where rupture will occur. The fimbriae position themselves to catch the ovum and prevent it from disappearing into the abdominal cavity. The soft folds in the mucous membrane of the fimbriae move unceasingly back and forth across the ovary's surface, apparently 'tasting' the chemical messenger substances there. The entire membrane is covered with tiny cilia, all beating in toward the interior of the Fallopian tube and creating a kind of suction for the fluid shed by the follicle. With this fluid comes further information in the form of chemical signals, which cause the muscles of the Fallopian tube to begin contracting rhythmically. These contractions help the cilia to trap the oocyte and direct it to the tube's lumen, where fertilization normally occurs within 1–2 days[26].

Before spermatozoa are able to fertilize an ovum, they must undergo the final maturation processes of capacitation (the loss of surface proteins and the glycoprotein coat covering their chromosomal region) and the acrosome reaction (the loss of acrosomal membrane and release of hyaluronidase, trypsin-like substance, and zona lysin[27]). After ejaculation, about 200 sperm reach their destination, the ovum surrounded by a porous sheath of nutrient cells. After a few hours, some of the outer layers are removed and the surface of the oocyte is exposed. As a small number of sperm begin to penetrate the ovum wall, a single one breaks all the way through, penetrating the inner plasma of the ovum. Following penetration of the corona radiata and zona pellucida, the spermatozoon and oocyte fuse. The oocyte resumes the second meiotic division immediately after spermatozoon entry, and the metabolic activity of the oocyte increases[26,27]. The fertilized zygote divides rapidly to form a cluster of cells called a morula. By menstrual day 20 the morula has differentiated into the blastocyst, a fluid filled sphere comprising an inner cell mass and an outer trophoblastic layer[13]. The inner cell mass eventually forms the fetus, yolk sac and allantois; the trophoblastic layer forms the placenta, chorion and amnion. The fertilized ovum has no direct contact with the mucous membrane of the Fallopian tube, but substances flowing through the membrane create a favorable habitat. On the surface of the mucous membrane millions of tiny cilia keep beating in the same direction – toward the uterus, and the muscles of the Fallopian tube contract periodically. In the transition between the wider and narrower parts of the Fallopian tube there is a sphincter muscle which is impassable to the fertilized ovum despite its small size. This sphincter relaxes in response to progesterone secreted by the corpus luteum, and the passage leading to the uterus opens. The blastocyst enters the uterus approximately 4–5 days after fertilization and remains free within the uterus for 2 days. The uterine lining, the endometrium, has been prepared by hormones from the ovary to receive the fertilized ovum. Implantation of the blastocyst occurs at approximately 21–23 days (a week following ovulation), and is complete by the 26th day of the menstrual cycle. At the time of its initial attachment the blastocyst is oriented with the inner cell mass aligned toward the endometrium[13]. Penetration and erosion of the uterine mucosa results from the action of proteolytic enzymes produced by the trophoblast. During implantation the trophoblast erodes adjacent maternal capillaries, and maternal blood comes into direct contact with the conceptus. This intercommunicating lacunar network becomes the intervillous space of the placenta. Trophoblastic invasion is controlled and supported by the decidual reaction of the endometrium, characterized by increased vascularity, edema and thickening[28]. There is some evidence to suggest that platelet activating factor is one of the messengers with unique vasodilating properties involved in this process. The passage from the uterus down to the cervix is sealed by a plug of mucus, and the muscles of the uterine wall become softer and more elastic.

The gestational sac, representing the chorionic cavity, is the first definitive sonographic sign of early pregnancy. This can be consistently visualized by transvaginal sonography by 33.8 ± 1.8 days after LMP (Figure 10). Although the gestational sac is very small, it is characteristically surrounded by an echogenic ring that represents the trophoblast and decidual reactions. Other normal features of the gestational sac include an eccentric position relative to the central endometrium, a location near the fundus, a round, oval or crescentic shape, and a smooth rounded contour (Figure 11).

Our study showed a mean constant growth rate of 1.2 mm/day for the gestational sac during early pregnancy (Figure 11). As the gestational sac enlarges, the embryonic disk and

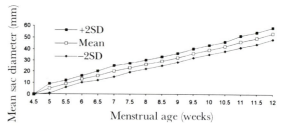

Figure 10 Gestational sac size related to postmenstrual age in 127 women in the first trimester of pregnancy

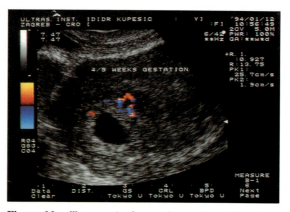

Figure 11 Transvaginal scan of an early gestational sac. Note its eccentric position, fundal location, oval shape and double contours. Color-coded 'hot' area represents increased vascularity

SONOGRAPHY IN THE FIRST 3 WEEKS

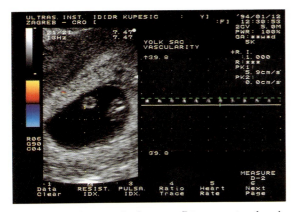

Figure 12 *Transvaginal scan at 7 post-menstrual weeks demonstrates a well-defined yolk sac within the gestational sac. The yolk sac, which is the embryo's first vascular organ, shows definite pulsations on real time ultrasound (right)*

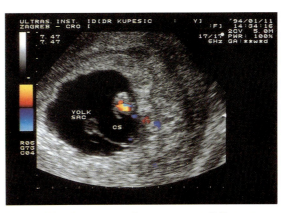

Figure 14 *Transvaginal sonogram at 7/8 post-menstrual weeks demonstrates living embryo, yolk sac and elongated yolk stalk*

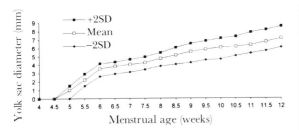

Figure 13 *Average yolk sac size related to post-menstrual age in 127 pregnant women*

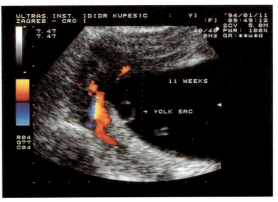

Figure 15 *Demonstration of an 11-week lasting gestation. Note increased peritrophoblastic flow and yolk sac localized between chorion and amnion, typical of this gestational age*

embryonic membrane undergo remarkable growth. The secondary yolk sac is the earliest embryonic landmark that can be recognized within the gestational sac, at the beginning of the fifth post-menstrual week[29]. This is the main supply line to the embryo prior to the development of the true intervillous circulation. The formation of the secondary yolk sac begins shortly after implantation, when the distal section of the primary yolk sac, enclosed by the embryonic disk and the exocelomic membrane, is 'pinched off'. This structure is the embryo's first vascular and hemopoietic organ (Figure 12), and it can be visualized when the gestational sac measures > 10 mm. Approximately 2 weeks following ovulation an extensive vascular system begins to develop in the wall of the yolk sac. Careful observation of the yolk sac contours permits the detection of early embryonic heart activity at 6 weeks of gestation. Average yolk sac diameter gradually increases between the 6th and 12th weeks after the last menstrual period from 3.5 mm (range 2.6–4.1) to 7.1 mm (range 6.0–8.5) (Figure 13). The yolk sac remains connected to the embryo by the yolk stalk, which contains the vitelline duct and vessels, until 8 weeks of gestation[30] (Figure 14). The amniotic cavity increases in size, and the yolk sac becomes solidified and clearly located between the amnion and chorion (Figure 15). The amnion is very thin, and is usually seen only when it lies perpendicular to the ultrasound beam (Figure 16). By the end of the first trimester, the exocelomic fluid has been absorbed and the amnion has fused with the chorion. Microscopic examination of the yolk sac obtained from

THE FETUS AS A PATIENT

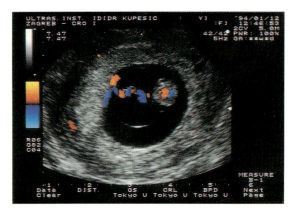

Figure 16 *Scan at 10 postmenstrual weeks shows a thin amnion surrounding the embryo. Full length of umbilical cord and both insertion are coded by color Doppler*

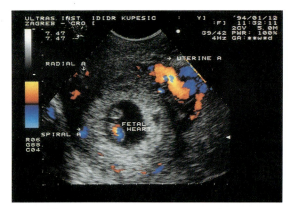

Figure 17 *Transvaginal scan at 7 post-menstrual weeks shows a well-defined yolk sac, and the embryo which measures 1 cm. Color signals simultaneously demonstrate cardiac activity and location of the uterine vessels (uterine, radial and spiral arteries)*

Table 4 *Discriminatory sac size by transvaginal sonography (gestational sac size in which living embryo can be demonstrated)*

Author	Reference	Discriminatory sac size (mm)
de Crepigni	34	12
Levi *et al.*	35	16
Bree *et al.*	36	9
Rempen	37	18
Cacciatore	38	18
Present study	–	16

early spontaneous abortions often reveals regression or cystic alteration[31]. The clinical use of ultrasound studies has proved to be disappointing[31,32]. In spontaneous abortion the size of the yolk sac measured by transvaginal ultrasound is usually within normal limits[29,32].

The size of the gestational sac in which a living embryo can be visualized has been reported in studies using either transabdominal or transvaginal ultrasound[33]. In our study using transvaginal sonography with color flow imaging, a living embryo could always be seen when the gestational sac was larger than 16 mm (Table 4). Other studies using the same technique have determined the discriminatory sac size to be between 9 and 18 mm[33-38]. High resolution ultrasound technology and Doppler measurements of small vessels in an early human being, vitelline artery, yolk sac and uteroplacental circulation (Figure 17) will open an unexplored scientific area at the beginning of human life.

UTERINE ENVIRONMENT – VASCULAR CHANGES

Implantation and the subsequent development of pregnancy in the human require complex changes of the main uterine arteries and its branches in the myometrium and endometrium. Changes that occur in the uterine vessels during the reproductive cycle are important in the process of implantation and the establishment of uteroplacental circulation. Transvaginal color Doppler provides a detailed visualization of the reproductive organs and enables the detection of most of these vasculatory circulatory changes[29]. The color signal from the main uterine arteries is seen laterally to the cervix (Figures 18 and 19). After passing through one-third of the thickness of the myometrium, the uterine arteries divide into an arcuate wreath encircling the uterus[30] (Figure 20). Radial arteries arising from this network are directed towards the uterine lumen (Figures 21 and 22). As radial arteries pass the myometrial – endometrial junction, they become the spiral arteries (Figure 23). Transvaginal color flow Doppler gives the physician an exciting opportunity to study blood flow velocity waveforms in radial and spiral arteries of the non-gravid uterus. The endometrium has an exceptional

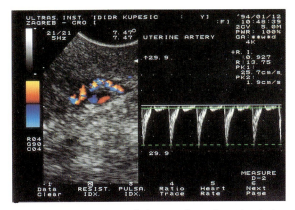

Figure 18 *Blood flow velocity waveforms from the uterine artery in the proliferative phase are characterized by a small amount of end-diastolic flow (resistance index = 0.92)*

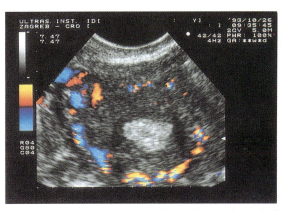

Figure 21 *Color signals are obtained from the radial arteries that are directed towards the uterine lumen*

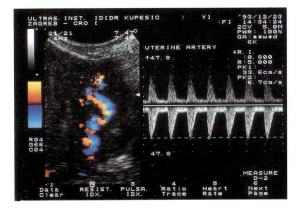

Figure 19 *Blood flow velocity waveforms from the uterine artery in the secretory phase are characterized by increased end-diastolic velocity (resistance index = 0.80)*

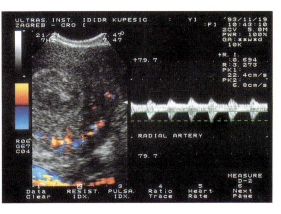

Figure 22 *Blood flow velocity waveforms of the radial arteries (right). Note the position of the gate on the left panel (within the myometrium) for sampling flow velocity waveforms*

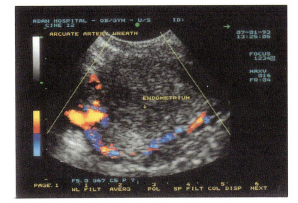

Figure 20 *Transvaginal color Doppler demonstrates arcuate artery wreath, encircling the uterus*

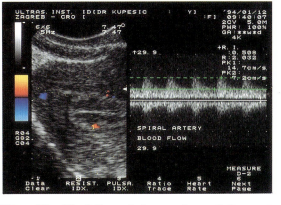

Figure 23 *Blood flow velocity waveforms of the spiral arteries during the periovulatory period. Decreased resistance index (0.51) and increased flow velocity occur during the day of ovulation*

capacity to undergo changes in structure and function during the menstrual cycle[30,32,39,40]. Histological changes include a striking development of blood vessels, the spiral arteries, which become much more developed during the menstrual cycle.

The increased endometrial vascularity depends on changes in uterine, arcuate and radial artery blood flow. Complex relationships exist between the concentration of ovarian hormones in peripheral venous plasma and uterine blood flow parameters[41,42]. In most women, there is a small amount of end-diastolic flow in the uterine arteries during the proliferative phase[9] (Figure 18). Uterine flow velocity has a RI of 0.88 ± 0.04 in the proliferative phase and starts to decrease the day before ovulation. During the normal ovulatory menstrual cycle there is a sharp increase in end-diastolic velocities between the proliferative and secretory phases (Figure 24). The resistance index reaches a nadir (0.84 ± 0.04) on day 18 and remains at that level for the rest of the cycle (Figure 19). These changes in flow velocity begin before ovulation, and may be a response to both angiogenesis and hormonal factors. Some authors[9,41,43,44] have found an absence of end-diastolic flow in uterine arteries of infertile patients: this may be associated with infertility or poor reproductive performance. It may also be a variant that disappears after a pregnancy[9]. Changes observed in normal ovulatory cycles do not occur in anovulatory cycles (Figure 24).

Transvaginal color Doppler makes it possible to study alterations of the radial and spiral arterial blood flows under physiologic and pathophysiologic conditions. A decrease of the resistance and pulsatility indices from the main uterine artery towards the spiral arteries can be demonstrated in the non-pregnant uterus. The radial artery blood flow resistance index in the proliferative phase is 0.78 ± 0.10. A significant decline begins at midcycle, reaching a nadir of 0.68 ± 0.04 in the midluteal phase (Figure 21). Spiral artery flow velocity has an RI of 0.54 ± 0.03 the day before ovulation, and a nadir of 0.49 ± 0.05 is reached approximately between days 16 and 18 (Figure 22). The changes in flow velocity patterns of the radial and spiral arteries in spontaneous ovulatory cycles parallel the blood flow dynamics of the uterine arteries. Transvaginal color Doppler may be used to predict implantation success rate, to reveal unexplained infertility problems and to select patients with abnormal myometrial and endometrial perfusion for appropriate treatment. A logical extension of this technology is to examine the effect of different medications on uterine perfusion[45]. Knowledge of such alterations in endometrial blood flow may play an important role in predicting the optimal time for implantation and embryo transfer. Transvaginal color Doppler may be used as non-invasive assay of uterine receptivity that would enable clinicians to cryopreserve the embryos if uterine conditions are adverse, and to reduce the number of transferred embryos when conditions are optimal.

CHANGES IN THE UTERINE PERFUSION ASSOCIATED WITH PLACENTATION

As soon as the blastocyst becomes attached to the endometrium, the migrating trophoblast encounters venous channels of increasing size, then superficial arterioles and eventually, during the 4th week, the spiral arteries[29,30]. The cytotrophoblastic cells reach the deciduo–myometrial junction between 8 and 12 weeks of gestation[46]. The trophoblastic invasion of the myometrium is progressive and restricted to the 8–18 week period[47]. During early pregnancy, the spiral arteries undergo morphological changes, including disruption of their architecture induced by the trophoblast, hypertrophy of the medial smooth vessels and swelling of the endothelium[47,48]. Erosion of the spiral arteries,

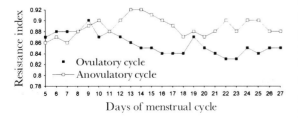

Figure 24 *Uterine artery blood flow velocity during the menstrual cycle*

as well as the changes in circulating steroid and protein and hormones, cause a significant fall in uterine vascular impedance. Low impedance turbulent flow is often detected near the placental implantation site[49] (Figure 25). Jaffe and Warsof[50] used Doppler techniques to study vascular changes associated with placentation as early as 5 weeks after the last menstrual period. Kurjack and co-workers[51] have shown Doppler changes in early pregnancy even before visualization of the gestational sac itself. These changes are characterized by the detection of low peak systolic and low impedance signals on the periphery of the endometrium. As the placenta develops, larger maternal blood vessels of higher pressure are invaded, resulting in higher velocity and a larger diastolic component of Doppler signals. The uteroplacental circulation has been extensively investigated throughout pregnancy[52–57]. The addition of color Doppler capabilities to transvaginal imaging will undoubtedly supplement morphological data with functional information, advancing our knowledge of fetal physiology[58,59]. Normal early human development depends on chromosomal structure, a functioning implantation mechanism and uterine perfusion. Poor implantation and poor uterine blood flow can be detected *in vivo* using non-invasive Doppler techniques. Transvaginal color Doppler could become the technique of choice for detection of hemodynamic abnormalities associated with early pregnancy failure. More detailed data are discussed in Chapter 35 on early pregnancy.

POTENTIAL DANGERS ON THE LONG JOURNEY OF THE FERTILIZED OVUM

One of the most critical phases of early development is the passage through the Fallopian tube. Sometimes the fertilized ovum becomes stuck in the tube and cannot proceed. Tubal abnormalities clearly play an important etiological role in tubal nidation. This is usually due to tubal inflammation (chlamydial infection, tuberculosis, shistosomiasis, etc.), tubal endometriosis, failed tubal sterilization and congenital abnormalities of the tube[60]. The process of placentation in an ectopic site appears to follow the same course as in an intrauterine gestation. The addition of color Doppler adds new information on perfusion and pathophysiologic changes associated with ectopic trophoblast implantation. Color Doppler exposes small and randomly dispersed vessels (Figure 26), while pulsed Doppler quantifies blood flow detected by color and gives information on trophoblastic vitality and invasiveness. Active trophoblasts show prominent and randomly dispersed flow inside the solid part of an adnexal mass or on the periphery of

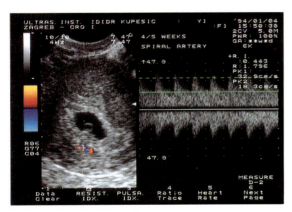

Figure 25 *Transvaginal color Doppler ultrasound and flow velocity waveforms obtained from the spiral arteries near the placental plate show a characteristic turbulent pattern and low resistance index (0.44)*

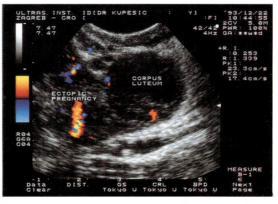

Figure 26 *Transvaginal scan of a highly vascularized adnexal mass suspected to be an ectopic pregnancy. Transvaginal color Doppler helps in the diagnosis of ectopic pregnancy by exposing small and randomly dispersed vessels within the solid part of an adnexal mass. The corpus luteum cyst is ipsilaterally situated and shows less prominent color signals*

a gestational ring (RI = 0.36 ± 0.04). Early pregnancy loss is the rule in an ectopic site: this occurs for mechanical and hemostatic reasons. A clinical impression of probable tubal abortion is obtained in patients with a high impedance signal (RI usually > 0.50) detected from the tubal arteries. Rarely, a fully adequate maternal blood supply to the placenta can be established even in such unlikely sites as the abdominal cavity or the uterine cervix. Using Doppler it is possible to identify the reactivity of the trophoblast to the feticidal agents which can provide a foundation for selective management of ectopic pregnancy.

Early miscarriages, before a woman is aware that she is pregnant, are very common. This is usually a result of abnormalities of chromosome structure or number[60]. If the uterine cavity is damaged or malformed the ovum may become implanted in various unfavorable sites, resulting in recurrent abortion, prematurity and intrauterine growth retardation.

CONCLUSIONS

While the problems surrounding the first trimester of pregnancy are better known, uncertainty still covers the most critical period of human development, the period between conception and implantation. Introduction of transvaginal color and pulsed Doppler and accumulation of experience from different centers has opened up new non-invasive possibilities for the precise assessment and measurement of many important events in this period. An important step forward has been made recently in the study of ovarian and uterine perfusion in nonpregnant patients. These results encourage development and scientific evaluation of a promising new field – the first days of human life.

References

1. Feichtinger, W. and Kemeter, P. (1989). Transvaginal sector sonography for needle guided transvaginal follicle aspiration and other applications in gynecologic routine and research. *Fertil. Steril.*, **45**, 722–5
2. Bourne, T., Jurkovic, D., Waterstone, J., Campbell, S. and Collins, W. P. (1991). Intrafollicular blood flow during human ovulation. *Ultrasound Obstet. Gynecol.*, **1**, 53–9
3. Collins, W. P., Jurkovic, D., Bourne, T. H., Kurjak, A. and Campbell, S. (1991). Ovarian morphology, endocrine function and intrafollicular blood flow during peri-ovulatory period. *Hum. Reprod.*, **6**, 319–24
4. Baber, R. J., McSweeney, M. B. and Gill, R. W. (1988). Transvaginal pulsed Doppler ultrasound assessment of blood flow to the corpus luteum in IVF patients following ET. *Br. J. Obstet. Gynaecol.*, **95**, 1226–30
5. Zalud, I. and Kurjak, A. (1990). The assessment of luteal blood flow in pregnant and nonpregnant women by transvaginal color Doppler. *J. Perinat. Med.*, **18**, 215–21
6. Hodgen, G. D. (1982). The dominant ovarian follicle. *Fertil. Steril.*, **38**, 281–300
7. Greenwald, G. S. and Terranova, R. F. (1988). Follicular selection and its control. In Knobil, E. and Neil, J. (eds.) *The Physiology of Reproduction*, p. 387. (New York: Raven Press)
8. Moor, R. M. and Seamark, R. F. (1986). Cell signaling, permeability and microvascular changes during follicular development in mammals. *J. Dairy Sci.*, **69**, 927–43
9. Kurjak, A., Kupesic-Urek, S., Schulman, H. and Zalud, I. (1991). Transvaginal color flow Doppler in the assessment of ovarian and uterine blood flow in infertile women. *Fertil. Steril.*, **56**, 870–3
10. Gosden, R. G. and Byat-Smith, J. G. (1986). Oxygen concentration across the follicular epithelium: model, prediction and implications. *Hum. Reprod.*, **1**, 65–8
11. Pierson, R. A. (1992). From ovulation to implantation. In Jaffe, R. and Warsof, S. L. (eds.) *Color Doppler Imaging in Obstetrics and Gynecology*, p. 35–46 (New York: McGraw Hill)
12. Harrison, R. J. (1962). The structure of the ovary. In Zuckerman, S., Mandl, A. M. and Eckstein, P. (eds.) *The Ovary*. p. 142–8. (London: Academic Press)
13. Nyberg, D. A. and Hill, A. (1992). Normal early intrauterine pregnancy: sonographic development and hCG correlation. In Nyberg, D. A., Hill, L. M., Bohm-Velez, M. and Mendelson,

E. B. (eds.) *Transvaginal Ultrasound*, p. 2–76. (St. Louis: Mosby)
14. Taylor, K. W. J., Burns, P. N., Wells, P. N. E., Conway, D. I. and Hull, M. G. R. (1985). Ultrasound Doppler flow studies of the ovarian and uterine arteries. *Br. J. Obstet. Gynecol.*, **92**, 240–6
15. Hata, K., Hata, T., Senot, D., Makihara, K., Aoki, S., Takamiya, O. and Kitao, M. (1990). Change in ovarian arterial compliance during the human menstrual cycle assessed by Doppler ultrasound. *Br. J. Obstet. Gynecol.*, **97**, 163–6
16. Kurjak, A., Zalud, I., Jurkovic, D., Alfirevic, Z. and Miljan, M. (1989). Transvaginal color Doppler in the assessment of pelvic circulation. *Acta Obstet. Gynecol. Scand.*, **68**, 131–5
17. Salim, A., Kurjak, A. and Zalud, I. (1992). Ovarian luteal flow in normal and abnormal early pregnancies. *J. Maternal Fetal Invest.*, **2**, 119
18. Soules, M. R., Bremner, W. J., Dahl, K. D., Rivier, J. E., Vale, W. and Clifton, D. K. (1991). The induction of premature luteolysis in normal women – follicular phase luteinizing hormone secretion and corpus luteum function in the subsequent cycle. *Am. J. Obstet. Gynecol.*, **164**, 989–96
19. Tulsky, A. S. and Koff, A. K. (1957). Some observations on the role of corpus luteum in early human pregnancy. *Fertil. Steril.*, **8**, 118–21
20. Adams, E. C. and Hertig, A. T. (1969). Studies on the human corpus luteum I and II. Observations on the ultrastructure of luteal cells during pregnancy. *J. Cell Biol.*, **41**, 496–8
21. Flint, A. P. F. and Scheldric, E. L. (1985). Ovarian peptides and luteolysis. In Edwards, R. G., Purdy, J. M. and Steptoe, P. C. (eds). *Implantation of Human Embryo*, p. 235–240 (London: Academic Press)
22. Csapo, A. I. and Pulkkinen, M. (1978). Indispensability of the human corpus luteum in the maintenance of early pregnancy. *Obstet. Gynecol. Surv.*, **33**, 69–81
23. Kratzer, P. G. and Taylor, R. N. (1990). Corpus luteum function in early pregnancies is primarily determined by the rate of change of human chorionic gonadotropin levels. *Am. J. Obstet. Gynecol.*, **163**, 1497–502
24. Taylor, K. J. W., Granum, P. T. and De Cherney, A. H. (1987). Research lessons for maternal-fetal research from reproductive system studies. In Maulik, D. and McNellis, D. (eds). *Reproductive and Perinatal Medicine. Doppler Ultrasound Measurement of Maternal Fetal Hemodynamics*, p. 192–8. (New York: Perinatology Press)
25. Nett, T. M. and Niswander, G. D. (1981). Luteal blood flow and receptors for LH during PGF2-alpha induced luteolysis: production of PGE2 and PGF2-alpha during early pregnancy. *Acta Vet. Scand.*, **77**, 117–30
26. Yanaginachi, R. (1988). Mammalian fertilization. In Knobil, E. and Neil, J. (eds.) *The Physiology of Reproduction*, p. 135–46 (New York: Raven Press)
27. Pedersen, R. A. (1988). Early mammalian embryogenesis. In Knobil, E. and Neil, J. (eds.) *The Physiology of Reproduction*, p. 187–98. (New York: Raven Press)
28. Timor-Tritsch, I. E., Peisner, D. B., and Rajn, S. (1990). Sonoembryology: an organ oriented approach using a high frequency vaginal probe. *J. Clin. Ultrasound*, **18**, 286–98
29. Jurkovic, D., Jauniaux, E., Kurjak, A., Hustin, J., Campbell, S. and Nicolaides, K. H. (1991). Transvaginal color Doppler assessment of uteroplacental circulation in early pregnancy. *Obstet. Gynecol.*, **77**, 365–9
30. Jauniaux, E., Jurkovic, D. and Campbell, S. (1991). *In vivo* investigation of the anatomy and the physiology of early human placental circulations. *Ultrasound Obstet. Gynecol.*, **1**, 435–45
31. Gonen, Y., Casper, R. F., Jacobson, W. and Blankier, J. Endometrial thickness and growth during ovarian stimulation: a possible predictor of implantation in *in vitro* fertilization. *Fertil. Steril.*, **52**, 446–50
32. Smith, B., Porter, R., Ahuja, K. and Craft, I. (1984). Ultrasonic assessment of changes in stimulated cycles in in vitro fertilization and ET program. *J. In Vitro Fertil. Embryo Transfer*, **1**, 233–8
33. Nyberg, D. A. and Hill, L. M. (1992). Threatened abortion and abnormal first trimester intrauterine pregnancy. In Nyberg, D. A., Hill, L. M., Bohm-Velez, M. and Mendelson, E. B. (eds). *Transvaginal Ultrasound*, p. 85–103. (St Louis: Mosby)
34. de Crepigni, L. S. (1988). Early diagnosis of pregnancy failure with transvaginal ultrasound. *Am. J. Obstet. Gynecol.*, **159**, 408–9
35. Levi, C. S., Lyons, E. A. and Lindsay, D. J. (1988). Early diagnosis of nonviable pregnancy with endovaginal ultrasound. *Radiology*, **167**, 383–5
36. Bree, L. R., Edwards, M. and Bohm Velez, M. (1989). Transvaginal sonography in the evaluation of normal early pregnancy: correlation with beta hCG level. *Am. J. Radiol.*, **153**, 75–9
37. Rempen, A. (1990). Diagnosis of viability in early pregnancy with vaginal sonography. *J. Ultrasound Med.*, **9**, 711–6
38. Cacciatore, B., Titinen, A., Stenman, U. H. and Ylostalo, P. (1990). Normal early pregnancy: serum hCG level and vaginal sonography findings. *Br. J. Obstet. Gynecol.*, **97**, 889–903
39. Glissant, A., de Mouzon, J. and Frydman, R. (1985). Ultrasound study of the endometrium during *in vitro* fertilization cycles. *Fertil. Steril.*, **44**, 786–90

40. Fleischer, A., Herbert, C. M., Hill, G. A., Keppler, D. M. and Worrell, J. A. (1991). Transvaginal sonography of the endometrium during induced cycles. *J. Ultrasound Med.*, **10**, 93–5
41. Goswamy, R. K. and Steptoe, P. C. (1988). Doppler ultrasound studies of the uterine artery in spontaneous ovarian cycles. *Hum. Reprod.*, **3**, 721–4
42. Long, M. C., Boultbee, J. E., Hanson, M. E. and Begent, R. H. J. (1989). Doppler time velocity waveform studies of the uterine artery and uterus. *Br. J. Obstet. Gynecol.*, **96**, 588–93
43. Goswamy, R. K., Williams, S. G. and Steptoe, P. C. (1988). Decreased uterine perfusion – a cause of infertility. *Hum. Reprod.*, **3**, 955–9
44. Steer, C. V., Mulls, C. L. and Campbell, S. (1991). Vaginal colour Doppler assessment on the day of embryo transfer accurately predicts patients in an *in vitro* fertilization programe with suboptimal uterine perfusion who fail to become pregnant. *Ultrasound Obstet. Gynecol.*, **1**, 79–80
45. Kupesic, S. and Kurjak, A. (1993). Uterine and ovarian perfusion during the preovulatory period assisted by transvaginal color Doppler. *Fertil. Steril.*, **60**, 439–43
46. Pijnenborg, R., Bland, J. M., Robertson, W. B., Dixon, G. and Brosens, I. (1990). The pattern of interstitial invasion of the myometrium in early human pregnancy. *Placenta*, **3**, 19–21
47. De Wolf, F. C., De Wolf-Peeters, C., Brosens, I. and Robertson, W. B. (1979). The human placental bed: electron microscopic study of trophoblastic invasion of spiral arteries. *Am. J. Obstet. Gynecol.*, **137**, 58–70
48. Pijnenborg, R., Bland, J. M., Robertson, W. B. and Brosens, I. (1983). Uteroplacental arterial changes related to interstitial trophoblast migration in early human pregnancy. *Placenta*, **4**, 397–414
49. Jauniaux, E., Jurkovic, D., Kurjak, A. and Hustin, J. (1991). Assessment of placental development and function. In Kurjak, A. (ed). *Transvaginal Color Doppler*, p. 53–60. (Carnforth: Parthenon Publishing)
50. Jaffe, R. and Warsof, S. L. (1991). Transvaginal color Doppler imaging in the assessment of uteroplacental blood flow in the normal first trimester of pregnancy. *Am. J. Obstet. Gynecol.*, **164**, 781–5
51. Kurjak, A., Kupesic-Urek, S. and Predanic, M. (1992). Transvaginal color Doppler in the study of early pregnancies associated with fibroids. *J. Maternal Fetal Invest.*, **2**, 81–3
52. Deutinger, J., Rudelstorfer, R. and Bernarschek, G. (1988). Vaginosonographic velocimetry of both main uterine arteries by visual vessel recognition and pulsed Doppler method during pregnancy. *Am. J. Obstet. Gyencol.*, **159**, 1072–4
53. Kurjak, A., Miljan, M. and Zalud, I. (1990). Transabdominal and transvaginal color Doppler in the assessment of fetomaternal circulation during all three trimesters of pregnancy. *Eur. J. Obstet. Gynecol. Reprod. Biol.*, **36**, 240–6
54. Schulman, H., Fleischer, A. and Farmakides, G. (1986). Development of uterine artery compliance in pregnancy as detected by Doppler ultrasound. *Am. J. Obstet. Gynecol.*, **155**, 103–5
55. Stabile, I., Bilardo, C. and Patella, M. (1988). Doppler measurement of uterine artery blood flow in the first trimester of normal and complicated pregnancies. *Trophoblast*, **3**, 301–4
56. Hustin, J. and Schaaps, J. P. (1987). Echographic and anatomic studies of the materno-trophoblastic border during the first trimester of pregnancy. *Am. J. Obstet. Gynecol.*, **157**, 162–3
57. Wladimiroff, J. W., Huisman, T. W. A. and Stewart, P. A. (1991). Fetal cardiac flow velocities in the late first trimester of pregnancy: a transvaginal Doppler study. *J. Am. Coll. Cardiol.*, **17**, 1357–9
58. Wladimiroff, J. W., Huisman, T. W. A. and Stewart, P. A. Intracerebral, aortic and umbilical artery flow velocity waveforms in the late first trimester fetus. *Am. J. Obstet. Gynecol.*, **166**, 46–9
59. Kupesic, S. and Kurjak, A. (1994). Development of an early human being from conception to implantation – transvaginal color Doppler study. In Kurjak, A. (ed). *Atlas of Transvaginal Color Doppler.*, pp.15–26 (Carnforth: Parthenon Publishing)
60. Nillson, L. (1990). Dangers on the way. In Nillson, L. (ed.) *A Child is Born*, pp. 69–71. (London: Transworld Publishers Ltd)

The use of transvaginal sonography in the dynamic evaluation of the uterine cervix in pregnancy

I. E. Timor-Tritsch, F. Boozarjomehri and A. Monteagudo

INTRODUCTION

Intensive studies aimed at preventing premature labor and delivery have yielded partial and disappointing progress. Uterine contractions detected by intermittent monitoring and subjective pelvic (digital) examination to detect the slightest changes in the qualities of the cervix, have had and will continue to have a low threshold for the initiation of immediate treatment. The rate of false-positive diagnosis is high. This treatment policy results in unnecessary hospitalization and wastes provider time and medication. The mother and fetus are also exposed to the potential adverse effects of medication.

The definition of premature labor relates to the perception of changes in the length (effacement) and in the dilatation of the cervix over a relatively short time, about 2 h, in the presence of detectable uterine activity. Palpation of the cervix was, and still is, the 'gold standard' for evaluation of the pregnant woman, using the scoring system developed by Bishop in 1964[1]. In spite of its low predictive value for inducibility as well as its subjectiveness and at times roughness, cervical examination is still widely used[2-4].

More objective evaluation of the cervix is required, since bimanual examination cannot evaluate the cervix above the vaginal vault and, even more importantly, cannot assess the shape of the internal os. Such evaluation may prove to be of importance in predicting impending labor or inducibility. During the last 8–10 years, transvaginal sonography (TVS) has become a valuable tool in the diagnostic and therapeutic armamentarium of the modern obstetrician and gynecologist. The vaginal ultrasound probe has the ability to furnish important information about the pelvic organs and their pathology. At times this information is more precise and objective than that provided by digital palpation. If the accuracy and the objectivity of anatomical investigations using transvaginal sonography is superior to the bimanual pelvic examination, why is it not used in labor and delivery suites or in obstetrical triage areas to evaluate the cervix? Possible answers may be that the relatively scant data in the literature are read and applied by few, and that vaginal transducer probes are not available in delivery suites. However, our feeling is that the use of ultrasound in the office and triage area is not sufficiently encouraged by those in charge of residency training.

This chapter reviews the available and pertinent literature and describes the technique of cervical evaluation by TVS in pregnancy. Some of our original work is also included, as well as discussion of the future applications of this technique.

BACKGROUND AND LITERATURE REVIEW

In spite of the fact that the Bishop score was developed to evaluate the cervix for inducibility[1], this chapter will deal with a more general aspect of cervical examination, the early detection of premature labor, as well as a more accurate prediction of inducibility of labor. Even prior to the articles published by Bishop[1] and Burnett[5] cervical effacement and 'ripeness' were found to be important in predicting the duration of labor[6].

Reading the pertinent literature in chronological order it is easy to detect the increasing dissatisfaction with the performance of these scoring systems. A constant search for better prognostic indices for patients in need of an efficient and successful induction of labor is also evident. Evaluating the predictive value of the Bishop score on the duration of labor, Lange and colleagues[7] found that the only significant factor was degree of dilatation. According to their study, dilatation should be weighted twice as high as station and effacement, while consistency and position should only given only half its present influence.

Ultrasonographic evaluation of the cervix was initiated as early as 1980[8-11]. However, the first studies comparing the transvaginal and the transabdominal sonographic approach were reported by Brown and co-workers in 1986[12]. In this study, it was stated that 'the transvaginal technique may be superior in obtaining an adequate evaluation of the lower uterine segment and cervix'. An added and special value of this article is that the terms of normal, Y-shaped, ballooning (U-shaped) and funneling (V-shaped) cervices were introduced. However, no clinical correlations with cervical shapes were attempted.

Kushnir and co-workers[13] measured cervical length using TVS in normal pregnancies at 8–37 weeks' gestation. The cervix was longest (4.8 cm) at 20–25 weeks and length then declined after 32 weeks. The main problem with their study is that cervical length measurements are not defined. Soneck and colleagues[14] compared TVS to measurements of the cervix derived from digital examination in pregnancy. In this double blind study, digital examination underestimated cervical length in the 2nd and 3rd trimester of the pregnancy by 1.0–1.4 cm in about 90% of cases, and overestimated length by 0.4 cm in about 10% of cases. They concluded that evaluation of cervical length by TVS is more objective.

Andersen and associates[15,16] made significant contributions to the application of TVS to the study of the pregnant uterine cervix to predict premature labor. Another important study is that of Paterson-Brown and co-workers[17], in which assessment of the Bishop score was compared to TVS. They found that patient discomfort was significantly less with TVS and determination of the posterior cervical angle by TVS predicted vaginal delivery better than digital examination. Better results can be achieved by combining the two methods.

In 1992, three important articles appeared. Smith and colleagues[18] concluded that cervical width increases but length does not change with gestational age. After 37 weeks, however, cervical length slightly decreases. A blinded study of the accuracy of ultrasound in measuring the cervix was undertaken in women before hysterectomy by Jackson and co-workers[19]. Digital, transabdominal and TVS results were compared to postoperative ruler measurements of the uterine cervix: digital examination underestimated the cervical length by 1.4 cm. Another study[20] prospectively compared TVS and digital examination of the cervix in the third trimester of pregnancy. Digital examination overestimated dilatation and underestimated cervical length. Okitsu and associates described funneling of the cervix as a predictor of premature delivery[21]. Transvaginal sonographic evaluation of the incompetent cervix was studied also by Quinn and co-workers[22]. In an original study, Guzman and colleagues used TVS to evaluate the risk of cervical incompetence by applying fundal pressure and observing the shape of the cervix[23]. They concluded that the application of transfundal pressure helped in the sonographic evaluation of the cervix detecting the assymptomatic incompetent cervix.

It is obvious that an abundance of articles have recently been published on the so far relatively neglected subject of the uterine cervix. Most of these studies have been directed towards the incompetent cervix in the late first and early second trimester and towards describing changes which may allow early detection of true premature labor.

ANATOMY AND TECIINIQUE

The sonographic anatomy of the cervix is simple. First, it is important to stress that the picture is obtained on the sagittal plane: images generated from coronal planes have not been found to be clinically useful.

Using TVS, which according to the available literature is the 'gold standard' for evaluation of the cervix, a sagittal picture is sought. If the apex of the 'slice' points upwards, that is, the transducer approaches the cervix from the top of the picture, the following ultrasound picture is obtained (Figure 1):

(1) The vagina (v) is flanked anteriorly by the ureter (u) leading to the bladder, and posteriorly by the hyperechoic rectum (r).

(2) The cervical canal is almost at a right angle to the vagina. The tip of the transducer will first touch the anterior lip of the cervix; however, both lips of the cervix are seen (c).

(3) The body of the anteverted uterus is situated below the urinary bladder. Different measurements of the cervical anatomy are possible:

   (a) cervical length, measured from the internal to the external os. Problems may arise in finding or defining the exact location of the internal os (this will be discussed later);

   (b) cervical width or thickness, measured from the outer boundaries of the anterior to the posterior cervical lips.

   (c) cervical dilatation, measured close to the external os.

The shape of the internal os can be determined by assessing the area of interest. Basically we agree to the previously proposed T-shaped (Figure 2), U-shaped (Figure 3) and V-shaped ('funneling') internal os (Figure 4).

When examining the cervix by TVS, the presence of relatively sonolucent cervical glands and at times the thick, echogenic mucous plug render a peculiar sonographic picture to this area. These structures have to be recognized and differentiated from the underlying true shape of the cervix.

It is imperative to find the optimal transducer tip location to produce the best possible image. The clearest picture with the greatest resolution will obviously be obtained if the cervix is within the focal range of the probe. If the transducer is not inserted deeply enough within the vagina

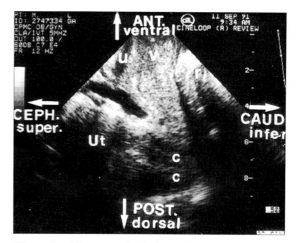

Figure 1 *The anatomical relationships seen by the transvaginal probe in the sagittal plane. The probe was situated in the lower 1/4 of the vagina. Note the three parallel structures: the urethra (u), vagina (v) and the rectum (r) at right angles to the uterus and cervical axis. The anterior and posterior cervical lips are seen (c). The arrows indicate the anatomical orientation of the image*

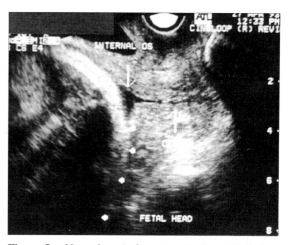

Figure 2 *Normal cervical anatomy in the sagittal plane on TVS*

a blurred image will result and the posterior cervical lip will probably not be imaged at all. Conversely, if the tip of the probe is placed deep into the vagina, past the cervix and into the posterior vaginal vault, only the bowel and its contents will be scanned.

The best image is usually obtained if the tip of the probe is about 1–2 cm from the anterior cervical lip or slightly touching it. The best position can be determined by a push-pull motion of the probe.

ONGOING RESEARCH

In a study including 53 patients scheduled for elective induction of labor, digital examination and TVS of the cervix in the sagittal plane were performed before induction (Boozarjomehri and colleagues, unpublished). The presence or the absence of cervical wedging at the level of the internal os were assessed, and the confounding effects of parity, previous dilatation and curettage and administration of prostaglandins were controlled for.

The results showed a significant association between the duration of the latent phase and the presence of wedging, as well as cervical length measured by TVS. There was no association between total labor duration and the results of digital examination of the cervical dilatation and effacement. A shorter total labor duration was associated with the presence of wedging (Table 1). We concluded that assessment of cervical length and wedging by TVS are better predictors of induction of labor and its duration than is initial digital assessment of cervical anatomy.

In another study (Timor-Tritsch and colleagues, unpublished) we addressed the problem of prematurity resulting from premature

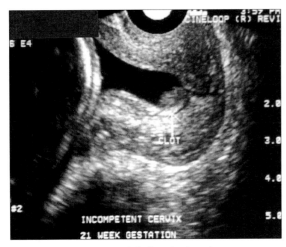

Figure 3 *The U-shaped 'ballooning' cervix*

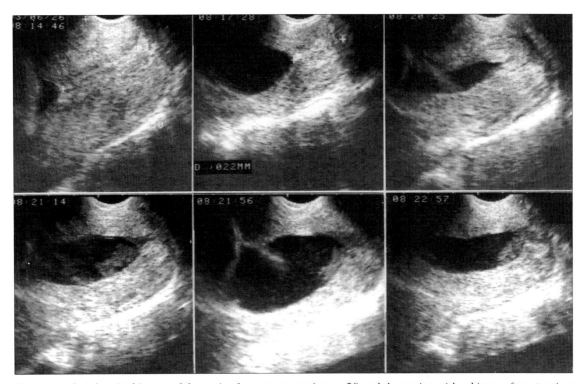

Figure 4 *Serial sagittal images of the cervix of a pregnant patient at 29 weeks' gestation with a history of two previous preterm deliveries. The six consecutive images, recorded within 9 min, show a progressive change in the cervical length from 35 mm (first image on the upper left) to 22 mm, and less during a uterine contraction. In spite of treatment the labor progressed and she delivered 10 h later*

Table 1 *Relationship between the presence of cervical wedging and duration of labor (h ± SEM)*

	Wedge	No wedge	p
Latent phase duration (h)	16.1 ± 1.7	32.9 ± 3.8	< 0.001
Total labor duration (h)	21.9 ± 1.9	37.9 ± 3.5	< 0.001

labor. Admission to hospital and treatment are usually based on a report of contractions by the patient herself, 'documented' contractions on an external monitor, and digital examination of the cervix. All of these assessments are either subjective or relative evaluations leading to overtreatment. The aim of the study was to identify a more objective method to discriminate between true and false premature labor. A sagittal section of the cervix was studied by TVS in 86 patients evaluated for threatened premature labor. This assessment was undertaken prior to therapy and the information was not used in determining treatment. The presence or absence of a wedge at the internal os as well as the cervical length were noted. Forty-five of the 86 patients had no wedge and 41 had a wedged configuration of the internal os. Forty-one of the 'non-wedged' group delivered at term, whereas 26 of the 'wedged' group delivered preterm and 15 at term. These preliminary results suggest that in patients with threatened premature labor the absence of cervical wedging was associated with term deliveries: these patients therefore had 'false labor'. The presence of wedging, on the other hand, was suggestive of true premature labor and these patients may require aggressive management. A 'snapshot' view of the cervix in the sagittal plane by TVS appeared a more reliable method of cervical evaluation than those currently used.

Figure 4 exemplifies the progress of cervical anatomy in a patient at risk for premature labor and the dynamic changes in the shape of the lower segment and the internal os.

COMMENTS

As seen from the literature and in our studies, evaluation of cervical anatomy by digital examination only is flawed by large errors. The error encountered in estimating cervical length and dilatation originates from two main sources. The first is the fact that digital palpation can probe only the outer half (vaginal portion) of the cervix and that all changes related to wedging and effacement start from the inner end of the cervical canal. Digital examination therefore cannot estimate true cervical length.

The second source of problems encountered in evaluating the cervix arises from the very fact that the fingers of the examiner are unable to determine the shape and configuration of the internal os and its adjacent structures, such as the lower uterine segment. The different shapes of the internal os described in the literature and observed in our studies, which are probably of importance in predicting inducibility or impending premature labor, cannot be perceived.

Towards the end of the latent phase of labor, at or after a dilatation of 3–4 cm and an 'effacement' of 90–100%, it becomes increasingly difficult to identify the cervix. At or after this stage in labor the digital pelvic examination is superior to TVS in its accuracy.

Technically, TVS of the cervix is easily applicable to all patients in the labor and delivery suites and takes a few minutes to perform. It is faster than any other routine ultrasound procedure performed in the labor and delivery rooms, such as fluid monitoring or confirming the presenting part of the fetus. It seems particularly useful in patients who are obese, or have cervices that are hard to reach, resulting in painful bimanual pelvic examinations. The procedure is well tolerated by the patients.

In a busy labor and delivery suite, where efficiency and a fast turnover are important, inappropriate evaluation for induction resulting from a subjective cervical examination results not only in improper use of resources and an eventual increase in the number of Cesarean sections but also in maternal exhaustion and frustration.

On the other hand, for more objective evaluation of the cervix in high-risk patients, sonographic evaluation has the potential to reduce the number of diagnoses of true premature labor. In doing so resources such as administration of potent drugs, hospitalization and use of various electronic and mechanical home monitoring devices can be undertaken more judiciously.

Based on the available literature on this subject and our experience in using TVS to determine cervical anatomy in a dynamic fashion, we recommend its use along with bimanual palpation.

References

1. Bishop, E. H. (1964). Pelvic scoring for elective induction. *Obstet. Gynecol.*, **24**, 266–8
2. Friedman, E. A., Niswander, K. R., Bayonet-Rievera, N. P. and Sachtleben, M. R. (1966). Relation of prelabor evaluation to inducibility and the course of labor. *Obstet. Gynecol.*, **28**, 495–501
3. Hughes, M. J., McElin, T. W. and Bird, C. C. (1976). An evaluation of pre-induction scoring systems. *Obstet. Gynecol.*, **48**, 635–41
4. Dhall, K., Mittal, S. C. and Kumar, A. (1987). Evaluation of pre-induction scoring systems. *Aust. NZ J. Obstet. Gynaecol.*, **27**, 309–11
5. Burnett, J. E. (1966). Preinduction scoring: An objective approach to induction of labor. *Obstet. Gynecol.*, **28**, 479–83
6. Calkins, L. A. (1941). On predicting the length of labor. *Am. J. Obstet. Gynecol.*, **42**, 802–6
7. Lange, A. P., Secher, N. J., Westergaard, J. G. and Skovgard, I. B. (1982). Prelabor evaluation of inducibility. *Obstet. Gynecol.*, **60**, 137–47
8. Fried, A. (1981). Bulging amnion in premature labor: spectrum of sonographic findings. *Am. J. Radiol.*, **136**, 181–5
9. Parulekar, S. G. and Kiwi, R. (1982). Ultrasound evaluation of sutures following cervical cerclage for incompetent cervix uteri. *J. Ultrasound Med.*, **1**, 223–8
10. Bowie, J. D., Andreotti, R. F. and Rosenberg, E. L. (1983). Sonographic appearance of the uterine cervix in pregnancy: The vertical cervix. *Am. J. Radiol.*, **140**, 737–40
11. Bartolucci, L., Hill, W., Katz, M., Gill, P. and Kitzmiller, J. (1984). Ultrasonography in preterm labor. *Am. J. Obstet. Gynecol.*, **149**, 52–6
12. Brown, J. E., Thiema, G. A., Shah, D. M., Fleischer, A. C. and Boehm, F. H. (1986). Transabdominal and transvaginal endosonography evaluation of the cervix and lower uterine segment in pregnancy. *Am. J. Obstet. Gynecol.*, **155**, 721–6
13. Kushnir, O., Vigil, D. A., Izquierdo, L., Schiff, M. and Curet, L. B. (1990). Vaginal sonographic assessment of cervical length changes during normal pregnancy. *Am. J. Obstet. Gynecol.*, **162**, 991–3
14. Soneck, J. D., Iams, J. D., Blumenfeld, M., Johnson, F., Landon, M. and Gabbe, S. (1990). Measurement of cervical length in pregnancy: comparison between vaginal ultrasonography and digital examination. *Obstet. Gynecol.*, **76**, 172–5
15. Andersen, H. F., Nugent, C. E., Wanty, S. D. and Hayashi, R. H. (1990). Prediction of risk for preterm delivery by ultrasonographic measurement of cervical length. *Am. J. Obstet. Gynecol.*, **163**, 859–67
16. Andersen, H. F. (1991). Transabdominal and transvaginal sonography of the uterine cervix during pregnancy. *J. Clin. Ultrasound*, **19**, 77–82
17. Paterson-Brown, S., Fisk, N. M., Rodeck, C. H. and Rodeck, E. Preinduction cervical assessment by Bishop's score and transvaginal ultrasound. *Eur. J. Obstet. Gynecol. Reprod. Biol.*, **40**, 17–23
18. Smith, C. V., Anderson, J. C., Matamoros, A. and Rayburn, W. F. (1992). Transvaginal sonography of cervical width and length during pregnancy. *J. Ultrasound Med.*, **11**, 465–7
19. Jackson, G. M., Ludmir, J. and Bader, T. J. (1992). The accuracy of digital examination and ultrasound in the evaluation of cervical length. *Obstet. Gynecol.*, **79**, 214–8
20. Lim, B. H., Mahmood, T. A., Smith, N. C. and Beat, I. (1992). A prospective comparative study of transvaginal ultrasonography and digital examination of cervical assessment in the third trimester of pregnancy. *J. Clin. Ultrasound*, **20**, 599–603
21. Okitsu, O., Mimura, T., Nakayama, T. and Aono, T. (1992). Early prediction of preterm delivery by transvaginal ultrasonography. *Ultrasound Obstet. Gynecol.* **2**, 402–9
22. Quinn, M. J. (1992). Vaginal ultrasound and cervical cerclage: A prospective study. *Ultrasound Obstet. Gynecol.*, **2**, 410–6
23. Guzman, E. R., Rosenberg, J. C., Houlihan, C., Ivan, J., Waldon, R. and Knuppel, R. (1993). A new method using vaginal ultrasound and transfundal pressure to evaluate the asymptomatic incompetent cervix. *Obstet. Gynecol.*, **83**, 248–52

Section 3

Assessment of the fetal condition

High-order multiple pregnancy

S. Mashiach, D. S. Seidman and S. Lipitz

The incidence of pregnancies with three or more fetuses has markedly increased over the past two decades. This change has been attributed to the introduction and widespread use of new techniques for ovulation induction and placement of multiple embryos during *in vitro* fertilization (IVF)[1–3]. This has been a matter of concern since triplet and higher multiple pregnancies have long been associated with an increased risk of maternal complications, and a high prevalence of perinatal and neonatal morbidity and mortality[4–8]. Furthermore, increased experience with multifetal pregnancy reduction offers a new option for the management of these pregnancies. This has increased the focus on the need to evaluate the management and outcome of these high-risk pregnancies.

INCIDENCE

The incidence of triplets or higher order multiple pregnancies depends to a large extent on the use of infertility agents in a given population. Petrikovsky and Vinzeleos[9] have stressed the influence of genetic and geographic factors. They reported an incidence of triplets that varied from 1/612 in the Yorube tribe in Western Nigeria to 1/7925 in the USA. In a recent series of 78 triplet pregnancies, we found an incidence of 1/849 deliveries[10]. This high incidence was due to the use of fertility treatment, as only 12% of the triplet pregnancies were conceived spontaneously. Ovulation was induced by human menopausal gonadotropin (hMG) and human chorionic gonadotropin (hCG) in 50% of the pregnancies. Clomiphene citrate administration accounted for 29% of pregnancies and the remaining 9% resulted from IVF. The prevalence of spontaneous triplet pregnancies that reached 20 weeks' gestation was 1/7358 deliveries[10]. Our data are in agreement with other recent studies. A report from the British Association of Perinatal Medicine[3] found that among 156 high-order multiple births in 1989 (143 triplets, 12 quadruplets and one quintuplet), 31% were conceived naturally, 34% had ovarian stimulation, (usually with clomiphene citrate or gonadotropins) and 35% had IVF. All quadruplet and quintuplet pregnancies were established after assisted reproduction.

The incidence of quadruplet pregnancies has been reported from 1/5370 to 1/600 000, while the birth of quintuplets is considered to be a rare event which occurs once in 15–20 million deliveries. In our recent series[11] we found an incidence of 1/9190 (eight of 73 527 deliveries) for quadruplet and 1/24 500 for higher multiple gestation (two quintuplets and one sextuplet). All pregnancies resulted from ovulation induction therapy with hMG and hCG.

Thus, it is evident that treatment of infertility has resulted in a dramatic increase in the number of triplets and high-order multiple births in developed countries; for example, in the United States, a 113% increase was observed from 1972 to 1989[12]. Ovulation stimulating drugs accounted for 50% of 1138 triplet pregnancies delivered in the United States[1]. Similarly, in Britain there has been a marked increase in the number of triplets born since the late 1970s, as well as a fourfold increase in the number of higher multiple births between 1971 and 1983, when compared with the 15-year period 1956–1970[3]. This marked increase in the numbers of high-order multiple births seems to be continuing[2,3].

Table 1 *Birth weight distribution and perinatal mortality in high-order multifetal pregnancies (quadruplets and more). (From Reference 11)*

Weight (g)	Number of fetuses	Stillbirth	Livebirth	Neonatal deaths	Perinatal deaths
< 500	7	6	1	1	7
500–749	5	3	2	0	3
750–999	10	0	10	1	1
1000–1499	16	0	16	0	0
1500–2000	10	0	10	0	0
Total	48	9	39	2	11

PRETERM LABOR

Preterm labor is the major complication of multifetal pregnancies. The risk of preterm labor and delivery rises with the number of fetuses in multifetal gestations[13]. The incidence of preterm labor in triplet pregnancies (< 37 completed gestational weeks) has been reported in recent studies to be as high as 66%[14], 80%[15] and 86%[10]. The risk is even greater still for higher multiple pregnancies. In our series of high-order multifetal pregnancies[11], only one pregnancy continued up to the 35th week of gestation. Similarly, in a review of eight sets of quintuplets, only one set completed 36 weeks of pregnancy[9]. As could be expected from the rate of preterm deliveries, the average gestational age of triplet pregnancies has been reported as 33.6 ± 3.0 weeks (mean ± SD)[14], 33.8 ± 2.8 weeks[1], and 33.2 ± 3.8 weeks[10], with a mean birth weight of 1871 ± 555 g[14], and 1911 ± 521 g[1]. For quadruplets, an average gestational age at the time of delivery was reported as 31.1 ± 6.8 weeks[9]. In our series, 74% of the 39 liveborn infants from high-order multifetal gestation weighed < 1500 g and 41% were below the tenth percentile for gestational age[11] (Table 1).

PERINATAL MORTALITY

Perinatal mortality rises progressively with the number of fetuses. Rates of 164, 200, 214 and 416 per 1000 births have been reported for triplets, quadruplets, quintuplets and sextuplets, respectively[16].

In our recent studies[10,11] we have found a perinatal mortality rate of 93 and 119 per 1000 deliveries for triplets and higher multiple births, respectively. These relatively low perinatal rates may reflect advances in perinatal and neonatal care. However, the mortality rates of extremely low birth weight infants have remained high, and in all likelihood could be reduced in the future. The mortality rates in our triplet series[10] were similar to those reported for twin gestations by the Oxford National Perinatal Epidemiology Unit[16] in England and Wales from 1975 to 1983, taking into account the exclusion of stillbirths before 28 weeks' gestation.

MANAGEMENT

The management of high-order multifetal pregnancies is controversial[5,6,10,14,17,18]. In view of the rarity of the condition and the complexity of the individual cases, it is unlikely that therapeutic regimens will be evaluated by randomized prospective studies. The basic aim of antenatal management is to prolong gestation. Early diagnosis of multiple pregnancy by routine ultrasound has been claimed to reduce the risk of preterm delivery and prenatal mortality[19]. Although many other factors could have contributed to the improved outcome, it is clear that early identification of these high-risk pregnancies could lead to improved diagnosis of early signs of preterm labor[13]. Prediction of preterm labor due to the detection of early ripening of the cervix through clinical or ultrasound examination has been attempted in twin pregnancies[13]. The commercially available home uterine activity monitor may aid in the identification of antepartum uterine contraction and thus provide an early warning of preterm labor[20,21]. However, their value in multiple pregnancies remains controversial[14]. An interesting observation in twin pregnancies was recently made by Neilson and Crowther[13]. They found that symphysis–fundal height measurements were inversely correlated with length of gestation. They concluded that their findings strongly suggest that the commonly accepted theory that preterm labor in twin pregnancies results simply from uterine over-distension is incorrect. The extent to which this observation can be implied to high-order multifetal gestations is not yet clear.

TREATMENT STRATEGIES

Three major treatment strategies have been tried in order to prevent preterm labor: rest, uterine tocolysis and cervical cerclage.

Rest

Hospitalization for rest in triplet and high-order multiple pregnancies has been routinely recommended at 27–28 weeks' gestation[5,10,11]. While the value of hospitalization for rest has been strongly questioned in studies investigating twin pregnancies[22–24], little data are available regarding high-order multifetal pregnancies. Newman and colleagues[14], in a contemporary series of 198 women, showed that outpatient triplet management results in a favorable outcome with a remarkable saving in hospital days through the avoidance of routine hospitalization. Crowther and co-workers[25] reported beneficial effects of hospitalization for bed rest. They observed a reduced incidence of preterm delivery, and a reduced incidence of very low and low birth weight. However, it should be noted that the study was a small trial of only 19 women with a triplet pregnancy, and thus the differences were compatible with chance variation. In our department, from 1970 to 1988, patients were routinely hospitalized in the high-risk pregnancy unit at 27–28 weeks' gestation. However, since 1989, home uterine monitoring was used and patients were not routinely hospitalized. Only a multicenter trial will ensure a sample size adequate for the full evaluation of the policy of routine hospitalization in the third trimester of triplet pregnancies[13].

Tocolysis

Tocolytics are commonly prescribed in high-order multifetal pregnancies[11,14]. The effectiveness of prophylactic tocolysis remains, however, a most controversial issue[13]. Seven randomized trials have been reported to date, examining a variety of oral β-mimetics in twin pregnancies. A meta-analysis of these trials showed no effect on the incidence of preterm delivery, birth weight or neonatal mortality, although a reduction in the risk of respiratory distress syndrome was evident[26]. To date, no randomized trials have been published regarding the use of prophylactic tocolysis in high-order multifetal pregnancies. Furthermore, it should be remembered that the use of β-mimetics in women with multifetal gestations is associated with a greater risk of complications, such as pulmonary edema[27]. One retrospective study[5] found no differences in the average length of triplet gestation between eight women who received β-adrenergic agents prophylactically, compared to six women who received no prophylactic tocolysis. Eleven other women with triplet pregnancies who received a combination of prophylactic oral β-mimetics and intramuscular progesterone actually shortened the pregnancy by almost 2 weeks[5]. Newman and colleagues[14] found that the use of prophylactic tocolysis was not associated with any clear improvement in either gestational age or birth weight at the time of delivery. These authors noted that their findings may be a result of a selection bias, as practitioners may have been more likely to use prophylactic tocolysis in cases which they perceived to be at greatest risk[14].

The role of tocolysis in preterm labor in triplet pregnancies has not been determined. Itzkowic[28] was successful in delaying delivery for more than 48 h in three of seven women. Holchberg and co-workers[6] achieved a similar delay in labor using tocolysis in four of five women. Newman and associates[14] reported a mean time gain *in utero* of almost 4 weeks for women with triplet pregnancies who received tocolysis.

The role of other tocolytic drugs such as the prostaglandin synthetase inhibitor, indomethacin, or the calcium antagonist, nifedipine, have not been evaluated yet for high-order multifetal pregnancies[29]. Our preliminary experience with nifedipine has revealed an apparent beneficial effect which is more pronounced in multiple pregnancies including twins (unpublished data). Controlled trials are needed to evaluate the use of these tocolytic agents in multifetal pregnancies.

Cervical cerclage

Two randomized trials have been undertaken to examine the value of cervical cerclage in twin pregnancies[30,31]. A meta-analysis of the two studies[32] was based on data from only 78 twin gestations, and failed to reveal a significant benefit of cervical cerclage in terms of prolongation of pregnancy or the improvement of fetal outcome. No randomized trials of the use of cervical cerclage have been reported to date in high-order gestations. In a retrospective study, Itzkowic[28] concluded that triplet pregnancies were not associated with cervical incompetence, and gestation did not appear to be prolonged by cervical ligation. Newman and colleagues[14] found that the seven women who received cerclage had a generally poor outcome with an average gestational age at delivery of 29.2 ± 4.2 weeks and a birth weight of 1271 ± 489 g. They suggested that the poorer obstetric performance of these women may be biased by the fact that most cerclages were placed only after the discovery of early cervical change.

In our series of 78 triplet pregnancies that reached a gestational age of 20 weeks or more, cervical cerclage was performed in 26 patients[10]. Elective cerclage was performed in 16 patients at the end of the first trimester, and in the remaining ten at between 17 and 27 weeks of gestation, because of progressive cervical dilatation. The length of gestation, the proportion of pregnancies that reached 26 weeks' gestation, and the total fetal and neonatal losses were similar in patients who underwent elective cerclage, as compared to all other patients. Three of the ten patients in whom late cerclage was performed did not achieve a gestation of 26 weeks; however, pregnancies were prolonged by 3–5 weeks in this group.

Since elective cervical cerclage was neither found to prolong gestation nor to decrease fetal loss, we no longer recommend elective cerclage in multifetal pregnancies.

MODE OF DELIVERY

The mode of delivery of triplet and higher multifetal pregnancies has never been examined in a randomized study. In a previous series of triplet pregnancies from the late 1970s and early 1980s[5–8,18,29,33] the vaginal route was the most frequently chosen mode of delivery. Cesarean sections were performed only in cases of obstetric complications. One of the major changes in contemporary care of high-order multifetal pregnancies has been the dramatic trend towards universal use of Cesarean delivery. Newman and colleagues[14] reported a Cesarean section rate of 94% in a series of 198 triplets delivered between 1985 and 1988. They suggested that Cesarean delivery may improve the prognosis for subsequent triplet births by avoidance of complications such as delivery trauma, intrapartum cord prolapse, placental abruption, and subtle alterations in uteroplacental blood flow.

An active policy decision to attempt delivery of all triplets of > 26 weeks' gestation by Cesarean section was taken in our department in 1979, and thereby ensured the presence of senior obstetric, neonatal and anesthesiology staff at all deliveries. In our recent series of 81 triplet pregnancies of 26 weeks' gestation or more, the Cesarean section rate was 93.8%[34]. We have previously reported an excess mortality in vaginally delivered triplet pregnancies which was attributable to fetuses delivered before 26 weeks' gestation[10]. Furthermore, our neonatal results, together with the follow-up data for very low birth weight infants, suggested an increased risk for infants delivered vaginally[10] (Table 2). We therefore believe that the low mortality and morbidity rates noted in our study[10] confirmed this approach, and we find little justification in

Table 2 *Mode of delivery and perinatal outcome in triplet pregnancies. (From Reference 10)*

	Vaginal		Cesarean section	
	n	%	n	%
Number of deliveries*	17**		60	
Total births†	40		182	
Stillbirths	7		2	
Livebirths	33		180	
Livebirths < 1000 g	3		14	
Perinatal deaths week of gestation†				
< 26	5/5	100.0	0/0	—
26–30	4/10	40.0	7/21	33.3
31–34	1/16	6.3	1/53	1.9
≥ 35	0/9	0.0	1/108	0.9
Total	10/40	25.0	9/182	4.9‡
Neonatal deaths	3	9.0	7	3.8

*One case excluded; **first fetus was delivered vaginally and the remaining two were delivered by Cesarean section; †excluding stillborn fetuses weighing < 500 g; ‡vaginal v.s. Cesarean section, $p < 0.001$

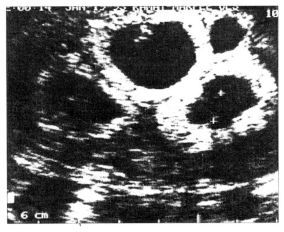

Figure 1 *Ultrasonography demonstrating four sacs of a 7-week quintuplet pregnancy*

attempting vaginal delivery in these high risk pregnancies.

Regarding high-order multifetal pregnancies, we recommend that a Cesarean section be performed in all cases[11]. An attempt should be made to schedule an elective Cesarean section in order to ensure the presence of an adequate number of experienced medical staff, especially neonatologists. However, in our series of high-order multifetal pregnancies[11], delivery was undertaken electively in only two patients. In the other seven women, timing of delivery was determined by the presence of active labor or rupture of membranes.

ANTENATAL ASSESSMENT OF INDIVIDUAL FETAL WELL-BEING

Antepartum care in multifetal pregnancies is complicated, since the monitoring techniques, including electronic fetal monitoring, ultrasonic estimation of fetal weight and growth, and measurement of umbilical blood flow are technically difficult and often not reproducible. Of the various modalities of antepartum fetal surveillance for triplet pregnancies, ultrasound seems to be the most appropriate (Figure 1). The non-stress test (NST), which was reported to be highly reliable for twin gestations[35], cannot reliably differentiate between the fetuses in high-order multifetal gestations.

The biophysical score (BPS) was used for fetal assessment in 35 triplet gestations in our department over a period of 6 years[36]. The results demonstrated that the specificity of the BPS for a 5-min Apgar score was high (94.9% per neonate). However, both sensitivity (14.3%), and positive predictive value (16.7%) of the BPS were found to be poor for the 5-min Apgar score. The sensitivity and specificity of the BPS for perinatal mortality were found to be 94.9% and 16.7%, respectively. These results are comparable to those reported by Manning and colleagues[37] for singleton pregnancies, in which a BPS of 6 had a positive predictive value of 9.16% for a low 5-min Apgar score, and 2.29% for neonatal death. According to our results, the BPS could not differentiate between distressed and normal fetuses from the same set of triplets. Three sets of triplets had an heterogenous outcome (normal and low 5-min Apgar scores) in the same set, and by using the BPS we could predict the outcome of these siblings.

Reports evaluating antepartum care in twin gestations have noted that fetal compromise can be detected using BPS and umbilical or uteroplacental Doppler techniques[38–40]. Lodeiro and associates, studying the relationship between last BPS before delivery and pregnancy outcome in twin gestation, reported sensitivity of 83.3%, specificity of 100%, false-positive rate of 0% and false-negative rate of 2.2%. These authors also reported that BPS could differentiate successfully between distressed and non-distressed siblings.

An important point to consider is whether an abnormal BPS in a single fetus in a triplet pregnancy is an indication to consider preterm delivery, thereby exposing the other fetuses with normal BPS to complications of prematurity. From our results, it seems that the discriminative potential of equivocal BPS is poor. Therefore, we suggest that consideration of preterm delivery should take place when the BPS of one fetus of a multifetal gestation is very abnormal (0–2), although this would have to be weighed against the degree of prematurity and other case-specific factors.

The overall value of the BPS in the management of triplet pregnancies appeared to be acceptable, although its sensitivity and specificity were lower than those reported for singleton and twin gestations.

Amniocentesis has been associated with an increase in the risk of pregnancy loss in cases of twin pregnancies[41]. Although no prospective study has examined the risk of amniocentesis in high-order multifetal pregnancies, this procedure is probably more hazardous in these gestations, and should be used with discretion for both prenatal diagnosis and antenatal evaluation of lung maturity.

THE EFFECT OF FERTILITY DRUGS AND IVF ON THE OUTCOME OF TRIPLET PREGNANCIES

The outcome of induced compared to spontaneous triplet pregnancies is a controversial subject. While some authors described a higher incidence of prematurity and low birth weight in babies born following induced conceptions[5,42], others have found these pregnancies to be associated with a more favorable outcome than spontaneous pregnancies[6,43,44].

Ron-El and associates[5] were among the first to observe that spontaneous triplet gestations lasted 2 weeks longer than induced pregnancies. Furthermore, in a more recent study, Mordel and colleagues[42] found that 17 triplets that were conceived following menotropin ovulation induction were delivered about 3–4 weeks earlier and weighed between 350 and 500 g less than seven impregnated spontaneously, or 12 following clomiphene citrate ovulation induction. In contrast to these disconcerting results, Holchberg and colleagues[6] compared nine induced triplet pregnancies to 12 spontaneous pregnancies, and observed that the latter were born 2.5 weeks earlier. It should be noted, however, that most of the above triplet gestations were induced with clomiphene citrate, rather than menotropins. One explanation for the discrepancies between the various studies has been put forward by Newman and co-workers[44]. They showed that the birth weight and gestational age advantage found in their large series for spontaneous triplets could be explained by the variance in fetal gender and maternal parity. Once these confounding factors were controlled for using a one-way analysis of variance (ANOVA), the advantage disappeared. Although the incidence of spontaneous triplets increases with age[1], among women undergoing IVF, multiple pregnancies are more common in younger patients[45]. Maternal age should therefore be considered as an additional confounding factor.

The outcome of triplet pregnancies following IVF has been subject to special concern[46]. In a recent study, we directly compared the results of IVF triplet pregnancies with spontaneous and ovulation-induced gestations[34]. Our results were reassuring with regard to the neonatal outcome. Despite the fact that a high rate of early pregnancy loss was observed in the IVF triplets (Table 3), the mean birth weight 1833 ± 458 g was comparable and the mean gestational age 33.9 ± 2.5 weeks was better than previously reported by Seoud and colleagues[45], 1666 ± 443 g and 31.8 ± 2.7 weeks, and by Kingsland and associates[47], 1850 g (range 720–2880 g) and 33.3 weeks (range 26–38 weeks). The still birth and prenatal mortality rates were also comparable to that previously reported regarding IVF trip-

Table 3 *Non-viable birth and perinatal mortality in triplet gestation according to conception mode. (From Reference 34)*

	Spontaneous		Clomiphene citrate		Menotropins		IVF	
	n	%	n	%	n	%	n	%
Non-viable birth (gestation ≤ 25 weeks) (n = no. of pregnancies)	1/7	14.3	3/16	18.8	12/56	21.4	9/27	33.3
Stillbirth* (n = no. of fetuses)	1/18	5.6	2/39	5.1	1/132	0.8	2/54	3.7
Neonatal mortality* (n = no. of fetuses)	1/17	5.9	4/37	108.1	5/131	3.8	1/52	1.9
Total fetal loss	5/21	23.8	15/48	31.3	42/168	25.0†	30/81	37.0†

*Pregnancies of 26 weeks' gestation or more; †$p < 0.01$ for comparison between groups IVF, *in vitro* fertilization

lets[48]. We concluded that induction of ovulation and IVF should not be considered a significant risk factor for the outcome of triplet pregnancies.

MULTIFETAL PREGNANCY REDUCTION

The procedure of multifetal pregnancy reduction has, in recent years, become both clinically and ethically accepted as a therapeutic option in pregnancies with four or more fetuses[49–55], and in multifetal pregnancies in which one or more of the fetuses have congenital abnormalities[50,56]. In cases of triplet gestations, however, this procedure remains controversial[49,55,57–59]. Reports of the improving outcome of triplet pregnancies[10,14], the failure to demonstrate an improvement in the outcome of triplet pregnancies reduced to twins as compared with those managed expectantly[57,58], and the procedure-related risk of losing the entire pregnancy[55,60] have complicated the clinical and ethical discussion surrounding this procedure in triplet gestations[51,53,54,56,57].

Consideration of the clinical options and the ethical issues involved in the management of triplet or high-order multifetal gestations must take into account the probability of achieving a successful pregnancy outcome if an expectant management policy is undertaken. Dickey and colleagues[61] reported that when three viable embryos were diagnosed at first trimester ultrasound, the probability of delivering triplets and twins was 68.4% and 21%, respectively. This outcome was influenced by the age of the mother.

Pregnancy loss subsequent to fetal reduction has been reported as ranging from 0 to 40%[62]. However, in three recent reports the reduction of triplets to twins resulted in a fairly consistent fetal loss of 8–10%[52,53,58]. In our experience, the four pregnancies lost following reduction occurred amongst the first seven patients[63]. The losses may have been due to a 'learning curve' associated with the introduction of a new procedure. Since 1900, all of the 27 patients in whom reduction was performed delivered viable fetuses[63]. Multifetal pregnancy reduction thus appears to be a safe procedure in triplet pregnancies and imposes a relatively small risk of losing the entire pregnancy[64]. Porreco and co-workers[58] did not, however, show an improvement in pregnancy outcome in 13 triplet pregnancies reduced to twins as compared with 11 triplet gestations managed expectantly.

In our prospective series, multifetal pregnancy reduction of triplets to twins was clearly associated with an improvement in the outcome of the pregnancies without an increased loss of the entire pregnancy[63]. A spontaneous pregnancy loss prior to 25 weeks' gestation of 20.7% of triplet gestations diagnosed soon after conception occurred as compared with a loss of 8.7% of the triplet pregnancies reduced to twins (Table 4). Furthermore, the mean gestational age of the reduced pregnancies was increased by approximately 3 weeks and the mean birth weight of the liveborn infants increased by 570 g, as compared to the triplet gestations (Table 5). The proportion of low birth weight (< 2500 g) infants, of very low birth weight (< 1500 g) infants and of premature infants (< 37 completed gestational weeks) were all

Table 4 *Outcome of triplet pregnancies with or without fetal reduction. (From Reference 63)*

	No intervention (n = 106)		Reduction to twins (n = 34)	
	n	%	n	%
Loss of entire pregnancy				
≤ 20 weeks	14	13.2	1	2.9
21–24 weeks	8	7.5	2	5.0
25–26 weeks	5	4.7	1	2.9
Total	27	25.5	4	11.8
Discharge home of at least one infant	79	74.5	30	88.2
Perinatal mortality rate	109/1000		48/1000	
Neonatal mortality rate	46/1000		0/1000	

Table 5 *Outcome of liveborn infants in triplet pregnancies with or without reduction. (From Reference 63)*

	No intervention		Reduction to twins	
	n	%	n	%
Number of liveborn infants	238		58	
Gestational age (weeks)	33.5 ± 3.6		36.7 ± 3.7*	
Birth weight (g)	1780 ± 470		2350 ± 670*	
< 1000	16	6.7	1	1.7
1000–1499	47	19.7	3	5.1*
1500–2499	171	71.8	30	51.7
> 2500	4	1.7	24	41.4
Respiratory disorders	69	28.9	4	6.9*
Sepsis	20	8.4	1	1.7
Necrotizing enterocolitis	5	2.1	1	1.7
IVH (only < 1500 g)	16/63	25.4	0/4	0.0
Neonatal mortality	11	4.6	0	0.0
Neonatal follow-up (birth weight < 1500 g)				
Severe disability	6/52	11.5	0/4	0.0
Mild disability	10/52	19.2	0/4	0.0
Normal	36/52	69.2	4/4	100.0

IVH, intraventricular hemorrhage; *$p < 0.001$ for the comparison between groups

significantly decreased following the reduction procedure. These results are comp[arable to those reported by others[52,53,57,59,64].

Although perinatal mortality rates for triplet pregnancies as low as 33–93/1000 deliveries have been reported[10,14,57], a review of 238 cases revealed a 20.5% perinatal mortality rate[9]. An extensive study from the Oxford National Perinatal Epidemiology Unit showed that 16% of the fetuses from triplet gestations died during the perinatal period, and 15% of liveborn infants did not survive infancy[16]. The incidence of premature delivery is approximately 80%, the mean gestational age is approximately 34 weeks, and a significant number of these prematurely born infants developed major neonatal and long-term complications[9,10,14].

Our data[63] suggest that the benefit of fetal reduction of triplets to twins exceeds the risk involved in the procedure *per se*; furthermore, all of the outcome measures evaluated were improved in the twin gestations as compared with triplet pregnancies managed expectantly. The increasing access to, and demand for assisted reproduction techniques will, in all likelihood, continue to result in an increasing incidence of iatrogenically induced triplet and high-order multifetal gestations[12]. In addition to the excess maternal morbidity and perinatal and neonatal morbidity and mortality, triplet and high-order multiple births are associated with socioeconomic difficulties and serious emotional and psychological disorders[65]. Although the ethical issues associated with the multifetal reduction procedure are complex, we believe that parents should be offered this therapeutic option in cases of triplet pregnancies.

Several methods for multifetal pregnancy reductions have been proposed: some authors have reported on the use of transcervical aspiration of the gestational sac[66,67]. This method, however, may be associated with an increased incidence of fetal loss due to infection caused by introduction of bacteria from the exocervix, or due to cervical incompetence brought about by cervical dilatation[55]. Multifetal pregnancy reduction using injection of potassium chloride into the embryo, by both the transabdominal and the transvaginal approaches, has been reported[49,50,52,60,66,68]. No method has yet been proven to be superior to others, due to a lack of comparative studies. Our results have also shown that both the transabdominal and the transvaginal routes are comparable, although we have not randomized the approaches[69]. We now prefer to use the abdominal approach which is performed at a more advanced gestational age. In doing so, cases that would have otherwise resulted in spontaneous abortions or spontaneous reduction in the number of fetuses by intrauterine demise are avoided. This approach and timing also allows early screening and diagnosis by vaginal sonography, in order to perform selective reduction when warranted.

Most studies previously published report only a few cases of high-order (quintuplets or more) multifetal pregnancy reductions (Wapner and colleagues[50]– seven cases, Lynch and associates[52]–ten cases, and Dommergues and co-workers[55]–13 cases). In most studies, little specific reference was made as to the outcome in such high-order multifetal pregnancies. This is regrettable because these patients are the best suited for the reduction procedure without which there is little hope for a favorable outcome. Moreover, it is clear that results of high-order multifetal pregnancy reductions are not comparable with those of triplet reductions. Our series[69] included 17 high-order multifetal pregnancies, with the abortion rate in these patients being relatively high (41.2%). However, perinatal outcome for those who did not abort was no worse as compared to those of lower-order multifetal pregnancies that were reduced, and certainly better than when non-intervention occurred[57,70]. Because these patients usually have longstanding infertility, it may seem wise to attempt reduction despite the high abortion rate. Moreover, most reductions were performed during the first period, when experience was still lacking. If the trend for improvement with experience is manifested in such high-order pregnancies as is true for triplets, then still better results may be expected.

References

1. Elster, A. D., Bleyl, J. L. and Craven, T. E. (1991). Birth weight standards for triplets under modern obstetric care in the United States 1984–1989. *Obstet. Gynecol.*, **77**, 387–93
2. Rein, M. S., Babieri, R. L. and Greene, M. F. (1990). The causes of high-order multiple gestation. *Int. J. Fertil.*, **35**, 154–6
3. Levene, M. I., Wild, J. and Steer, P. (1992). Higher multiple births and the modern management of infertility in Britain. *Br. J. Obstet. Gynaecol.*, **99**, 607–13
4. Gonen, R., Heyman, E., Asztalos, E. V., Ohlsson, A., Pitson, L. C., Shennan, A. T. and Milligan, J. E. (1990). The outcome of triplet, quadruplet and quintuplet pregnancies managed in a perinatal unit: obstetric neonatal and follow-up data. *Am. J. Obstet. Gynecol.*, **162**, 454–9
5. Ron-El, R., Caspi, E., Schreyer, P. *et al.* Triplet and quadruplet pregnancies and management. *Obstet. Gynecol.*, **57**, 458–63
6. Holchberg, G., Biale, Y., Lewenthal, H. and Insler, V. (1982). Outcome of pregnancy in 31 triplet gestations. *Obstet. Gynecol.*, **59**, 472–6
7. Loucopoulos, A. and Jewelewicz, R. (1982). Management of multifetal pregnancies: sixteen

years' experience at the Sloane Hospital for Women. *Am. J. Obstet. Gynecol.*, **143**, 902–5
8. Deale, C. J. C. and Cronje, H. S. (1984). A review of 367 triplet pregnancies. *S. Afr. Med. J.*, **66**, 92–4
9. Petrikovsky, B. M. and Vintzeleos, A. M. (1989). Management and outcome of multiple pregnancy of high fetal order: Literature review. *Obstet. Gynecol.*, **44**, 578–84
10. Lipitz, S., Reichman, B., Paret, G., Lipitz, S., Reichman, B., Panet, B., Modan, M., Shaler, J., Senn, D., Mashiach, S. and Frenkel, Y. (1989). The improving outcome of triplet pregnancies. *Am. J. Obstet. Gynecol.*, **161**, 1279–84
11. Lipitz, S., Frenkel, Y., Watts, C., Lipitz, S., Frenkel, Y., Waltes, C., Ben-Rafael, Z., Bonkai, G. and Reichman, B. (1990). High-order multifetal gestation – management and outcome. *Obstet. Gyncecol.*, **76**, 215–18
12. Kiely, J. L., Kleinman, J. C. and Kiely, M. (1992). Triplets and higher-order multiple births. *Am. J. Dis. Child.*, **146**, 862
13. Neilson, J. P. and Crowther, C. A. (1993). Preterm labor in multiple pregnancies. *Fetal Maternal Med. Rev.*, **5**, 105–19
14. Newman, R. B., Horner, C. and Miller, M. C. (1989). Outpatient triplet management: a contemporary review. *Am. J. Obstet. Gynecol.*, **161**, 547–55
15. Sassoon, D. A., Castro, L. C., Davis, J. L. *et al.* (1990). Perinatal outcome in triplet versus twin gestations. *Obstet. Gynecol.*, **75**, 817–20
16. Botting, B. H., McDonald-Davis, I. and McFarlane, A. J. (1987). Recent trends in the incidence of multiple births and associated mortality. *Arch. Dis. Child.*, **62**, 941–50
17. Daw, E. (1978). Triplet pregnancy. *Br. J. Obstet. Gynaecol.*, **85**, 505–9
18. Syrop, C. H. and Varner, M. W. (1985). Triplet gestation: maternal and neonatal implications. *Acta Genet. Med. Gemellol. (Roma)*, **34**, 81–8
19. Persson, P. and Grennert, L. (1979). Towards normalisation of outcome of twin pregnancy. *Acta Genet. Med. Gemellol. (Roma)*, **28**, 341–6
20. Mon, S. M., Sunderji, S. G., Gall, S. *et al.* (1991). Multicenter randomized clinical trial of home uterine activity monitoring for detection of preterm labor. *Am. J. Obstet. Gynecol.*, **165**, 858–66
21. Grimes, D. A. and Schultz, K. F. (1992). Randomized controlled trials of home uterine monitoring: a review and critique. *Obstet. Gynecol.*, **79**, 137–42
22. McLennan, A. H., Green, R. C., O'Shea, R. *et al.* (1990). Routine hospital admission in twin pregnancy between 26 and 30 weeks' gestation. *Lancet*, **335**, 267–9
23. Crowther, C. A., Verkuyl, D. A. A., Neilson, J. P. *et al.* (1990). The effects of hospitalization for rest on fetal growth, neonatal morbidity and length of gestation in twin pregnancy. *Br. J. Obstet. Gynaecol.*, **97**, 872–7
24. Crowther, C. A., Neilson, J. P., Verkuyl, D. A. A. *et al.* (1989). Preterm labor in twin pregnancies: can it be prevented by hospital admission. *Br. J. Obstet. Gynaecol.*, **96**, 850–3
25. Crowther, C. A., Verkuyl, D. A. A. and Ashworth, M. (1991). The effects of hospitalization for bed rest on duration of gestation, fetal growth and neonatal morbidity in triplet pregnancy. *Acta Genet. Med. Gemellol. (Roma)*, **40**, 63–8
26. Keirse, M. J. N. C. (1992). Prophylactic oral betamimetics in twin pregnancies. In Chalmers, I. (ed.) *Oxford Database of Perinatal Trials*, version 1.3, disk issue 7, record 3462. (Oxford: Oxford University Press)
27. Katz, M., Robertson, P. A. and Creasy, R. K. (1981). Cardiovascular complications associated with terbutaline treatment for preterm labor. *Am. J. Obstet. Gynecol.*, **139**, 605–8
28. Itzkowic, D. (1979). A survey of 59 triplet pregnancies. *Br. J. Obstet. Gynaecol.*, **86**, 23–8
29. Keirse, M. J. N. C. (1990). Indomethacin tocolysis in preterm labor. In Chalmers, I. (ed.) *Oxford Database of Perinatal Trials*, version 1.2, disk issue 4, record 4383. (Oxford: Oxford University Press)
30. Dor, J., Shalev, J., Mashiach, S. *et al.* (1982). Elective cervical suture of twin pregnancies diagnosed ultrasonically in the first trimester following induced ovulation. *Gynecol. Obstet. Invest.*, **13**, 55–60
31. MRC cervical cerclage trial. MRC/RCOG Working Party on cervical cerclage. Interim report of the Medical Research Council/Royal College of Obstetricians and Gynaecologists multicentre randomised trial of cervical cerclage. *Br. J. Obstet. Gynaecol.*, **95**, 437–45
32. Grant, A. (1992). Cervical cerclage in twin pregnancy. In Chalmers, I. (ed.) *Oxford Database of Perinatal Trials*, version 1.3, disk issue 8, record 3280. (Oxford: Oxford University Press)
33. Pheiffer, E. L. and Golan, A. (1979). Triplet pregnancy: a 10-year review of cases at Baragwanath Hospital. *S. Afr. Med. J.*, **55**, 843–6
34. Lipitz, S., Seidman, D. S., Alcalay, M., Lipitz, S., Seichman, D. S., Alcalay, M., Achison, R., Masiach, S. and Reichman, B. (1993). The effect of fertility drugs and *in vitro* methods on the outcome of 106 triplet pregnancies. *Fertil. Steril.*, **60**, 1031–4
35. Barke, J. D., Knuppel, R. A., Ingardia, C. J. *et al.* (1984). Evaluation of non-stress fetal heart rate testing in multiple gestations. *Obstet. Gynecol.*, **63**, 528–32
36. Alcalay, M., Lipitz, S., Ben-Rafael, Z. *et al.* (1993). Fetal biophysical profile score in triplet pregnancies. *J. Reprod. Med.*, in press

37. Manning, F. A., Morrison, M. B., Harman, C. R. et al. (1990). The abnormal biophysical profile score. V. Predictive accuracy according to score composition. *Am. J. Obstet. Gynecol.*, **162**, 918–25
38. Lodeiro, J. R., Vinzileos, A. M., Freinstein, S. J. et al. (1986). Fetal biophysical profile in twin gestations. *Obstet. Gynecol.*, **67**, 824–7
39. Giles, W. B., Trudinger, B. J. and Cook, C. M. (1985). Umbilical waveforms in twin pregnancy. *Acta Genet. Med. Gemellol. (Roma)*, **34**, 233–8
40. Gerson, A. G., Wallace, B. M., Bridgens, N. K. et al. (1987). Duplex Doppler ultrasound in the evaluation of growth in twin pregnancies. *Obstet. Gynecol.*, **70**, 419–23
41. Anderson, R. L., Goldborg, S. D. and Golbus, M. S. (1991). Prenatal diagnosis in multiple gestation: 20 years' experience with amniocentesis. *Prenatal Diagnosis*, **11**, 263–70
42. Mordel, N., Laufer, N., Zajicek, G., Dorembus, D., Benshushan, A., Schenker, J. G. and Sadorsky, E. (1991). Menotropins as a possible risk factor for premature deliveries in triplet pregnancies. *Gynecol. Endocrinol.*, **5**, 197–201
43. Pons, J. C., Mayenga, J. M., Plu, G., Forman, R. G. and Papiernik, E. (1988). Management of triplet pregnancy. *Acta Genet. Med. Gemellol. (Roma)*, **37**, 99–103
44. Newman, R. B., Jones, J. S. and Miller, M. C. (1991). Influence of clinical variables on triplet birth weight. *Acta Genet. Med. Gemellol. (Roma)*, **40**, 173–9
45. Seoud, M. A. F., Toner, J. P., Kruithoff, C. and Muasher, S. J. (1992). Outcome of twin, triplet and quadruplet *in vitro* pregnancies: the Norfolk experience. *Fertil. Steril.*, **57**, 825–34
46. Botting, B., MacFarlane, A. and Price, A. M. (1991). Triplet and higher order multiple births. *The Sixth Report of the Interim Licensing Authority for Human In Vitro Fertilization and Embryology*, 32–7
47. Kingsland, C. R., Steer, C. V., Pampliglione, J. S., Mason, B. A., Edwards, R. G. and Campbell, S. (1990). Outcome of triplet pregnancies resulting from IVF at Bourn Hallam 1984–1987. *Eur. J. Obstet. Gynecol. Rep. Biol.*, **34**, 197–203
48. Rizk, B., Doyle, P., Tan, S. L., Rainsbury, P., Betts, J., Brinsden, P. and Edwards, R. (1991). Perinatal outcome and congenital malformations in *in vitro* fertilization babies from the Bourn-Hallam Group. *Hum. Reprod.*, **6**, 1259–64
49. Berkowitz, R. L., Lynch, L., Chitakara, U., Wilkins, J. A., Mehalek, K. E. and Alvarez, E. (1988). Selective reduction of multifetal pregnancies in the first trimester. *N. Engl. J. Med.*, **318**, 1043–7
50. Wapner, R. J., Davis, G., Johnson, A., Weinblatt, V. J., Fischer, R. G., Jackson, L. G. and Chervenak, F. A. (1990). Selective reduction in multifetal pregnancies. *Lancet*, **335**, 90–3
51. Evans, M. I., Fletcher, J. C., Zador, I. E. et al. (1988). Selective first trimester termination in octuplet and quadruplet pregnancies: clinical and ethical issues. *Obstet. Gynecol.*, **71**, 289–96
52. Lynch, L., Berkowitz, R. L., Chitakara, U. et al. (1990). First trimester transabdominal multifetal pregnancy reduction: a report of 85 cases. *Obstet. Gynecol.*, **75**, 735–8
53. Boulot, P., Hedon, B., Pelliccia, G., Deschaps, F., Benos, P., Andibert, F., Humeau, C., Mares, P., Laffargne, F. and Viala, J. R. (1990). Obstetrical results after embryonic reductions performed on 34 multiple pregnancies. *Hum. Reprod.*, **5**, 1009–13
54. Evans, M. I., May, M., Drugan, A., Flecher, J. C., Johnson, M. P. and Sokol, R. J. (1990). Selective termination: clinical experience and residual risks. *Am. J. Obstet. Gynecol.*, **162**, 1568–75
55. Dommergues, M., Nisand, I., Mandelbrot, L., Isfer, E., Radunovic, N. and Donnez, J. (1991). Embryo reduction in multifetal pregnancies after infertility therapy: obstetrical risks and perinatal benefits are related to operative strategy. *Fertil. Steril.*, **55**, 805–11
56. American College of Obstetrics and Gynecology. (1991). Multifetal pregnancy reduction and selective fetal termination. *ACOG Committee Opinion*, **94**
57. Melgar, C. A., Rosenfeld, D. L., Rawlinson, K. and Greenberg, M. (1991). Perinatal outcome after multifetal reduction to twins compared with non-reduced multiple gestations. *Obstet. Gynecol.*, **78**, 763–6
58. Porreco, R. P., Burke, M. S. and Hendrix, M. L. (1991). Multiple reduction of triplets and pregnancy outcome. *Obstet. Gynecol.*, **78**, 335–9
59. Vauthier-Brouzes, D. and Lefebvre, G. (1992). Selective reduction in multifetal pregnancies: technical and psychological aspects. *Fertil. Steril.*, **57**, 1012–16
60. Shalev, J., Frenkel, Y., Goldenberg, M., Shaler, E., Lipitz, S., Barkai, G., Nebel, L. and Mashiach, S. (1989). Selective reduction in multiple gestations: pregnancy outcome after transvaginal and transabdominal needle-guided procedures. *Fertil. Steril.*, **52**, 416–20
61. Dickey, R. P., Olar, T. T., Curole, D. N., Taylor, S. N., Rye, P. M. and Matulich, E. M. (1990). The probability of multiple births when multiple gestational sacs or viable embryos are diagnosed at first trimester ultrasound. *Hum. Reprod.*, **5**, 880–2
62. Itskovitz-Eldor, J., Drugan, A., Levron, J., Thaler, I. and Brandes, J. M. (1992). Transvaginal embryo aspiration – a safe method for selective reduction in multiple pregnancies. *Fertil. Steril.*, **58**, 351–5
63. Lipitz, S., Reichman, B., Ural, J. et al. (1993). A prospective comparison of the outcome of trip-

let pregnancies managed expectantly or by multifetal reduction to twins. *Am. J. Obstet. Gynecol.*, in press
64. Tabsh, K. M. (1990). Transabdominal multifetal pregnancy reduction: report of 40 cases. *Obstet. Gynecol.*, **75**, 739–41
65. Garel, M. and Blondel, B. (1992). Assessment at 1 year of the psychological consequences of having triplets. *Hum. Reprod.*, **7**, 729–32
66. Salat-Baroux, J., Aknin, J., Antoine, J. M. and Alamowitch, R. (1988). The management of multiple pregnancies after induction for superovulation. *Hum. Reprod.*, **3**, 399–401
67. Itskovitz, J., Boldes, R., Thaler, I., Levron, J., Rottem, S. and Brandes, J. M. (1990). First trimester selective reduction in multiple pregnancy guided by transvaginal sonography. *J. Clin. Ultrasound*, **18**, 323–7
68. Gonen, Y., Blankier, J. and Casper, R. F. (1990). Transvaginal ultrasound in selective embryo reduction for multiple pregnancy. *Obstet. Gynecol.*, **75**, 720–2
69. Lipitz, S., Yaron, Y., Shalev, J., Lipitz, S., Yaron, Y., Shaler, J., Achison, K., Zolti, M. and Masiach, S. (1994). Improved results in multifetal pregnancy reduction: a report of 72 cases. *Fertil. Steril.*, **61**, 59–61
70. Alvarez, M. and Berkowitz, R. L. (1990). Multifetal gestation. *Clin. Obstet. Gynecol.*, **33**, 79–87

Computerized evaluation of cardiotocography and its clinical role

18

G. P. Mandruzzato, G. S. Dawes and Y. J. Meir

INTRODUCTION

Auscultation of the fetal heart was described more than 200 years ago, but attempts at continuous registration of fetal heart activity were only begun in 1892 by Pestalozza, in 1903 by Seitz, and in 1908 by Hofbauer and Weiss. The instantaneous fetal heart rate (FHR, 'beat-to-beat') was first registered, by means of external (transabdominal) electrocardiogram (ECG) by Hon and Wolgemuth in 1961. In 1962, Hammacher described the oscillatory characteristics of time intervals between adjacent fetal heart cycles, giving the theoretical and practical basis for a correct registration. In 1963, Hon proposed transvaginal introduction of an electrode to be placed on the fetal scalp and with this method continuous registration of FHR entered clinical routine. The introduction of ultrasound in the mid-1960s by Donald, Kratochwill and others opened the modern era of obstetrics offering new possibilities for the measurement of fetal heart rate. Applying the Doppler effect, Mosler (1969) developed the first equipment for the registration of FHR based on beat-to-beat impulses[1-3]. Most of the electronic fetal monitors developed were based on the principle of 'peak detection' until the early 1980s. The main problem with these instruments was low signal : noise ratio with frequent signal loss and artifacts with consequent erroneous or doubtful interpretation. Since 1981, a new generation of instruments was provided with autocorrelation, a method of processing ultrasound signals to derive the best estimate of pulse intervals, and range gates that lowered the signal : noise ratio and improved record quality.

At first, continuous electronic fetal monitoring was used mainly in labor. The principles of interpretation was based on this experience. Previously, evaluation of fetal state and uterine contractions was derived from discontinuous auscultation and palpation, which were simple and comprehensive methods, but clinically unreliable. With the introduction of cardiotocography (CTG), the identification of the distressed infant improved, but various complications emerged for the obstetrician. The quantity and quality of information continuously produced required both constant attention and familiarity with the different CTG patterns for accurate interpretation. More recently, the CTG has been introduced as a method of antepartum fetal monitoring, especially in high-risk pregnancies. It soon appeared that application of the intrapartum rules for CTG interpretation was inappropriate antepartum; this added further perplexities. Scoring systems were designed by Kubli (1971), Hammacher (1974), Fischer (1976), Myer-Menk (1976), Pearson and Weaver (1978) and Lyons (1979). Other authors (Sill and Wilson (1975), Flynn and Kelly (1977), Martin and Schifrin (1977)) tried to simplify interpretation by using descriptive terms such as 'reactive' and 'non-reactive' or 'normal, abnormal and pathological' or 'normal, suspect and ominous'. The reliability of the test did not improve significantly. Although several studies have reported good correlation between CTG data and perinatal outcome, reliable assessment of CTG is by no means easy. Borgatta and colleagues (1988) have commented that '. . . if a non-reactive test is to reliably predict an individual infant who will be distressed, a repetition of the reading of the test must also give the same unfavorable interpretation . . .'. Intra- and interobserver variability investigated by Trimbos[4], Lotgering[5], Flynn (1982), Nielsen (1987), Borgatta (1988) and other authors[6-11] led to the conclusion that visual assessment of the antepartum CTG, considered in isolation of other clinical data, leads either to unnecessary intervention or to unwarranted conservation in a large proportion of cases. The initial enthusiasm based on the use of an instrumental test of fetal health was soon invaded by doubt due to its poor reproducibility. At the beginning of the 1980s, four prospective randomized clinical trials were carried out to examine the utility of antepartum FHR monitoring[12-15]. In spite of the fact that each trial used monitors designed before 1980 with poor signal : noise ratio, visual analysis, poor selection of patients, and few records per patient, Nielson[16] concluded that there was no evidence of the usefulness of the antepartum non-stress test (NST) in high-risk pregnancies.

One of the major dilemmas encountered by obstetricians today is how to monitor fetal health in high-risk pregnancies, especially in those associated with disturbances in the feto-maternal circulation, which compromise, sooner or later, fetal oxygen delivery. When the first signs of hypoxemia appear, the same question always arises: when is it safe to leave the infant in the uterus? It is essential to have methods available that provide information about small changes in fetal oxygenation. These tools should provide precise methods for the evaluation of the risk of acidemia and intrauterine death so the clinician can assess the benefit of leaving the baby *in utero*, or alternatively, of delivering the infant.

Dawes and collaborators started work on the development of a computerized system to analyze human FHR patterns in 1978. Initially, their motivation was derived from animal experiments which demonstrated that heart rate was modulated by many rhythms of breathing associated with sleep states, with age and the time of day[17,18,19] and because of their expectation that there could be more information to be gained by an accurate analysis in the human fetus[20-24]. Subsequently, with the increasing number of studies that recognized the lack of reproducibility of visual evaluation of CTG, a numerical on-line analysis of FHR patterns was found to be essential, not only for research, but as a more accurate tool in the assessment of fetal conditions. Since 1983, a computerized on-line CTG system entered clinical use in Oxford and soon after in several other departments of obstetrics and gynecology in Europe and Canada.

PRINCIPLES OF COMPUTERIZED CARDIOTOCOGRAPHY

To date, the largest experience with computerized analysis of CTG has been achieved by the Oxford group (Dawes, Redman, Moulden and colleagues[10,11,18-34]). Other authors[35-38] have published variations of the methods for acquiring and elaborating data produced by the electronic fetal monitor. The principles are more or less the same, but there are important small differences.

In a computerized CTG system, results of analysis are given on-line continuously both in graphic and written form on a monitor. Warnings are usually displayed or heard when signal loss is too high, when fetal movements are deficient and when the trace is abnormally flat or decelerative. A print-out of the record with the results of analysis is available (Figure 1). So far as the program is concerned the authors will refer mainly to the one developed by Dawes and co-workers[25] at the Nuffield Institute in Oxford. The system acquires data continuously up to 60 min. The fetal monitor is set up to monitor the autocorrelation function, the tocodynamometer reading and fetal movements. The measurement of fetal pulse interval is controlled by error algorithms. Valid pulse intervals are averaged over an epoch of 1/16 min (3.75 s) and stored (the software developed by Van Geijn[39,40] averages pulse intervals over 2.5 s.). The first analysis is done after 10 min and every 2 min thereafter. The principal parameters calculated are fetal movements, the basal FHR, the number of accelerations and decelerations and the variation and the episodes of high and low FHR variation[22-27].

FETAL MOVEMENTS

During the registration the mother signals all fetal movements with a hand-held event marker.

COMPUTERIZED CARDIOTOCOGRAPHY

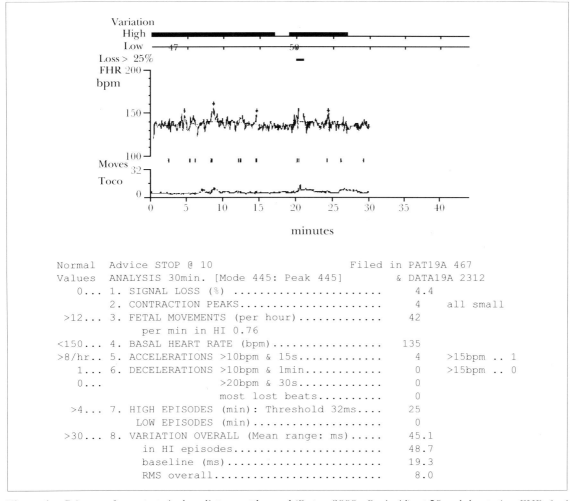

Figure 1 *Printout of a computerized cardiotocograph record (System 8000 – Sonicaid), at 39 weeks' gestation. FHR, fetal heart rate; bpm, beats per minute*

Each epoch containing one or more perceived movements is identified.

FHR BASELINE AND BASAL HEART RATE

The baseline has been defined as a running average of heart rate in the absence of accelerations and decelerations. The baseline is derived using a digital filter (autoregressive to avoid phase changes) and from the frequency distribution of pulse intervals. The basal FHR is recorded in beats per min (bpm), averaged from episodes of low FHR variation, or otherwise from the frequency distribution of pulse intervals.

ACCELERATIONS AND DECELERATIONS

Accelerations and decelerations are occasional deviations from the baseline with a certain amplitude and duration. In the Oxford system there are two types of decelerations: type I, amplitude > 10 bpm and duration > 1 min; and type II, amplitude > 20 bpm, duration > 30 s. Large decelerations are defined by area greater than 20 beats below the basline. Accelerations are identified when the FHR deviates above the baseline by more than 10 bpm for more than 15 s.

VARIATION AND EPISODES OF HIGH AND LOW VARIATION

With the present instruments there is no point in measuring very short-term beat-to-beat variation because it is normally so low (about 2 ms) and too near to the limit of accuracy. It is underestimated if autocorrelation is used, and overestimated by conventional Doppler detector systems (Lawson and colleagues 1982–1983). Moreover, the amount of data to be stored and the time required for analysis would be 8–10 times greater. The Oxford system considers two types of variations – long- and short-term, both excluding decelerations. Long- or medium-term variation is expressed as the mean 1-min range of pulse intervals. Short-term variation is calculated as the mean of successive epochal (1/16 min) pulse interval differences. Short-term variation is more useful when low-frequency sinusoidal rhythms are present. To minimize the effects of gestational age, episodes of high or low variation are identified when, during consecutive minutes of a trace, the long-term variation exceeds or falls below a certain threshold, defined as the first centile of measurements at 30–33 weeks.

Over the past 10 years, more than 40 000 clinical records have been collected from different centers (Oxford, Luton, Southampton and Trieste). The first records were registered in normal pregnancies to established the limits of normality of the different parameters calculated by the system. Later they were made for clinical purposes, predominantly for monitoring fetal conditions in pregnancies complicated by fetal growth retardation or known maternal disease.

LIMITS OF NORMALITY

It took several years and thousands of records to elaborate normal tables for the different patterns of the CTG. It must be stressed that for most of the parameters there is a wide range of normality within the same gestational age. The reason for this is that FHR varies greatly with

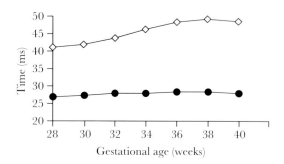

Figure 2 Median and lower 5th percentile of mean minute range in normal pregnancies from 28 weeks' gestation to term

fetal behavioral states after 28 weeks' gestation, and with gestational age[36,37,41,42]. The fetal basal heart rate decreases with gestational age; the normal range appears to be between 120 and 160 bpm and not between 110 and 150 bpm as suggested in the conclusions of a FIGO consensus meeting in 1987[43].

The number of accelerations increases with gestational age from 28 to 40 weeks by more than threefold, but FHR accelerations may be absent in many traces of normal fetuses[44]. Yet, at least one episode of high FHR variation is always present (> 99%) from 28 weeks on in normal fetuses if the duration of the CTG is sufficient. Episodes of low variation may last for up to 50 min in normal fetuses near term. This is why there is no constant length of recording recommended; the length should depend on the fulfilment of certain criteria, i.e. the presence of an episode of high variation of sufficient amplitude, and no evidence of large decelerations or a sinusoidal rhythm. Decelerations are present in some normal fetuses near term, and even when associated with low FHR variation they are poor guides to outcome. The diagnostic importance of both accelerations and decelerations has been overstated, probably because exact measurements were difficult without computers. Even though variation demonstrates a wide band of values in the normal fetus (Figures 2–3), it seems that this is the best measure for the evaluation of the fetal condition. Long-term variation (mean minute range in the Oxford system) tends to increase with gestational age. Values above 30 ms are considered normal, between 20–30 ms are questionable and below 20 ms are considered abnormal (Table 1).

Short-term variation is highly correlated with long-term variation. In the presence of low frequency (1 in 2–5/min) sinusoidal rhythms, short-term variation in the absence of an episode of high FHR variation is a better guide to outcome.

Clinical applications of computerized cardiotocography

One of the major issues in obstetrics, today as in the past, consists in the evaluation of relative risks. On one side of the scale we find the risk of fetal death or severe damage *in utero*, and on the other, neonatal death or severe morbidity as a result of prematurity. Improvements in neonatal care have lowered neonatal mortality and morbidity, but for the obstetrician the problem remains, the difference being that he has to resolve it at an earlier gestational age. The introduction of computerized CTG offers a new means of assessing relative risk. As for all the other methods used for the evaluation of the fetal condition, it must be stressed that computerized CTG should be used in conjunction with other biological measurements. Before reviewing clinical experiences with computerized CTG, some concepts should be kept in mind:

(1) Antepartum CTG is used as an intermittent examination. The identification of acute events, like sudden fetal death not preceded by progressive deterioration (e.g. abruption or placental infarction), are excluded;

(2) CTG is not useful for the detection of growth retardation in itself, but it is useful in detecting hypoxemia and alterations of metabolic status, whether or not associated with placental vascular disease or growth retardation;

(3) Gross changes in FHR are late signs of fetal hypoxemia;

(4) In a distressed fetus, it is necessary to have reliable means of detecting small progressive changes in metabolic status; and

(5) All instrumental and biochemical parameters used today to monitor fetal condition give a numerical measurement. The only

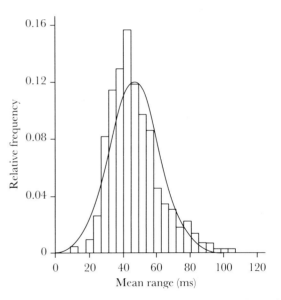

Figure 3 *Frequency distribution histogram – values of mean range of fetal heart rate variation during 32–33 weeks' gestation in normal pregnancies*

Table 1 *Changes in long-term fetal heart rate variation (mean range) at different gestational ages in normal pregnancies*

Gestational age (weeks)	Number of traces	Mean range (ms)				Lower 3rd centile
		Average	Median	SEM	SD	
28–29	293	42.3	40.9	0.6	10.9	25.5
30–31	405	44.5	42.6	0.7	14.1	24.2
32–33	466	46.5	44.0	0.7	14.8	24.6
34–35	491	48.6	46.2	0.7	15.3	25.9
36–37	572	49.5	47.4	0.6	14.8	27.9
38–39	568	50.6	48.4	0.7	16.5	26.8
40–41	434	50.1	48.2	0.8	16.5	25.3

one based on an opinion is 'eye ball' evaluation of CTG, which is highly unreliable.

Clinical and experimental experience with antepartum CTG have shown that the most reliable single parameter of the fetal condition is variation[28–33,45–49]. Absence of accelerations, the presence of decelerations, reduction of movements, and changes in basal FHR are all likely to occur occasionally in normal fetuses. On the other hand, they may be absent in hypoxemic or anemic fetuses. Some authors[45,50–52] have shown that the presence of repetitive late decelerations is almost constantly present in advanced stages of fetal deterioration, but the problem is that they may not be present or be so small they are overlooked by visual assessment.

As far as terminal traces are concerned, computerized CTG improves reproducibility by supplying numerical thresholds. Numerical analysis of the CTG detects fetal deterioration at an early stage and enables the obstetrician to follow longitudinally fetuses at risk. A constant, progressive reduction in variation has been shown to be associated with progressive deterioration of fetal oxygenation. We emphasize 'progressive' because, as mentioned by Smith and colleagues[46], there is a small proportion of fetuses that exhibit persistently low heart rate variation and neither their outcome, nor their postnatal FHR features differ from those of controls with a higher FHR variation before birth. This provides further evidence that the 'unreactive' trace is not a reliable indication of fetal compromise.

The best way to demonstrate a relationship between FHR patterns and fetal biochemical status is to find a significant correlation between numerical CTG measurements and numerical values of fetal blood gas analysis. Although it is easy and non-invasive to perform fetal electronic monitoring, if necessary more than once or twice a day, it is too invasive and too risky to perform fetal blood sampling (cordocentesis) in the same way. However, a sample of blood may be acquired after Cesarean section in the absence of labor. Smith and co-workers[48] studied the correlation between FHR patterns and biochemical measurements in cord samples obtained in three groups of patients delivered by Cesarean section

(1) Group 1: for fetal compromise between 28 and 36 weeks' gestation;

(2) Group 2: for urgent maternal reasons between 28 and 36 weeks' gestation; and

(3) Group 3: electively at 38–40 weeks.

The comparison between Groups 1 and 2 in this study is not between abnormal and normal, but

Table 2 Analysis of fetal movements and heart rate by a group of patients delivered by Cesarean section for different indications. (From Reference 48)

	Group 1 (fetal indication) ($n = 21$)	p^*	Group 2 (maternal indication) ($n = 20$)	p^*	Group 3 (other) ($n = 30$)
Fetal movements/h	11.7 (2.2)	< 0.01	44.0 (9.1)		78.4 (15.0)
Basal heart rate (bpm)	143.5 (2.3)		139.6 (2.0)	< 0.01	131.7 (1.6)
FHR variation					
Mean range	20.6 (1.2)	< 0.001	35.0 (1.5)	< 0.001	58.1 (3.3)
Number of accelerations					
> 10 bpm and 15 s	2.0 (0.5)	< 0.01	8.0 (1.6)	< 0.001	20.2 (1.5)
> 15 bpm and 30 s	0.5 (0.2)	< 0.05	3.9 (1.3)	< 0.001	15.7 (1.4)
Number of decelerations					
> 10 bpm and 60 s	0.6 (0.2)	< 0.01	0.05 (0.05)		0.2 (0.1)
> 20 bpm and 30 s	1.9 (0.3)	< 0.001	0.3 (0.2)		0.3 (0.2)
Minutes of high variation	4.2 (1.2)	< 0.001	24.4 (3.0)	< 0.001	40.3 (1.9)

*Significance of difference between Groups 1 and 2 and between Groups 2 and 3 (Mann–Whitney). FHR, fetal heart rate; bpm, beats per minute

Table 3 *Umbilical cord blood gas values in groups of patients by reasons for delivery. (From Reference 48)*

	Group 1 (fetal indication) (n = 21)	p*	Group 2 (maternal indication) (n = 20)	p*	Group 3 (other) (n = 30)
Umbilical artery					
pH	7.23 (0.01)		7.26 (0.01)		7.27 (0.010)
pO_2 (mmHg)	6.1 (1.6)	< 0.001	10.0 (1.0)		13.0 (0.9)
pCO_2 (mmHg)	58.4 (1.7)		55.8 (1.0)	< 0.05	49.7 (1.2)
Base deficit	5.2 (0.6)		4.0 (0.4)	< 0.001	4.6 (0.3)
Umbilical vein					
pH	7.27 (0.01)		7.29 (0.01)	< 0.001	7.33 (0.01)
pO_2 (mmHg)	16.9 (1.1)		20.1 (1.4)	< 0.01	25.9 (1.2)
pCO_2 (mmHg)	47.7 (1.7)		46.4 (1.1)	< 0.001	40.0 (0.8)
Base deficit	5.5 (0.4)		4.5 (0.4)		4.8 (0.3)

*Significance of difference between Groups 1 and 2 and between Groups 2 and 3 (Mann–Whitney)

between compromised fetuses with and without marked fetal heart rate abnormalities.

The authors showed that fetuses with abnormal FHR patterns (Group 1) exhibited lower umbilical arterial pO_2 values than those at a corresponding gestational age but with normal or suboptimal traces (Group 2) (Tables 2 and 3). When Groups 1 and 2 were combined there was a significant correlation between the mean minute range of FHR variation and umbilical artery pO_2. The results demonstrate that measurement of FHR variation can help identify fetuses which are becoming hypoxemic without acidemia. They suggest that a mean range of < 20 ms is abnormal, and a value of > 20–30 ms is probably abnormal, especially if associated with decelerations.

The next step was to investigate the clinical implications of very low FHR variation. Street and co-workers[30] studied retrospectively the outcome of pregnancies in which at least one computerized CTG record displayed a long-term variation (mean range) < 20 ms. They found a mean range < 20 ms in 78 women (961 traces) out of 2582 (7396 traces) that had computerized CTG between 1983 and 1987. They considered as the index trace the first trace with a mean range < 20 ms. Most of the pregnancies were complicated by proteinuric hypertension (73%) or by intrauterine growth retardation (19%). There were five intrauterine deaths and four neonatal deaths for a total perinatal mortality rate of 11.5%. Of the liveborn, eight were acidemic at delivery and 30 had hyaline membrane disease. All deaths occurred when the index trace was taken before 32 weeks. One of the most interesting features is that 27 fetuses were < 30 weeks' gestation when the index trace was taken; nevertheless, pregnancy was safely prolonged in 17 (63%) by an average of 17 days. This fact outlines the value of having measures in order to quantify longitudinally the state of fetal compromise even when ominous signs are already present. While processing their data the authors found that the long-term variation in a sinusoidal FHR pattern superimposed on an otherwise flat trace is normal or high. Moreover, one of nine terminal traces is sinusoidal. This led the authors to examine measurements of short-term variation. As mentioned above, beat-to-beat variation cannot be measured accurately with present Doppler-based instruments. Therefore, they defined a new measure of short-term variation as that of successive epochs (3.75 s) during which valid FHR values are averaged. Of the 78 fetuses in the study, 44 had a short-term variation < 3 ms in at least one record. Four of these fetuses died *in utero*. All four had short-term variations between 0.9 and 2.5 ms in the last trace within 24 h of death. Of the remaining 40 liveborn babies, those who showed short-term variation < 2.6 ms had a decreased arterial pH and an increased base deficit suggesting that they were becoming acidotic and that the trace might have been preterminal.

Table 4 Decelerative records of fetuses studies for 5 days or more without decelerations, with decelerations only on the last day before Cesarean section, or with many decelerative records. Values are mean (with range). (From Reference 31)

	No decelerations	Decelerations on last day only before Cesarean section	Multiple decelerations (40%) range, (21–58%)
No. of fetuses	6	14	15
Days studied	11.8 (5–26)	15.6 (5–32)	17 (5–48)
Records/day	0.94 (0.5–1.3)	0.9 (0.3–1.5)	3.4 (1.5–4.8)
Short-term FHR variation in last record (ms)	2.8 (2.4–3.1)	2.6 (2.1–2.9)	3.4 (1.5–4.8)
Delivery data			
Umbilical artery base deficit (mmol/l)	5.4 ± 1.6	7.7 ± 3.2	4.0 ± 2.0
Gestation (week)	33.3 (27–36)	32.6 (26–37)	28.9 (27–31)

FHR, fetal heart rate

Another important study about short-term variation and its relation with decelerations and umbilical flow velocity waveforms was published in 1992 by Dawes and colleagues[32]. They studied 89 patients demonstrating at least one record with short-term variation < 3 ms. If the fetus did not die *in utero*, umbilical artery blood gases were sampled at Cesarean section in the absence of labor. When short-term variation fell below 2.6 ms, there was a high incidence of metabolic acidemia and intrauterine death (34% combined). On the other hand, there were also eight fetuses in which short-term variation fell transiently below 2.6 ms, and within 24 h was above 3 ms, all without acidemia at delivery. In our opinion, the main feature of this study is the relationship between low variation, decelerations and outcome.

The authors showed that the presence of decelerations did not predict metabolic acidemia or loss of other vital signs. As for the temporal relationship, decelerations usually appeared late as compared with the fall in FHR variation below the lower limit of normality (5.7 msec) (Table 4).

Visser and associates[52] have studied FHR patterns in relation to blood gas values in small-for-gestational-age babies obtained at cordocentesis and found that a repetitive decelerative trace, rather than a low variation trace, is associated with hypoxemia, acidemia or both. Their evaluation of CTG traces was based on visual interpretation and not on numerical analysis. In a more recent study, Snijders and colleagues[49] studied 13 fetuses with intrauterine growth retardation over a period of 25 days. FHR records were analyzed numerically. They found that, on average, long-term FHR variation fell below the normal limits at about the same time that decelerations appeared and concluded that a decrease in long-term variation is rather a late sign of fetal impairment that coincides with the occurrence of late decelerations. It is not so clear to which kind of decelerations Snijders and co-workers refer, because sometimes they refer to 'late decelerations' and other times generally to decelerations. It is known that the appearance of isolated decelerations during the third trimester is quite common and has little to do with fetal chronic hypoxemia while late decelerations or constant repetitive variable decelerations are commonly associated with hypoxemia and acidemia. There is an obvious inconsistency between the results of Visser and colleagues[52] and those of Dawes and associates[31] that probably depends on the number of subjects studied and on gestational age at first observation.

CONCLUSION

CTG is continuously used in clinical practice although it has been shown that visual reading of a CTG trace reduces markedly its accuracy. Computerized CTG analysis offers new perspectives for a more reliable assessment of 'at risk' fetuses and for the interpretation of FHR patterns. The advantages of computerized CTG may be summarized as follows:

(1) Predefined criteria to be satisfied are always interpreted in the same way, obtaining an

objective reading of the FHR trace which eliminates the observer variability;

(2) Numerical measurements of FHR patterns are available and can be stored in large databases. This allows statistical evaluation of the different parameters of FHR introducing a better scientific approach for the definition of normality and abnormality;

(3) The quality of the record is improved;

(4) The time required for the test is reduced;

(5) Computerized systems can be programmed to be interactive and give necessary warning signals when necessary;

(6) By accumulating sufficient data it is possible to extrapolate the measure of FHR that gives the best estimate of fetal wellbeing. Until now, the best single measure to be taken into consideration seems to be variation (long- or short-term);

(7) A more accurate comparison between FHR patterns and other biological measurements is possible; and

(8) Computerized CTG enables the detection of small changes in FHR occurring in time, so when initial deterioration signs arise, the single fetus can be followed up longitudinally.

In conclusion, computerized analysis of CTG as offered by System 8000 and other systems, greatly improves the reliability of FHR evaluation in clinical practice. It is, in fact, possible to distinguish, with a good accuracy, fetuses that are truly jeopardized because of hypoxemia or acidemia from those that are not. Therefore, the timing of delivery, when necessary can be established in an objective way.

References

1. Martin, C. B. and Schifrin, B. S. (1976). Prenatal fetal monitoring. In Aadjem, S. and Brown, A. K. (eds.) *Perinatal Intensive Care*, pp. 1–17. (St Louis: Mosby)
2. Evertson, L. R., Gauthier, R. J., Schifrin, B. S. and Paul, R. H. (1979). Antepartum fetal heart rate testing I. Evolution of the non-stress test. *Am. J. Obstet. Gynecol.*, **133**, 29–37
3. Wulf, K.-H. (1985). History of fetal heart rate monitoring. In Kunzel, W. (ed.) *Fetal Heart Rate Monitoring*, pp. 3–15. (Berlin: Springer Verlag)
4. Trimbos, J. B. and Keirse, M. N. J. C. (1978). Observer variability in assessment of antepartum cardiotocograms. *Br. J. Obstet. Gynaecol.*, **85**, 900–6
5. Lotgering, F. K., Wallenburg, H. C. S. and Schouten, H. J. A. (1982). Interobserver and intra-observer variation in the assessment of antepartum cardiotocograms. *Am. J. Obstet. Gynecol.*, **144**, 701–5
6. Schneider, E., Schulman, H., Farmakides, G. and Paksima, S. (1991). Comparison of the interpretation of antepartum fetal heart rate tracings between a computer program and experts. *J. Maternal Fetal Invest.*, **1**, 205–8
7. Van Geijn, H. P., Donker, D. K. and Hasman, A. (1992). How objective is visual evaluation of antepartum and intrapartum cardiotocograms? In Saling, E. (ed.) *Perinatology, Nestlé' Nutrition Workshop Series*, Vol 26, pp. 67–77. (Vevey NY: Raven Press)
8. Gagnon, R., Campbell, M. K. and Hunse, C. (1993). A comparison between visual and computer analysis of antepartum fetal heart rate tracings. *Am. J. Obstet. Gynecol.*, **168**, 842–7
9. Cheng, L. C., Gibb, D. M. F., Ajayi, R. A. and Soothill, P. W. (1992). A comparison between computerised (mean range) and clinical visual cardiotocographic assessment. *Br. J. Obstet. Gynaecol.*, **99**, 817–20
10. Dawes, G. S., Moulden, M. and Redman, C. W. G. (1990). Limitations of antenatal fetal heart rate monitors. *Am. J. Obstet. Gynecol.*, **162**, 170–3
11. Dawes, G. S., Lobb, M., Moulden, M., Redman, C. W. G. and Wheeler, T. (1992). Antenatal cardiotocogram quality and interpretation using computers. *Br. J. Obstet. Gynaecol.*, **99**, 791–7
12. Flynn, A. M., Kelly, J., Mansfield, H., Needham, P., O'Conor, M. and Viegas, O. (1982). A randomized trial of non-stress test antepartum cardiotocography. *Br. J. Obstet. Gynaecol.*, **89**, 427–33

13. Brown, V. A., Sawers, R. S., Parsons, R. J., Duncan, S. L. B. and Cooke, I. D. (1982). The value of antenatal cardiotocography in the management of high risk pregnancy: a randomized controlled trial. *Br. J. Obstet. Gynaecol.*, **89**, 716–22
14. Lumley, J., Lester, A., Anderson, I., Renou, P. and Wood, C. (1983). A randomized trial of weekly cardiotocography in high-risk obstetric patients. *Br. J. Obstet. Gynaecol.* **90**, 1018–26
15. Kidd, L. C., Patel, N. B. and Smith, R. (1985). Non-stress antenatal cardiotocography – a prospective randomized clinical trial. *Br. J. Obstet. Gynaecol.*, **92**, 1156–9
16. Nielson, J. P. (1992). Cardiotocography for antepartum fetal assessment. In Chalmers, I. (ed.) *Oxford Database of Perinatal Trials*. version 1.3, disk issue 7, record 3881
17. Dalton, K. J., Dawes, G. S. and Patrick, J. E. (1977). Diurnal, respiratory and other rhythms of fetal heart rate in lambs. *Am. J. Obstet. Gynecol.*, **89**, 276–84
18. Dawes, G. S., Visser, G. H. A., Goodman, J. D. S. and Levine, D. H. (1981). Numerical analysis of the human fetal heart rate: modulation by breathing and movement. *Am. J. Obstet. Gynecol.*, **140**, 535–44
19. Visser, G. H. A., Dawes, G. S. and Redman, C. W. G. (1981). Numerical analysis of the normal human antenatal fetal heart rate. *Br. J. Obstet. Gynaecol.* **88**, 792–802
20. Dawes, G. S., Visser, G. H. A., Goodman, J. D. S. and Redman, C. W. G. (1981). Numerical analysis of the human fetal heart rate: the quality of ultrasound records. *Am. J. Obstet. Gynecol.*, **141**, 43–51
21. Visser, G. H. A., Goodman, J. D. S., Levine, D. H. and Dawes, G. S. (1982). Diurnal and other cyclic variations in human fetal heart near term. *Am. J. Obstet. Gynecol.*, **142**, 535–44
22. Dawes, G. S., Houghton, C. R. S. and Redman, C. W. G. (1982). Baseline in human fetal heart rate records. *Br. J. Obstet. Gynaecol.*, **89**, 270–5
23. Dawes, G. S., Houghton, C. R. S., Redman, C. W. G. and Visser, G. H. A. (1982). Pattern of the normal human fetal heart rate. *Br. J. Obstet. Gynaecol.*, **89**, 276–84
24. Lawson, G. W., Dawes, G. S. and Redman, C. W. G. (1984). Analysis of fetal heart rate on-line at 32 weeks' gestation. *Br. J. Obstet. Gynaecol.*, **91**, 542–50
25. Dawes, G. S., Redman, C. W. G. and Smith, J. (1985). Improvements in the registration and analysis of fetal heart rate records at the bedside. *Br. J. Obstet. Gynaecol.* **92**, 317–25
26. Dawes, G. S., Moulden, M. and Redman, C. W. G. (1990). Criteria for the design of fetal heart rate systems. *Int. J. Biomed. Comput.*, **25**, 287–94
27. Dawes, G. S., Moulden, M. and Redman, C. W. G. (1991). System 8000: computerized antenatal FHR analysis. *J. Perinatal Med.*, **19**, 47–51
28. Henson, G. L., Dawes, G. S. and Redman, C. W. G. (1983). Antenatal fetal heart rate variability in relation to fetal acid-base status at cesarean section. *Br. J. Obstet. Gynaecol.*, **90**, 516–21
29. Henson, G. L., Dawes, G. S. and Redman, C. W. G. (1984). Characterization of the reduced heart rate variation in growth retarded fetuses. *Br. J. Obstet. Gynaecol.*, **91**, 751–5
30. Street, P., Dawes, G. S., Moulden, M. and Redman, C. W. G. (1991). Short-term variation in abnormal antenatal fetal heart rate records. *Am. J. Obstet. Gynecol.*, **165**, 515–23
31. Dawes, G. S., Moulden, M. and Redman, C. W. G. (1992). Short-term fetal heart rate variation, decelerations, and umbilical flow velocity waveforms before labor. *Obstet. Gynecol.*, **80**, 673–80
32. Dawes, G. S., Lobb, M. O., Mandruzzato, G., Moulden, M., Redman, C. W. G. and Wheeler, T. (1993). Large fetal heart rate decelerations at term associated with changes in fetal heart rate variation. *Am. J. Obstet. Gynecol.*, **168**, 105–11
33. Dawes, G. S., Serra-Serra, V., Moulden, M. and Redman, C. W. G. (1993). Dexamethasone and fetal heart rate variation. *Proc. Soc. Study Fetal Physiol.*, **20**, 30
34. Dawes, G. S. (1993). The fetal ECG: accuracy of measurements. *Br. J. Obstet. Gynaecol.*, Suppl. 9, 15–17
35. Searle, J. R., Devoe, L. D., Phillips, M. C. and Searle, N. S. (1988). Computerized analysis of resting fetal heart rate tracings. *Obstet. Gynecol.*, **71**, 407–11
36. van Vliet, M. A. T., Martin, C. B., Nijhuis, J. R. and Prechtl, H. F. R. (1985). Behavioural states in the fetuses of nulliparous women. *Early Human Dev.*, **12**, 121–35
37. Mantel, R., Van Geijn, H. P., Ververs, I. A. P. and Copray, F. J. A. (1991). Automated analysis of near term antepartum fetal heart rate in relation to fetal behavioural states: the Sonicaid System 8000*. *Am. J. Obstet. Gynecol.*, **165**, 57–65
38. Schneider, E. P., Schulman, H., Farmakides, G. and Chan, L. (1992). Clinical experience with antepartum computerized fetal heart monitoring. *J. Maternal Fetal Invest.*, **2**, 41–4
39. Mantel, R., Van Geijn, H. P., Caron, F. J. M., Swartjes, J. M., van Worden, E. E. and Jongsma, H. W. (1990). Computer analysis of antepartum fetal heart rate. I. Baseline determination. *Int. J. Biomed. Comput.*, **25**, 261–72
40. Mantel, R., Van Geijn, H. P., Caron, F. J. M. *et al.* (1990). Computer analysis of antepartum fetal heart rate. II. Detection of accelerations and decelerations. *Int. J. Biomed. Comput.*, **25**, 273–86

41. Ribbert, L. S. M., Fidler, V. and Visser, G. H. A. (1991). Computer-assisted analysis of normal second trimester fetal heart rate patterns. *J. Perinatal Med.*, **19**, 53–9
42. Arduini, D. and Rizzo, G. (1990). Quantitative analysis of fetal heart rate: its application in antepartum clinical monitoring and behavioural pattern recognition. *Int. J. Biomed. Comput.*, **25**, 247–52
43. Rooth, G., Huch, A. and Huch, R. (1987). Guidelines for the use of fetal monitoring. *Int. J. Gynaecol. Obstet.*, **25**, 159–67
44. Patrick, J., Carmichael, L., Chess, L., Probert, C. and Staples, C. (1985). The distribution of accelerations of the human fetal heart rate at 38 to 40 weeks' gestational age. *Am. J. Obstet. Gynecol.*, **151**, 283–7
45. Beckedam, D. J., Visser, G. H. A., Mulder, E. J. H. and Poelmann, Weesjes, G. (1987). Heart rate variation and movement incidence in growth retarded fetuses: the significance of antenatal late heart rate decelerations. *Am. J. Obstet. Gynecol.*, **157**, 126–33
46. Smith, J. H., Dawes, G. S. and Redman, C. W. G. (1987). Low human fetal heart rate variation in normal pregnancy. *Br. J. Obstet. Gynaecol.*, **94**, 656–64
47. Economides, D. L., Selinger, M., Ferguson, P. J. *et al.* (1992). Computerized measurement of heart rate variation in fetal anemia caused by rhesus alloimmunization. *Am. J. Obstet. Gynecol.*, **167**, 689–93
48. Smith, J. H., Anand, K. J. S., Cotes, P. M., Dawes, G. S., Harkness, R. A., Howlett, T. A., Rees, L. H. and Redman, C. W. G. (1988). Antenatal fetal heart rate variation in relation to the respiratory and metabolic status of the compromised human fetus. *Br. J. Obstet. Gynaecol.*, **95**, 980–9
49. Snijders, R. J. M., Ribbert, L. S. M., Visser, G. H. A. and Mulder, E. J. H. (1992). Numeric analysis of heart rate variation in intrauterine growth retarded fetuses: a longitudinal study. *Am. J. Obstet. Gynecol.*, **166**(1), 22–7
50. Visser, G. H. A., Bekedam, D. J. and Ribbert, L. S. M. (1990). Changes in antepartum heart rate patterns with progressive deterioration of the fetal condition. *Int. J. Biomed. Comput.*, **25**, 239–46
51. Ribbert, S. L. M., Snijders, R. J. M., Nicolaides, K. H. and Visser, G. H. (1991). Relation of fetal blood gases and data from computer-assisted fetal heart rate patterns in small for gestational age fetuses. *Br. J. Obstet. Gynaecol.*, **98**, 820–3
52. Visser, G. H. A., Sadovsky, G. and Nicolaides, K. H. (1990). Antepartum heart rate patterns in small-for-gestational-age third-trimester fetuses: correlations with blood gas values obtained at cordocentesis. *Am. J. Obstet. Gynecol.*, **162**, 698–703

Universal intrapartum external monitoring and improved outcome

K. Maeda

Improved fetal outcome was expected at the introduction of intrapartum electronic fetal monitoring because the fetus with an abnormal heart rate would be managed with early delivery. However, electronic fetal monitoring has not been shown to result in an improvement of fetal outcome compared to intermittent auscultation[1]. There has been no reduction in the occurrence of infantile cerebral palsy after the introduction of electronic fetal monitoring[2]. Since cerebral palsy is caused by intrapartum asphyxia in only 10% of cases, this frequency is believed to be too small for electronic fetal monitoring to reduce its overall occurrence[3].

Perinatal mortality has, however, markedly dropped in Japan from 46.6 per 1000 in 1950 to 5.3 per 1000 in 1991[4]. Before 1980, this reduction was thought to be due partly to improved socioeconomic status, but later improvement is believed to be caused by perinatal medical efforts, including the wide use of fetal monitoring. The author was concerned that the incidence of cerebral palsy might be increased because of the increased survival rate, but this was not shown[5]. Tsuzaki[6] and Takeshita[7] also studied this occurrence.

Initially, fetal monitoring was performed by the auscultation of fetal heart sounds with a stethoscope. However, this method often results in counting errors[8]. Subsequently, the monitoring has been changed to electronic examination. Augmented auscultation of the heart sounds with the use of a microphone, amplifier and loudspeaker was our original electronic method of counting the fetal heart rate. External electronic fetal monitoring was a natural extension of augmented auscultation. An instantaneous heart rate meter was used and a scalp electrode was used in the second stage of labor, if necessary.

After the widespread use of monitoring of fetal heart sounds, an ultrasonic real-time autocorrelation heart rate meter was introduced into our monitoring of the fetal heart rate in the late 1970s. As the fetal heart rate tracing improved markedly, the scalp electrode was rarely necessary. This external method was universally employed because of its non-invasive nature, reducing concern about injury to the fetus. As the ultrasound intensity was very low in the fetal monitor, there was no bioeffect. Therefore, the external method was used both before and during labor, whereas the internal scalp–electrode method could be used only after the rupture of the membrane.

Long- and short-term outcome after external fetal monitoring was reported by Tsuzaki and colleagues[6] from Yohka General Hospital of Japan. Monitoring in all stages of labor in all women was universal during the study period from 1977 to 1986. The results were compared with those of 1975 and 1976, when no monitoring was used. The number of births was 661 in the control period, 3147 in 1977–1982, when the non-stress test (NST) was carried out in less than 20% of pregnancies, and 2903 in 1983–1986, when the NST was carried out in more than 20% of pregnancies. The following were recorded: stillbirths in fetuses weighing 1000 g or more, early neonatal deaths, number of anencephalic infants, 'rough' perinatal mortality rate, 'corrected' perinatal mortality rate excluding referred anencephalic infants and fetal deaths diagnosed before admission, infants of low birth weight, premature labor, immature labor in pregnancies of less than 34 weeks,

Table 1 Introduction and outcome of full intrapartum fetal monitoring[6]. Period A, no fetal monitoring, periods B and C, full intrapartum monitoring

	Period A (1975–76)	Period B (1977–82)	Period C (1983–86)	Statistics A–B	B–C	A–C
Births (n)	661	3417	2903			
Non-stress test (%)	0	< 20	> 20			
Perinatal mortality (per 1000 births)	6.1	6.1	3.1	NS	S	S
Neonatal depression (%)	7.3	5.2	4.3	S	NS	S
Registered cerebral palsy (per 1000 births)	2.2	0.2	0.3	S	NS	S
Infants of very low birth weight (%)	0.9	0.6	0.6	NS	NS	
Cesarean sections (%)	7.0	11.7	9.8	S	S	S

NS, not statistically significant; S, statistically significant ($p < 0.05$)

infants of very low birth weight, infants of extremely low birth weight, large babies weighing more than 4000 g, number of births with Apgar score less than 7 and those of 7 or more, number of Cesarean sections, number of births, frequency of cerebral palsy registered in the regional governmental health center, and the frequency of the NSTs in the outpatient clinic.

The rough perinatal mortality rate was 6.1 per 1000 in the control period (period A) and no difference was observed in the period of low NST frequency (period B), whereas the rate in the period of high NST frequency (period C) showed a significant reduction to 3.1 per 1000. The corrected perinatal mortality rate showed the same tendency. Premature labor was 2.7% in A, 2.1% in B, and 1.8% in C. The frequency of infants with very low birth weight was 0.9% in A, 0.6% in B, and 0.6% in C, without significant differences. Macrosomia was 2.0% in A, 2.8% in B and 1.9% in C. Neonatal depression diagnosed by an Apgar score of less than 7 was 7.3% in A, 5.2% in B, and 4.3% in C. There was a significant reduction of neonatal depression between periods A and B, and also between periods A and C. The registered cerebral palsy rate was 2.2 per 1000 births in A, 0.2 in B, and 0.3 in C. There was a significant reduction between periods A and B, and also between periods A and C. The rate of Cesarean sections was 7.0% in A, 11.7% in B and 9.8% in C, with significant differences between A and B, A and C, and also between B and C[6]. Important findings were the reduction of perinatal mortality, neonatal depression, and cerebral palsy. The Cesarean section rate increased from A to B periods but decreased from the B to C periods[6] (Table 1).

Table 2 Incidence of cerebral palsy in the Tottori area[7]

	1971–74	1975–80
Fetal monitoring	rare	widespread use
Births (n)	35 707	50 814
Cerebral palsy (per 1000 births)	1.428	0.571*

*Significant difference ($p < 0.0005$)

According to the pediatric neurology report of Takeshita and associates[7], the cerebral palsy incidence in all births of the Tottori prefecture was 1.428 per 1000 (among 35 707 births) in the years from 1971 to 1974, when fetal heart rate monitoring was rarely used in the area, whereas the incidence was 0.571 per 1000 (among 50 814 births) in the following years 1975 to 1980, when the use of fetal heart rate monitoring in the area was widespread. There was a significant decrease of the occurrence of cerebral palsy between the two periods ($p < 0.0005$) (Table 2). They concluded that the widespread use of fetal monitoring was responsible for the reduction of the incidence of cerebral palsy in the Tottori area.

Others have not confirmed the above results. The Dublin trial showed the outcome of pregnancy was the same, whether intrapartum fetal monitoring was continuous with a scalp clip, or performed by intermittent auscultation[1]. The technique was used in the Dublin trial with the combination of the instantaneous heart rate meter, which provided an accurate tracing of

Table 3 Sampling interval of changes in fetal heart rate

	Frequency (cpm)	Frequency × 4 (cpm)	Interval (s)
Bradycardia	DC	DC	∞
Deceleration	2	8	8
Variable deceleration			
slope	1.5	6	10
bottom	1	4	15
Sinusoidal fetal heart rate	3	12	5
Acceleration	4	16	4
Long-term variability	8	32	2

cpm, cycles/min

the fetal heart rate, but the electrode was attached to the scalp only after the rupture of membranes. Consequently, the fetal monitoring was limited to the period after the rupture of membranes. The early stage of labor, directly after the onset of contractions, was excluded in the Dublin trial. We experienced fetal deaths that showed abnormal fetal heart rate findings before the onset of labor[9]. Using a cardiotocograph (CTG) on admission has resulted in improved outcome[10]. Fetal deterioration was also experienced in the early stage of labor during induction, maternal shock, various cord complications, abruption and other complications. Therefore, in the author's view, fetal monitoring is indispensable immediately after the onset of labor in order to improve fetal outcome. The fetus should be monitored continuously during labor because of various abnormalities of sudden occurrence, including cord complications (prolapse, descent, coiling, vasa previa), abruption, maternal shock, prolonged labor and excessive contractions. Intermittent monitoring may overlook the sudden appearance of the abnormalities and may lead to fetal damage. An appropriate sampling interval is needed for correct fetal heart rate diagnosis. Particularly abrupt fetal heart rate changes occur in decelerations in the decreasing and recovering slopes. The sampling interval, therefore, must be less than 10 s. Long-term variability is a parameter in the diagnosis of chronic fetal hypoxia, and the sampling interval should be less than 2 s in the case of long-term variability of 8 cycles per minute (Table 3). Therefore, intermittent auscultation, of which the main purpose is the detection of changes in fetal heart rate, with a 15-min interval, is inappropriate for correct fetal heart rate diagnosis. The sampling interval longer than 1 min is suitable only for continuous bradycardia, which may be a sign of already-established fetal damage.

Although the incidence of cerebral palsy was reduced by 60–90% after the introduction of universal intrapartum monitoring, mainly by the rescue of the hypoxic fetus from deterioration into irreversible brain damage due to anoxia, by the detection of signs of hypoxic fetal heart rate and by rapid delivery, there still remain 0.2–0.3 cases of cerebral palsy in 1000 births[6,7]. Further reduction of cerebral palsy is a challenge for the future.

According to recent reports, there are many causes of the development of cerebral palsy. Congenital anomalies of the central nervous system, antepartum brain injuries, and intrapartum and postpartum hypoxic damage develop at various stages of pregnancy. Pathologically, conditions such as hypoxic ischemic damage, including direct neuronal necrosis, delayed neuronal death, parasagittal injury, focal or multiple infarction, periventricular leukomalacia, and intraventricular hemorrhage are causes of cerebral palsy. Diagnostic efforts include using ultrasound and magnetic resonance imaging (MRI), fetal behavioral studies and Doppler flow studies. Fetal pulse oxymetry or near-infrared spectroscopy may be useful in the future.

There have been reports of antepartum brain injuries with intraventricular hemorrhage, periventricular leukomalacia and infarction.

Recently, we diagnosed fetal intraventricular hemorrhage by ultrasonography and MRI. Antepartum periventricular leukomalacia development is diagnosed when the cysts are detected within a week after the delivery[11]. Antepartum development of brain infarction is diagnosed by the lack of a unilateral wedge-shaped brain image, when the change is detected immediately after the birth.

Gross congenital brain anomalies, including anencephaly, hydrocephaly, Dandy–Walker malformation and holoprosencephaly, are diagnosed during the antepartum period by ultrasound. Motor function abnormality, caused by a minor structural injury, or for which antenatal diagnosis is difficult, is detected by fetal behavioral studies[12].

After exclusion of these antepartum causes of cerebral palsy, and the rescue of the fetus with pathological fetal heart rate findings from falling into severe anoxia, there still remains the cerebral palsy caused by hypoxic brain injuries developed by very acute and unavoidable anoxia in the intrapartum stage. Various cord complications, or abruption, excessive uterine contraction, or maternal shock, may cause unavoidable intrapartum fetal damage, mainly by hypoxic fetal neuronal injuries, including direct neuronal necrosis and delayed neuronal death. The latter will be the main cause of intrapartum damage, and it cannot be cured by intrapartum reoxygenation, or the reoxygenation and conventional hypoxia treatment after delivery, because the delayed neuronal death advances rapidly after the triggering of the damage, which is caused by the increase of glutamate, calcium ions and free radicals[13]. Fortunately, the treatment of delayed neuronal death is the subject of studies in neonates, with the use of blockers of glutamate and calcium ions, and scavengers of free radicals[14]. These experimental modalities may be of value after the occurrence of severe anoxia that triggers delayed neuronal death.

Some fetal heart rate patterns, such as severe fetal bradycardia less than 60 bpm lasting for 16 min or more, will result in fetal damage, regardless of management[15], confirmed by increases in levels of glutamate, calcium ions and free radicals in the fetal blood. Even in this case, the damage may be lessened by rapid delivery, and neonatal treatment by specific therapy with blockers and scavengers[14].

There may be further methods to detect periventricular leukomalacia by Doppler blood-flow studies in high-risk patients with such conditions as prematurity, multiple pregnancy, hypoxic signs, infection and vaginal hemorrhage. Disturbed fetal movement, suspected by maternal perception, or by our actocardiogram, will be a further sign of fetal abnormality. We showed the decrease of cerebral arterial blood flow by intrapartum transvaginal color Doppler in normal mature fetuses in labor. Blood flow reduction or collapse may result in periventricular leukomalacia. The detection of blood flow changes may lead to early detection of the fetus in jeopardy and the prevention of periventricular leukomalacia and cerebral palsy, in the future.

Fetal intracranial blood volume and an increase in the intrapartum period was reported by the use of near-infrared spectroscopy[16]. This modality may be useful to predict intraventricular hemorrhage in the future, with the potential for prevention of cerebral palsy caused by hemorrhage. From these reports, the author believes that a further reduction of the occurrence of cerebral palsy will be possible in the future.

In conclusion, perinatal mortality, neonatal depression, and the occurrence of cerebral palsy have decreased after the introduction of universal intrapartum fetal monitoring using external fetal monitoring. A marked reduction in the frequency of cerebral palsy in Japan has been reported with a low rate of Cesarean sections. There remain cases of cerebral palsy such as congenital anomaly, antepartum brain injuries and unavoidable intrapartum anoxia. New techniques may be useful for the detection of antepartum periventricular leukomalacia and intraventricular hemorrhage. Delayed neuronal death caused by unavoidable anoxia will be further studied, and new pharmacological treatments of delayed neuronal death may be of value to the fetus exposed to severe anoxia.

References

1. MacDonald, D., Grant, A., Sheridan-Perenia, M., Boyland, P. and Chalmers, I. (1985). The Dublin randomized controlled trial of intrapartum fetal heart rate monitoring. *Am. J. Obstet. Gynecol.*, **152**, 524–39
2. Havercamp, A. D. (1976). The evaluation of continuous fetal heart rate monitoring in high-risk pregnancy. *Am. J. Obstet. Gynecol.*, **125**, 310–17
3. Naeye, R. I., Peters, E. C., Bartholomew, M. and Landis, J. R. (1989). Origins of cerebral palsy. *Am. J. Dis. Child.*, **143**, 1154–61
4. Ministry of Health and Welfare, Japan. (1992). *Maternal and Child Health Statistics in Japan*, pp.14–15. (Tokyo: Mothers' & Children's Health Organization)
5. Oguta, H. (1976). Studies on the relation between fetal distress at birth and developmental sequelae. *J. Yonago Med. Assoc.*, **27**, 488–502
6. Tsuzaki, T., Morishita, K., Takeuchi, Y., Mizuta, M., Minagawa, Y., Nakajima, K. and Maeda, K. (1990). The survey on the perinatal variables and the incidence of cerebral palsy for 12 years before and after the application of the fetal monitoring system. *Acta Obstet. Gynaecol. Jpn.* **42**, 99–105
7. Takeshita, K., Ando, Y., Ohtani, K. and Takashima, S. (1989). Cerebral palsy in Tottori, Japan. *Neuroepidemiology*, **8**, 184–92
8. Hon, E. H. (1968). *An Atlas of Fetal Heart Rate Pattern*, pp.25–7. (New Haven: Harty Press)
9. Maeda, K., Kimura, S., Fukui, Y., Ozawa, S., Kosaka, W., Wong, F., Tamura, M., Takata, D. and Nakano, H. (1969). *Pathophysiology of the Fetus*, pp.45–51. (Fukuoka: Fukuoka Printing)
10. Ingemarsson, I., Ingemarsson, E. and Spencer, J. A. D. (1993). *Fetal Heart Rate Monitoring, a Practical Guide*, pp.274–81. (Oxford: Oxford University Press)
11. Sher, M. S., Belfar, H., Martin, J. and Painter, M. J. (1991). Destructive brain lesions of presumed fetal onset: antepartum causes of cerebral palsy. *Pediatrics*, **88**, 898–906
12. Horimoto, N., Koyanagi, T., Maeda, H., Satoh, S., Takashima, T., Minami, T. and Nakano, H. (1993). Can brain impairment be detected by *in utero* behavioral patterns? *Arch. Dis. Child.*, **69**, 3–8
13. Espinoza, M. I. and Parer, J. T. (1991). Mechanisms of asphyxial brain damage, and possible pharmacologic interventions, in the fetus. *Am. J. Obstet. Gynecol.*, **164**, 1582–91
14. Kochhar, A., Zivin, J. A., Lyden, P. D. and Mazzarella, V. (1988). Glutamate antagonist therapy reduces neurologic deficits produced by focal central nervous system ischemia. *Arch. Neurol.*, **45**, 148–53
15. Phelan, J. P. (1992). Quo vadis intrapartum monitoring? *2nd World Congression Perinatal Medicine*, Rome. Discussion. (Abstr. 53)
16. Naruse, H., Imanishi, M., Sumimoto, K., Kanayama, N., Ooi, H., Maehara, K., Itou, M., Maeda, M., Inukai, K. and Terao, T. (1992). Near infrared spectroscopy in perinatal period. *Jpn. J. Obstet. Gynecol. Neonatal Hematol.*, **2**, 79–87

Domiciliary fetal heart rate monitoring by telephone

S. Uzan, T. Harvey, B. Guyot and M. Uzan

INTRODUCTION

Current evaluation of fetal well-being in high-risk pregnancies or suspicion of chronic fetal distress relies on the use of scores that take into account different parameters. The most useful of these is Manning's score[1], but recently Arabin[2] has proposed a new score that includes maternal and fetal blood velocimetry. However, all of these scores include fetal heart rate monitoring (FHRM), which is the parameter most widely used for the diagnosis and for establishment of the prognosis of chronic fetal distress.

The use of FHRM in antepartum care has increased. A technical evaluation reported by ANDEM[3], including six University obstetrics units in France, showed that 30–50% of patients underwent cardiotocography at least once before delivery (excluding those who were recorded systematically during emergency care in the last month of the pregnancy).

Fetal heart rate monitoring may be performed in two types of situations: first, during admission to hospital for an obstetric problem (sometimes more than once a day), in which case FHRM is performed with classical cardiotocography, and second, when hospital admission is not really necessary but FHRM is desirable. Hospitalization is costly in terms of materials and staff, but to leave a classical cardiotocograph at the patient's home and perform FHRM by a midwife is also expensive.

Provision of a smaller and less expensive system allows the patient to perform fetal monitoring herself. The results are transmitted to the central maternity unit over the telephone line. The development of such systems has been possible thanks to their miniaturization and simplification: patients require only a short period of training.

We will now describe the system. Our experience concerns two sorts of monitor: the first can only record the FHRM – domiciliary fetal monitoring (DFM), while the second can simultaneously record FHRM and uterine contractions (CTT 2000). Although the idea of telephone-transmitted FHRM is not new[4] current utilization of these autonomous systems is more recent[5–7].

MATERIALS AND RECORDING

The domiciliary fetal monitor

The equipment consists of a portable case containing an ultrasound transducer and hand-held event marker (to record fetal movements

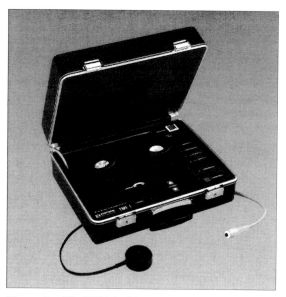

Figure 1 *The DFM fetal heart rate monitor*

or uterine contractions). In the middle of the case (Figure 1) are rubber cups which hold the telephone handset used for transmission (acoustic modem). The case weighs 9.9 pounds (4.5 kg). The other half of the equipment comprises a central unit with a hard disk PC-type microprocessor, screen, printer and electronic modem.

Practically, self-monitoring is very easy and instruction in its use takes only 1 h. In our experience less than 10% of patients are unable to perform this self-recording. The patient, after placing the transducers on her abdomen, tries to obtain the best audible signal from the FHRM. When the quality is sufficient, recording is undertaken for 30 min, after which the system is switched to a stand-by position. The data obtained are stored by the microprocessor until transmitted by telephone. This telephone transmission is performed simultaneously with clinical information to the midwife at the hospital. During this discussion the midwife asks the woman about symptoms, and the results of urine or blood tests performed at home.

A perfect signal is theoretically transmitted over the telephone network within 45 s. We will discuss this point further. At the end of the transmission, the trace is displayed on the screen and the midwife assesses its normality. She then gives instructions to the patient for the next recording and telephone transmission. The last step consists in printing the record for inclusion in the medical file. Most of the software has a computerized medical file that automatically includes the FHRM recordings. These systems can also recall earlier recordings to allow comparison. After the delivery, all these data can be stored on a hard disk.

Description of a trace

Figure 2 shows a trace. Parameters included for clinical reference are time of transmission, recording duration, and decision of the clinician receiving the trace. In this system, the acceptance rate is calculated with the percentage of time for which data are available.

The traces are easily legible and their representation on A4 paper leads to no loss of information. Under the trace appear arrows made by the event marker (fetal movements or uterine contractions). In this case the events are active fetal movements accompanied by fetal heart rate accelerations.

The CTT 2000

This is the most recent system, allowing simultaneous recording of FHRM and uterine contractions. This system is smaller than the DFM (Figure 3). The remote unit consists of two different transducers and its use is very simple. It permits 45 min of recording. One of its most important differences is that it is plugged directly into the telephone network, increasing the proportion of successful transmissions.

The base until is still a PC with a modem. The trace obtained with this system is a little different, since FHRM and uterine contractions are combined on the recording.

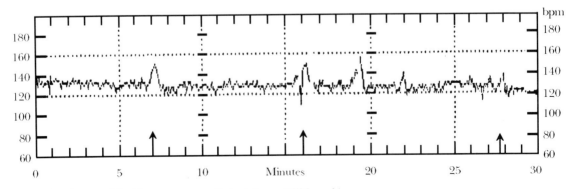

Figure 2 *A normal fetal heart rate trace obtained from a DFM machine*

MAIN RESULTS

Domiciliary fetal monitoring is unlikely to produce results significantly different from those obtained with conventional cardiotocography, since both methods use the same technology.

We compared FHRM using the DFM with direct fetal ECG monitoring by a scalp electrode in 14 women in labor. Superimposition (Figures 4 and 5) of the traces is completely satisfactory, and gives clinically useful information. This correlation has also been examined by Gonen and co-workers[8] and by Lindsay and colleagues[9]. Most comparisons have been made with a conventional Hewlett-Packard cardiotocograph monitor. More indirectly, Reece and associates[14] have studied traces obtained in hospital less than 1 h after monitoring with a DFM. The correlation between the two traces was excellent.

The homologation of this system (as a conventional monitor) is now in progress in France.

Acceptance rate

Figure 6 represents a trace with many arrows indicating many active fetal movements. This phenomenon has brought about only a 62% success rate. This rate is inadequate to allow the trace to be defined as acceptable.

During a meeting on telephone monitoring of fetuses, held in Paris in 1991[11] most of the speakers reported a minimum success rate of > 70%. We performed a prospective study in 402 patients with 816 traces[7,8] and studied the success rate according to several factors supposed to influence FHRM. The most important factors in our experience are the term of the pregnancy and the use of the recorder by women at home or in the hospital. Globally, about 80% of the traces are interpretable, varying from 73% to 86%. The ANDEM inquiry[3] found the global rate of technically successful traces to vary between 79% and 93%. One of the

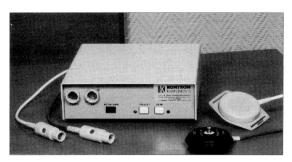

Figure 3 *CCT 2000 fetal heart rate recorder*

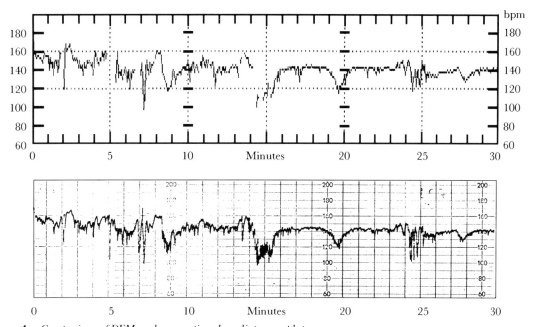

Figure 4 *Comparison of DFM and conventional cardiotocograph traces*

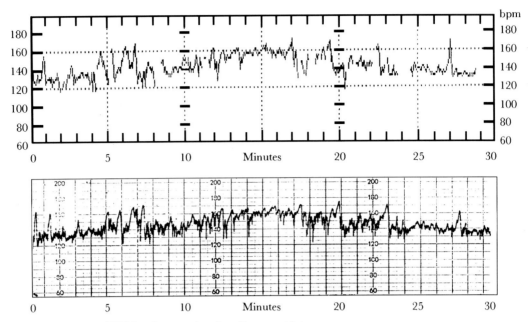

Figure 5 *Comparison of DFM and conventional cardiotocograph traces*

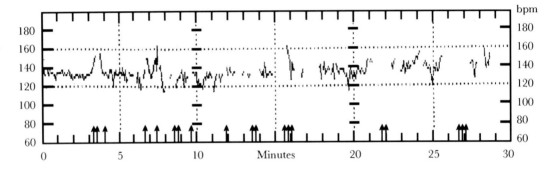

Figure 6 *Suitability of traces according to recording circumstances*

most important factors influencing the success rate is the gestational age at which recording is performed. According to the ANDEM inquiry, a majority of obstetricians begin recordings in cases of suspected chronic fetal distress between 28 and 30 weeks. However, 25% start recording at 27 weeks or even earlier: it is likely that at these gestational ages (not evaluated in our prospective study) the success rate may be lower.

Transmission of traces

A summary of results relating to transmission and interpretation of traces, from data presented at the 1991 Paris meeting[11], is shown is Figure 7. A total of 70% of traces are successfully transmitted at the first attempt and this reaches, 80% after a second attempt. Of the remaining 20%, half are difficult to interpret and half are uninterpretable.

These data correspond to the first system using the telephone's handset, and better results have been obtained since the utilization of direct telephone line transmission. More than 80% of the traces are now successfully transmitted at the first attempt.

Acceptability and psychological impact

The most specific study has been performed by Dawson and colleagues[12], who analyzed anxiety and depression felt by 40 women involved in prenatal care. The group with DFM surveillance showed less anxiety during the study than during conventional surveillance. The authors attribute this result to factors linked to the more personal care associated with domiciliary surveillance. Our results of a prospective study of womens' reactions are shown in Figure 8. The proportions in which use of the DFM failed for technical reasons, or was not undertaken because of initial refusal or later withdrawal are displayed. A simple enquiry showed that 65% of the patients were reassured, 20% were reassured but worried and 15% were anxious. However more than 85% of the patients would like to use the system again in another pregnancy. We must ask ourselves about the usefulness of such surveillance in anxious pregnant women.

Moore and colleagues[13] and Pasquier and associates[14] sent postal questionnaires to women after delivery. In Moore's study (75% responses) 95% of women found DFM reassuring and 28% commented that DFM had reduced the need for frequent hospital visits or admissions. Five of 75 women judged the experience to be unsatisfactory. Pasquier and co-workers did not mention the rate of responses, but found that 81% of patients considered the surveillance reassuring, and here 19% thought it reassuring but worrying or restricting.

Economic study

This has been studied by very few authors. The cost of this system is very variable between countries, and the topic it is too long to discuss here. Several authors have studied the influence of the DFM on the need for attendance at hospital. Prato[15] found a highly significant reduction in journeys to hospital.

PRESENTATION OF CLINICAL CASES

Clinical case 1 (Figure 9)

This case seemed interesting because, on the same record, it shows for the first 15 min a normally fluctuating and reactive trace and in the next 15 min a poorly fluctuating, non-reactive trace. This proves the ease of interpretation.

Clinical case 2 (Figure 10)

This trace was obtained at 34 weeks' gestation in a pregnancy complicated by maternal hypertension. The reduced variability and absent reactivity indicate the need for monitoring to be repeated immediately in hospital.

Clinical case 3 (Figure 11)

This record was obtained in a woman bearing a twin pregnancy who felt reduced fetal movements for one twin. A recording lasting only 20 min shows an abnormal trace requiring admission to hospital. Persisting abnormality necessitated a Cesarean section.

Clinical case 4 (Figure 12)

Basic heart rate is elevated at 160 beats/min but with normal fluctuations and accelerations. Further traces were normal.

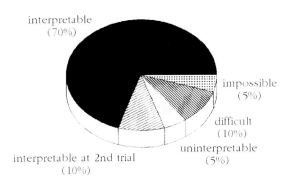

Figure 7 *Transmission and interpretability of traces*

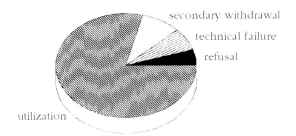

Figure 8 *Patients' reactions*

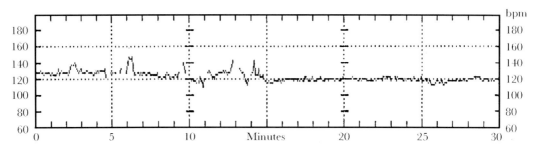

Figure 9 *Clinical case 1: a normal trace for 15 min followed by a poorly fluctuating, non-reactive trace*

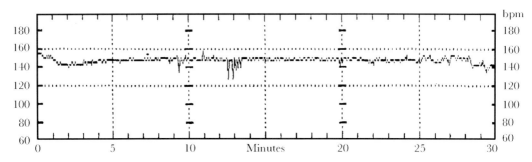

Figure 10 *Clinical case 2: absent reactivity in a fetus at 34 weeks' gestation, in a pregnancy complicated by hypertension*

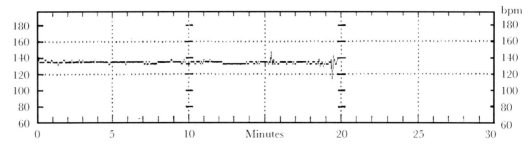

Figure 11 *Clinical case 3: twin pregnancy with abnormal movements for one fetus*

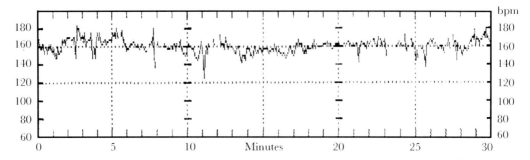

Figure 12 *Clinical case 4: elevated heart rate*

Clinical case 5 (Figure 13)

This record in a woman at 30 weeks of gestation shows a deceleration followed by transient tachycardia and a normal trace at the end of record. The patient was immediately admitted to hospital for further monitoring. More abnormalities appeared, and immediate delivery was performed.

Clinical case 6 (Figure 14)

This recording shows an abnormality similar to that in case 5, but a with a normal trace and active movements in the second part of the trace. A trace obtained in hospital did not confirm these abnormalities and labor was induced a few days later.

Clinical case 7 (Figure 15)

The basic heart rate is < 120 beats/min (abnormal). The rate is however strictly normal. The patient had autoimmune thrombocytopenia.

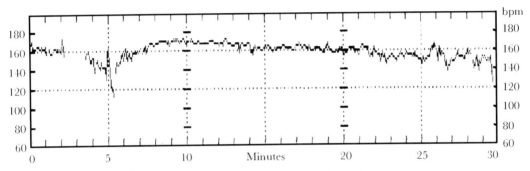

Figure 13 *Clinical case 5: deceleration and transient tachycardia at 30 weeks' gestation*

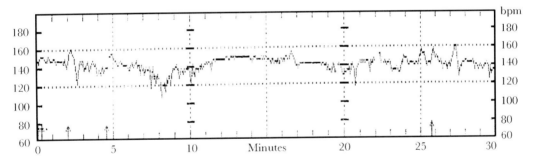

Figure 14 *Clinical case 6*

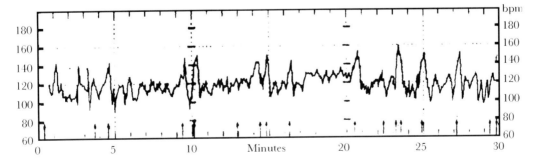

Figure 15 *Clinical case 7: maternal thrombocytopenia*

Clinical case 8 (Figure 16 and 17)

These recordings were obtained from a fetus with a poorly reactive heart rate. Immediate hospital admission was planned, but refused by the patients, who had insulin-dependent diabetes. Next day she transmitted a pathological trace.

Clinical case 9 (Figure 18)

This patient had a history of two totally unexplained intrauterine fetal deaths. This systematic record shows tachycardia and pseudosinusoidal recording. After immediate admission to hospital another cardiotocograph was still abnormal. A Cesarean section was performed. The fetus was anemic (The Kleihauer–Betke test was positive).

PERFORMED TRIALS

The Paris meeting in 1991 summarized the French experience[11]. During this meeting, traces corresponding to 2547 patients recorded over an average period of 3 weeks (an average of 15 records per patient) were pooled. In 50%

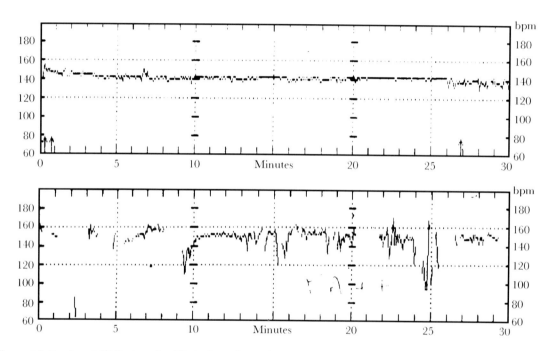

Figure 16 (top) and 17 (bottom) *Clinical case 8: poorly reactive heart rate in a fetus of a diabetic mother*

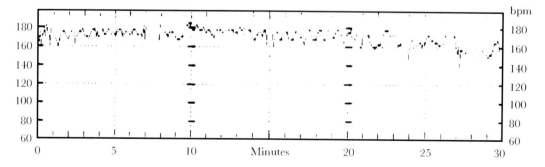

Figure 18 *Clinical case 9: tachycardia in a fetus whose mother suffered two previous unexplained intrauterine deaths*

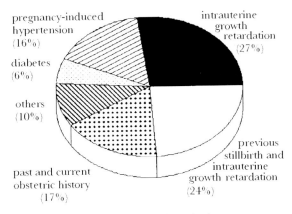

Figure 19 *Indications for fetal monitoring*

of patients recordings were made on a daily basis, and in 40% recording was performed every other day. Problems of success rate and transmission are discussed above. The most common indications for DFM are shown in (Figure 19). Other pathologies which were found less frequently included gestational cholestasis, premature labor, infection and other maternal diseases. Most patients (63%) were instructed in the use of the system during a hospital stay; 29% received instruction during a one-day hospitalization and 8% were instructed after a routine visit.

The consequences of the procedure were also studied in this meeting. A total of 10.9% of the traces were considered uninterpretable or pathological, and needed a mean of 7.7% hospital admissions. This admission rate varied from 5.2% to 12% between units. While in two-thirds of cases traces became normal during hospital admission, the traces remained abnormal in one-third, necessitating delivery within 48 h.

Among all the cases presented two cases of intrauterine death were observed in patients undergoing such surveillance. One followed a refusal of hospital admission, and the other one was due to misinterpretation of the tracing. In two cases complicated by pre-eclampsia fetal distress was observed within 48 h of a normal trace being obtained. Unfortunately these data do not correspond to an exhaustive prospective study and do not permit formal conclusions on the sensitivity and specificity of this method to be reached. It would be very difficult to evaluate or judge the sensitivity or specificity of FHRM.

Many studies have been published of surveillance using these systems. Some have been cited above. James and colleagues[16] studied 368 recordings made from 85 women. The data transmission time varied between 40 and 60 s. The median telephone time (including data transmission and conversation) with a dedicated direct line was 7 min. Mean success rates for the four centers were between 70 and 80%. Ten recordings were abnormal. The women and midwives were equally proficient in using the DFM.

Dawson and associates[12] undertook a randomized study and appeared to demonstrate a reduction in duration of hospital admission from 50 to 16%.

Moore and co-workers[13] performed DFM on 100 patients with suspected intrauterine growth retardation or reduced fetal movements. Thirty-one were abnormal, and nine of these were abnormal when cardiotocography was repeated in hospital. All such patients were delivered within seven days. Forty-nine percent of infants were small for gestational age. The number and duration of hospital admissions for fetal surveillance were reduced by 29% and 52%, respectively.

Gonen and colleagues[8] studied two series of patients: 38 high-risk hospitalized pregnant women performed DFM in their room and 34 undertook home monitoring. Ninety-three percent of recordings were transmitted successfully and 98% were considered interpretable.

Lindsay and colleagues[9] studied 134 pregnant women who were at moderate risk for fetal distress. All abnormal fetal heart-rate patterns were detected during the study. They were no intrauterine or neonatal deaths and no overall increase in pathology. There appeared to be a significant reduction in the inconvenience suffered by the patient and family compared with conventional monitoring. FHRM performed by patients was of high quality and reduced the demand on midwife resources.

A prospective trial is being undertaken in Lyon, France, using the CTT 2000 with an FHRM transducer and a uterine contraction captor. It also includes patients presenting with premature labor. Although the definitive results of this study have not yet been published, intermediate results seem to demonstrate the efficiency of the system and a reduced duration of hospitalization with cheaper, cost-effective surveillance.

Trials of different systems, using the telephone network only for retransmission of a conventional cardiotocograph or systems transmitting a record from one unit to another to obtain advice from different clinicians are outside the scope of this review.

DISCUSSION AND CONCLUSIONS

The reliability of this system seems to be good, particularly since the technology used is often the same as that employed in conventional cardiotocography. Their simplicity makes these systems' easily used by over 80% of patients. There are no definitive data to demonstrate a reduction in hospital admission with the use of these systems. However, for women who do not need admission, but who require ambulatory medical care, these systems reduce journeys to clinics and subsequent fatigue. These systems also significatively increase medical supervision without increasing the medical staff's workload.

These systems have several inconveniences, in addition to the lack of undertaking to reimburse medical expenses by the Social Security. Anxiety may be produced in patients and also among medical staff when major abnormalities appear on monitoring. However, patients in whom such problems are detected would not be in hospital and would come for recording much later than is the case with recording done at home.

The most common indications for FHRM at home are systematic recording in women with a previous adverse obstetrical history (for example intrauterine death, unexplained acute fetal distress) and pregnancies complicated by isolated intrauterine growth retardation, hypertension or pre-eclampsia. Other indications include velocimetric abnormalities detected on uterine artery Doppler studies, and other maternal conditions such as isolated gestational thrombocytopenia, diabetes and cholestasis.

Patients admitted with preterm labor are increasing being systematically monitored. Recording at admission and every other day during hospitalization ensures detection of atypical abruptio placentae and fetal complications of prematurity. The most recent system, CTT 200, theoretically allows complete monitoring of these patients (uterine contractions and FHRM). Although its use for domiciliary antenatal care is being evaluated, the complete results are not yet available. Whatever the indication for domiciliary surveillance, patients must have a moderate and stable form of pathology which does not require emergency hospitalization.

In the future this system may be integrated into a network of FHRM surveillance techniques. Patients admitted to hospital may be given recording units for FHRM and uterine contractions. Recording can be performed early in the morning and transmitted directly through the telephone network from the patient's room. At her arrival in the unit the midwife would then analyze the recordings of the majority of patients and could immediately determine which women required attention. Women unable to perform their own monitoring who have classical cardiotocography undertaken by the midwife. The small system could be used to obtain recordings from patients hospitalized in other care units in the hospital, such as intensive care, cardiology or nephrology. All the traces are stored in the central unit after interpretation; they also can be printed or stored on backup units. This system is also indicated for use in outpatients, either in the context of domiciliary hospitalization (this is a special home case with midwives and nurses), as part of home care undertaken by a midwife or prenatal care performed by the patient herself. The traces transmitted from these sources are also stored in patients' files in the computer and a secondary archive can also be established.

All things considered, although this system does not change significantly the antenatal care of high-risk women, it simplifies some problems of recording for outpatients or for those in long-term hospitalization.

References

1. Manning, F. A., Platt, F. D. and Sipos, L. (1980). Antepartum fetal evaluation: development of a fetal biophysical profile. *Am. J. Obstet. Gynecol.*, **136**, 787–97
2. Arabin, B., Snyjders, R., Mohnhaupt, A., Ragosch, V. and Nicolaides, K. (1993). Evaluation of the fetal assessment score in pregnancies at risk for intrauterine hypoxia. *Am. J. Obstet. Gynecol.*, **169**, 549–54
3. ANDEM (Agence Nationale pour le Développement de l'Evaluation Médicale). (1992). *Le télémonitorage foetal: état des connaissances et recommandations.* Service des Etudes, Novembre 1992
4. Dalton, K. J., Dawson, A. J. and Gough, N. A. (1983). Long distance telemetry of fetal heart rate from patients homes using public telephone network. *Br. Med. J.*, **286**, 1545
5. Dawson, A. J., Middlemiss, C., Jones, E. M. and Gough, N. A. (1988). Fetal heart rate monitoring by telephone. I. Development of an integrated system in Cardiff. *Br. J. Obstet. Gynecol.*, **95**, 1018–23
6. Uzan, S. and Uzan, M. (1988). Premiers essais et résultats concernant un système de transmission à distance par téléphone du R.C.F. *Gynécol. Obstet. Pratique*, **3**, 1–2
7. Uzan, S., Uzan, M., Salat-Baroux, J. and Sureau, C. (1989). Telemonitoring fetal. *J. Gynecol. Obstet. Biol. Reprod.*, **18**, 871–8
8. Gonen, R., Braithwaite, N. and Milligan, J. E. (1990). Fetal heart rate monitoring at home and transmission by telephone. *Obstet. Gynecol.*, **75**, 464–8
9. Lindsay, P. C., Beveridge, R., Tayob, Y., Irvine, L. M., Vellacott, I. D., Giles, J. A., Hussain, S. Y. and O'Brien, P. M. (1990). Patient-recorded domiciliary fetal monitoring. *Am. J. Obstet. Gynecol.*, **162**, 466–70
10. Reece, E. A., Hagay, Z., Garofalo, J. and Hobbins, J. C. (1992). A controlled trial of self-non-stress test versus assisted nonstress test in the evaluation of fetal well-being. *Am. J. Obstet. Gynecol.*, **166**, 489–492
11. Colloque sur le monitoring du rythme cardiaque foetal par téléphone Paris, Maison de la Recherche, Juin 1991
12. Dawson, A. J., Middlemiss, C., Coles, E. C., Gough, N. A. and Jones, M. E. (1989). A randomized study of a domiciliary ante natal care scheme: the effect on hospital admissions. *Br. J. Obstet. Gynaecol.*, **96**, 1319–22
13. Moore, K. H. and Sill, R. (1990). Domiciliary fetal monitoring in a District maternity unit. *Aust. N.Z. J. Obstet. Gynaecol.*, **30**, 36–40
14. Pasquier, J. L. (1991). Surveillance des grossesses à risque par télémonitoring foetal à domicile. Créteil, Faculté de Médecine, Thesis
15. Prato, E. (1990–1991). Le télémonitorage foetal à domicile: analyse des aspects médicaux organisationnels et budgétaires. Liège, Faculté de Médecine, Dept Gynécologie et Obstétrique, Mémoire, 174 p.
16. James, D., Peralta, B., Porter, S., Darvill, D., Walker, J., McCall, M., Calder, A., O'Brien, S., Beveridge, R. and Liu, D. (1988). Fetal heart rate monitoring by telephone. II. Clinical experience in four centres with a commercially produced system. *Br. J. Obstet. Gynaecol.*, **95**, 1024–9

Assessment of fetal well-being with the actocardiogram and fetal response to acoustic and photic stimuli

K. Maeda

Fetal movement is a good indicator of fetal well-being in pregnancy. Many studies have reported its importance in maternal perception and ultrasonic image observation. However, the percentage of fetal movements detected by maternal perception was only 67% of actographic movement bursts, and showed large personal variations. Ultrasonic observation is also subjective, since it relies on visual observation. Fetal well-being assessment by the reactive or non-reactive fetal heart rate should be based on objective fetal movement documentation in the non-stress test (NST).

THE PRINCIPLE OF THE ACTOCARDIOGRAM

The sounds of gross fetal movements can be heard when they occur during ultrasonic fetal monitoring. In addition, some miscounts appear in the charts recording fetal heart rate in some older ultrasonic monitors. The sounds are caused by ultrasonic Doppler signals. The author has endeavored to convert these sounds into meaningful signals of fetal movement.

As the Doppler frequency is lower than that of the fetal heart, the original Doppler signals were separated by an acoustic filter into the signals higher than 100 Hz, and lower-frequency signals of 20–80 Hz, which included signals of fetal movement. The ultrasound frequency used was 2 MHz. Maternal movement signals of very low frequency and large amplitude were rejected by filtering. Fetal movement Doppler signals were changed into spike signals and recorded on the chart of a cardiotocograph (CTG). The synchronization of the spike with the fetal movement was confirmed by the M-mode record.

Fetal movement signals and fetal heart rate were simultaneously recorded on the chart in order to compare the two phenomena. This is termed the 'actocardiogram'. This method of fetal surveillance was developed and a machine invented by the author, modifying the TN-400 fetal monitor in 1984[1]. The Toitu Company has produced several models of actocardiographs. Ultrasound was changed into a 1-MHz pulse in order to improve fetal heart rate detection. Twin fetal monitors are composed of two channel actograms. Automatic dot-marking was initially prepared in the Toitu models. The Hewlett Packard model records only the dots and fetal heart rate, and this is termed a 'kinetocardiogram'. The Sonicaid model, however, records the movement signals in a similar manner to those recorded by the author. The recording of original movement signals is important in estimating the amplitude of fetal movements, cyclic movements synchronized with physiological sinusoidal fetal heart rate, and the analysis of the motion of fetal hiccuping.

The transducer is the same as in a CTG, and a single transducer is used for fetal movement and fetal heart rate. It is placed on the maternal abdomen, fetal heart beats are detected and fetal heart rate is recorded. At the same time, the transducer detects the movement of the fetal trunk. Uterine contractions can be recorded by switching the channel from the movement to the contraction, or by overlapping the movement to the contraction curve. An augmented actogram is under further investigation by the author, using a multichannel recorder.

ANALYSIS OF THE ACTOCARDIOGRAM

A spike of the actogram shows a single fetal movement, but the movement signals usually form a group of 10 s to 1 min, starting from a small spike, which gradually enlarges, reaching a peak then becomes smaller and finally ceases. The grouping is called an 'FM burst', which frequently appears in an active fetal state (Figure 1). The active state lasts for 50 min to several hours. Sudden and abrupt FM bursts were observed in an anencephalic fetus.

A close relationship of FM bursts and fetal heart rate acceleration is clearly noted in the normal active state, and the FM burst synchronizes with the accelerations of the fetal heart rate. Cross-correlation analysis of the fetal heart rate and the movement show a high correlation coefficient in the two phenomena after several seconds' delay of the movement signal in the active fetal state.

In the resting fetal state, fetal movement and acceleration of the fetal heart rate are absent, the baseline of the fetal heart rate is low, and the variability of the baseline of the fetal heart rate is decreased. The resting state lasts for 10–40 min (Figure 1).

Fetal hiccuping was confirmed by B-mode, and it was represented by very regular spikes with the interval of 2–3 s. Pregnant women perceived the motion of fetal hiccuping, but there was no acceleration if the fetus was resting. There may be erroneous interpretation of the non-reactive NST in that case. Fetal hiccuping signals are more clearly demonstrated in the augmented record (Figure 2). Low but continuous and regular spikes are recorded on the appearance of fetal breathing on the B-mode screen (Figure 1).

DIAGNOSIS OF FETAL WELL-BEING

Fetal well-being is assessed usually by a NST with the use of CTG. Ultrasonic Doppler blood flowmetry and the biophysical profile are also used in antepartum fetal assessment. A false-positive non-reactive NST is frequent in the use of the common simple CTG. Teshima[2] reported that a false-positive NST was found in 71% of the cases when no fetal movement was taken into account, and only fetal heart rate was observed.

The false-positive NST is caused first by the incorrect interpretation of absent acceleration in the resting fetal state that is clearly separated

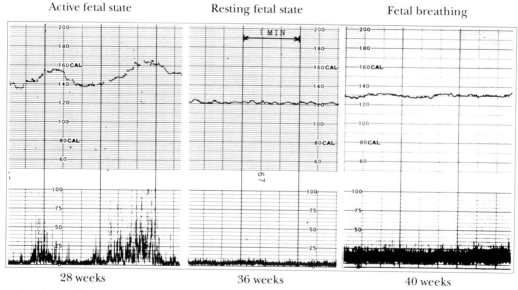

Figure 1 Actocardiograms in an active fetal state, resting fetal state, and in fetal breathing (upper panels, fetal heart rate; lower panels, fetal movement)

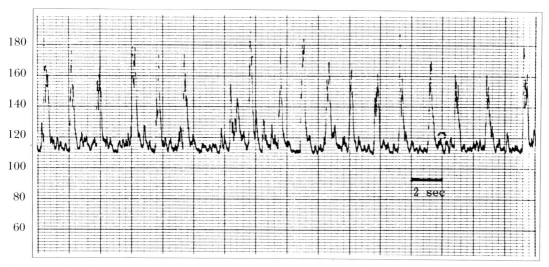

Figure 2 *Fetal hiccup movements recorded by augmented actocardiogram (chart speed 10 times, and amplitude about 10 times larger than the records in Figure 1). Regular spikes with 2–3 seconds' interval show fetal hiccups*

from the true non-reactive fetal heart rate by the use of the actocardiogram. As the motion of fetal hiccups results in no acceleration in the resting fetal state, its recognition contributes to a reduction in the false-positive non-reactive NSTs. Sinusoidal fetal heart rate is usually an ominous sign, however. The pattern is not ominous when the change synchronizes with cyclic fetal movements and is associated with a normal reactive fetal heart rate before and after the pattern (Figure 3). A characteristic fetal movement is suggestive of cyclic fetal breathing, by its regular appearance and frequency (Figure 3).

After exclusion of false-positive cases and pseudosinusoidal changes, truly non-reactive cases were diagnosed by the actocardiogram. Truly non-reactive fetal heart rate is diagnosed by the actocardiogram by the loss of acceleration or its severe decrease in spite of the presence of active fetal movements. The baseline level is normal, as is the long-term variability. There is no deceleration (Figure 4). The truly non-reactive NST is frequently followed by severe changes in the fetal heart rate (fetal distress) within a few days.

We experienced many cases, examples of which are shown in Figure 4. Teshima[2] reported 25 cases of truly non-reactive tracings by the actocardiogram. There were 20 cases of intrauterine growth retardation, 14 with oligohy-

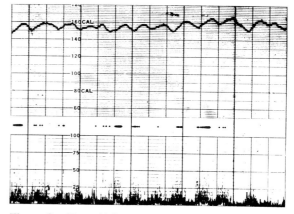

Figure 3 *Sinusoidal pattern of fetal heart rate synchronized with cyclic fetal movements (supposedly cyclic fetal breathing movements). Normal reactive fetal heart rate was recorded before and after the pseudo-sinusoidal pattern, and the outcome was normal*

dramnios, and 11 with pre-eclampsia in the truly non-reactive cases. Of the 25 cases, 19 (76%) developed fetal distress in antepartum and intrapartum periods, and received emergency Cesarean section.

Intrauterine growth retardation was common among the 25 cases. We therefore collected 20 control fetuses with intrauterine growth retardation that showed normal reactive fetal heart rates. The outcome was compared in the two groups. Seventeen truly non-reactive fetuses

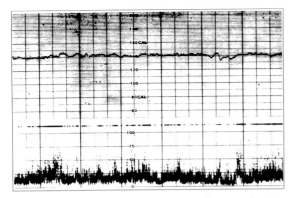

Figure 4 *Truly non-reactive actocardiogram showing frequent fetal movements but no definite acceleration of fetal heart rate. The patient showed fetal distress immediately after the record, and received Cesarean section*

Table 1 *Fetal distress in actocardiographically diagnosed cases that were reactive and truly non-reactive. (From reference 2)*

		Fetal distress		
	n	Positive	%	Negative
Reactive				
All stages	20	4	20	16
Antepartum	17	1	6	16
Truly non-reactive				
All stages	20	17	85	3
Antepartum	18	15	84	3

with intrauterine growth retardation developed signs of fetal distress, including bradycardia, late deceleration, severe variable deceleration or the loss of variability in antepartum of intrapartum periods, but only four fetuses with intrauterine growth retardation and reactive fetal heart rate developed fetal distress. The sensitivity of the truly non-reactive tracing in the fetuses with intrauterine growth retardation to predict fetal distress was 81%, the specificity was 84%, the positive predictive value was 85%, the negative predictive value was 80%, and the accuracy was 83%.

As antepartum fetal distress was frequent in the study, we compared the two groups in the antepartum period, so that the influence of labor stress could be excluded. Fifteen cases developed fetal distress during pregnancy among the 18 with truly non-reactive tracings, whereas only one case developed antepartum fetal distress in the 17 with reactive tracings. Therefore, the sensitivity to predict antepartum fetal distress was corrected to 94% in the truly non-reactive tracings in fetuses with intrauterine growth retardation (Table 1).

The interval before development of signs of fetal distress after the truly non-reactive diagnoses was 0–15 days.

Other clinical outcomes are compared between the reactive and truly non-reactive cases. In the cases with truly non-reactive actocardiograms, gestational age was decreased, birth weight was decreased, fetal distress was increased, and neonatal depression was increased, compared to the reactive cases with intrauterine growth retardation.

The frequency of the umbilical arterial Doppler flow wave showed the loss of end-diastolic flow or reverse flow in the truly non-reactive cases. As the actocardiogram is mainly related to function of the central nervous system, and the Doppler flow wave to circulatory function, combined use of these techniques should further improve the assessment of fetal well-being.

DIAGNOSIS OF FETAL DISTRESS

In the cases of fetal distress diagnosed by changes in fetal heart rate, fetal movement was reduced, or disappeared. Cases with mild distress showed the decrease of fetal movement and severe fetal distress immediately before fetal death showed absent movement. Therefore, the disappearance of fetal movement is a late sign of fetal deterioration. The fetus should be carefully examined and treated if necessary when there is reduction of fetal movement. Complete loss of fetal movement will often be too late to prevent hypoxic damage.

ACOUSTIC AND PHOTIC FETAL STIMULATION

In the author's view, the purpose of acoustic and photic stimulation of the fetus is to detect the threshold of the stimuli needed to develop a fetal response, in order to reduce the intensity of stimulation, and also to study fetal sensitivity to sound and light.

The vibroacoustic stimulator (VAST or FAST) was not used in the author's experience, but instead the sound used was pure sine-wave sound, with a frequency of 250, 500 or 1000 Hz. The intensity was 80 dB or less. Sound intensity gradually increased until the appearance of fetal response, which was acceleration of fetal heart rate and/or fetal movement (Figure 5). The actocardiogram was used in the recording of fetal response.

Fetal photic stimulation was carried out by the exposure of the maternal abdomen to photographic flash light. The light was weakened and changed into red color after passing through pork of 3 cm in diameter. Therefore, the stimulation would be safe due to the reduction of intensity and ultraviolet light. The fetal response was the same as to acoustic stimulation.

The intensity threshold of 1000 Hz pure sound to develop a fetal response was 80 dB at 28 weeks of pregnancy, reduced to 60 dB at 40 weeks. This suggests that the sound intensity which was necessary to develop a fetal response was reduced by 20 dB (10%). In other words, fetal sensitivity increased tenfold in late pregnancy, compared to 28 weeks (Figure 6). The technique can be used for a test of fetal auditory function or the total response in the cases of anatomical or functional abnormality of the central nervous system.

The fetal response to photic stimulation appeared after 22 weeks of pregnancy, and gradually increased. Visual function of the fetus also increased in the late stage of pregnancy.

CONCLUSION

In conclusion, the actocardiogram is useful not only in fetal behavioral studies but also in the evaluation of fetal well-being, reducing false-positive non-reactive tests or false sinusoidal patterns. It is a valuable tool to predict fetal distress in the antepartum period. The results obtained by intrapartum monitoring should be further improved by the careful application of antepartum monitoring.

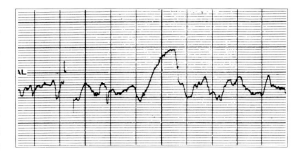
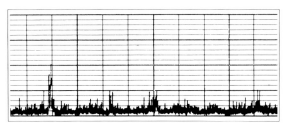

Figure 5 *Fetal response with acceleration of heart rate to acoustic stimulation with 1000 Hz and 72 dB pure sound for 2 s*

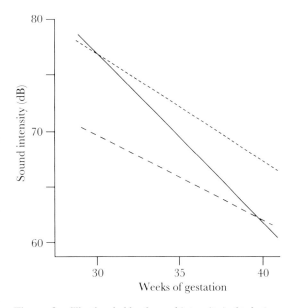

Figure 6 *The thresholds of sound intensity in fetal stimulation with pure sinewave sound of 250 (– – –) 500 (- - -) and 1000 Hz (———). Only sound of 1000 Hz showed a significant linear correlation with weeks of gestation*

The truly non-reactive fetus diagnosed by the actocardiogram can be treated by admission of the mother to the hospital and giving her bedrest, oxygen inhalation, or treatment of an underlying condition, or, when necessary, by early termination of pregnancy.

This strategy should improve fetal outcome, and also reduce maternal morbidity due to the reduction of Cesarean deliveries. For example, Cesarean delivery was reduced after the widespread use of antepartum NSTs in Yohka Hospital[4]. This may be due to detection of fetal abnormality and the capability of its treatment before the onset of labor, reducing intrapartum Cesarean delivery due to fetal distress. Actocardiographic NSTs should be more useful for this purpose than the simple CTG.

Actocardiographic fetal response to pure sound and flash light is valuable not only in evaluating fetal well-being, but also in evaluating the function of the central nervous system, particularly the auditory and visual capability of the fetus.

References

1. Maeda, K. (1984). Studies on new ultrasonic Doppler fetal actograph and continuous recording of fetal movement. *Acta. Obstet. Gynaecol. Jpn.*, **36**, 280–8
2. Teshima, N. (1993). Non-reactive pattern diagnosed by ultrasonic Doppler fetal actocardiogram and outcome of the fetuses with non-reactive pattern. *Acta Obstet. Gynaecol. Jpn.*, **45**, 423–30
3. Maeda, K. and Tatsumura, M. (1993). Antepartum development of fetal behavior and fetal sensitivity to acoustic and photic stimuli: actocardiographic studies. *Asian Med. J.*, **36**, 277–88
4. Tsuzaki, T., Sekijima, A., Morishita, K., Takeuchi, U., Mizuta, M., Mimagawa, Y., Nakajima, K. and Maeda, K. (1990). The survey on the perinatal variables and the incidence of cerebral palsy for 12 years before and after the application of the fetal monitoring system. *Acta Obstet. Gynaecol. Jpn.*, **42**, 99–105

The fetal biophysical profile 22

J. M. Carrera, J. Mallafré and M. Torrents

INTRODUCTION

The progressive introduction of new methods for antepartum fetal surveillance has allowed the obstetrician over the past 20 years to view and assess the fetus as a patient. Advances in biophysical techniques, particularly electronic fetal heart rate monitoring, real-time ultrasound scanning and Doppler velocimetry, have provided clinicians with the ability to examine the unborn patient directly. Indirect tools of fetal surveillance, such as biochemical monitoring of hormone and enzyme levels, have fallen into disuse, because of low sensitivity and specificity. Moreover, biophysical assessment of the fetus allows an immediate evaluation of the current fetal condition, and has proven to be preferable.

Biophysical techniques are used in obstetric practice to assess the generalized and specific biophysical activities of the fetus, including gross body movements, breathing movements, tone, heart rate, reflex activities, sucking, swallowing and micturition, fetal growth and development, rest/activity cycles, fetal responses after vibroacoustic stimulation or direct tactile scalp stimulation, flow in the uteroplacental and fetal umbilical vessels, and the intrauterine environment, including amniotic fluid volume and placental location and grade.

Monitoring of a single biophysical variable as a tool for fetal risk assessment has been shown to present unacceptably high false-positive rates. In contrast, data provided by the evaluation of multiple biophysical variables are difficult to integrate for diagnosing and predicting fetal outcome in a given patient. Several authors have, therefore, contributed to the development of 'biophysical profiles' that include the most significant biophysical variables and that offer an overall assessment of fetal condition with an acceptable sensitivity and specificity.

In this chapter, following an overview of the biophysical variables most useful for antepartum fetal surveillance, a description is given of the biophysical profiles that have proved most successful in predicting perinatal outcome. A new alternative scheme, the so-called 'progressive biophysical profile', is also reported.

FETAL BIOPHYSICAL PARAMETERS USEFUL IN CLINICAL DIAGNOSIS

The biophysical approach to antenatal fetal surveillance is based on the assessment of the same basic functions that the Apgar test evaluates in neonates, i.e. respiratory function, by measuring uteroplacental blood flow (Doppler velocimetry); hemodynamic function, by determining fetal heart rate activity and fetal blood flow distribution (Doppler velocimetry in fetal blood vessels); and neuromuscular function, both intrinsic (ultrasound monitoring of fetal tone and fetal movements) and extrinsic (fetal startle response evoked by vibroacoustic stimulation) (Table 1). However, the number of potentially useful biophysical variables that may be assessed during sonographic and cardiotocographic examinations is, in fact, much larger.

Biometric studies

Ultrasound fetal biometric measurements are not usually included in surveys of biophysical variables, since it is assumed that these data have been obtained prior to biophysical profile scoring. When the fetal biophysical profile is going to be used to follow pregnancies at risk for uteroplacental insufficiency[1], the assessment of fetal growth should be included in the survey.

Table 1 *Relationship between methods of neonatal evaluation and antenatal surveillance*

	Neonatal evaluation (Apgar score)	Antenatal surveillance (biophysical approach)
Respiratory function	breathing movements	uteroplacental blood flow (Doppler velocimetry)
Hemodynamic function		
heart	fetal heart rate	fetal heart rate patterns (cardiotocographic monitoring)
perfusion	color	fetal blood flow distribution (Doppler velocimetry in fetal blood vessels)
Neuromuscular function		
intrinsic	tone	tone and gross body movements (real-time ultrasound)
extrinsic	reflex activities	fetal responses after vibroacoustic stimulation

Despite the fact that many different parameters exist, the most commonly used are cephalometric measurements (biparietal and fronto-occipital diameters, head circumference, cephalic area, etc.), abdominal measurements (transverse and anteroposterior diameters, abdominal circumference, abdominal area, etc.), and the measurements of long bones (length of femur, length of humerus, etc.).

If such variables are to be included in the fetal biophysical profile, only those with the greater degree of diagnostic accuracy should be considered. It would seem reasonable to include a cephalometric measurement (head circumference or cephalic area, for example) and an abdominal measurement (abdominal circumference or abdominal area). In cases of intrauterine growth retardation, the correlation between both parameters would allow determination of the type of retardation involved.

Amniotic fluid volume

When chronic fetal hypoxia occurs, there is an impairment of the balance between amniotic fluid formation and reabsorption. The reason for this may be found in decreased renal activity as a result of hypoperfusion of the kidneys, due to blood flow redistribution[2]. It has been shown that oligohydramnios is associated with a significant increase in perinatal morbidity and mortality[3-7]. The decrease in amniotic fluid volume is, therefore, considered a clear marker of the compromised fetus.

Although several methods, some of them highly sophisticated, have been proposed to assess quantitatively the volume of amniotic fluid[3,8-10], semiquantitative techniques based upon measurement of the largest pocket of amniotic fluid are preferred by most authors[6-11]. Manning[7] has shown a close correlation between the vertical diameter of the largest pocket of amniotic fluid and perinatal mortality. Oligohydramnios is sonographically diagnosed when the depth of the largest pocket measures less than 1 or 2 cm. Because amniotic fluid volume varies considerably in later pregnancy – the depth of pockets is greater at 30–33 weeks (> 3 cm) that at term (> 2 cm) or post-term (> 1 cm) – the definition of oligohydramnios should probably be adjusted to gestational age.

The four-quadrant assessment of amniotic fluid volume, described by Phelan and colleagues[12], is a very useful method. The landmarks used to divide the uterine cavity into four sections are the umbilicus (upper and lower halves) and the linea nigra (right and left halves). The total depth of the amniotic fluid pockets in all four quadrants is determined and called the amniotic fluid index (normal score at term 12.9 ± 4.6 cm)[13]. An amniotic fluid index of less than 6.0 cm has been associated with a higher incidence of meconium, intrapartum fetal distress, and a low 5-min Apgar score.

Placental grading

Technical advances in the field of ultrasonography have permitted the observation of textural changes in the placenta. Grannum and associates[14] have developed a practical classification of placental maturity changes. This classification grades placentas from 0 to III according to specific ultrasonic changes at the basal layer,

Table 2 *Classification of placental maturity changes. (Modified from Reference 14)*

	Grade 0	Grade I	Grade II	Grade III	Grade IV
Basal layer	devoid of densities	devoid of densities	basal stippling	irregular densities	irregular densities with acoustic shadowing
Placental substance	homogeneous	linear, echogenic densities	comma-like densities	fall-out areas	echo-spared areas surrounded by calcified rings
Chorionic plate	smooth	undulating	subtle indentations	large indentations	'skeletal' indentations

placental substance and chorionic plate. We have described a fifth pattern of placental maturation (Table 2). The grade IV placenta manifests extensive echo-spared areas surrounded by clearly defined calcified rings that occupy the whole placental substance, giving a 'skeletal appearance', as if only the structure of intercotyledonary septa had been left untouched. These pathological maturational changes have been documented in 59% of cases of placenta-related intrauterine growth retardation. Vintzileos and colleagues[15] suggest that a grade III placental score has a significant association with abnormal intrapartum fetal heart rate patterns.

Fetal movements

Fetal movements are indirect evidence of activity of the central nervous system (CNS). Progressive maturation of the CNS increases the complexity of patterns of fetal movement, which are at present well defined[16,17].

The quantification of fetal movements, whether gross body movements or breathing movements, has been considered for a long time to be a reliable method of assessing fetal condition[18-20]. Although fetal behavior patterns based on fetal eye and body movements and fetal heart rate recordings have been established[17], most biophysical profiles include assessment of fetal movement in only a semi-quantitative manner.

Gross fetal activity is easily observed by simple cardiotocographic or ultrasound monitoring. Different types of gross fetal body movements at 30–41 weeks and normal daily patterns of fetal activity were reported by our group in 1981[21]. In a group of 216 patients with high-risk pregnancies, Manning and associates[22] showed that decreased (abnormal) gross body movements were associated with a significantly higher occurrence of fetal distress and perinatal mortality as compared with fetuses with normal body movements.

With respect to fetal breathing movements, Platt and colleagues[23], by means of the real-time B-scan method, showed that the presence of fetal breathing movements was a valuable sign of fetal well-being, while reduced breathing activity was consistently associated with neonatal asphyxia. Since fetal breathing movements are a periodic phenomenon, a long observation period is required in order to differentiate the abnormal fetus from the fetus whose length of apnea corresponds to a normal resting cycle.

Fetal tone

The fetal tone center (cortex–subcortical area) is the earliest to function during intrauterine life and is the last to disappear during asphyxia[24]. The absence of fetal tone is associated with a perinatal death rate of 45–50%[15,22,25]. Normal fetal tone is considered to be active flexion–extension of the fetal limbs or opening and closing of the fetal hands[22].

Fetal heart rate activity

Although antepartum cardiotocographic monitoring of fetal heart activity may not seem to be useful as a routine procedure in all pregnancies[26], it provides useful information on possible respiratory compromise in high-risk pregnancies, particularly in cases of intrauterine growth retardation[26-28] and cord accidents[29,30]. The relatively high false-positive rate is the main disadvantage of the procedure[31], while simplicity is its greatest advantage.

An important feature to be assessed is the relationship between fetal movements and/or spontaneous contractions and the occurrence of accelerations and decelerations in fetal heart rate. The induction of accelerations by a reflex feedback mechanism is associated with favorable perinatal outcome[32,33]. Two movement-related accelerations in a 20-min span are needed to deem the heart rate reactive.

Our group uses the Dexeus scoring system[19], which assesses the baseline fetal heart rate, variability of the baseline trace, fetal body movement, and reactivity of fetal heart rate in relation to fetal body movements and spontaneous uterine contractions (Table 3).

Vibroacoustic stimulation

Over the past decade fetal vibroacoustic stimulation, using an electronic artificial larynx, has been used to improve the efficiency of the non-stress test by reducing the incidence of non-reactive tests and the prolonged test time[34-36]. In addition, it has been shown that fetal vibroacoustic stimulation reliably predicts fetal pH in labor[34,37].

The stimulus, lasting 3 s, is equivalent to 75–96 dB at a frequency of 81–110 Hz, depending on the equipment used. The stimulus is usually applied to the maternal abdomen at the level of the fetal head, and responses are evaluated by sonographic or cardiotocographic monitoring. At our institution, changes in cardiotocographic recordings are assessed using a scoring system that takes into account fetal movement, baseline fetal heart rate, variability of heart rate, and duration of accelerations and decelerations (Table 4).

Table 3 Dexeus scoring system. (From Reference 19)

	Score		
	0	1	2
Baseline FHR (beats/min)	< 100 or > 180	100–120 or 160–180	120–160
Variability of FHR (beats/min)	< 5	5–10 or > 25	10–25
Fetal body movements	absence	< 20 movements/h	> 20 movements/h
Reactivity of FHR in relation to fetal body movements	without change	lambda or elliptic accelerations	omega or periodic accelerations
Reactivity of FHR in relation to spontaneous uterine contractions	late decelerations	non-reactive or with early decelerations	accelerations

FHR, fetal heart rate. Total scores: 9–10, normal; 7–8, equivocal; < 7, abnormal

Table 4 Evaluation of changes in cardiotocographic recordings used our scoring system

	Score		
	0	1	2
Baseline FHR	absence of changes	increase < 15 beats/min or < 1 min	increase > 15 beats/min or > 1 min
Fetal movements	absence of movements	slow movements	quick movements
Variability of FHR	absence of changes	increase < 15 beats/min	increase > 15 beats/min
Accelerations	absence	increase < 15 beats/min or < 15 s	increase > 15 beats/min or > 15 s
Decelerations (duration)	> 15 s	0–15 s	absence

FHR, fetal heart rate. Total scores: 9–10, normal (reactive); 7–8, equivocal (incomplete); < 7, abnormal

Doppler velocimetry

Umbilical artery velocity waveforms have been valuable in the early assessment of the compromised fetus[38–40]. These are obtained by means of continuous-wave Doppler instruments in combination, if necessary, with evaluation of blood flow in specific blood vessels (descending aorta, common carotid artery, middle cerebral artery), using more sophisticated Doppler systems (e.g. pulsed and color Doppler). Changes in blood flow velocity waveforms have also been documented in direct relationship with ominous biochemical patterns in fetal blood, obtained by puncture of the umbilical cord, and unfavorable perinatal outcome[41,42].

In our experience, abnormal umbilical artery velocity waveforms were associated, in 43.7% of cases, with changes in fetal blood flow, which evidenced peripheral redistribution of blood by the hypoxic fetus. Because changes in umbilical artery velocity waveforms usually precede changes that occur in the other fetal blood vessels, a normal examination would obviate an in-depth hemodynamic study of the fetus.

Although it is now possible to visualize and monitor the velocity of waveforms in the main fetal blood vessels using color Doppler, for obvious reasons the use of this technique should be limited to only a small number of vessels. In 1989, we designed the 'hemodynamic profile' which was based on data from one maternal artery (arcuate artery) and four fetal arteries (umbilical artery, descending aorta, common carotid artery, and middle cerebral artery)[43]. From the results obtained, a 'normal hemodynamic pattern' and a 'pathological hemodynamic pattern' were established (Table 5). Since normal curves had not as yet been developed, qualitative or semiquantitative criteria were used to assign results to one category or the other. Gestational age was not taken into consideration. Today, with the availability of percentile curves of the pulsatility of these vessels, quantitative criteria are used (Table 6).

FACTORS INFLUENCING BIOPHYSICAL VARIABLES

Most biophysical variables used in antepartum fetal surveillance reflect the condition of the fetal CNS and, more particularly, the degree of oxygenation. Several experimental studies have shown a decrease in or the abolition of these variables when animals suffered hypoxemia, which more or less severely affected their CNS and their biophysical activities[44–46]. The order in which biophysical variables are affected in the presence of asphyxia and the type of response

Table 6 Hemodynamic profile II. Pulsatility indexes. (From Reference 54)

	Normal	Abnormal
Umbilical artery	< 95th centile	> 95th centile
Thoracic aorta	< 95th centile	> 95th centile
Common carotid artery	> 5th centile	< 5th centile
Middle cerebral artery	> 5th centile	< 5th centile

Table 5 Hemodynamic profile I. Flow velocity waveforms. (From References 43 and 54)

	Hemodynamic patterns	
	Normal	Pathological
Arcuate artery (CI)	> 10th centile	< 10th centile
Umbilical artery (CI)	> 10th centile	< 10th centile
Thoracic aorta (PI)	1.5–2.5	> 2.5
Common carotid artery	absent end-diastolic velocity	diastolic flow
Middle cerebral artery (PI)	poor diastolic flow	< 1.25

CI, conductance index ($\frac{D}{S}.100$); PI, pulsatility index ($\frac{S-D}{V_m}$); D, diastolic velocity (minimum); S, systolic velocity (maximum); V_m, mean velocity

Table 7 *Fetal centers of the central nervous system and the effects of hypoxia. (From Reference 15, with permission)*

Biophysical variable	Center	Embryogenesis (weeks)	Hypoxia
Fetal tone	cortex (subcortical area?)	7.5–8.5	↑
Fetal corporal movements	cortex (nuclei)	9	
Fetal breathing movements	ventral surface of 4th ventricle	20–21	
Fetal heart rate activity	posterior hypothalamus, medulla	24–26	↓

to a hypoxemic stimulus varies according to the onset, extent and duration of the insult.

Order in which biophysical variables are affected

Vintzileos and colleagues[24] have shown that the order in which hypoxia affects different biophysical variables is the inverse of the order in which they become active in fetal development, although in the case of sufficiently severe asphyxia all parameters are impaired (Table 7). Thus, fetal tone, whose hypothetical center (subcortical area) is the first to function (7.5 to 8.5 weeks) is the last function to disappear in the presence of progressively worsening asphyxia. It has already been mentioned that the absence of fetal tone is associated with a very high perinatal mortality rate (40–45%). In contrast, the fetal heart rate reactivity center that matures late (28 weeks) is the first variable to be affected and may be considered to be the biophysical variable most sensitive to asphyxia.

Type of response

Fetal biophysical response patterns in the presence of asphyxia may, depending upon the duration and the severity of the insult, be of two types:

(1) Acute response pattern. As a result of an insult that is equally acute, rapid changes are brought about which affect CNS-regulated biophysical activities: reactivity of fetal heart rate, gross body movements, fetal breathing movements, fetal tone, etc.

(2) Chronic or subacute response pattern. Chronic fetal asphyxia results in decreased amniotic fluid volume, deceleration of fetal growth and redistribution and centralization of blood flow. In this case, there is a substantial increase in neonatal complications.

The pattern of response produced depends upon the cause of asphyxia. Acute response patterns usually occur in cases of abruptio placenta or sudden drop in uterine perfusion (e.g. maternal cardiorespiratory arrest) or umbilical perfusion (e.g. cord prolapse), whereas chronic response patterns are more frequent in cases of intrauterine growth retardation associated with progressive placental failure. In general terms, and in the absence of medical intervention, approximately 10% of perinatal deaths are the result of an acute asphyxial insult, 30% are the result of anomalies in fetal growth, and 60% are due to chronic sustained asphyxia[47].

Interpretation of individual biophysical variables

Biophysical variables are affected not only by CNS hypoxia but also by other pharmacological and physiological factors. Pharmaceutical products that depress the CNS, such as analgesics, sedatives and anesthetics, effectively reduce and can even abolish some fetal biophysical activities, while drugs used to stimulate the CNS may enhance fetal biophysical variables. On the other hand, rest/activity cycles and changes in blood levels of glucose may exert a physiological influence upon biophysical parameters.

Thus, while normal biophysical activity indicates that the area of the CNS which controls this type of activity is intact, and is not subject to hypoxemia, a decrease in or absence of biophysical activity is difficult to interpret. It may be due to hypoxemia, but also to a phase of physiological sleep, or to the effects of a particular drug. For this reason, Manning and colleagues developed a biophysical profile designed to minimize false-positive results by combining the simultaneous assessment of a number of variables (all variables can be affected by physiological or pharmaceutical factors) over a period of time that was greater than the usual sleep–wake periods.

It is well known that the study of a series of variables of different pathophysiological significance increases the predictive capacity of the test. The assessment of single biophysical variables has shown a high number of abnormal tests (10–15%) with a high rate of false-negative results (36/1000) and, more particularly, an unacceptably high rate of false-positive results (30–70%). In contrast, fetal biophysical profiles show a high number of normal results (97%), a much lower rate of false-positive results with greater specificity and positive predictive value (Table 8).

THE BIOPHYSICAL PROFILE PROPOSED BY MANNING AND COLLEAGUES

Manning and colleagues[11,22,47,50] developed a fetal biophysical profile based on a series of five basic variables: fetal breathing movements, gross body movements, fetal tone, fetal heart rate reactivity, and amniotic fluid volume (Table 9).

Equipment

A linear array real-time ultrasound method with a 3.5-MHz transducer together with a two-channel cardiotocograph was used to assess fetal heart rate and intrauterine activity (contractions, gross body movements, etc.).

Scoring

Each variable is assigned a score of 2, if considered normal, or 0, if considered abnormal.

The absence (abnormal) or presence (normal) of fetal breathing movements is assessed by ultrasound scanning longitudinally of the fetal thorax and diaphragm. Evidence of at least one episode of fetal breathing of 30-s duration, during a 30-min period of observation, scores 2 points. The absence of fetal breathing scores 0.

Gross body movements, defined as single or multiple, are assessed and counted by monitoring the fetal thorax and upper and lower limbs. Detection of at least three movements of the

Table 8 *Efficacy of individual and combined tests to predict fetal acidosis, for a total of 62 patients. (From Reference 49, with permission)*

Definition of abnormal test	Patients (n)	Sensitivity	Specificity*	PPV†	NPV	Overall efficiency‡	p (Fisher exact test)
Non-reactive NST	30	100% (9/9)	60% (32/53)	30% (9/30)	100% (32/32)	66% (41/62)	< 0.005
Biophysical score ≤ 7	13	89% (8/9)	91% (48/53)	62% (8/13)	98% (48/49)	90% (56/62)	< 0.001
High S/D**	37	66% (6/9)	42% (22/53)	16% (6/37)	88% (22/25)	45% (28/62)	NS
Non-reactive NST and high S/D	24	66% (6/9)	66% (35/53)	25% (6/24)	92% (35/38)	66% (41/62)	
Non-reactive NST or high S/D	41	100% (9/9)	40% (21/53)	22% (9/41)	100% (21/21)	48% (30/62)	
Biophysical score ≤ 7 and high S/D	8	56% (5/9)	94% (50/53)	63% (5/8)	92% (50/54)	88% (55/62)	
Biophysical score ≤ 7 high S/D	37	100% (9/9)	47% (25/53)	24% (9/37)	100% (25/25)	55% (34/62)	

PPV, positive predictive value; NPV, negative predictive value; NST, non-stress test; S/D, systolic/diastolic ratio; NS, not significant; *2 vs. 3, $p < 0.001$, Fisher exact test; †2 vs. 3, $p < 0.01$, Fisher exact test; ‡2 vs. 3 $p < 0.001$, Fisher exact test; **According to the nomogram by Schulman and colleagues[48]

Table 9 *Biophysical profile scoring: technique and interpretation (proposed by Manning and colleagues[22])*

Biophysical variable	Normal (score = 2)	Abnormal (score = 0)
Fetal breathing movements	≥ one episode of ≥ 30 s in 30 min	absent or no episode of ≥ 30 s in 30 min
Gross body movements	≥ discrete body/limb movements in 30 min (episodes of active continuous movement considered)	< 2 episodes of body/limb movements in 30 min as single movement
Fetal tone	≥ one episode of active extension with return to flexion of fetal limb(s) or trunk. Opening and closing of hand considered normal tone	either slow extension with return to partial flexion movement of limb in full extension or absent fetal movement
Reactive fetal heart rate	≥ two episodes of acceleration of ≥ 15 bpm and of > 15 s associated with fetal movement in 20 min	> 2 episodes of acceleration of fetal heart rate or acceleration of < 15 bpm in 20 min
Qualitative amniotic fluid volume	≥ one pocket of fluid measuring 1 cm in two perpendicular planes	either no pockets or largest pocket < 1 cm in two perpendicular planes

bpm, beats per min

body/limbs during a 30-min period of observation scores 2 points. The absence of body movements scores 0. Fetal eye movements, sucking, swallowing, etc. are also monitored, but are not included in the profile. On the other hand, episodes of uninterrupted movement are assessed as one movement.

Fetal tone is assessed through ultrasound imaging of the trunk, limbs and hands of the fetus. Each episode of flexion/extension of the trunk or limbs scores 2 points, as does the opening and closing of the fetal hand. The absence of these movements scores 0.

Amniotic fluid volume is calculated by measuring the vertical diameter of the largest pocket detected. Although in the initial description, in 1980, Manning and associates[22] considered the largest pocket of fluid greater than 1 cm in two perpendicular planes to be normal (score 2), later, in 1985, a vertical diameter of 2 cm was considered to be normal[50].

Fetal heart rate reactivity is assessed by continuous cardiotocographic monitoring of fetal heart rate during a period of 20 min. The observation of two or more fetal heart rate accelerations of at least 15 beats per minute in amplitude and at least 30-s duration associated with fetal movement(s) in a 20-min period, scores 2 points; otherwise, 0 points are scored. If, during the first 20 min of monitoring, the trace is non-reactive, examination will continue for another 20 min.

Manning and co-workers[47] believe that if the first four variables are normal, the biophysical profile test is complete. Only in those cases in which one or more variables are abnormal, is monitoring of fetal heart rate reactivity required.

Results

It has been shown that both the positive and the negative predictive value of the test are higher when variables are assessed in combination rather than individually[11,22,47,51] (Table 10). The false-negative rate was < 1% (between 0.5% and 0.8%) and, therefore, similar to the oxytocin challenge test. With its use, however, the number of false-positive results is considerably reduced.

Perinatal mortality was 10/1000 with scores of 10, rising to 600/1000 with scores of 0[17]. In the experience of Baskett and colleagues[52], the percentage of perinatal death was 0.3/1000 with scores of 8–10 and 292/1000 with scores of 0–4. The incidence of morbid perinatal outcome also increased when scores of the fetal biophysical profile were low (Table 11).

Although there are no statistically significant differences in sensitivity and specificity between the fetal biophysical profile and the non-stress test, the positive predictive value of the biophysical profile is clearly higher. Moreover, the num-

Table 10 Cumulative results of fetal biophysical profile for antepartum fetal assessment. (From Reference 50, with permission)

Study population	Patients (n)	High risk (%)	Tests Number	Normal (%)	Equivocal (%)	Abnormal (%)	Crude PNM n	Crude PNM Rate	Corrected PNM* n	Corrected PNM* Rate	False-negatives n	False-negatives Rate
Manitoba general population 1979–82	65 979	20	—	—	—	—	943	14.1	586	8.81	—	—
Manitoba prospective study	12 260	100	26 257	97.92	1.72	0.75	93	7.37	24	1.90	8	0.643
From reference 52	2 400	100	5 618	97.1	1.70	1.2	23	9.20	11	4.40	1	0.500
From reference 23	286	100	1 112	94.0	3.5	2.4	4	14.00	2	7.00	2	7.400
From reference	150	100	342	94.9	2.0	3.1	5	33.00	4	26.60	0	0
Total	15 614	>90	33 569	>95	2.0	1.0	132	8.40	43	2.70	12	0.770

PNM, perinatal mortality; *Corrected to exclude death due to lethal anomaly or Rh disease

Table 11 Last biophysical profile scoring result and normal perinatal outcome variable. (From Reference 53, with permission)

	Last biophysical profile scoring result					R^2 value	p^*
	Normal	6	4	2	0		
Number of patients	6 500	512	228	117	28		
Fetal distress (%)	12.8	24.3**	58.1	66.7	100**	0.9670	< 0.003
Admission to neonatal intensive care unit (%)	4	11.4**	28.8	40.2	83**	0.90 0.92	< 0.01 < 0.01
Intrauterine growth retardation (%)	3.4	4.4	28.8	41	75		
5-min Apgar score < 7 (%)	3.7	11.4**	18**	30.8**	60.7**	0.89	< 0.02
pH recorded† (%)	4	14	27	26.5	53.6	0.98	< 0.001
Cord pH < 7.20† (%)	2.2	14.5**	26**	32.3	40**	0.98	< 0.002
Mean pH	7.36	7.34**	7.26**	7.22**	7.17**	0.97	< 0.01
Meconium (%)	8.7	20.3**	23.4	19.7	21.4	—	NS
Anomaly (%)	3.7	3.8**	4.1	4.3	14.3**	—	NS

*Calculated as linear regression of y or x as outcome variable; **significant increase compared with next highest score; †not a complete sample of all patients

ber of false-negative results registered is four to six times greater in the non-stress test.

MODIFICATIONS TO THE BIOPHYSICAL PROFILE PROPOSED BY MANNING AND COLLEAGUES

The biophysical profile developed by Vintzileos and associates

In 1983, Vintzileos and associates[15] introduced a series of modifications to the biophysical profile proposed by Manning and co-workers[22], largely consisting of the addition of a sixth parameter – placental grading – and the institution of three, as opposed to two scores for each biophysical variable (0, 1, or 2 points) (Table 12).

The ultrasound imaging of the placenta, graded according to the classification proposed by Grannum and co-workers[14], provides a new parameter for the fetal biophysical profile, which is not usually difficult to obtain and which, although there is a divergence of opin-

Table 12 *Criteria for scoring biophysical variables according to Vintzileos and colleagues. Maximal score 12; minimal score 0. (Reprinted with permission from the American College of Obstetricians and Gynecologists[15]*

Non-stress test (NST)
Score 2 (NST 2): Five or more fetal heart rate accelerations of at least 15 beats/min in duration associated with fetal movements in a 20-min period

Score 1 (NST 1): Two to four accelerations of at least 15 beats/min in amplitude and at least 15 s in duration associated with fetal movements in a 20-min period

Score 0 (NST 0): One or fewer accelerations in a 20-min period

Fetal movements (FM)
Score 2 (FM 2): At least three gross (trunk and limbs) episodes of fetal movements within 30 min. Simultaneous limb and trunk movements are counted as a single movement

Score 1 (FM 1): One or two fetal movements within 30 min

Score 0 (FM 0): Absence of fetal movements within 30 min

Fetal breathing movements (FBM)
Score 2 (FBM 2): At least one episode of fetal breathing at least 60 s in duration within a 30-min observation period

Score 1 (FBM 1): At least one episode of fetal breathing lasting 30–60 s within 30 min

Score 0 (FBM 0): Absence of fetal breathing or lasting less than 30 s within 30 min

Fetal tone (FT)
Score 2 (FT 2): At least one episode of extension of extremities with return to position of flexion, and also one episode of extension of spine with return to position of flexion

Score 1 (FT 1): At least one episode of extension of extremities with return to position of flexion, or one episode of extension of spine with return to position of flexion

Score 0 (FT 0): Extremities in extension. Fetal movements not followed by return to flexion. Open hand

Amniotic fluid volume (AF)
Score 2 (AF 2): Fluid evident throughout the uterine cavity. A pocket that measures 2 cm or more in vertical diameter

Score 1 (AF 1): A pocket that measures less than 2 cm but more than 1 cm in vertical diameter

Score 0 (AF 0): Crowding of fetal small parts. Largest pocket less than 1 cm in vertical diameter

Placental grading (PG)
Score 2 (PL 2): Placental grading 0, 1 or 2

Score 1 (PL 1): Placenta posterior difficult to evaluate

Score 0 (PL 0): Placental grading 3

ions in the literature, we believe to be useful in antepartum fetal surveillance.

Vintzileos and associates[24,56,57] have also contributed by providing pathophysiological support to the fetal biophysical profile, validating the variables used and establishing that the order in which hypoxemia affects different biophysical variables is the inverse of the order in which biophysical activities become active in fetal development. Thus, fetal heart rate reactivity is the first variable to be affected and should therefore be a fundamental element in any biophysical profile.

The modified biophysical profile proposed by Eden and colleagues

In the modified biophysical profile developed by Eden and colleagues[58], particular importance is given to non-stress testing and ultrasound evaluation of amniotic fluid volume. Ultrasound assessment of fetal breathing and body movements is performed only to evaluate the non-reactive non-stress test. When the non-stress test is non-reactive, any of the following are considered an indication for delivery: decreased amniotic fluid volume, spontaneous fetal heart rate decelerations, or abnormal fetal breathing or body movements.

The modified scheme for biophysical profile scoring proposed by Shah and associates

In contrast to the proposal of Eden and colleagues[58], Shah and associates[59] developed a modified method for biophysical profile scoring based exclusively on real-time ultrasonographic evaluation, and including expanded scores for fetal movement and fetal breathing, and only qualitative assessment for decreased fetal tone, subjective oligohydramnios and accelerated placental maturation, without score assignment for the latter three components. The maximum total score is 8. Perinatal outcome is considered to be favorable if a total score between 6 and 8 is obtained. The aim of this scoring method is to screen for acute fetal asphyxia.

THE PROGRESSIVE BIOPHYSICAL PROFILE SCORING METHOD

New technological advances for use in antepartum fetal surveillance (vibroacoustic stimulation, Doppler velocimetry, etc.) which were not included in the fetal biophysical profile proposed by Manning and associates[22] in 1980, together with the aim to develop an integrated system of fetal monitoring applicable to all pregnancies, prompted us to design an alternative profile, the so-called 'progressive biophysical profile'[60]. In the modified scheme proposed by our group, different testing procedures are carried out according to the characteristics of each pregnancy. The higher the risk, the more sophisticated the procedure used.

The progressive biophysical profile consists of three profiles (baseline, functional and hemodynamic), each of which varies in the degree of sophistication of the equipment used and experience required of the examiner (Table 13). While the baseline biophysical profile is based on the results of conventional ultrasound imaging only, the functional biophysical profile requires the use of cardiotocographic monitoring and Doppler ultrasound equipment (continuous or pulsed) for the assessment of umbilical artery velocity waveforms. At the final step, the hemodynamic biophysical profile requires the use of high-resolution ultrasound equipment, including a pulsed Doppler, in order to assess velocity waveforms in fetal and uteroplacental blood vessels[55].

Altogether, the progressive biophysical profile includes all the biophysical variables that have been shown to be useful in screening for pregnancies that require special management and predicting fetal condition, thereby enabling a prognosis and a management program to be established. Biophysical variables, however, are not determined simultaneously, as in the case of the fetal biophysical profiles proposed by Manning and colleagues[22] and Vintzileos and associates[24], but rather consecu-

Table 13 *Progressive biophysical profile (PBP)*

	Baseline profile (PBP-B)	Functional profile (PBP-F)	Hemodynamic profile (PBP-H)
Methods	ultrasound	ultrasound cardiotocography umbilical Doppler	ultrasound umbilical Doppler fetal Doppler
Parameters	fetal biometry amniotic fluid volume placenta grading	fetal movements tone cardiotocography patterns reflex activities (vibroacoustic stimulation) umbilical Doppler (pulsatility index)	uteroplacental hemo- dynamic pattern fetal hemodynamic pattern

tively, depending upon the risk factors involved in each case. It is thus possible to institute a progressive, rational adaptation of the procedures available to the needs of each case. The greater the risk, the more complex the procedures used, the more time is spent on examination, the greater the experience required of the examiner, and, inevitably, the higher the cost. The use of this strategy simplifies the patient's care and reduces the cost of medical attention without impairing the quality.

The baseline biophysical profile

Concept

The baseline biophysical profile includes the sonographic assessment of five variables: two provide fetal biometric data (cephalic area and abdominal area), another two provide data on the fetal environment (placental structure and amniotic fluid volume), and the fifth assesses the evoked fetal startle response or fetal movements in response to vibroacoustic stimulation (Table 14).

Indications

The baseline biophysical profile has been design to be carried out at 33–35-weeks' gestation in order to monitor fetal condition in all pregnancies. In low-risk pregnancies, normal testing results make any subsequent examination unnecessary, unless the evolution of the pregnancy makes this necessary. An abnormal baseline profile indicates the need to carry out a functional biophysical profile.

Equipment

The baseline biophysical profile may be carried out at the first level of the health-care system, using ordinary equipment for conventional ultrasound imaging. The examiner needs only to have adequate expertise in obstetric ultrasound scanning. Vibroacoustic stimulation is carried out using an electronic artificial larynx.

Scoring

The five components of the biophysical profile are scored on a range from 0 to 2.

As far as biomorphic data are concerned, both the cephalic and the abdominal areas are classified according to their location on the normal curve in both parameters (score 0, < mean − 2 SD; score 1, > mean − 2 SD and < mean − 1 SD; score 2, > mean − 1 SD and < mean + 2 SD). In the event of the equipment not being able to plot a line, but a curve, identical criteria may be used for the head and abdominal circumference[54,61].

Amniotic fluid volume is assessed using the amniotic-fluid index in the four-quadrant method (score 0, amniotic fluid index < 5; score 1, amniotic fluid index between 5 and 8; score 2, amniotic fluid index ≥ 8.

Placental grading is carried out using the classification modified from Grannum and colleagues[14] (Table 2) to which the grade IV placenta (a more severe stage than grade III) has been added (score 0, grade IV placenta; score 1, grade III placenta; score 2, grades I or II placentas).

Table 14 Baseline biophysical profile. (From Reference 54)

	Score		
	0	1	2
Cephalic area	$< \bar{x} - 2$ SD	$< \bar{x} - 1$ SD and $> \bar{x} - 2$ SD	$> \bar{x} - 1$ SD and $< \bar{x} + 2$ SD
Abdominal area	$< \bar{x} - 2$ SD	$< \bar{x} - 1$ SD and $> \bar{x} - 2$ SD	$> \bar{x} - 1$ SD and $< \bar{x} + 2$ SD
Amniotic fluid index	< 5	5–8	> 8
Placental grading	IV	III	I–II
Acoustic stimulation*	non-reactive (< 7)	incomplete (7–8)	reactive (9–10)

*Scoring system, see Table 4; total score: 9–10, normal; 7–8, equivocal; < 7, abnormal

Gross body movements in response to vibroacoustic stimulation are detected by monitoring fetal movements, especially in the trunk and upper limbs, after one vibroacoustic stimulation of 3-s duration. If there is no response to the first stimulation, the test cannot be considered concluded until two further stimulations of identical characteristics have been given, slightly modifying the position of the larynx and the transducer (score 0, no appreciable response; score 1, slight or low movements limited to the fetal limbs; score 2, rapid, numerous movements of the limbs with flexion of the trunk; opening and closing of the fetal hand is also a sign of favorable fetal outcome).

Interpretation

A total score of 9 or 10 is indicative of normal fetal condition, with the appropriate growth rate, compatible with a normal placenta. A score of < 7 is associated with a greater or lesser degree of chronic fetal compromise. In these circumstances, a functional biophysical profile should be performed immediately in association with any other examinations that would be required. Delivery will probably be indicated. Finally, a score of 7 or 8 should be considered equivocal, thus requiring a functional biophysical profile. A score of 0 in any of the five biophysical variables should be considered particularly suspicious, particularly in the case of oligohydramnios.

The functional biophysical profile

Concept

Of the five variables included in the functional biophysical profile, two are assessed by cardiotocographic monitoring (cardiotocographic pattern evaluated by means of the Dexeus test, and evoked fetal startle reflex after vibroacoustic stimulation), two using real-time ultrasonographic imaging (fetal tone and gross body movements) and the last using Doppler continuous wave ultrasound equipment capable of monitoring umbilical artery velocity waveforms (Table 15). Cardiotocography and ultrasound monitoring should take place over a time period of at least 20 min.

Indications

The functional profile has been designed as a second step in fetal biophysical assessment. It should routinely be carried out in all high-risk pregnancies in which there is either suspicion or evidence of intercurrent disease. In low-risk pregnancies, however, it should only be used when the result of the baseline biophysical profile are equivocal or abnormal.

Equipment

Assessment of variables included in the functional biophysical profile should be carried out in hospital services (at level II of the healthcare system). High-resolution real-time ultra-

Table 15 *Functional biophysical profile. (From References 54 and 60)*

	Score		
	0	1	2
Cardiotocographic pattern (Dexeus score)	< 7	7–8	9–10
Reflex activity (scoring system for vibroacoustic stimulation)	< 7	7–8	9–10
Fetal tone	absence	slow extension/flexion movements	rapid extension/flexion movements
Gross body movements	absence	poor movements	rapid and numerous body movements
Umbilical Doppler (pulsatility index)	absent end-diastolic velocity/reverse flow	> 95th centile	< 95th centile

Total scores: 9–10, normal; 7–8, equivocal; < 7, abnormal

sound imaging, a two-channel cardiotocograph (with Doppler transducer, if possible), and Doppler continuous wave ultrasound equipment are needed. As in the case of the baseline biophysical profile, an electronic artificial larynx is required for vibroacoustic stimulation.

In addition to adequate experience in ultrasound imaging, appropriate knowledge of fetal medicine is required on the part of the examiner.

Scoring

The cardiotocographic pattern is assessed using the Dexeus test (score 0, < 7; score 1, between 7 and 8; score 2, > 8). Gross body movement in response to vibroacoustic stimulation is carried out as described in the baseline biophysical profile. As in the Dexeus test, a value of < 7 is considered to be abnormal and scores 0; a value between 7 and 8 scores 1; and a value between 9 and 10 scores 2.

Fetal tone is assessed by ultrasound monitoring of the fetus, particularly of upper and lower limbs (score 0, virtual absence of tone with permanent extension of the limbs and open hands; score 1, slow or incomplete extension/flexion movements; score 2, rapid extension/flexion movements of limbs and trunk).

Monitoring of fetal movement is limited to gross body movements although fetal breathing movements are also taken into consideration, if they appear (score 0, total absence of movement; score 1, fewer than three gross body movements of the trunk and limbs during the period of observation and/or fetal breathing movements of less than 30–60-s duration; score 2, rapid, numerous body movements – three or more during the period of observation – in association with fetal breathing movements of more than 60-s duration).

The umbilical artery velocity waveforms may be evaluated using any of the different parameters for assessing the flow velocity waveforms (FVW): pulsatility index, resistance index, conductance index, etc. In our group, the pulsatility index is currently being used (score 0, absence of diastole, and the 'reverse flow'; score 1, pulsatility index over the 95th centile; score 2, pulsatility index under the 95th centile).

Interpretation

As in the case of the baseline biophysical profile, a total score of < 7 suggests probable fetal asphyxia and a hemodynamic biophysical profile is required. This is also the case in scores of 7 or 8, when results are equivocal. In contrast, a total score of 9 or 10 is considered normal.

The hemodynamic biophysical profile

Concept

The hemodynamic biophysical profile includes the Doppler ultrasound assessment of velocity waveforms in the umbilical artery, descending aorta, common carotid artery and middle cerebral artery (Table 6).

Indications

The hemodynamic biophysical profile should be carried out in pregnant women with previous abnormal scores on the functional profile and pregnancy-induced hypertension. In cases of pregnancy-induced hypertension, early referral for fetal assessment by the hemodynamic biophysical profile is mandatory, no matter what the result of the other two biophysical profiles.

Equipment

High-resolution ultrasound equipment, including a duplex system for connecting B-mode (sectorial) to Doppler (pulsed and continuous, and, if possible, in color) is required to establish this profile. The biophysical basis for this technique and the methods used have been previously reported[43,62,63].

Given the sophisticated technology and the high cost of the equipment required, this procedure should be carried out in hospital services

Interpretation

Centile curves for the pulsatility index of each of the arteries monitored are currently available (discriminant values are given for each week of gestation). Quantitative evaluation of results is therefore possible when determining whether or not a hemodynamic pattern is normal or abnormal.

If the Doppler examination confirms normal distribution of fetal blood flow, it should be concluded that there is no evidence of fetal asphyxia. On the other hand, an abnormal hemodynamic pattern suggests a redistribution of cardiac output with centralization of fetal blood flow, which should be interpreted as evidence of fetal asphyxia. In this case delivery should be performed if the minimal conditions for fetal survival are present.

Clinical application of fetal biophysical profiles

Indications

The fetal biophysical profile has been used for different purposes, as follows:

(1) Screening for high-risk pregnancies. This is possible with the progressive biophysical profile but is practically impossible with Manning's biophysical profile, which is very time-consuming.

(2) For use only when the non-stress test[58] or results of other testing procedures are abnormal (e.g. grade III placenta)[24,56,57].

(3) Monitoring of high-risk pregnancies[25] (e.g. intrauterine growth retardation[22], premature rupture of membranes[64,65], uteroplacental insufficiency including pregnancy-induced hypertension, diabetes mellitus, previous obstetric complications, maternal disease, etc.[1], twin gestations[66] and post-term pregnancies with or without fetal macrosomia[67].

Table 16 Interpretation of fetal biophysical profile score results and recommended clinical management. (From Reference 50, with permission)

Test score result	Interpretation	PNM within 1 week without intervention	Management
10 of 10 8 of 10 (normal fluid) 8 of 8 (NST not done)	risk of fetal asphyxia extremely rare	< 1/1000	intervention only for obstetric and maternal factors. No indication for intervention for fetal disease
8 of 10 (abnormal fluid)	probable chronic fetal compromise	89/1000	determine that there is functioning renal tissue and these are intact membranes. If so, deliver for fetal indications
6 of 10 (normal fluid)	equivocal test, possible fetal asphyxia	variable	if the fetus is mature, deliver. In the immature fetus, repeat test within 24 h. If < 6/10, deliver
6 of 10 (abnormal fluid)	probable fetal asphyxia	89/1000	deliver for fetal indications
4 of 10	high probability of fetal asphyxia	91/1000	deliver for fetal indications
2 of 10	fetal asphyxia almost certain	125/1000	deliver for fetal indications
0 of 10	fetal asphyxia certain	600/1000	deliver for fetal indications

PNM, perinatal mortality; NST, non-stress test

Interpretation and recommended management

In 1985, Manning and colleagues[50,68] standardized the interpretation of his fetal biophysical profile score results and recommended clinical management (Table 16).

Although there is controversy over the frequency with which profiles should be determined[24,56,57], in high-risk pregnancies, even when the results are acceptable (scores 8–9), at least one testing of the biophysical profile per week should be carried out. In the opinion of Manning and associates[47], in some cases such as those of post-term pregnancies, insulin-dependent diabetes mellitus and Rh-sensitization, two testings of the biophysical profile per week are required. In this way, a clear difference can be established between fetuses that are normal and those that are at risk of suffering intrauterine hypoxemia. Indeed, the frequency with which testings of the biophysical profile are repeated should conform to the requirements of each individual case.

In progressive biophysical profiles, algorithms vary according to whether a pregnancy is considered low- or high-risk (Figures 1 and 2). The baseline fetal biophysical profile is designed to be carried out at approximately 33–35 weeks' gestation and provides information on fetal condition in all pregnancies. Normal results in low-risk pregnancies obviate the need for further testing unless the subsequent evolution of the pregnancy makes this necessary. When abnormal results are found in the baseline biophysical profile, a functional biophysical profile should be obtained.

In high-risk pregnancies and, in particular, in those in which intrauterine growth retardation is suspected, a baseline biophysical profile should be carried out between 30 and 31 weeks and another at 34–35 weeks, the latter in combination with a functional biophysical profile. The hemodynamic biophysical profile should be carried out only when abnormal results have been obtained in the functional biophysical profile, particularly when the umbilical pulsatility index is abnormal.

In a hospital service with a 20–30% rate of high-risk pregnancies, functional testing of the

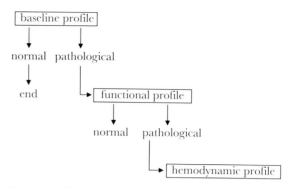

Figure 1 *Use of the progressive biophysical profile in low-risk pregnancies*

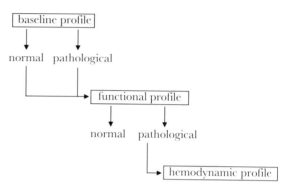

Figure 2 *Use of the progressive biophysical profile in high-risk pregnancies*

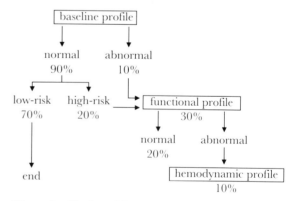

Figure 3 *Testing of the progressive biophysical profile in a hospital service with a 20–30% rate of high-risk pregnancies*

biophysical profile should be performed in approximately 30% of cases (Figure 3), and testing of the hemodynamic profile in 10% of cases. The frequency with which testing of the functional biophysical profile is repeated

Table 17 *Progressive biophysical profile: interpretation and recommended clinical management*

Test result	Interpretation			Management
	Baseline profile	Functional profile	Hemodynamic profile	
9–10	normal fetus	normal fetus		conservative management
7–8	possible chronic fetal compromise	possible fetal asphyxia		determine functional and/or hemodynamic profile; if normal, serial testing
< 7	probable chronic fetal compromise	probable fetal asphyxia		determine hemodynamic profile
Abnormal hemodynamic pattern			redistribution of fetal blood; fetal asphyxia certain	deliver for fetal indication

Table 18 *Efficacy of progressive biophysical profile to predict fetal distress*

	Baseline profile (%) n = 810	Functional profile (%) n = 224	Hemodynamic profile (%) n = 93
Sensitivity	63	81	90
Specificity	87	100	100
Positive predictive value	58	100	100
Negative predictive value	89	95	90

depends upon the circumstances of each case, but high-risk pregnancies are usually tested every week.

With regard to interpretation and recommended clinical management of the three stages of the progressive biophysical profile, whereas abnormal results in the baseline profile suggest chronic fetal compromise, a similar score in the functional biophysical profile probably suggests fetal asphyxia, which is confirmed by abnormal results in the hemodynamic profile (Table 17). The efficacy of the progressive biophysical profile to predict fetal distress is shown in Table 18.

References

1. Sachs, B. P. (1987). Biophysical profile. In Friedman, E. A., Acker, D. B. and Sachs, B. P. (eds.) *Obstetrical Decision Making*, 2nd edn., p.70. (Toronto: B.C. Decker Inc.)
2. Saunders, P. and Rhodes, P. (1973). The origin and circulation of amniotic fluid. In Fairweather, D. I. V. and Eskes, T. K. A. B. (eds.) *Amniotic Fluid Research in Clinical Applications*. (Amsterdam: Excerpta Medica Foundation)
3. Gohari, P., Berkowitz, R. L. and Hobbins, J. C. (1977). Prediction of intrauterine growth retarding by determination of total intrauterine volume. *Am. J. Obstet. Gynecol.*, **127**, 255–60
4. Pritchard, J. A. and McDonald, P. C. (1980). *Williams Obstetrics*, pp. 578–81. (New York: Appleton-Country Crofts)
5. Rayburn, W. T., Motley, M. E., Stempel, L. E. and Gendreau, R. M. (1982). Antepartum prediction of the postmature infant. *Obstet. Gynecol.*, **60**, 148–53
6. Chamberlain, P. F., Manning, F. A., Morrison, I., Harman, C. R. and Lange, I. R. (1984). Ultrasound evaluation of amniotic fluid volume. I. The relationship of marginal and decreased amniotic fluid volumes to perinatal outcome. *Am. J. Obstet. Gynecol.*, **150**, 245–9

7. Manning, F. A. (1989). General principles and application of ultrasound. In Creasy, R. and Resnick, P. (eds.) *Maternal–Fetal Medicine*, 2nd edn., pp. 195–243. (Philadelphia: W.B. Saunders Company)

8. Geirson, R. T., Christie, A. D. and Patel, N. B. (1982). Ultrasound volume measurement comparing a predate ellipsoid method with a parallel planimetric area method against a known volume. *J.V.C.*, **10**, 329–32

9. Geirson, R. T., Patel, N. B. and Christie, A. D. (1984). *In vivo* accuracy of ultrasound measurement of intrauterine volume in pregnancy. *Br. J. Obstet. Gynaecol.*, **91**, 37–40

10. Kirkinen, P. (1978). Ultrasonic assessment of polyhydramnios. In Kurjak, A. (ed.) *Advances in Ultrasound Diagnosis*, pp. 209–12. (Amsterdam: Excerpta Medica)

11. Manning, F. A., Hill, L. M. and Platt, L. D. (1981). Qualitative amniotic fluid volume determination by ultrasound: antepartum detection of intrauterine growth retardation. *Am. J. Obstet. Gynecol.*, **139**, 254–8

12. Phelan, J. P., Smith, C. V., Broussard, P. and Small, M. (1987). Amniotic fluid volume assessment with the four-quadrant technique at 36–42 weeks' gestation. *J. Reprod. Med.*, **32**, 540–2

13. Rutherford, S. E., Phelan, J. P., Smith, C. V. and Jacobs, N. (1987). The four-quadrant assessment of amniotic fluid volume: an adjunct to antepartum fetal heart rate testing. *Obstet. Gynecol.*, **70**, 353–6

14. Grannum, P. A. T., Berkowitz, R. L. and Hobbins, J. C. (1979). The ultrasonic changes in the maturing placenta and their relation to fetal pulmonic maturity. *Am. J. Obstet. Gynecol.*, **133**, 915–22

15. Vintzileos, A. M., Campbell, W. A., Ingardia, C. J. and Nochimson, D. J. (1993). The fetal biophysical profile and its predictive value. *Obstet. Gynecol.*, **62**, 271–8

16. De Vries, J. I. P., Visser, G. H. A. and Prechtl, H. F. R. (1982). The emergence of fetal behavior. I. Quantitative aspects. *Early Hum. Dev.*, **7**, 301–22

17. Nijhuis, J. G., Prechtl, H. F. R., Martin, C. B. and Bots, R. S. M. G. (1982). Are there behavioural states in the human fetuses? *Early Hum. Dev.*, **6**, 177–95

18. Timor-Tritsch, I., Zador, I., Hertz, R. R. H. and Rosen, M. G. (1976). Classification of fetal movement. *Am. J. Obstet. Gynecol.*, **126**, 70–7

19. Carrera, J. M. (1979). Evaluación del cardiotocograma anteparto mediante el test de Dexeus. *Prog. Obstet. Ginecol.*, **22**, 17–26

20. Sadovsky, E. and Polishuk, W. Z. (1977). Fetal movements *in utero*. *Obstet. Gynecol.*, **50**, 49–54

21. Carrera, J. M., Padula, C. and Alegre, M. (1981). Cinética fetal. In Carrera, J. M. (ed.) *Biología y Ecología Fetal*, pp.459–74. (Barcelona: Salvat Editores)

22. Manning, F. A., Platt, L. D. and Sipos, L. (1980). Antepartum fetal evaluation: development of a fetal biophysical profile. *Am. J. Obstet. Gynecol.*, **136**, 787–95

23. Platt, L. D., Manning, F. A., Lemay, M. and Sipos, L. (1978). Human fetal breathing: relationship to fetal condition. *Am. J. Obstet. Gynecol.*, **132**, 514–19

24. Vintzileos, A. M., Campbell, W. A., Nochimson, D. J. and Weinbaum, P. J. (1987). The use and abuse of the fetal biophysical profile. *Am. J. Obstet. Gynecol.*, **156**, 527–33

25. Brar, H. S., Platt, L. D. and Devore, G. R. (1987). Antepartum fetal surveillance: the biophysical profile. *Clin. Obstet. Gynecol.*, **30**, 936–47

26. Tacker, S. B. and Berkelman, R. L. (1986). Assessing the diagnostic accuracy and efficacy of selected antepartum fetal surveillance techniques. *Obstet. Gynecol. Surv.*, **41**, 121

27. Kubli, F. and Rüttgers, H. (1972). Semiquantitative evaluation of antepartum fetal heart rate. *Int. J. Gynaecol. Obstet.*, **10**, 180

28. Lee, C. Y., Di Loreto, P. C. and Logrand, B. (1976). Fetal activity acceleration determination for the evaluation of fetal reserve. *Obstet. Gynecol.*, **48**, 19–26

29. Fisher, W. M. (1980). Valoración del cardiotocograma prenatal. In Carrera, J. M. (ed.) *Monitorización Fetal Anteparto 1*. (Barcelona: Salvat Editores)

30. Losa, F. and Ruiz, J. (1984). Predicción anteparto de la patología funicular mediante monitorización biofísica. In *VI Reunión Nacional de Medicina Perinatal*, Barcelona (Abstr.) p. 26.

31. Evertson, L. R., Gauthier, R. R. J., Schifrin, B. S. and Paul, R. H. (1979). Antepartum fetal heart rate testing. I. Evolution of the nonstress test. *Am. J. Obstet. Gynecol.*, **133**, 29–33

32. Timor-Tritsch, I. E., Dierker, L. J., Zador, I., Hertz, R. H. and Rosen, M. G. (1978). Fetal movements associated with fetal heart rate accelerations and decelerations. *Am. J. Obstet. Gynecol.*, **131**, 276–80

33. Phelan, J. P. (1981). The nonstress test: a review of 3,000 tests. *Am. J. Obstet. Gynecol.*, **139**, 7–10

34. Edersheim, T. G., Hutson, J. M., Druzin, M. L. and Kogut, E. A. (1987). Fetal heart rate response to vibratory acoustic stimulation predicts fetal pH in labor. *Am. J. Obstet. Gynecol.*, **157**, 1557–60

35. Smith, C. V., Phelan, J. P., Platt, L. D., Broussard, P. and Paul, R. J. (1986). Fetal acoustic stimulation testing. II. A randomized clinical

comparison with the nonstress test. *Am. J. Obstet. Gynecol.*, **155**, 131–4

36. Gagnon, R., Hunse, C., Carmichael, L., Fellows, F. and Patrick, J. (1987). Human fetal responses to vibratory acoustic stimulation from twenty-six weeks to term. *Am. J. Obstet. Gynecol.*, **157**, 137–81
37. Polzin, G. B., Blakemore, K. J., Petrie, R. H. and Amon, E. (1988). Fetal vibro-acoustic stimulation: magnitude and duration of fetal heart rate accelerations as a marker of fetal health. *Obstet. Gynecol.*, **72**, 621–6
38. Fleischer, A., Schulman, H., Farmakides, G., Bracero, L., Blattner, P. and Randolph, G. (1985). Umbilical artery velocity waveforms and intrauterine growth retardation. *Am. J. Obstet. Gynecol.*, **151**, 502–5
39. Gill, R. W., Trudinger, B. J., Garrett, W. J., Kossoff, G. and Warren, P. S. (1981). Fetal umbilical venous flow measured *in utero* by pulsed Doppler and B-mode ultrasound. I. Normal pregnancies. *Am. J. Obstet. Gynecol.*, **139**, 720–5
40. Trudinger, B. J., Giles, W. B. and Cook, C. M. (1985). Flow velocity waveforms in the maternal uteroplacental and fetal umbilical placental circulations. *Am. J. Obstet. Gynecol.*, **152**, 155–63
41. Soothill, P. W., Nicolaides, K. H., Rodeck, C. H. and Campbell, S. (1986). Effect of gestational age of fetal and intervillous blood gas and acid-base value in human pregnancy. *Fetal Ther.*, **1**, 168–75
42. Rizzo, G., Arduini, D., Pennestri, F., Romanini, C. and Mancuso, S. (1987). Fetal behaviour in growth retardation: its relationship to fetal blood flow. *Prenat. Diagn.*, **7**, 229–38
43. Carrera, J. M., Mortera, C., Alegre, M., Pérez-Ares, C., Torrents, M. and Salvador, M. J. (1989). Fluxometría Doppler en la preeclampsia. *Prog. Obstet. Gynecol.*, **32**, 7–23
44. Manning, F. A., Martin, C. B., Murata, Y., Miyaki, K. and Danzler, G. (1979). Breathing movements before death in the primate fetus (*Macaca mulatta*). *Am. J. Obstet. Gynecol.*, **135**, 71–6
45. Boddy, K., Dawes, G. S., Fische, R., Pinter, S. and Robinson, J. S. (1974). Fetal respiratory movements, electrocortical and cardiovascular responses to hypoxemia in sheep. *J. Physiol. (London)*, **243**, 599–608
46. Natale, R. R., Clelow, F. and Dawes, G. S. (1981). Measurement of fetal forelimb movements in the lamb *in utero*. *Am. J. Obstet. Gynecol.*, **140**, 545–51
47. Manning, F. A., Harman, C. R., Menticoglou, S. and Morrison, I. (1991). Assessment of fetal well-being with ultrasound. *Obstet. Gynecol. Clin. N. Am.*, **18**, 891–905
48. Schulman, H., Winter, D., Farmakides, G., Ducey, J., Guzmán, E., Coury, E. and Penny, B. (1989). Pregnancy surveillance with Doppler velocimetry of uterine and umbilical arteries. *Am. J. Obstet. Gynecol.*, **160**, 192–6
49. Vintzileos, A. M., Campbell, W. A., Rodis, J. F., Mclean, D. A., Fleming, A. D. and Scorza, W. E. (1991). The relationship between fetal biophysical assessment, umbilical artery velocimetry and fetal acidosis. *Obstet. Gynecol.*, **77**, 4, 622–6
50. Manning, F. A. (1985). Assessment of fetal condition and risk: analysis of single and combined biophysical variable monitoring. *Sem. Perinatal.*, **9**, 168–83
51. Manning, F. A., Baskett, T. F., Morrison, I. and Lange, I. (1981). Fetal biophysical profile scoring: a prospective study in 1,184 high-risk patients. *Am. J. Obstet. Gynecol.*, **140**, 289–94
52. Baskett, T. F., Gray, J. H., Prewett, S. J., Young, L. M. and Allen, A. C. (1984). Antepartum fetal assessment using fetal biophysical profile score. *Am. J. Obstet. Gynecol.*, **148**, 630–3
53. Manning, F. A., Harman, C. R., Morrison, I., Menticoglu, S. M., Lange, I. R., and Johnson, J. M. (1990). Fetal assessment based on fetal biophysical profile scoring. An analysis of perinatal morbidity and mortality. *Am. J. Obstet. Gynecol.*, **162**, 3, 703–9
54. Cerrera, J. M., Mortera, C., Torrents, M. and Serra, B. (1993). Estudio de la redistribución del flujo vascular fetal mediante Doppler y su relación con la hipoxia fetal. In de Miguel, J. R. and Gómez-Ullate, J. (eds.) *Libro de Abstracts del XIV Congreso Nacional Español de Medicina Perinatal.*, pp. 309–28
55. Carrera, J. M., Mallafré, J., Torrents, M., Carreras, E. and Salvador, M. J. (1992). Perfil biofísico progresivo. In Carrera, J. M. (ed.) *Doppler en Obstetricia*, pp. 369–81. (Barcelona: Salvat)
56. Vintzileos, A. M., Campbell, W. A., Feinstein, S. J., Lodeiro, J. G., Weinbaum, P. J. and Nochimson, D. J. (1987). The fetal biophysical profile in pregnancies with grade III placentas. *Am. J. Perinatol.*, **4**, 90–3
57. Vintzileos, A. M., Gaffney, S. E., Salinger, L. M., Kontopoulos, V. G., Campbell, W. A. and Nochimson, D. J. (1987). The relationships among the fetal biophysical profile, umbilical cord pH, and Apgar scores. *Am. J. Obstet. Gynecol.*, **157**, 627–31
58. Eden, R. D., Seifert, L. S., Kodack, L. D., Trofatter, K. F., Killam, A. P. and Gall, S. A. (1988). A modified biophysical profile for antenatal fetal surveillance. *Obstet. Gynecol.*, **71**, 365–9
59. Shah, D. M., Brown, J. E., Salyer, S. L., Fleischer, A. C. and Boehm, F. H. (1989). A modified scheme for biophysical profile scoring. *Am. J. Obstet. Gynecol.*, **160**, 586–91
60. Carrera, J. M., Mallafré, J., Torrents, M., Carrera, E., Salvador, M. J. and Alegre, M. (1990). Perfil

biofísico progresivo. *Prog. Obstet. Ginecol.*, **33**, 2, 31–46

61. Carrera, J. M. and Alegre, M. (1981). Curso sobre ecobiometía fetal. *Abstracts of the Symposium on fetal Medicine*, p. 46. (Barcelona: Instituto Dexeus)

62. Carrera, J. M., Alegre, M., Pérez-Ares, C., Mortera, C. and Torrents, M. (1986). Evaluación de las resistencias vasculares úteroplanentarias mediante el análisis espectral de la onda de velocidad de flujo. *Prog. Obstet. Ginecol.*, **29**, 397–404

63. Carrera, J. M., Alegre, M., Pérez-Ares, C., Mortera, C. and Torrents, M. (1986). Evaluación de las resistencias vasculares umbílico-placentarias mediante el análisis espectral de la onda de velocidad de flujo. *Prog. Obstet. Ginecol.*, **29**, 321–9

64. Vintzileos, A. M., Campbell, W. A., Nochimson, D. J. and Weinbaum, P. J. (1985). The use of real-time scanning in antepartum fetal evaluation: the fetal biophysical profile. In Sanders, R. C. and Hill, M. C. (eds.) *Ultrasound Annual*, p. 251. (New York: Raven Press)

65. Vintzileos, A. M. and Tsapanos, V. (1992). Biophysical assessment of the fetus. *Ultrasound. Obstet. Gynecol.*, **2**, 133–43

66. Lodeiro, J. G., Vintzileos, A. M., Feinstein, S. J., Campbell, W. A. and Nochimson, D. J. (1986). Fetal biophysical profile in twin gestations. *Obstet. Gynecol.*, **67**, 824–7

67. Johnson, J. M., Harman, C. R., Lange, I. R. and Manning, F. A. (1986). Biophysical profile scoring in the management of the postterm pregnancy: an analysis of 307 patients. *Am. J. Obstet. Gyncol.*, **154**, 269–73

68. Manning, F. A., Morrison, I., Lange, I. R., Harman, C. R. and Chamberlain, P. F. (1985). Fetal assessment based on fetal biophysical profile scoring: experience in 12,620 referred high-risk pregnancies. I. Perinatal mortality by frequency and etiology. *Am. J. Obstet. Gynecol.*, **151**, 343–50

Intrauterine growth retardation

J. M. Carrera and J. Mallafré

INTRODUCTION

Intrauterine growth retardation (IUGR) undoubtedly constitutes one of the most challenging areas of research for obstetricians today. With other obstetric problems of concern having been solved, or well on the way to being solved, the finding of a solution to the problem of nutrient supply deficiency would appear to be our next goal if we are to continue to reduce, slowly but inexorably, the rate of perinatal mortality and the risk of mental and psychomotor retardation.

Despite marked progress made over the past decade in both diagnostic procedures and management strategies, the question of what causes growth retardation still remains unanswered in 40% of all cases of IUGR. On the other hand, IUGR continues to be associated with a three-fold to ten-fold increase in perinatal mortality; an increase in early perinatal morbidity due to congenital abnormalities, perinatal asphyxia and other neonatal processes (persistent fetal blood flow, hypothermia, hypoglycemia, polycythemia, etc.); and an increase in long-term morbidity (learning problems, abnormal behavior patterns, neurological deficits, etc.)[1-4].

FETAL GROWTH CHARACTERISTICS

'Growth' is usually defined as the process whereby the body mass of a living being increases in size as a result of the increase in number (hyperplasia) and size (hypertrophy) of its cells and intracellular matrix. 'Development', on the other hand, should be understood as the process by which organs and their regulatory mechanisms gradually assume their functions in living beings. Broadly speaking, the term 'growth' is preferred when referring to measurable anatomical changes; 'development' is used to refer to the gradual acquisition of certain specific physiological functions.

The fetal growth rate is mainly determined by the intrinsic potential of fetal growth, which is primarily genetically controlled ('genetic factor'). However, the influence of this genetic factor is considerably modified by two other intrauterine regulating factors of fetal growth, the 'hormone factor', fetal and growth promoting, and the 'environmental factor', maternal and usually growth-restraining.

The fetal growth curve during gestation and ultimately the weight at birth are, therefore, the result of the interaction between growth restraining and promoting factors in the fetal genotype. The human fetus may be considered to be the result of the interaction of its genetic potential, its possibility of 'being', and the circumstances surrounding its attempt to 'be' – the environment, which limits or favors it.

The genetic factor, which imposes fairly narrow limits of variability, dominates during the first half of pregnancy, whereas hormone and environmental factors exert their greatest influence during the second half of pregnancy, resulting in a widening of the limits of variability in fetal growth and development. For this reason the fetal growth rate is not constant during pregnancy but rather shows a progressive, sustained transition from the exponential rate – in the first weeks of pregnancy – to the linear rate – in late pregnancy[5].

CONCEPTS

A clear distinction should be made between the meaning of three different terms – low birth weight, small-for-dates, and IUGR – that tend to be considered as synonymous.

Low birth weight

This term refers only to newborn infants weighing less than 2500 g independently of gestational age[6]. A distinction is made between low birth weight in newborns delivered before 37 weeks (preterm), low birth weight in newborns delivered between 37 and 42 weeks (full term) and low birth weight in newborns delivered after 42 weeks (post-term). On the other hand, low birth weight may also be subdivided into 'very low birth weight' (1000 to 1499 g) and 'extremely low birth weight' (500 to 999 g).

Small-for-dates

This term is based on a statistical definition which includes all newborn infants found below the lower confidence limit of a normal weight–weeks-of-gestation curve. Depending upon the type of curve, the lower confidence limit may be the third, fifth or tenth centile or −1 or −2 SD.

Thus, in 1963, Gruenwald[7] proposed that growth-retarded newborns were those whose weight was 1 SD (probable or likely growth retardation) or 2 SD (growth retardation) below the mean weight for their age. In the same year, basing their calculations on a growth curve using the centile system, Lubchenko and associates[8] considered newborns below the 25th centile to be small, although some years later, they agreed to term newborn infants below the 10th centile as small for gestational age or small-for-dates (Figure 1). Newborn infants between the 10th and 90th centile were considered to be appropriate for gestational age, and those over the 90th centile large for gestational age. In 1966, Gruenwald[9] proposed using the 5th centile as an alternative limit, admitting that his first criterion of −2 SD was too strict.

Finally, in 1970, in the final recommendations of the II European Congress of Perinatal Medicine, it was suggested that these newborn infants should be referred to as thin for their gestational age, since they were thin, rather than small or short.

Intrauterine growth retardation

IUGR refers to any process that is capable of limiting intrinsic fetal growth potential *in utero*. It is thus a heterogeneous entity with a variety of possible etiologies.

The term 'intrauterine growth retardation' was introduced by Warkani and colleagues[10] in 1961. The first obstetrician who stated that weight and age were not necessarily related was in fact Pierre Budin[11] in 1907, although it was not until McBurney[12] in 1947, that proofs of intrauterine growth retardation were provided.

The distinction between IUGR and small-for-dates is important, since (1) some newborn infants may be termed small-for-dates (below the 5th or 10th centile) without having suffered IUGR. In this case, there are normal genetic reasons for their low birth weight (constitutional); and (2) many cases of IUGR are not considered to be small-for-dates at birth. This is the case in fetuses that, given their high intrinsic growth potential, should weigh, for example, 4 kg at term but, as a result of an unfavorable gestational environment (IUGR), weigh only 3 kg. In this case, they are considered to be 'normal for their gestational age'.

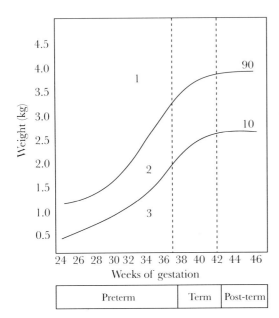

Figure 1 *Statistical definitions of weight centiles for gestational age. 1, large for gestational age; 2, appropriate for gestational age; 3, small for gestational age*

An evaluation of the postnatal ponderal index may help to establish which fetuses really have suffered deficiencies in intrauterine nutrient supply, independent of their weight at birth. Apparently, and in agreement with this index, 40% of fetuses termed small-for-dates should not be considered as intrauterine growth-retarded[13].

INCIDENCE

The incidence of IUGR varies greatly in the literature, with reports of figures ranging from 1.1% to 10.8%[14]. The reason for this may be found in different factors, including:

(1) The definition of birth weight, such as low birth weight, growth retardation with respect to gestational age, mixed categories, etc.;

(2) Different ways in which standard curves are drawn (centiles, standard deviations, etc.);

(3) Different criteria used for discrimination (10th centile, 5th centile, −1 SD, −2 SD, etc.);

(4) Different geopolitical situations (while some northern countries have a very low rate of IUGR, some underdeveloped countries have very high rates. The factors influencing standard values in each country vary, and include height above sea level, degree of development of the country, ethnic characteristics, etc.); and

(5) Social and economic status of the population under study in each country.

It is therefore difficult to compare the figures obtained in environments and countries that are very different, even when similar yardsticks are used. It is for this reason that each community (country, region, etc.) is encouraged to develop its own standard curve.

In our environment, the 10th centile has generally been accepted as the distinguishing criterion. If suitable, up-to-date curves are used for each community studied, the incidence of IUGR will obviously be 10%. However, this hardly ever occurs and figures reported usually range between 3% and 7%[15,16]. For obvious reasons, it is easier to compare figures obtained for low weight at birth. In Spain, during the 10-year period between 1980 and 1989, the figure obtained was 5.7%[17], which is similar to 5.57% found in Catalonia in 1991.

According to gestational age, the majority of cases of IUGR occur at term, during weeks 38 to 42, followed by post-term and preterm pregnancies. The last account for only 0.9% of all neonates (Figure 2).

ETIOLOGY

Innumerable factors are supposedly associated with variations in fetal birth weight. In the multicentric study carried out by Niswander and Gordon[18], 32 associated factors were identified, and it is clear from an overall review of the literature that many more may be recognized. The etiological factors usually associated with IUGR may be divided into three groups: maternal factors, fetal factors and uteroplacental factors.

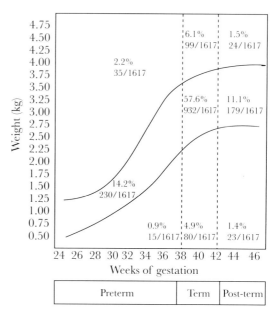

Figure 2 *Incidence of intrauterine growth retardation according to gestational age, 1967–68 (Colorado University)*

Maternal factors

This group includes the largest number of variables. The most common are as follows:

Constitutional factors

Maternal height It has been reported that for each centimeter by which maternal height exceeds normal values, fetal weight at birth is increased by 16 g. When the weight factor is corrected, however, maternal height has little influence on the weight of the fetus[19].

Maternal weight at birth Ounsted and Ounsted[20] have found a significant relationship between neonatal birth weight and maternal birth weight and have suggested a strong hereditary influence on fetal variables.

Maternal weight prior to pregnancy Simpson and associates[21] have shown a clear correlation between maternal and fetal weights. Fetal growth retardation is particularly associated with mothers weighing less than 54 kg.

Maternal age The incidence of neonates with low weight at birth in women under the age of 20 is double that in women between the ages of 25 and 30[22]. There is also a greater relative risk of fetal malnutrition, vascular and metabolic disorders, and a larger number of fetal chromosomal abnormalities in older women.

Social and economic status Unfavorable socioeconomic conditions clearly increase the incidence of neonates with low weight at birth. This is particularly true in developing countries. Factors responsible for this situation include diet, social and family environment, education, type of work, teenage pregnancies, and marital status, among others.

Toxic habits

Smoking, alcohol use and drug consumption are included in this group. Different studies have demonstrated that, after excluding other variables, the weight at birth is reduced by an average of 170 to 200 g in infants born to mothers who smoke more than 10 cigarettes a day[1,23,24].

Ulleland[25], in 1972, reported for the first time that IUGR was particularly common among children born to alcoholic mothers. Subsequently, other authors[26] described the characteristics of these children and established the concept of fetal alcoholic syndrome, in which weight, size and head circumference of neonates are below the 3rd centile.

Finally, infants born to heroin-addicted mothers weigh significantly less than do those born to mothers who do not consume opioids[24], independent of maternal nutrition during pregnancy.

Maternal diseases

Chronic renal disease Chronic renal diseases most frequently associated with IUGR include chronic pyelonephritis, glomerulosclerosis, chronic glomerular disease and lupus nephritis[27–29].

Chronic hypertension This is one of the most frequent causes of IUGR. It usually affects multiparas, giving rise to early growth retardation and microsomic neonates with learning and psychomotor problems.

Chronic cardiopulmonary disease IUGR has been reported in patients with heart or lung disease causing hypoxemia, such as congenital cardiopathies, coarctation of the aorta, pulmonary atresia, reduced cardiac output, etc. and pulmonary diseases, such as bronchial asthma, bronchiectasis, etc.

Dysglycemias Long-standing, poorly-controlled insulin-dependent diabetes associated with diabetic retinopathy, hypertension and nephritis may cause placental microvascular disorders that give rise to an increase in IUGR. In pregnancy-induced diabetes, a marked decrease in fetal weight may be due to an excessive caloric reduction.

Autoimmune diseases The association between systemic lupus erythematosus and IUGR is well known, although it is usually difficult to distinguish between the effects of high doses of glucocorticoids and azathioprine, and vasculitis caused by the disease[30]. On the other hand, antiphospholipid (lupus-like) syndrome has been associated with an increase in the number of cases of miscarriage, IUGR, and intrauterine death[31-34].

Anemia Whilst low levels of hemoglobin (less than 6 g/dl) are associated with an increase in perinatal mortality, moderate anemia (6–10 g/dl) is associated with a significant decrease in fetal weight[35]. This may be due to a decrease in oxygen transport (sickle cell anemia, etc.) or it may simply be related to poor maternal nutrition.

Urinary tract infection It has been generally accepted that pyelonephritis during pregnancy causes IUGR[27].

Fetal factors

Chromosome abnormalities Chromosome abnormalities, in particular trisomy 13, 18 and 21, as well as the Turner syndrome (45,X), sex chromosomal trisomy (XXX, XYY, XXY) or segmental chromosome imbalances (4p–short arm, 5p–cri-du-chat syndrome, 18p, 18q, etc.) are accompanied by a high incidence of IUGR, which occurs early in pregnancy (IUGR type I) (Figure 3). It is for this reason that antenatal ultrasonographic diagnosis of growth retardation of this type should be followed by a study of fetal karyotype using the most appropriate method in each case (amniocentesis, chorionic villus biopsy or cordocentesis).

Inherited syndromes A variety of diseases of bone and cartilage have been called dysplasias, e.g. dwarfism (achondroplasia, hypochondro-

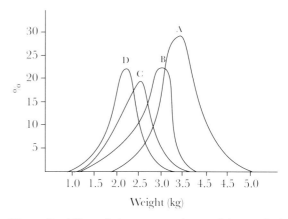

Figure 3 *Effect of chromosome abnormalities on fetal weight. A, control group; B, trisomy 13; C, trisomy 21; D, trisomy 18*

plasia, Russell–Silver syndrome, etc.), chondrodystrophies, osteogenesis imperfecta, etc. Placental sulfatase deficiency has also been cited.

Fetal infection As a result of the epidemic of rubella in 1963, it was established that transplacental infection of the fetus can cause IUGR. Since 1963, numerous reports have appeared associating low fetal weight with intrauterine infections such as rubella, cytomegalovirus, herpes simplex, toxoplasmosis, paludism, congenital syphilis, and other acute bacterial infections. Unfortunately, most reports make no distinction between premature and small-for-dates neonates.

Twin pregnancies This is one of the most frequent and well-known causes of IUGR. In all series of IUGR, twin pregnancies account for 20–30% of the cases. The intrauterine growth curve of twin pregnancies is similar to that of singleton pregnancies until week 33 of gestation; from then on, the curve for monozygotic twins diverges whilst that of dizygotic twins does so between weeks 35–36.

Fetal order at birth IUGR occurs more often in first-born neonates, particularly when the mother is very young or old. The second or third child of the same mother usually weighs more than the first child. What happens after the fourth child on is not clear, as the series studied are small. In most countries, women who have more than three children belong to the lower social classes. This may be a factor in decreased fetal weight.

Uteroplacental factors

Uterine anomalies Congenital uterine anomalies, in particular uterus bicornis and septate uterus, are consistently associated with IUGR, accounting for approximately 1–3% of the cases.

Poor adaptation of maternal circulation There is growing evidence that poor circulation prior to pregnancy, with or without deficiencies in uterine vasculature, can give rise to repeated miscarriages and very early growth retardation[36]. Inadequate vascular supply, whether anatomical or functional, prevents correct placental implantation and circulatory anchorage. Color Doppler imaging is currently being used to study placental blood supply. It may well provide the key to the early diagnosis of pregnancies in which these conditions occur.

Poor adaptation of maternal circulation may also be associated with immunological factors[37,38]. This would seem to be particularly so in the case of early IUGR in the presence of anti-phospholipid antibodies (lupus anticoagulant and anti-cardiolipin antibodies). In this case, the cause may lie in an early inhibition of the production of prostacyclin at the level of vascular endothelium[33]. However, more specific immunological studies are required to determine the mechanism linking poor vascular support with immunological rejection, very early growth retardation and possible fetal death.

Placental mosaicism Numerous cases of placental aneuploidies have been described, particularly trisomies 2, 7, 9, 10, 12, 13, 15, 16 and 18, that have been associated with miscarriages, growth retardation and fetal death, despite the fact that fetuses were chromosomally normal[39–45]. Kalousek and Dill[39] have suggested that the occurrence of non-disjunction at random in the very early stages after conception could have given rise to mosaicism in the placenta or in the fetus, but not necessarily in both. According to Kalousek and co-workers[41], three types of placental mosaicism may be defined:

(1) Type I, which is the most common, and may be found in cytotrophoblastic cells by carrying out a karyotype chorionic villus biopsy using the direct method of Simoni; fetal outcome is good;

(2) Type II, in which the abnormal karyotype is confined to mesenchymal cells. Diagnosis by chorionic villus biopsy can only be made when a prolonged cell culture is done. It is not as common as Type I and usually causes quite severe IUGR;

(3) Type III, in which aneuploidy is present not only in the cytotrophoblast but also in mesenchymal cells. It occurs rarely and very often causes severe IUGR and fetal death.

There is a high correlation between the number of aneuploid cells detected using chorionic villus biopsy and the number confirmed in studies of the placenta at term. These data are also relevant to fetal outcome. Thus, growth retardation (80% of cases) and fetal death (20–30% of cases) normally need only be feared in cases of high levels of mosaicism (more than 45% of cells involved)[46–49]. For this reason, it has been suggested[41] that, at least in part, the length of gestation and fetal survival depends upon the ratio of euploid cells to aneuploid cells in the placenta. Many other conceptions are, however, aborted before 22 weeks' gestation. There are nevertheless case reports of normal fetuses[50,51].

PATHOGENESIS

Three basic etiopathogenic mechanisms are currently recognized.

Decrease in intrinsic fetal growth potential

Different etiological factors, such as those of genetic and/or chromosomal origin, toxic habits or infectious diseases, cause a decrease in intrinsic fetal growth potential. The pathological factors begin to exert their influence from the time of conception or, at least, from the embryonic stage.

In certain chromosome abnormalities, such as those involving sex chromosomes, a progressive, linear decrease in fetal weight has been detected in relation to an excess number of chromosomes in the karyotype. Thus, for every extra X chromosome, fetal weight loss would be equivalent to 300 g[51].

Embryopathic infectious processes may influence intrinsic fetal growth potential in several ways, either by first affecting the mother, thereby directly affecting the fetus, or by negatively affecting both. When they directly affect the fetus during the stages of organ differentiation, they are capable of causing permanent reductions in the number of cells, thereby causing more or less severe damage to most of the fetal organs. Rubella and cytomegalovirus infection are the most significant. Cytomegalovirus, in particular, would appear to be responsible for a large number of cases of IUGR that are often considered idiopathic.

Uteroplacental insufficiency

This includes all factors capable of affecting maternal–placental–fetal exchange, usually as a result of deficiencies in placental microcirculation. Uteroplacental insufficiency usually occurs in the presence of favorable conditions (primiparity, insertion anomalies of the placenta, uterine blood-flow impairment, etc.) as well as determining factors (pre-eclampsia, hypertension prior to pregnancy, renal disease, diabetes, post-term pregnancy, etc.). None of these factors usually comes into play unless the fetus requires the reserve capacity of the placenta.

The main pathological finding is a significant decrease in the number of arterioles of the tertiary villi[52], which may be the result of two basic pathogenetic mechanisms: (a) lack of formation of arterioles, due to interference in the process of placental maturational angiogenesis[53], or (b) obliteration, secondary to a thromboembolic or angiopastic phenomenon[54]. In both cases, the cause of these changes may ultimately lie in a decrease in uterine perfusion, or in the fetus itself.

Impaired uterine perfusion causes hypoxic ischemia in the intervillous space, with secondary constriction of villi arterioles[55]. In this case, changes in uterine blood flow velocity waveforms may be detected in Doppler studies before changes are detected in umbilical velocity waveforms, as occurs for example in patients with pre-eclampsia[56,57].

Evidence currently exists of the fact that the fetus itself, through poorly-understood reflex or biochemical mechanisms, may induce changes in villous microcirculatory resistance. This occurs, for example, in fetuses with certain chromosome or morphological anomalies[54,58–61].

The study of the placenta in the fetus with autosomal trisomy reveals a decreased vasculature in tertiary villi[62], which accounts for the reduced umbilical conductance indices and frequent episodes of distress observed in this type of fetus. Exactly how chromosome anomalies act on the placenta to cause these anomalies is still unknown. It has been suggested, in the case of trisomy 21 in particular, that these anomalies make the placenta more susceptible to disrupting environmental influences[58,60], a concept known as 'enhanced development of instability'[60]. It is, however, still not clear how this 'susceptibility' is mediated at the cellular or subcellular level, thereby causing deficient cell proliferation, changing the cell cycle or modifying cell DNA or rRNA content.

Other researchers[53,54] have shown that, in a statistically significant percentage of placentas from fetuses with certain abnormalities, there was a significant decrease in the number of arterioles in tertiary villi. The most commonly occurring malformations in this group are those affecting the central nervous system.

Current research is focused on identifying the teleological mechanism by which the embryo or fetus affects the placenta, thereby causing placental insufficiency. The fact is that under these circumstances, although the umbilical velocity waveforms may be affected, uteroplacental velocity waveforms remain unaffected[53,63–66].

Fetal malnutrition secondary to maternal malnutrition

The physiopathological cause of low fetal birth weight may be found in the unsuitable composition of maternal blood, which causes an almost constant nutritional and metabolic deficiency in the fetus throughout pregnancy. Etiological factors include maternal nutritional deficits, poor living conditions, anemia, severe placental dystrophy, maternal hyperinsulinism (pregnant women with baseline and postprandial hypoglycemia), poor weight gain as a result of unbalanced diets, etc.

CLASSIFICATION OF IUGR

Classifying cases of IUGR constitutes not only an attempt to understand the etiopathogenesis of the process, but also, and more particularly, a means of predicting outcome and determining appropriate obstetric management strategies.

Attempts to classify IUGR

The first classification of IUGR that was widely used was the one proposed by Winick and colleagues[67-72]. Based on experimental studies in rats, two types of IUGR were proposed: (a) 'intrinsic', caused by a decrease in fetal growth potential, and (b) 'extrinsic', caused by placental insufficiency (asymmetrical IUGR), or maternal protein restriction (symmetrical IUGR). This classification was accepted, with only slight variations, by the majority of Anglo-Saxon authors[73,74] and has come to be taken for granted in most texts on the subject.

On the basis of sonographic features, Campbell and associates[75-77] proposed a classification of IUGR largely based on the profile of the fetal biparietal-diameter curve. These authors distinguished between IUGR with an 'early low profile' in the cephalometric curve and IUGR with a downturn or 'late flattening' of the curve. This classification, adopted by most specialists in ultrasonography, was later added to by Levi and colleagues[78,79], who also took into account the head circumference/abdominal circumference (HC/AC) index. Following this classification, IUGR was divided into 'harmonious' or 'proportionate' (normal HC/AC ratio) and 'disharmonious' or 'disproportionate' (HC greater than AC). Experience soon showed that cases of IUGR classified as harmonious were usually intrinsic and exhibited an early low cephalometric profile; in contrast, cases of IUGR classified as disharmonious were extrinsic and exhibited a late flattening of the cephalometric curve.

Most Anglo-Saxon specialists[80] subsequently adopted the classification of symmetrical or asymmetrical IUGR, with some[81] adding a third category known as symmetrical IUGR with 'femur sparing', characterized by femur length appropriate for gestational age but out of proportion to all other biometrical parameters.

From the point of view of the characteristics of the newborn infant (presence or absence of malformations, biometrical data, trophism, etc.), several classifications have been proposed. Rosso and Winick[82] identified IUGR accompanied by congenital malformations, and IUGR without congenital malformations. The latter group is subdivided into type I (extrinsic symmetrical) and type II (extrinsic asymmetrical). In 1977, Sieroszewski[83] and Holtorff each proposed their own, very similar, classifications. The first divided fetuses that were small-for-gestational age into hypoplastic and hypotrophic, and the second divided them into eutrophic (genetically small), hypoplastic, hypotrophic, and with multiple congenital malformations.

In practice, most pediatric departments classify cases of IUGR as proportionate (or symmetrical) and disproportionate (or asymmetrical) by calculating the ponderal index of Rohrer (fetal weight divided by fetal length (crown–rump), raising to the cube and multiplying by 100). If the index is normal (≥ 2.20), IUGR is considered symmetrical; if it is abnormally low, IUGR is considered asymmetrical[84-88].

Based on the time-course of fetal growth during pregnancy, Salvadori[89] identified 'primary' IUGR (constant throughout gestation), 'secondary' (early or late, depending on when the adverse factor begins to affect the fetus), and 'transitory' (when recovery takes place after deceleration in fetal growth).

Depending upon the severity of IUGR, it has been classified as slight, moderate, and severe[7,90].

Integrated classification of IUGR

This classification has been proposed by our group[90–96] since 1976, and takes into account all the basic aspects of IUGR, such as onset (early or late), etiology (intrinsically abnormal developmental process, etc.), anthropometric data of the newborn infant (weight, length, head circumference), general morphology (proportionate, disproportionate, semiproportionate), trophism (eutrophic, hypotrophic, dystrophic), etc. In accordance with these characteristics, three types of IUGR have been recognized (Table 1).

Type I implies a decrease in intrinsic fetal growth potential and is also known as intrinsic, harmonious, proportionate, symmetrical or early. In this case, the adverse factor exerts its influence from the time of conception, or at least from the embryonic stage (hyperplastic stage) (Figure 4). Due to the early onset of the process, the three parameters that are usually assessed to determine IUGR are uniformly affected: fetal weight, length and head circumference. Newborn infants are hypoplastic or microsomic, but their appearance is clearly eutrophic. The incidence of congenital malformations is very high (aneuploidy in 25% of fetuses with severe growth retardation in the early stages of gestation)[97].

It is thus advisable to carry out routine studies of fetal karyotype. Approximately 20–30% of cases of IUGR are of this type[90,98,99].

Type II is known as extrinsic, disharmonious, disproportionate, asymmetrical or late, and uteroplacental insufficiency is the etiopatho-

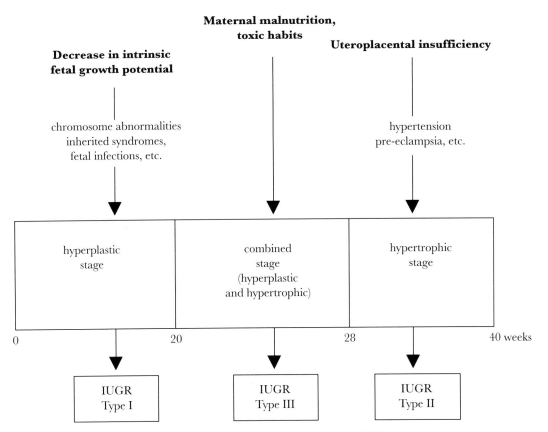

Figure 4 *Pathogenesis and classification of intrauterine growth retardation (IUGR)*

Table 1 Types of intrauterine growth retardation

	Type I	Type II	Type III
Anthropometrical parameters	weight, size and heart perimeter	weight	weight and size
General morphology	harmonious	non-harmonious	semi-harmonious
Origin	intrinsic	extrinsic pathological	extrinsic (deficiency)
Starting	early	late	semi-early
Trophism	hypoplastic eutrophic	dystrophic underfed	hypotrophic badly fed

genetic mechanism. Since factors involved in uteroplacental insufficiency are particularly common during the last trimester of pregnancy (hypertrophic stage), only fetal weight is affected, whilst little or no effect is evident in fetal length or head circumference. The physical appearance of the neonate is characteristic, with a disproportionately large head and dystrophic, undernourished body. Cases of *in utero* fetal death and fetal distress during delivery are most often found in this group. Approximately 70–80% of cases of IUGR are thought to be of this type[90,100].

Type III is somewhat mixed in comparison with the other two types. While the factors at work are apparently extrinsic and appear relatively early on in pregnancy (nutrient deficiency), the consequences are more akin to those associated with intrinsic IUGR, where fetal weight and length, in particular, are modified. Neonates in this group are characterized by semi-harmonious morphology and a hypotrophic, undernourished appearance.

ANTENATAL DIAGNOSIS OF IUGR

Diagnosis of the risk of IUGR

Pregnancies at risk for IUGR may be diagnosed on the basis of previous history (low fetal birth weight in earlier pregnancies, etc.), associated disorders (autoimmune diseases, high blood pressure, etc.), and toxic habits (regular smoker, etc.). Previous history of IUGR is the most important risk factor[101]. Pregnancies with a two-fold or three-fold increased risk should be given special attention and fetal growth should be closely monitored[94,95].

Attempts have been made to predict the risk of IUGR, in particular in association with pregnancy-induced hypertension, using Doppler velocimetry in maternal uterine arteries. Campbell and associates[56] assessed arcuate artery velocity waveforms in low-risk pregnancies between weeks 16 and 18 of gestation, and reported a positive predictive value of 42%, negative predictive value of 87%, sensitivity of 68% and specificity of 69%. Steele and colleagues[102] obtained similar results. Nevertheless, other groups[103] have reported less encouraging data.

Diagnosis of presumed or suspected IUGR

This is perhaps the most important and the most difficult diagnosis to make, when we consider that more than 50% of pregnancies are free of any associated conditions that would alert obstetricians to the possibility of IUGR. Apart from the patient's previous history, underlying diseases, poor weight gain or toxic habits, the discrepancy between gestational age and the size of the uterus is the most clearly indicative sign of IUGR.

Serial symphysis fundal height (SFH) is the most acceptable method used for initial screening for IUGR. Westin[104] has developed diagrams of the increase in the height of the uterus from week 18 to 43 of gestation. It has been shown that at about week 28 of gestation, the height of the uterus in the IUGR group (1.2 ± 0.4 cm) differed significantly ($p < 0.01$) from that in the group of neonates with adequate weight at birth, and these differences increased from week 36 on.

Effer[105] drew up a centile curve divided into six areas. If a value fell within area 5 (between the 25th and the 10th centile), this could be indicative of incipient IUGR and the patient was

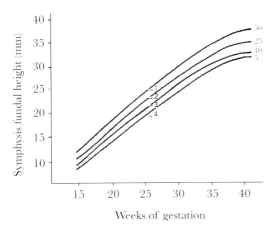

Figure 5 *Centile curve of symphysis fundal height*

submitted to close surveillance. If values fell within area 6 (below the 10th centile) IUGR was likely.

Since 1976, we have used a similar curve drawn up from our own data (positive predictive value, 60%; negative predictive value, 96%). The results of this measurement are particularly useful before week 37 of gestation. Clearly this method is not applicable to cases of twin pregnancies, hydramnios, etc. (Figure 5).

Campbell and Soothill[106] compared the sensitivity of SFH with fetal abdominal circumference measurements (76% vs. 83%) and found that there was no statistically significant difference. These authors concluded that basic screening for IUGR should be done using SFH, a procedure which, moreover, had the advantage of being able to be carried out at each control visit, reserving ultrasound biometrical data for those cases in which the SFH fell below the 5th centile.

Errors occur most frequently during the last 8 weeks of pregnancy, given the variability of the results obtained and the possibility of the fetus being deeply embedded. This would explain differences of up to 6 cm in the SFH.

Diagnosis of probable IUGR (ultrasound diagnosis)

The diagnosis of IUGR is based on biometrical parameters recorded during ultrasound scanning. For data to be useful, however, measurements must be standardized (precisely-defined cross-sections for ultrasound imaging, clear reference points, etc.), discrimination consistent (identical cut-off points to differentiate fetuses and neonates), and appropriate curves used for the populations under study, which should then be correctly interpreted. It should be borne in mind that the independent variable used to calculate the dependent variable is located in the abscissa. On the other hand, in order to reduce misreadings to a minimum, gestational age should be precisely determined. If it is not clinically reliable, it must be determined by using measurements of fetal structures that are affected either little or not at all by fetal growth retardation, such as transverse cerebellar diameter[107–111].

Although there are multiple standardized measurements of fetal parameters for which tables or curves showing normal values have been developed, the following parameters are those used in clinical practice.

Crown–rump length

This is a particularly sensitive biometric parameter that can be measured in the early stages of gestation[112] (Figure 6). Technically, the only limitation is the progressive bending of the embryo, which makes measurements less reliable after weeks 10–12 of gestation. Between weeks 6–12 of gestation, there is an exponential increase in crown–rump length, although this increase later appears to be linear. The maximum error obtained when calculating this parameter with respect to gestational age is ± 5 days in 95% of cases (between weeks 6 and 14 fetal growth is rapid and the limits of confidence are very narrow). If an embryo falls well outside the normal curve, the presence of chromosome anomalies or dysmorphism should be suspected. Fetal surveillance using ultrasound imaging should be instituted and the karyotype determined.

Biparietal diameter

This is the most reproducible parameter and it may be determined from weeks 13–14 of gestation. The sonographic section, from front to

Table 2 Comparison of several biometric parameters, for detection of the small-for-gestational-age infants at 34 or 36 weeks of gestation

	Sensitivity	Specificity	Predictive value Positive	Negative
Biparietal diameter	45	74.5	23	81.5
Cephalic circumference	52	80	26	94.3
Cephalic area	60	80	23	95.2
Abdominal circumference	83	87.7	43	97.8
Abdominal area	85	88	44	98.1
Femur length	58	81	23.3	95

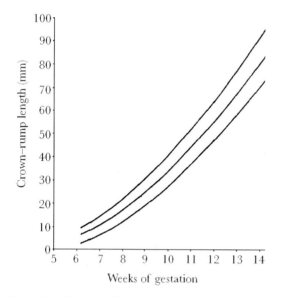

Figure 6 Mean ± 2 SD fetal crown–rump length for gestational age 6–14 weeks

back, includes the most anterior portion of the longitudinal fissure[113], the cavum of the septum pellucidum, the thick line of the third ventricle, and quadrigeminal cisterna with the punctiform echo on the pineal body. Frontal horns of lateral ventricles and thalami on either side of the third ventricle should be visible[113,114].

Until week 30 of gestation, increases in biparietal diameter are reasonably linear, with weekly increases of 3 mm, which are approximately equal to the standard deviation of mean values for this period[115,116]. From week 30 to 38, the rate of change gradually slows, with weekly increases of about 1.5 mm[115,116]. From week 38 to term, weekly increases are 1 mm, and virtually nil from week 42. The sum of the different rates of increase in biparietal diameter causes standard deviations to increase as pregnancy reaches term (Figure 7).

Campbell and Dewhurst[117] reported that when the biparietal diameter was lower than the 5th centile, IUGR was confirmed in 68% of cases. Most errors occurred when values fell between the 5th and the 10th centile; in these circumstances, weight at birth was within the normal range in 69% of newborns.

The sensitivity of biparietal diameter as the only cephalometric parameter does not exceed 50%[118] (varying from 26.9% to 48%[119–121]) when determining small-for-dates below the 10th centile. In our experience, the sensitivity of biparietal diameter between weeks 34 and 36 of gestation is 45% (Table 2).

Given the variability of biparietal diameter (at least three different weeks may theoretically be ascribed to each value), serial measurements are recommended. Sabbagha and associates[122] proposed that the so-called 'growth-adjusted sonar age' should be determined in order to determine sonar age precisely and to improve the prediction of IUGR. The ideal evolution of the 226 cases in which serial measurements of biparietal diameter were made (the first within the 24th week and the last after the 30th) on an original percentile curve is shown in Figure 8.

An analysis of these data shows interesting findings:

(1) It would be exceptional for biparietal diameter values to fall, between weeks 21 and 30, below the fiducial limits, provided that there are no date errors, and the age is adjusted to biparietal-diameter growth according to the method described by Sabbagha and colleagues[122];

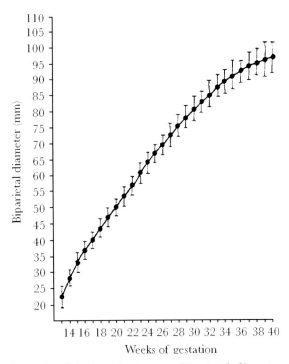

Figure 7 *Relationship between biparietal diameter (mean ± 1 SD) and fetal age*

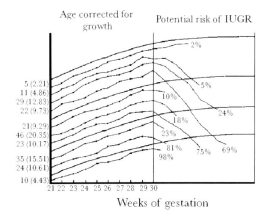

Figure 8 *Potential risk of intrauterine growth retardation (IUGR) according to the evolution of biparietal diameter (BPD). Curves are shown for the 5th, 25th, 75th and 95th centiles, with 'small', 'medium' and 'large' BPD between them. Numbers of cases analyzed by Sabbagha and colleagues[121] are shown on the left, with percentage incidence of IUGR in parentheses*

(2) Only in 34.9% of all growth-adjusted-sonar age did the biparietal diameter fall below the 5th centile at some stage during pregnancy. Only by raising the band to the 25% mark does it prove possible to discriminate 83.62% of confirmed cases of IUGR;

(3) In 16.7% of cases, the biparietal diameter measurements were found above the 25% mark; and

(4) Theoretically, it is possible to determine fetal growth models. Each model has a determined relative incidence (on the left of the figure) and a different potential risk of IUGR (on the right of the figure).

At present, despite the fact that it continues to be the most frequently used biometrical parameter, biparietal diameter is not considered to be a reliable indicator of IUGR. This is because head size is rarely affected in many cases of IUGR (in particular type II, the most commonly occurring) and, moreover, because in the last weeks of pregnancy it is very difficult to determine whether or not the fetus is really growing or not, since weekly gains in fetal weight are minimal. On the other hand, biparietal diameter should only be used when the cephalic index (fronto-occipital diameter divided by biparietal diameter and multiplied by 100) falls between 70 and 85.

Head circumference or cephalic area

Measuring the head circumference or cephalic area is a more complex procedure than measuring biparietal diameter, since, for measurements to be correct, the sonographic section should include both the biparietal and fronto-occipital diameters. These parameters, however, have some advantages over biparietal diameter, since they avoid the errors that occur in biparietal diameter measurements as a result of brachycephaly or dolichocephaly (e.g. craniosynostosis), and in cases of breech presentation, which often accompanies a fundic placenta, biparietal-diameter measurements in normally-developed fetuses are abnormally small, while head circumference or cephalic area are within normal limits.

The sensitivity of head circumference measurements is 52% and, therefore, somewhat

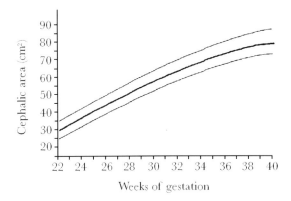

Figure 9 *Relationship between cephalic area (mean ± 2 SD) and fetal age*

higher than that of biparietal diameter. Specificity, however, is similar (80%). Predictive values do not seem to differ greatly whether head circumference or cephalic area are used (Figure 9). In our experience (using our own curve) the sensitivity of cephalic area is 60% and specificity 80% (Table 2).

Abdominal diameters

Both transverse and anteroposterior abdominal diameters have been used to assess fetal development. Some authors consider[123] that measurement of abdominal diameters has the advantage over abdominal circumference or abdominal area of being much simpler and open to fewer errors. To ensure the reproducibility of abdominal diameter measurements, a cross-sectional view should be obtained from the appropriate site – the site of choice is the level at which the umbilical vein leads into the canal of Arantius (ductus venosus). At this point, the diameter of the fetal liver and, therefore, of the abdomen is at its greatest. The section should be as orthogonal as possible, and the measurement should be made during a moment of fetal apnea.

Macler and co-workers[123], correlating false-positive and false-negative results from biparietal diameter, thoracic diameter and abdominal diameter, have shown that figures were particularly low, throughout gestation, when abdominal diameters were used,

Abdominal circumference or abdominal area

Measurement of abdominal circumference or abdominal area of the fetus is facilitated by the cylindrical shape of this body segment and the existence of an excellent point of reference (the umbilical vein). The curve of values for the abdominal circumference during pregnancy shows an almost linear increase until week 36, with a slight decrease from this time on. The tendency for values to fall off suddenly at term, typical of cephalometric parameters is, therefore, not detected.

If measurements of abdominal circumference are compared with those of head circumference is may be observed that, although mean abdominal circumference measurements are at first smaller than mean head circumference measurements, they equal out at week 36, and from then on the mean abdominal circumference measurements are greater than those of head circumference. According to Campbell and Wilkin[76] the diagnostic accuracy of this parameter in cases of IUGR is remarkable; using a single measurement at week 32 of gestation, 86.7% of newborns who fell below the 5th centile, could be identified. Results are less favorable, however, as pregnancy progresses. At weeks 35 to 36, Campbell and Soothill[106] have reported a sensitivity of 83%, specificity of 79%, positive predictive value of 39%, and negative predictive value of 87%. Similar results have been reported by other authors[124,125]. In our experience this parameter shows an overall sensitivity of 83% with a specificity of 87.7%; in the case of abdominal area, the sensitivity and specificity are 85% and 88%, respectively[93] (Figure 10, Table 2).

It should be noted that sensitivity and positive predictive value increase with gestational age, so that week 34 ± 1 of pregnancy is considered to be the best time for differentiating fetuses with IUGR[80].

Unfortunately, measurements of both head circumference and head area are subject to greater inter- and intra-observer variations than biparietal diameter, due to the changes that take place in measurements as a result of fetal breathing movements and fetal position[77].

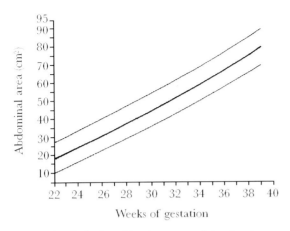

Figure 10 *Relationship between abdominal area (mean ± 2 SD) and fetal age*

Length of femur

The femur is the easiest long bone to identify and measure. Its typical 'golf club'-like appearance and moderate curvature from week 18 on are unmistakable. The normal curve for length of femur, similar to that of abdominal parameters, does not suffer the sudden flattening out characteristic of cephalic parameters (Figure 11).

O'Brian and Queenan[126] show that values for fetal femur length in 60% of cases of IUGR fall below the lower confidence limit. This parameter, just like cephalic parameters, is affected in cases of symmetrical fetal growth retardation (type I) but is hardly or not at all affected in cases of asymmetrical fetal growth retardation (type II). Hadlock and colleagues[127] have emphasized the usefulness of the femur length/abdominal circumference ratio, which not only presents acceptable levels of sensitivity (63%) but also has the advantage of being independent of gestational age. Indeed, this ratio remains constant (22 ± 2%) from week 22 of gestation. Its predictive value, however, is less than 30%[128].

Total intrauterine volume

Gohari and associates[129] have measured maximum longitudinal (L), transverse (T) and anteroposterior (AP) diameters of the uterus to calculate total intrauterine volume (TIUV:

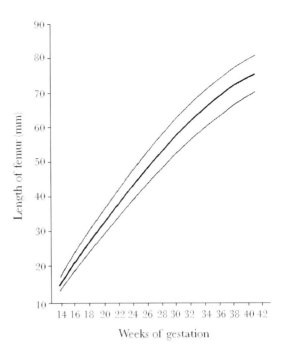

Figure 11 *Relationship between length of femur (mean ± 2 SD) and fetal age*

TIUV = L × T × AP × 0.5233). Using measurements obtained from 100 pregnancies at different stages of gestation, they calculated a normal curve. In a series of 96 cases of suspected IUGR (with postnatal confirmation in 28 cases), it was concluded that IUGR is likely when the total intrauterine volume corresponds to −1.5 SD of the mean, equivocal when figures fall between −1 and −1.5 SD of the mean (one third of cases of IUGR), and should be excluded when they are over −1 SD. The only errors recorded were those caused by severe oligohydramnios. Results of some later studies, however, are less encouraging (sensitivity 60%, positive predictive value 30%)[130,131].

Diagnosis of type of IUGR

Profile of the curve of cephalometric parameters

These data (biparietal diameter, head circumference or cephalic area) provide information on the moment when adverse factors began to affect fetal cranial structures, thus allowing a distinction to be made between fetal growth retardation of early (type I), late (type II) or semi-early (type III) onset.

In the case of type I IUGR (symmetrical or intrinsic), the curve of the mean values falls below −2 SD of the mean values of the normal population early on in pregnancy and evolves largely parallel to the latter. This is due to the fact that the factors responsible for fetal growth retardation negatively influence, early and simultaneously, the three parameters that define growth − fetal length, fetal weight and head circumference.

In contrast, in type II IUGR (asymmetrical or extrinsic), the mean curve of biparietal diameter or head circumference coincides with mean values for the normal population until approximately week 30 of gestation, when it falls below the mean. Nevertheless, although the difference continues to increase till the end of pregnancy, at no time does the mean of the affected group fall below −2 SD of mean values of the normal population. In this case, factors causing IUGR have exerted their influence late in the second trimester of pregnancy and, therefore, although they have had sufficient time to affect fetal nutrition, cranial structures that are much less susceptible to undernourishment are affected little and late. In contrast, the rest of the fetal body soon suffers from undernourishment with weight, height and thoracic and abdominal perimeters being primarily affected.

Finally, in type III IUGR (semi-harmonious), which usually results from maternal malnutrition, the biparietal diameter profile shows an intermediate pattern.

Calculation of the head/abdominal circumference ratio

The study of this ratio provides data on overall fetal morphology helping to define fetal growth as proportionate (type I), disproportionate (type II) or semi-proportionate (type III). A relationship may be established between head and abdominal circumferences, diameters or areas.

The head/abdominal circumference ratio decreases throughout pregnancy[117] (values > 1.2 at 14 to 16 weeks, < 1 after 36 weeks, and between 0.9 and 1 at term) due to the rapid accumulation of fat in subcutaneous and soft tissue in the fetal thorax and abdomen during the last trimester.

Kurjak and Breyer[132] have correlated head/abdominal circumference ratio with the position of the newborn on the centile curve at 36 weeks. When this method was reproduced by our group, similar results were obtained, with the only difference that in the group of neonates below the 10th centile, one-third of cases showed a ratio of < 1, whereas in the experience of Kurjak and Breyer[132] this occurred in only 5% of infants in this group (Figure 12).

It may be concluded that head/abdominal circumference ratio is inverted after week 36 of gestation (from > 1 to < 1). Only 7% of normal fetuses do not fulfil this pattern[22,91].

Fetuses small-for-gestational-age behave differently, depending upon the causes of growth retardation. If the ratio is inverted and, therefore, values are within the confidence interval of the normal curve, it is safe to assume that the case is one of fetal growth retardation of the proportionate or symmetrical type (type I IUGR). The neonate that is small-for-gestational-age is hypoplastic, but not hypotrophic. Only 11.76% of infants do not fulfil this pattern. Fetal growth retardation, however, will not go unnoticed at the time of sonographic examination, since, as we have already

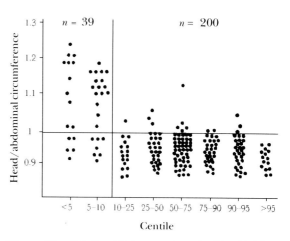

Figure 12 *Relationship between the ratio of head/abdominal circumference and the position of the newborn on the centile curve at 36 weeks of gestation*

mentioned, biparietal diameter is markedly affected. On the other hand, when the ratio is above the upper limit of the confidence interval of this curve and consequently is not inverted, the case is probably one of growth retardation of asymmetrical, disproportionate, or extrinsic type (IUGR type II), as a result of which newborn infants will be small-for-gestational-age, hypotrophic and, in some cases, dystrophic. Only 7.14% of infants do not fulfil this pattern[22,91]. Finally, in the case of IUGR type III (semiproportionate), the ratio is > 1 in 41.7% of cases, < 1 in 52.94%, and equal to 1 in 5.82%.

Assessment of fetal condition

The degree of fetal well-being or distress may be determined by the evaluation of various biophysical and biochemical parameters.

Ultrasonographic parameters

Cephalometric curve It is obvious that the greater the deceleration in increases in biparietal diameter or head circumference measurements, the greater the likelihood of placental insufficiency. This is particularly evident in cases in which these parameters show normal curves during the second trimester of pregnancy.

Fetal urine production rate This is a parameter developed by Campbell and associates[133] which, based on fetal urine production, determines the amount of urine passed by the fetus during a specific period of time. In cases of IUGR, a decrease in perfusion in the area supplied by the aorta, and, in particular, in the renal vessels, reduces renal filtration and, as a result, fetal urine production. Wladimiroff and Campbell[134] have shown that in some cases of IUGR values fall below confidence intervals expected for a specific week. We have obtained similar results in 56 cases of IUGR and 11 normal pregnancies (Figure 13).

In cases of IUGR type I and type III, usually without marked fetal hypoxia, the value of fetal urine production rate fell below the lower limit

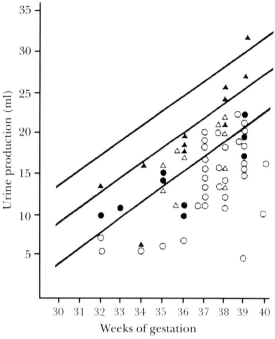

Figure 13 *Fetal urine production rate in cases of intrauterine growth retardation (IUGR). Filled triangles, control group; filled circles, IUGR type I; open circles, IUGR type II; open triangles, IUGR type III*

of the confidence interval in only 33.33% and 30% of cases, respectively, while 70.58% of cases of IUGR type II, in which fetal hypoxia is common, did so.

Amniotic fluid volume The importance of the quantitative determination of amniotic fluid volume in order to assess fetal condition has already been established. In cases of IUGR, a decrease in amniotic fluid volume indicates blood-flow redistribution, which in turn leads to hypoperfusion of the kidney and decreased renal activity.

Fetal kinetics Real-time ultrasound methods can help to determine the characteristics of fetal kinetics. When growth retardation is sufficiently marked to cause respiratory insufficiency, ultrasound imaging together with cardiotocographic monitoring usually detects decreases in fetal gross body movements and fetal breathing movements. These signs, however, appear long after abnormal cardiotocographic recordings have been detected[135–137]. Changes in the type of fetal body movements occur earlier. Apparently, before there is a quantitative decrease in fetal body movements, an increase in so-called 'individual' movements is observed to the detriment of more complex, stronger movements (rolling movements)[138].

Placental grading Technical advances in the field of ultrasonography have permitted the observation *in vivo* of textural changes in the placenta. Sonolucent areas have been considered of particular interest in the assessment of fetal well-being in cases of IUGR[139–141]. Since 1980, placental images have been classified according to the classification of placental maturity changes developed by Grannum and colleagues[142]. The appearance of echo-spared or 'fallout' areas in the placental substance (grade III) are particularly relevant.

Ultrasonographic signs of a grade III placenta before week 35 were detected in 14.49% of cases of IUGR as compared to 6% in normal pregnancies. These differences were statistically significant in IUGR type II (17.64%; $p < 0.005$) and IUGR type III (14.28%; $p < 0.01$). As from week 35, the occurrence of echo-spared areas was also twice as common in cases of IUGR (43% vs. 24% in normal pregnancies) although this finding was only statistically significant in IUGR type II (58.82%; $p < 0.005$). Kazzi and co-workers[143] also considered that the presence of a grade III placenta prior to week 35 should alert obstetricians to the possibility of IUGR. These authors reported a sensitivity of 62% and positive predictive value of 59%.

These images undoubtedly reflect pathological maturation changes.

Cardiotocographic parameters

The usefulness of the non-stress test in the assessment of fetal condition in cases of IUGR has been documented in numerous studies[144–148].

In 1982, our group reported a study of 358 cardiotocographic recordings which were

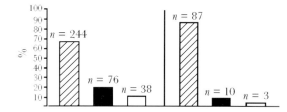

Figure 14 *Distribution of classifications according to the Dexeus test of 358 fetuses with intrauterine growth retardation (on the left of the figure) and 100 controls (on the right). The two groups showed statistically significant differences ($\chi^2 = 14.08$, $p < 0.001$).* ▨, normal; ■, prepathological; □, pathological

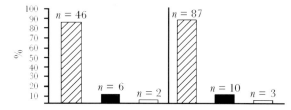

Figure 15 *Distribution of classifications according to the Dexeus test of 54 fetuses with intrauterine growth retardation type I (on the left of the figure) and 100 controls (on the right). The two groups were not significantly different ($\chi^2 = 0.1$).* ▨, normal; ■, prepathological; □, pathological

obtained during the week before delivery and were evaluated using the Dexeus test. Results were classified as normal (Dexeus test 9–10), pre-pathological (Dexeus test 7–8) and pathological (Dexeus test < 7) and then compared with those of a control group of 100 recordings of normal pregnancies with appropriate fetal growth. There were statistically significant differences between the two groups ($p < 0.001$) (Figure 14). In order to determine whether different IUGR types behaved in the same way, the three types of IUGR were statistically compared. Although there were no significant differences in IUGR types I and III, statistically significant differences were found in IUGR type II ($p < 0.001$) (Figures 15, 16, 17).

In an attempt to establish the predictive value of non-stressing prenatal monitoring assessed using the Dexeus test, these results were correlated with Apgar scores, umbilical cord pH, and antenatal fetal mortality. The occurrence of an Apgar score of < 7 was significantly more

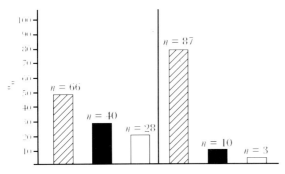

Figure 16 Distribution of classifications according to the Dexeus test of 134 fetuses with intrauterine growth retardation type II (on the left of the figure) and 100 controls (on the right). The two groups showed statistically significant differences ($\chi^2 = 36.88$, $p < 0.001$). ▨, normal; ■, prepathological; ☐, pathological

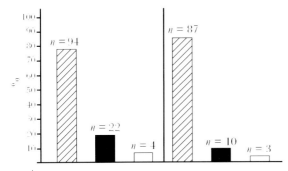

Figure 17 Distribution of classifications according to the Dexeus test of 120 fetuses with intrauterine growth retardation type III (on the left of the figure) and 100 normal controls (on the right). The two groups were not significantly different ($\chi^2 = 3.12$). ▨, normal; ■, prepathological; ☐, pathological

frequent ($p < 0.0001$) when antepartum assessment using the Dexeus test was < 7 (Figure 18). Likewise, when antenatal cardiotocographic recordings evaluated using the Dexeus test scored < 7, the umbilical cord pH was, in the majority of cases, lower than 7.25, thus confirming a highly significant difference ($p < 0.0001$) (Figure 19). Finally, there was a very good correlation ($p < 0.0001$) between antenatal cardiotocographic recordings and antepartum mortality (Figure 20).

The sensitivity reported by different authors varies between 69% and 80%, although specificity is low (< 60%); the positive predictive value is high, between 90% and 96%.

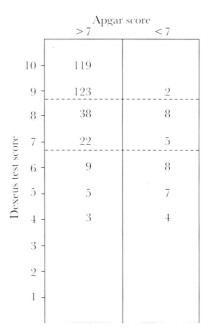

Figure 18 Comparison of Apgar scores with the Dexeus test

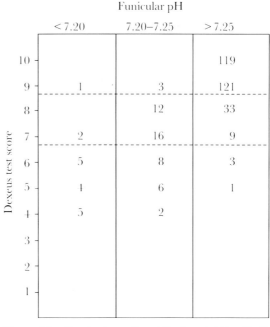

Figure 19 Comparison of umbilical cord pH with the Dexeus test

Late decelerations in fetal heart rate are associated with significantly lower levels of pO_2 in the umbilical artery than in the control group,

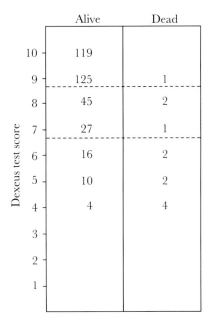

Figure 20 *Comparison of mortality with the Dexeus test. Alive, neonates alive in the 1st week of life; dead, perinatal mortality*

or in the IUGR group with a normal heart-rate pattern[149,150]. Chronologically, however, hypoxemia is associated first with late decelerations and, subsequently, with a decrease in the variability of fetal heart-rate activity[149,151,152]. This would indicate that the non-stress test may be carried out too late to detect deterioration in fetal pO_2 levels. Slomka and Phelan[153], combining the non-stress test with the oxytocin challenge test, have shown that when results of both procedures are abnormal, 90% of fetuses with IUGR present fetal compromise; in these cases, Cesarean section should be carried out.

Doppler velocimetry

Umbilical artery velocity waveforms have been used to diagnose and even prospectively to predict all types of IUGR. Disappointing results have generally been obtained, since not all cases of IUGR originate from placental insufficiency, which can theoretically be detected using Doppler velocimetry[154–156]. Ultrasonographic biometric parameters are the most useful diagnostic tools in cases of IUGR[157], and it must be agreed that the sensitivity of Doppler velocimetry is lower than that of biometric data[158–161].

Nevertheless, when IUGR has already been diagnosed on the basis of biometric data, then the assessment of umbilical artery velocimetry waveforms is a useful procedure to determine whether IUGR is harmonious (type I) or disharmonious (type II). Whereas in the first case, umbilical perfusion will be normal, in the second, pathologic values will often be found in indices of flow velocity waveforms. As Burke and associates[156] have indicated, however, the confirmation of normal umbilical artery velocity waveforms in cases of IUGR is not associated with an increase in fetal risk; in contrast, abnormal umbilical artery velocity waveforms in fetuses with IUGR are associated with a statistically significant increase in perinatal mortality (fetal and neonatal), fetal distress, and the need for urgent delivery[162–168].

Finally, in cases of IUGR with decreased umbilical perfusion, Doppler velocimetry of fetal blood vessels, referred to as the 'hemodynamic profile' in previous studies[36,169], allows us to monitor the different stages of fetal compromise and redistribution of blood flow, so that delivery can promptly be indicated.

Fetal biophysical profile

One of the main reasons for using fetal biophysical profile schemes is the suspicion or evidence of IUGR. The combined use of different biophysical parameters both increases the sensitivity and the predictive value, and greatly reduces false-positive rates.

Biochemical parameters

At the end of the 1960s, and more particularly during the 1970s, a number of biochemical parameters was widely used to study fetal metabolic functions, a decrease in which was associated with different conditions, including IUGR. Biochemical monitoring of levels of hormones (estriol, human placental lactogen)[170,171] and enzymes (cystinoaminepeptidase)[172,173] have fallen into disuse, because of low sensitivity and specificity.

NATURAL HISTORY OF FETAL COMPROMISE IN IUGR: CHRONOLOGY OF PATHOGENETIC CHANGES AND BIOPHYSICAL AND BIOCHEMICAL CORRELATION

The reduction in the number of functional arterioles in the tertiary villi gradually increases umbilical artery resistance with a subsequent decrease in pO_2 in the umbilical vein. Both facts, at a specific moment in time, give rise to redistribution of blood flow, i.e. centralization of blood flow. The best oxygenated blood is distributed through vital organs (brain, heart, adrenal glands), while, as a result of vasoconstriction, blood flow to organs that are considered to be less vital is restricted (digestive system, lungs, skin, skeleton, etc.).

The redistribution or centralization of blood flow has been studied in experimental animals, in particular by Rudolph and Heymann[174] and Reuss and colleagues[175] in sheep, and by Behrmann and associates[176] in fetal primates. In most cases, blood flow redistribution was assessed by injecting radioactive-labelled microspheres, and hypoxemia and acidosis were induced by different procedures, such as maternal breathing of a mixture low in oxygen, hypotension, partial umbilical compression using clamps, microembolization of the umbilical arteries, etc. In all cases the aforementioned pattern of redistribution of blood flow was confirmed. It is, however, worth pointing out that when fetal hypoxemia occurred as a result of maternal hypoxemia, not only did cardiac and cerebral blood perfusion increase but umbilical artery blood flow also increased significantly. This did not occur when fetal asphyxia was induced by microembolization of umbilical arteries, a condition similar to that encountered in human fetuses with placental lesions[177].

Four stages with relatively well-defined hemodynamic, biophysical and biochemical patterns can be distinguished by ultrasound Doppler studies in the compromised fetus with IUGR.

Silent stage of increase in vascular resistance

Physiopathological basis

The progressive impairment of microcirculation in the villi is reflected in Doppler velocimetry of the umbilical artery (changes in the pulsatility index) only when more than 50% of villi arterioles are affected[178]. Until then, the theoretical deficit in gas exchange is maintained by the reserve capacity of the placenta, as long as the maternal blood supply continues to be acceptable[179]

Doppler hemodynamic profile

For a period of time, usually 3 to 6 weeks, fetal hemodynamic profiles are normal. Umbilical artery velocity waveforms show a positive blood-flow pattern throughout the cardiac cycle and pulsatility, resistance or conductance values are within the confidence intervals. These are the umbilical artery velocity waveforms described by Laurin and associates[163,164] as type 0, with strictly passive diastolic flow (Figure 21). Doppler velocimetry of the remaining fetal blood vessels (descending aorta, common carotid artery, middle cerebral artery) also shows morphologically normal velocity waveforms with pulsatility indices within safety margins of each centile curve.

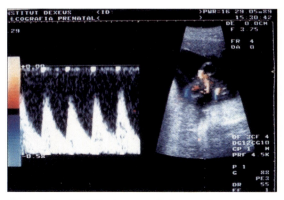

Figure 21 *Umbilical artery velocity waveforms type 0*

Doppler velocimetry in 82 cases of IUGR confirmed at birth showed that in 36 cases (43.9%) the pulsatility index of the umbilical artery was normal. In none of these cases did the study of other fetal blood vessels show any abnormalities. For this reason, an in-depth fetal hemodynamic study, when umbilical waveforms are normal, seems to be unnecessary (Table 3).

Biophysical correlation

Both cardiotocographic recordings and other parameters included in the fetal biophysical profile are normal.

Biochemical correlation

The analysis of fetal blood gases obtained at cordocentesis is normal. In our experience, this type of study is unwarranted when Doppler velocimetry gives normal results. Normal standardized curves have been developed using data obtained at protocolized cordocentesis, which has been indicated in circumstances other than those intervening in fetal distress (study of fetal karyotype, diagnosis of fetal infection, etc.).

Obstetric outcome

There is no increase in perinatal mortality rate and the percentage of IUGR is still not significantly high.

Decrease in umbilical blood flow

The decrease in umbilical blood flow is the first objective sign of chronic fetal compromise as a result of placental insufficiency.

Physiopathological basis

As Trudinger[178] has shown in a mathematical model, the functional obstruction of over 50% of placental blood vessels causes umbilical artery velocity waveforms that are clearly abnormal (Figure 22).

Although it has been stated that the umbilical artery is not always the first vessel to be affected, in our experience and in that of other authors[180,181], the increase in umbilical artery resistance is usually the first apparent hemodynamic sign when there are placental lesions affecting the microcirculation of the villi. In only 15–20% of fetuses with IUGR of placental origin can the sudden increase in pO_2 cause an increase in the aortic and/or cerebral pulsatility index (mediated by aortic and carotid chemore-

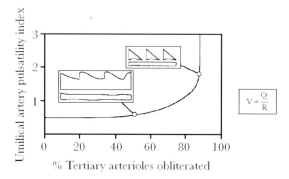

Figure 22 *Mathematical model of Trudinger*[178]

Table 3 *Doppler velocimetry of umbilical-artery pulsatility index (PI) and fetal hemodynamic profile (FHP) in 82 cases of intrauterine growth retardation confirmed at birth, with fetal mortality and pH of blood from the umbilical artery*

	Cases		Fetal mortality		pH < 7.20	
	n	%	n	%	n	%
PI normal, FHP normal	36	43.9	0	0.0	6	16.6
PI normal, FHP abnormal	0	0.0	–	–	–	–
PI abnormal, FHP normal	22	26.8	0	0.0	8	36.4
PI abnormal, FHP abnormal	24	29.2	6	25.0	15	83.3
Total	82	100	6	7.3	29	38.2

ceptors) that precedes and/or is greater than that observed in the umbilical artery. On the other hand, it is also possible to detect abnormal values of the pulsatility index in the aorta or cerebral arteries prior to changes in umbilical blood flow, when the cause of fetal compromise is to be found in anomalies in the maternal environment (hypoxemia due to cardiopulmonary disease, severe nutrient deficiency, severe anemia, etc.) or in maternal circulatory hemodynamics (acute hypertensive episodes, etc.). In these cases, even umbilical conductance may increase.

Experimental studies have provided irrefutable evidence that a placental lesion is followed by decreased umbilical artery blood flow. In the studies of Morrow and associates[177], sheep fetuses were subjected to embolization of villi microcirculation (plastic microemboli of 50 μm in diameter). Gradual changes in umbilical artery velocity waveforms, similar to those detected in human fetuses with IUGR, caused by placental insufficiency (decrease in diastolic blood flow, diastole 0, and, finally, reverse flow) were observed. The cause of the deterioration in umbilical artery velocity waveforms, therefore, must be found in the increase in villi microvasculature resistance. At the same time as this causes the flow of primarily the umbilical artery to decrease, it also causes a gradual decrease in pO_2 in the umbilical vein. Hypoxemia is, therefore, the result, not the cause, of umbilicoplacental hemodynamic changes. For this reason, a decrease in pO_2 in the absence of placental insufficiency does not produce any changes in umbilical artery waveforms[177,182,183], nor are they affected by increased blood viscosity or an increase in maternal blood pressure[177].

Doppler hemodynamic profile

For a certain period of time, the length of which largely depends on the rate at which placental lesion occurs, a moderate increase in umbilical vascular resistance is the only sign of the onset of chronic fetal compromise (Figure 23). During this period, Doppler velocimetry of other fetal blood vessels (including the descending aorta) is usually normal. In our ex-

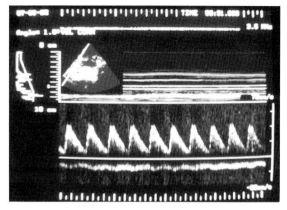

Figure 23 *Pathological flow velocity waveform of the umbilical artery showing diastolic flow, but increase in the pulsatility index*

perience, 56% of fetuses with IUGR present an abnormal pulsatility index of the umbilical artery, although in only 52% of these cases is an 'abnormal fetal hemodynamic pattern' found.

Doppler velocimetry of the umbilical artery shows positive flow velocities throughout the cardiac cycle, but the pulsatility index (or conductance) falls outside the acceptable range for the gestational age. A patent ductus venosus is the only hemodynamic compensatory mechanism – blood is moved from the liver to the heart – that can be observed by color Doppler. This shunting mechanism may delay centralization of blood flow for a period of a few weeks, but induces IUGR of the asymmetrical type[181].

Biophysical correlation

All parameters of the fetal biophysical profile, including cardiotocographic recordings, are normal. Results of the vibroacoustic stimulation test and even stress tests are also normal. These parameters are only affected when cerebral and/or fetal heart hypoxia occurs.

Biochemical correlation

The oxygen supply to fetal tissue is normal. In our experience it is not necessary to carry out cordocentesis if the onset of centralization of blood flow is not confirmed.

Obstetric outcome

According to our statistics for this group, there are no cases of fetal death due to chronic fetal compromise, although there is a significant increase in the percentage of newborn infants that are small-for-dates. For this reason, 38% of newborns have pH levels < 7.20 (Table 3). In fact, there is a three-fold increase in the number of cases of intrapartum fetal distress, thus indicating a greater vulnerability of the fetus. Delivery is by Cesarean section in 30–40% of cases.

Centralization of blood flow

Physiopathological basis

As umbilical artery resistance increases, there is a decrease in pO_2 in the umbilical vein; when a certain level of pO_2 is reached, in addition to dilatation of the ductus venosus, redistribution of fetal blood flow occurs, so as to maintain oxygen supply to the fetal structures most sensitive to hypoxia. Redistribution of blood flow consists of the 'centralization' of blood flow as a result of selective vasodilatation of cerebral, cardiac or adrenal blood vessels and vasoconstriction of pulmonary, intestinal, cutaneous, renal or skeletal vessels. Doppler velocimetry reveals progressive increases in the pulsatility indices of the descending aorta and renal arteries, and decreases in the pulsatility indices of the common carotid and intracranial arteries.

These changes in arterial perfusion are mainly mediated by neuronal stimulation, either directly through stimulation of the vagal centre or through chemoreceptors in the aorta and carotid arteries. Dawes and co-workers[184], in 1969, demonstrated that aortic chemoreceptors were sensitive to small reductions in oxygen levels in fetal lambs. It is likely, however, that vasoconstriction would be modulated by other factors, such as the direct effect of hypoxemia and acidemia on certain tissues through release of vasoactive compounds or catecholamines, increase in the overall activity of the autonomic nervous system, etc.

Although the chronology of these changes has not yet been established, it would appear that the first vessel affected, after the umbilical artery and ductus venosus, is the aorta. Increases in the vascular resistance of the descending aorta are probably the result of the combined effect of several factors, such as increase in vascular resistance of umbilicoplacental vessels, reflex arterial vasoconstriction, due to progressive hypoxemia, and ultimately a decrease in myocardial contractility[185]. Lingman and colleagues[186] have suggested that there is an inverse relationship between myocardial contractility and pulsatility indices of the umbilical and aortic arteries.

Hemodynamic Doppler profile

Doppler velocimetry reveals an increase in the pulsatility index of the umbilical artery but also of the descending aorta and renal artery[73,187–189]. When vascular resistance reaches a certain level, a gradual decrease in diastolic velocity waveforms occurs in both vessels. A parallel decrease in pulsatility indices in the common carotid and cerebral arteries occurs as a result of vasodilatation.

In our experience in 46 cases of IUGR with an abnormal pulsatility index of the umbilical artery, 52% of fetuses also showed abnormal increases in the pulsatility index of the descending aorta and 41.1% showed a decrease in vascular resistance of the middle cerebral artery.

Three stages in the process of centralization of fetal blood flow are frequently observed.

Initial stage The pulsatility index of the umbilical artery is elevated, but Doppler velocimetry frequency values continue to be positive throughout the cardiac cycle, even during the end-diastolic phase. On the other hand, common carotid artery velocimetry waveforms, for which diastolic frequencies are absent until week 32 to 34[190], recover diastolic velocity flow shortly after a moderate increase in vascular intracranial perfusion occurs. This suggests that the decrease in the pulsatility index of the common carotid is largely due to the reduction in vascular resistance of cerebral blood vessels.

During this initial stage, the assessment of the pulsatility index ratio of the umbilical artery and

INTRAUTERINE GROWTH RETARDATION

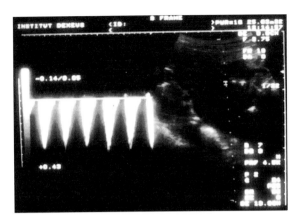

Figure 24 *Umbilical artery flow velocity waveforms with absence of end-diastolic velocities*

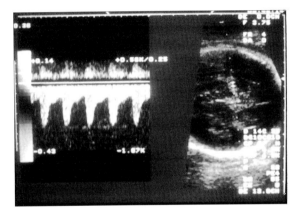

Figure 25 *Middle cerebral artery flow velocity waveforms with pulsatility index decreased by vasodilatation and reduction in vascular resistance*

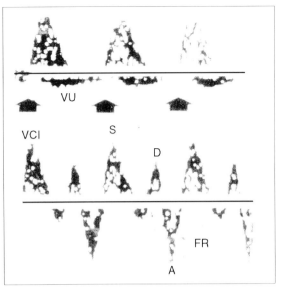

Figure 26 *Venous signs of heart failure. Upper figure, venous pulsations in the umbilical vein (VU) coinciding with the absence of diastole in the umbilical artery; lower figure, elevated reverse flow in the inferior vena cava (VCI)*

of the common carotid artery and middle cerebral artery are at their lowest as a result of concurrent maximal vasodilatation of cerebral blood vessels (Figure 25).

Terminal stage In addition to arterial hemodynamic changes, signs of heart failure become apparent in the Doppler velocimetry of fetal venous blood flow, in particular in elevated reverse blood flow in the vena cava (which coincides with atrial contraction) and venous pulsation in the umbilical vein (Figure 26).

An elevated reverse flow in the inferior vena cava indicates impairment of blood flow in the right atrium, which may be attributed to abnormalities in fetal heart rate or deficient atrial contractility[192–194]. Standardized normal curves of reverse flow in the inferior vena cava for each week of gestation[194] allows the differentiation of normal from pathological cases. Venous pulsation in the umbilical vein with apparent cyclical decreases in venous blood flow, which coincides with the absence of diastole in umbilical artery velocity waveforms, is also considered a sign of heart failure.

the middle cerebral artery (cerebral/umbilical Doppler ratio) could be particularly useful in showing the centralization of blood flow. Several authors believe that this is the best blood flow index for screening for IUGR[180,191].

Advanced stage Umbilical artery velocity waveforms show absence of diastolic frequencies; end-diastolic frequency disappears first, but subsequently the lack of blood flow is apparent in the whole of diastole (Figure 24). According to Trudinger[178], this occurs when 80% of villi arterioles are occluded. Aortic velocity waveforms also exhibit absence of diastolic frequencies. At the same time, pulsatility indices

Venous signs of heart failure have the advantage over parameters that are exclusively assessed by ultrasonography, in that they are independent of the angle at which pulses of ultrasound are transmitted into the vessels, and do not require the calculation of the diameter or cross-sectional areas of large blood vessels.

Biophysical correlation

In the initial stage of the centralization of blood flow, cardiotocographic recordings may still be apparently normal, and results of Manning's fetal biophysical profile considered to be normal or equivocal (scores 5 to 7). Changes in rest/activity cycles and a decrease in multiple fetal body movements ('rolling') are early detected[195,196]. Although there is an increase in abnormal results of non-stress tests in comparison with the previous stage, statistically significant differences between both stages have not been encountered.

In the advanced stage of the centralization of blood flow, there is a progressive impairment of fetal heart-rate activity with the occurrence of late decelerations. An abnormal pulsatility index of the umbilical artery usually precedes, by 9 to 60 days[165,197] (mean 2 to 3 weeks[198,199]), the occurrence of late decelerations in the fetal heart rate. Moreover, ultrasonography also shows a clear decrease in gross fetal movements, fetal breathing, and fetal tone. The amniotic liquid volume can also decrease markedly (amniotic fluid index between 5 and 8)[200]. If all these parameters are evaluated according to Manning's fetal biophysical profile, a total score of less than 7 is usually obtained. At this stage, the number of positive results obtained in oxytocin challenge tests is clearly significant, as are the results obtained in stress tests and vibroacoustic stimulation tests. Chronic fetal compromise, for which up this point there was thought to be compensation, is now seen to be uncompensated.

Finally, in the late stage of the centralization of blood flow, cardiotocographic recordings reveal not only late decelerations in fetal heart rate but also a notable decrease in heart rate reactivity. These ominous recordings probably do not appear until 2–3 weeks after minimal values for the pulsatility index of the middle cerebral artery have been recorded. The time lapse depends on the ability of the fetus to compensate for the reduction in its metabolic supply[198].

Total scores of the fetal biophysical profile are very low (always < 5), due to abnormal results for each individual variable (marked decrease in fetal movements, fetal tone, etc. and increasingly severe oligohydramnios (amniotic fluid index < 5).

Biochemical correlation

When abnormal Doppler arterial velocity waveforms are registered not only in the umbilical artery but also in the remaining fetal arteries (descending aorta, common carotid, middle cerebral artery, etc.), low pO_2 and pH levels are to be expected in fetal blood samples obtained at cordocentesis[63,180,196,201,202]. In fact, redistribution of blood flow only begins when fetal hypoxemia and acidosis occur.

In the initial stage, in which diastolic frequencies are still present in the aorta and umbilical arteries, there are usually nor more than 25–30% of cases of hypoxemia. The situation changes dramatically in the advanced stage, coinciding with the disappearance of diastolic frequencies in Doppler velocimetry of the aorta and umbilical artery; in this case, 80% of fetuses present clear signs of hypoxemia and 43% of acidosis[202]. Similar figures have been reported by Montenegro and co-workers[180]: fetal hypoxemia in 70.3% of cases, fetal acidosis in 66.6%, and fetal asphyxia in 74%. In fact, most authors[203–205] consider that the absence of diastolic flow at this stage of redistribution of blood flow is synonymous with abnormal acid–base balance in fetal blood. In the late stage, pO_2 values in almost all fetuses are about −2 to −4 SD of the mean[206].

Obstetric and neonatal outcome

A large number of fetal (250/1000) and neonatal deaths are found in this group, with a significant increase in the number of newborn infants with pH < 7.20 (83.3%). In our experience, the rate of Cesarean deliveries was 100%. The fetuses that survived showed a high incidence of complications (necrotizing colitis, hemorrhages, etc.) as a result of persistent vasoconstriction in specific organs[207].

Different authors[164,208] have reported that the absence of diastolic values in the aortic velocity waveforms significantly predicts neonatal morbidity. Thus, whilst the group of fetuses in which diastolic flow was absent suffered necrotizing enterocolitis (27% of cases) and hemorrhages in different organs (23% of cases) after delivery, these complications did not occur when diastolic frequencies were present[208].

Decentralization of blood flow

This is the term used by Montenegro and associates[180] to refer to the irreversible hemodynamic changes that take place after the centralization of fetal blood flow and that precede fetal death.

Physiopathological basis

If hypoxia persists, a generalized phenomenon of vasomotor paralysis occurs. It may be postulated that the resulting condition may be similar to that described in experimental animals subjected to sustained and severe hypoxemia[209,210]. The cerebral blood flow is mechanically restricted, due to the appearance of cerebral edema and the resulting increase in intracranial pressure. Cerebral edema is probably caused by local accumulation of lactic acid, as a result of sustained anaerobic metabolism, which affects the permeability of the cell membrane, increases intracellular osmotic pressure and, finally, leads to edema and tissue necrosis.

In addition to hypoxia of cerebral centers, irreversible interference with control mechanisms of vascular tone in arterial vessels also occurs (usually in extreme cases of hypoxemia, with more than − 4SD of the mean)[206,211].

Doppler hemodynamic profile

Mari and Wasserstrum[212], who have reported the results of Doppler velocimetry of this condi-

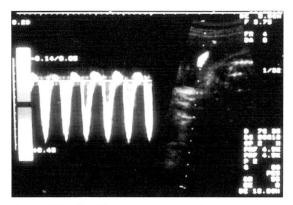

Figure 27 Umbilical artery flow velocity waveforms, showing reverse diastolic flow

tion, indicated that diagnosis is largely based on confirmation of vascular resistance in umbilical and peripheral circulation (aorta, renal, etc.) in the presence of reverse diastolic flow (Figure 27), and increases, after a brief period of stability, in pulsatility indices of intracranial arteries. These values may appear to be normal and cerebral artery velocity waveforms may be observed with no diastoles or with reverse flow. How much time lapses between the onset of the process and intrauterine fetal death is not known, although it probably does not exceed 2 to 3 days and in many cases is a matter of only a few hours. This explains the difficulties found in detecting all these changes by Doppler velocimetry.

Biophysical correlation

If, at this time, a cardiotocographic examination is carried out, a terminal pattern known as 'intrauterine fetal brain death' will be observed[213-217]. The recordings invariably show fixed fetal heart-rate activity with no variability, and total absence of accelerations or decelerations, even when contractions are provoked by the oxytocin challenge test or vibroacoustic stimulation of the fetus. The fetal biophysical profile shows an immobile, atonic fetus with very little amniotic fluid, although some cases with hydramnios have been reported[217,218]. The total score of the fetal biophysical profile is < 2. Cystic periventricular brain lesions (porencephalic cyst) or marked dilatation of the ventricles as a result of hypoxic necrosis are only occasionally observed by ultrasonography[213,217,219,220].

Biochemical correlation

As has already been mentioned, if cordocentesis is carried out, extreme hypoxia is confirmed (pO_2 values less than -4 SD of the mean) as is severe acidosis.

Obstetric outcome

This is the phase that precedes death, so that fetal or neonatal death, when delivery is initiated, is the rule. Cesarean delivery is therefore considered to be unnecessary[217].

MANAGEMENT OF IUGR: TIMING OF DELIVERY

The decision as to when and how to deliver should be taken while bearing in mind:

(1) The objective data concerning fetal well-being (type of IUGR, absence or presence of congenital malformations, onset of centralization of blood flow, etc.);

(2) The degree of fetal lung maturity; and

(3) The clinical features of each case (parity, underlying diseases, etc.).

In the case of IUGR of type I (intrinsic or harmonious), with evidence, or likelihood, of fetal anomalies (trisomy, congenital malformations, etc.), whatever the results of tests to determine lung maturity, fetal hemodynamics, etc., normal delivery may be contemplated. If the presence of congenital malformations has not been confirmed, the procedure to follow is that of extrinsic IUGR.

In the case of IUGR of type II (extrinsic or disharmonious), different tests currently used in antepartum fetal surveillance should help to determine the most suitable time for delivery. Present knowledge and diagnostic possibilities afford two alternative approaches with regard to timing of delivery.

The first is delivery when cardiotocographic recordings are abnormal and/or signs of chronic fetal distress are evident (decrease in fetal tone and fetal body movements, meconium staining of amniotic fluid, etc.). In this case, a high rate of asphyxia and perinatal morbidity and mortality may be expected[221,222].

The second is delivery at the onset of centralization of blood flow, in which case a high rate of premature infants is expected. In order to minimize this risk, particularly if gestational age is less than 30 weeks, cordocentesis should be carried out to study fetal blood gases. This decision should be taken especially when pulsatility indices in the aorta and umbilical artery are clearly abnormal, but diastolic frequencies are still recorded. If diastolic flow is absent, and more particularly if reverse diastolic flow exists, fetal outcome is poor and cordocentesis is of little use.

In the case of mature fetuses or fetuses in transitional stages of maturity, delivery should always be instituted before disappearance of diastolic frequencies. Delivery when diastolic flow is absent may be too late, given the high percentage of acidosis (70%) and the high rate of perinatal mortality present in this group.

References

1. Butler, N. R. and Alberman, E. D. (1969). *Second Report of British Perinatal Problems.* (Edinburgh: Churchill Livingstone)
2. Bard, H. (1970). Intrauterine growth retardation. *Clin. Obstet. Gynecol.*, **13**, 511–25
3. Ounsted, M., Moar, V. and Scott, W. A. (1981). Prenatal morbidity and mortality in small-for-dates babies: the relative importance of some maternal factors. *Early Hum. Dev.*, **5**, 367–75
4. Teberg, A. J., Walther, F. J. and Pena, I. C. (1988). Mortality, morbidity, and outcome of the small-for-gestational age infants. *Semin. Perinatol.*, **12**, 84–94

5. Creasy, R. (1986). *Maternal–Fetal Medicine.* (London: Churchill Livingstone)
6. World Health Organization (1961). Aspects of low birth weight. Report of the Expert Committee of maternal child health. *WHO Technical Report*, **217**, 3–16
7. Gruenwald, P. (1963). Chronic fetal distress and placental insufficiency. *Biol. Neonate*, **5**, 215–21
8. Lubchenko, L. O., Hansman, C., Dressler, M. and Boyd, E. (1963). Intrauterine growth as estimated from liveborn birth weight at 24 to 42 weeks of gestation. *Pediatrics*, **32**, 793–800
9. Gruenwald, P. (1966). Growth of the human fetus. I. Normal growth audits variation. *Am. J. Obstet. Gynecol.*, **94**, 1112–19
10. Warkani, J., Monroe, B. and Ystherland, B. S. (1961). Intrauterine growth retardation. *Am. J. Dis. Child,*, **102**, 249–79
11. Budin, P. (1907). *The Nursling. The Feeding and Hygiene of Premature and Full Term Infants.* Maloney, W. J. (transl.). (London: Caxton Publishing)
12. McBurney, R. D. (1947). The undernourished full term infant. *West. J. Surg. Obstet. Gynecol.*, **55**, 363–74
13. Weiner, C. P. and Robinson, D. (1989). The sonographic diagnosis of intrauterine growth retardation using the postnatal ponderal index and the crown–heel length as standards of diagnosis. *Am. J. Perinatol.*, **6**, 380–3
14. Branconi, F., Faldi, P., Mello, G., Cariati, E., Nannini, C., Paladini, S. and Gerli, P.(1977). The poor endouterine growth of the fetus in treated diabetic patients. Possible role of diet and insulin. In Salvadori, B. and Bacchi-Modena, A. (eds.) *Poor Intrauterine Fetal Growth*, pp.151–4. (Parma, Italy: Minerva Medica)
15. Berkowitz, R. L. and Hobbins, J. C. (1977). Ultrasonography in the antepartum patient. In Bolognese, R. J. and Schwartz, R. (eds.) *Perinatal Medicine Management in the High-Risk Fetus and Neonate*, pp. 85–112. (Baltimore: Williams)
16. Galbraith, R. S., Karchmar, E. J., Pievey, W. N. and Low, J. A. (1979). The clinical prediction of intrauterine growth retardation. *Am. J. Obstet. Gynecol.*, **133**, 281–6
17. Fabre, E., González de Agüero, R., De Agustín, J. I.., Repollés, S. and Tajada, M. (1993). Epidemiology of intrauterine growth retardation. *Rev. Iberoam. de Fertilidad*, **X**, 15–20
18. Niswander, K. R. and Gordon, M. (1972). *The Women and Their Pregnancies.* (Philadelphia: Saunders)
19. Love, E. J. and Kinch, R. A. M. (1965). Factors influencing the birth weight in normal pregnancy. *Am. J. Obstet. Gynecol.*, **91**, 342–9
20. Ounsted, M. and Ounsted, C. (1968). Maternal regulation of intrauterine growth. *Nature (London)*, **87**, 777–81
21. Simpson, J. W., Lawless, R. W. and Cameron, A. (1975). Responsibility of the obstetrician to the fetus. *Obstet. Gynecol.*, **45**, 481–7
22. Carrera, J. M. (1977). Diagnóstico prenatal del retardo de crecimiento fetal. *Clín. Ginecol.*, **5**, 86–94
23. Goldstein, H. (1973). Smoking and pregnancy. *Nature (London)*, **245**, 277–83
24. Naeye, R. L., Blanc, W., Leblanc, W. and Khatamee, M. A. (1973). Fetal complications of maternal heroin addiction: abnormal growth, infections, and episodes of stress. *J. Pediatr.*, **83**, 1055–61
25. Ulleland, C. N. (1972). The offspring of alcoholic mothers. *Ann. NY Acad. Sci.*, **197**, 167–9
26. Palmer, R. H., Oullette, E. M., Warner, L. and Leichtman, S. R. (1974). Congenital malformations in offspring of a chronic alcoholic mother. (1974). *Pediatrics*, **53**, 490–6
27. Katz, A. I., Davison, J. M., Hayslett, J. P., Singson, E. and Lindheimer, M. D. (1980). Pregnancy in women with kidney disease. *Kidney Int.*, **18**, 192–206
28. Surian, M., Imbasciate, E., Cosci, P., Banfi, G., Brancaccio, D., Barbiano, D. I., Belgiojoso, G., Minetti, L. and Ponticelli, C. (1984). Glomerular disease and pregnancy: a study of 123 pregnancies in patients with primary and secondary glomerular disease. *Nephron*, **36**, 101–5
29. Jungers, P., Forget, D., Hovillier, P., Henry-Amar, M. and Grunfeld, J. P. (1987). Pregnancy in IgA nephropathy, reflux nephropathy and focal glomerular sclerosis. *Am. J. Kidney Dis.*, **9**, 334–8
30. Fine, L. G., Barnett, E. V., Danowitch, G. M., Nissenson, A. R., Conolly, M. E., Lieb, S. M. and Barrett, C. T. (1981). Systemic lupus erythematosus in pregnancy. *Ann. Intern. Med.*, **94**, 667–77
31. Farquharson, R. C., Pearson, J. F. and John, L. (1984). Lupus anticoagulant and intrauterine death in the absence of systemic lupus. *Lancet*, **2**, 228–8
32. Branch, D. W., Scott, J. R., Kochenoor, N. K. and Hershgold, E. (1985). Obstetric complications associated with the lupus anticoagulant. *N. Engl. J. Med.*, **313**, 1322–6

33. Lubbe, W. F. and Liggins, G. (1985). Lupus anticoagulant and pregnancy. *Am. J. Obstet. Gynecol.*, **153**, 322–7
34. Lockwood, C. J., Romero, R., Feinberg, R. F., Clyne, L. P., Coster, B. and Hoobins, J. C. (1989). The prevalence and biological significance of lupus anticoagulant and anticardiolipin antibodies in a general obstetric population. *Am. J. Obstet. Gynecol.*, **161**, 369–73
35. Beischer, N. A. (1971). The effects of maternal anemia upon the fetus. *J. Reprod. Med.*, **6**, 262–74
36. Carrera, J. M., Mallafré, J., Otero, F., Rubio, R. and Carrera, M. (1992). Síndrome de mala adaptación circulatoria materna: Bases etiopatogénicas y terapéuticas. In Carrera, J. M. (ed.) *Doppler en Obstetricia*, pp. 335. (Barcelona: Masson Salvat)
37. Mowbray, J. F. and Underwood, J. C. (1985). Immunology of abortion. *Clin. Exp. Immunol.*, **60**, 1–7
38. Scott, J. B., Rote, N. S. and Branoh, D. W. (1987). Immunologic aspects of recurrent abortion and fetal death. *Obstet. Gynecol.*, **70**, 645–56
39. Kalousek, D. K. and Dill, F. J. (1983). Chromosomal mosaicism confined to the placenta in human conceptions. *Science*, **221**, 665–7
40. Kalousek, D. K., Dill, F. J., Pantzar, J. J., McGuilliuray, B. C., Yong, S. L. and Wilson, R. D. (1987). Confined chorionic mosaicism in prenatal diagnosis. *Hum. Genet.*, **77**, 163–7
41. Kalousek, D. K., Barret, I. and McGuilliuray, B. C. (1989). Placental mosaicism and intrauterine survival for trisomies 13 and 18. *Am. J. Hum. Genet.*, **44**, 338–43
42. Kalousek, D. K., Howard-Peebles, P. N., Olsons, S. B., Barret, I. J., Dorfmann, A., Black, S. H., Schulman, J. D. and Wilson, R. D. (1991). Confirmation of CVS mosaicism in term placental and high frequency of intrauterine growth retardation association with confined placental mosaicism. *Prenat. Diagn.*, **11**, 743–50
43. Verp, M. S. and Unger, N. L. (1988). Placental chromosome abnormalities and intrauterine growth retardation (IUGR). In *Proceedings of the 35th Annual Meeting of the Society for Gynecologic Investigation*, p. 143, (Baltimore, MD, 17–20 March)
44. Stioui, S., De Silvestris, M., Molinari, A., Stripparo, L., Ghisoni, L. and Simoni, G. (1989). Trisomic 22 placenta in a case of severe intrauterine growth retardation. *Prenat. Diagn.*, **9**, 673–6
45. Holzgreve, B., Exeler, R., Holzgreve, W., Wittwer, B. and Miny, P. (1992). Nonviable trisomies confined to the placenta leading to poor pregnancy outcome. *Prenat. Diagn.*, **12** (Suppl.), S95
46. Hashish, A. F., Mouk, N. A., Lovell-Smith, M. P., Bardwell, L. M., Fiddes, T. M. and Gardner, R. J. (1989). Trisomy detected at chorionic villus sampling. *Prenat. Diagn.*, **9**, 427–32
47. Williams, J., Wang, B., Rubin, C., Clark, R. and Oblandas, T. (1989). Apparent non mosaic trisomy 16 in chorionic villi: diagnostic dilemma or clinically significant findings. *Prenat. Diagn.*, **12**, 163–8
48. Reddy, N. S., Blakemore, K. J., Stetten, G. and Corson, U. (1990). The significance of trisomy 7 mosaicism in chorionic villus cultures. *Prenat. Diagn.*, **10**, 417–23
49. Appelman, Z., Rosensaft, J., Chemke, J., Caspi, B., Ashkenazi, M. and Mogilner, M. B. (1991). Trisomy 9 confined to the placenta: prenatal diagnosis and neonatal follow up. *Am. J. Med. Genet.*, **40**, 464–6
50. Tharapel, T., Elias, S., Shulman, L. P., Seely, L., Emerson, D. S. and Simpson, J. L. (1989). Resorbed co-twin as an explanation for discrepant chorionic villus results: non mosaic 47, XX, +16 in villi (direct and culture) with normal (46XX) amniotic fluid and neonatal blood. *Prenat. Diagn.*, **9**, 467–72
51. Barlow, P. (1973). The influence of inactive chromosomes on human development: anomalous sex chromosome complements and the phenotype. *Hum. Genet.*, **17**, 105–9
52. Giles, W. B., Trudinger, B. J. and Baird, P. J. (1985). Fetal umbilical artery flow velocity waveforms and placental resistance: a pathological correlation. *Br. J. Obstet. Gynaecol.*, **92**, 31–8
53. Trudinger, B. J. and Cook, M. (1985). Umbilical and uterine artery flow velocity waveforms in pregnancy associated with major fetal abnormality. *Br. J. Obstet. Gynaecol.*, **92**, 666–70
54. Meizner, I., Katz, M., Lunenfeld, E. and Insler, V. (1987). Umbilical and uterine flow velocity waveforms in pregnancies complicated by major fetal anomalies. *Prenat. Diagn.*, **7**, 491–3
55. Rankin, J. H. G. and McLaughlin, M. K. (1979). The regulation of placental blood flow. *J. Dev. Physiol.*, **1**, 3–30
56. Campbell, S., Pearce, J. M. F., Hackett, G., Cohen-Overbee, T. and Hernández, C. (1986). Qualitative assessment of uteroplacental blood

flow: early screening test for high-risk pregnancies. *Obstet. Gynecol.*, **68**, 649–53

57. Khons, Y. T. and Pearce, J. M. F. (1987). Development and investigation of the placenta and its blood supply. In Lavery, J. P. (ed.) *The Human Placenta*, pp. 25–46. (Rockville, Maryland: Aspen)

58. Shapiro, B. L. (1983). Down syndrome: a disruption of homeostasis. *Am. J. Med. Genet.*, **14**, 241–69

59. Jones, C. T. (1985). Reprogramming of metabolic development by restriction of fetal growth. *Biochem. Soc. Trans.*, **13**, 84–91

60. Kornguth, S. E., Bersn, E. T., Anerbach, R., Sobkowicz, H. M., Schutta, H. S. and Scott, G. L. (1986). Trisomy 16 mice: neural, morphological and immunological studies. *Ann. NY Acad. Sci. USA*, **477**, 160–8

61. Meizner, I., Katz, M., Lunenfeld, E. and Insler, V. (1987). Umbilical and uterine flow velocity waveforms in pregnancies complicated by major fetal anomalies. *Prenat. Diagn.*, **7**, 491–3

62. Rochelson, B., Kaplan, C., Guzman, E., Arato, M., Hansen, K. and Trunca, C. (1990). A quantitative analysis of placental vasculature in the third trimester fetus with autosomal trisomy. *Obstet. Gynecol.*, **75**, 59–63

63. Hsieh, F. J., Chang, F. M., Ko, T. M., Chen, T. M. and Chen, Y. P. (1988). Umbilical artery flow velocity waveforms in fetuses, dying with congenital anomalies. *Br. J. Obstet. Gynaecol.*, **95**, 478–82

64. Hata, K., Hata, T., Senom, D., Aoki, S., Takamiya, O. and Kitao, M. (1989). Umbilical artery blood flow velocity waveforms and association with fetal abnormality. *Gynecol. Obstet. Invest.*, **27**, 179–82

65. Gaziano, E., Knox, E., Wager, G. P., Bendel, R. P. and Olsen, J. D. (1990). Pulsed Doppler umbilical artery waveforms: significance of elevated artery systolic/diastolic ratios in the normally grown fetus. *Obstet. Gynecol.*, **75**, 189–93

66. Carrera, J. M. and Mortera, C. (1991). Estudio Doppler de los defectos congénitos. *Primer Congreso Mundial de Obstetricia y Ginecología*, London, December

67. Winick, M. and Noble, A. (1966). Cellular response in rats during malnutrition at various ages. *J. Nutr.*, **89**, 300–8

68. Winick, M., Coscia, A. and Noble, A. (1967). Cellular growth in human placenta. *J. Pediatr.*, **39**, 248–51

69. Winick, M. (1968). Changes in nucleic acid and protein content of the human brain during growth. *Pediatr. Res.*, **2**, 352–5

70. Winick, M. and Rosso, P. (1969). The effect of severe early malnutrition on cellular growth of human brain. *Pediatr. Res.*, **3**, 181–4

71. Winick, M. (1971). Cellular changes during placental and fetal growth. *Am. J. Obstet. Gynecol.*, **109**, 166–76

72. Winick, M., Brasel, J. A. and Velasco, E. G. (1973). Effects of prenatal nutrition upon pregnancy risk. *Clin. Obstet. Gynecol.*, **16**, 184–92

73. Holtorff, J. (1977). Poor intrauterine fetal growth. An intrauterine nomenclature approach. In Salvadori, B. and Bacchi-Modena, A. (eds.) *Poor Intrauterine Fetal Growth*, pp. 23–7. (Parma, Italy: Minerva Médica)

74. Hobbins, J. C., Berkowitz, R. L. and Grannum. P. A. T. (1978). Diaagnosis and antepartum management of intrauterine growth retardation. *J. Reprod. Med.*, **21**, 319–22

75. Campbell, S. and Newman, G. B. (1971). Growth in the fetal biparietal diameter during normal pregnancy. *J. Obstet. Gynecol. Br. Commonw.*, **78**, 513–19

76. Campbell, S. and Wilkin, P. (1975). Ultrasonic measurement of fetal abdominal circumference in the estimation of fetal weight. *Br. J. Obstet. Gynaecol.*, **82**, 689–97

77. Campbell, S. and Thoms, A. (1977). Ultrasound measurement of the fetal head to abdominal circumference ratio in the assessment of growth retardation. *Br. J. Obstet. Gynaecol.*, **84**, 165–74

78. Levi, S. and Flamme, P. (1970). Relation entre divers paramètres foetomaternels et le diamètre biparietal mesuré par les ultrasons. *Fonds National de la Recherche Scient. Med. Group de Perinatologie*, pp. 324–5. (Brussels)

79. Levi, S. and Maamari, R. (1977). Echographic diagnosis of PIFG. In Salvadori, B. and Bachhi-Modena, A. (eds.) *Poor Intrauterine Fetal Growth*, p. 251. (Parma, Italy: Minerva Médica)

80. Warsof, S. L., Cooper, D. J., Little, D. and Campbell, S. (1986). Routine ultrasound screening for antenatal detection of intrauterine growth retardation. *Obstet. Gynecol.*, **67**, 33–9

81. Clark, S. L. (1992). Patterns of intrauterine growth retardation. *Clin. Obstet. Gynecol.*, **35**, 194–201

82. Ross, P. and Winick, M. (1974). Intrauterine growth retardation. A new systematic approach based on the clinical and biometrical charac-

teristics of this condition. *J. Perinat. Med.*, **42**, 147

83. Sieroszewski, J. (1977). Poor intrauterine fetal growth. A classification system for the fetus. In Salvadori, B. and Bachhi-Modena, A. (eds.) *Poor Intrauterine Fetal Growth*, p. 3. (Parma, Italy: Minerva Médica)

84. Miller, R. C. and Hassanein, K. (1971). Diagnosis of impaired fetal growth in newborn infants. *Pediatrics*, **48**, 511–22

85. Villar, J. and Belizan, J. M. (1982). The timing factor in the pathophysiology of the intrauterine growth retardation syndrome. *Obstet. Gynecol. Surv.*, **37**, 499–506

86. Balcazar, H. and Haas, J. (1990). Classification schemes of small-for-gestational age and type of intrauterine growth retardation and its implications to early neonatal mortality. *Early Hum. Dev.*, **24**, 219–30

87. Grauw, T. J. and Hopkins, B. (1991). Severity of growth retardation and physical condition at birth in small for gestational age infants. *Biol. Neonate.*, **60**, 176–83

88. Tudehope, D. I. (1991). Neonatal aspects of intrauterine growth retardation. *Fetal Med. Rev.*, **3**, 73–85

89. Salvadori, B. (1977). Poor intrauterine fetal growth: an attempt to make out an intrauterine classification. In Salvadori, B. and Bachhi-Modena, A. (eds.) *Poor Intrauterine Fetal Growth.*, pp.29–30. (Parma, Italy: Minerva Médica)

90. Carrera, J. M. (1976). Intrauterine growth retardation. *VIII World Congress of Gynecology and Obstetrics (FIGO)*, Mexico, D. F., October 17–22

91. Carrera, J. M. and Barri, P. N. (1977). Diagnosis of the intrauterine growth retardation. In Salvadori, B. and Bachhi-Modena, A. (eds.) *Poor Intrauterine Fetal Growth.*, pp.277–81. (Parma, Italy: Minerva Médica)

92. Carrera, J. M. (1978). Concepto, selección y clasificación de los recién nacidos pequeños por retardo de crecimiento intrauterino. *Prog. Obstet. Ginecol.*, **21**, 197–208

93. Carrera, J. M. and Mallafré, J. (1980). Tratamiento '*in utero*' del retardo de crecimiento fetal. In Esteban Altirriba, J. (ed.) *Perinatología Clínica 3*. (Barcelona: Salvat Editores)

94. Carrera, J. M. (1981). Regulación del crecimiento fetal. In Carrera, J. M. (ed.) *Biología y Ecología Fetal*, p. 217. (Barcelona: Salvat Editores)

95. Carrera, J. M. (1981). *Clasificación del Crecimiento Intrauterino Retardado*, Tesis doctoral, Santiago de Compostela

96. Carrera, J. M. (1985). *Ecografía Obstétrica*, 2nd edn. (Barcelona: Salvat Editores)

97. Weiner, C. P. and Williamson, R. A. (1989). Evaluation of severe retardation using cordocentesis – hematologic and metabolic alterations by etiology. *Obstet. Gynecol.*, **73**, 225–9

98. Lockwood, C. J. and Weiner, S. (1986). Assessment of fetal growth. *Clin. Perinatol.*, **13**, 3–35

99. Mintz, M. and Landon, M. (1988). Sonographic diagnosis of fetal growth disorders. *Clin. Obstet. Gynecol.*, **31**, 44–52

100. Brar, H. S. and Rutherford, S. E. (1988). Classification of intrauterine growth retardation. *Semin. Perinatol.*, **12**, 2–10

101. Scott, M., Moar, V. and Ounsted, M. (1981). The relative contributions of different maternal factors in small-for-gestational age pregnancies. *J. Obstet. Ginecol. Reprod. Biol.*, **12**, 157–64

102. Steele, S. A., Pearce, J. M. and Chamberlain, G. V. (1988). Doppler ultrasound of the uteroplacental circulation as a screening test for severe preeclampsia with intrauterine growth retardation. *Eur. J. Obstet. Gynecol. Reprod. Biol.*, **28**, 279–87

103. Jacobson, S. L., Imhof, R., Manning, N., Mannion, V., Little, D., Rey, E. and Redman, C. H. (1989). The value of Doppler assessment of the uteroplacental circulation in predicting preeclampsia or intrauterine growth retardation. *Am. J. Obstet. Gynecol.*, **162**, 110–14

104. Westin, B. (1977). Gravidogram and poor intrauterine fetal growth. In Salvadori, B. and Bacchi-Modena, A. (eds.) *Poor Intrauterine Fetal Growth*, pp.44–7. (Parma, Italy: Minerva Médica)

105. Effer, S. B. (1969). Management of high-risk pregnancy: report of a combined obstetrical and neonatal intensive care unit. *Can. Med. Assoc. J.*, **101**, 389–404

106. Campbell, S. and Soothill, P. (1993). Detection and management of intrauterine growth retardation. A British approach. In Chervenak, F. A., Isaacson, J. and Campbell, S. (eds.) *Ultrasound in Obstetrics and Gynecology*, p. 1431. (London: Little Brown)

107. Goldstein, I., Reece, E. A., Pilu, G., Bovicelli, L. and Hobbins, J. C. (1987). Cerebellar measurements with ultrasonography in the evaluation of fetal growth and development. *Am. J. Obstet. Gynecol.*, **156**, 1065–9

108. Reece, E. A., Goldstein, I., Pilu, G. and Hobbins, J. C. (1987). Fetal cerebellar growth unaffected by intrauterine growth retardation: a

new parameter for prenatal diagnosis. *Am. J. Obstet. Gynecol.*, **157**, 632–8

109. Reece, E. A. and Hagay, Z. (1992). Prenatal diagnosis of deviant fetal growth. In Reece, A. E., Hobbins, J. C., Mahoney, M. J. and Petrie, R. H. (eds.) *Medicine of the Fetus and Mother*, pp.671–85. (Philadelphia: Lippincott, Co.)

110. Duchatel, F., Mennesson, B., Berseneff, H. and Oury, J. F. (1989). Antenatal echographic measurement of the fetal cerebellum. Significance in the evaluation of fetal development. *J. Gynecol. Obstet. Biol. Reprod.*, **18**, 879–83

111. Campbell, W. A., Narci, D., Vintzileos, A. M., Rodis, J. F., Turner, C. W. and Egan, J. F. (1991). Transverse cerebellar diameter/abdominal circumference ratio throughout pregnancy: a gestational age independent method to assess fetal growth. *Obstet. Gynecol.*, **77**, 893–6

112. Robinson, H. P. and Fleming, J. E. F. (1973). A critical evaluation of sonar 'crown-rump-length' measurements. *Br. J. Obstet. Gynaecol.*, **82**, 702–10

113. Shepard, M. J., Richards, V. A., Berkowitz, R. L., Warsof, S. L. and Hobbins, J. C. (1982). An evaluation of two equations for predicting fetal weight by ultrasound. *Am. J. Obstet. Gynecol.*, **142**, 47–54

114. Johnson, M. L. and Dunne, M. C. (1980). Evaluation of fetal intracranial anatomy by static and real-time ultrasound. *J. Clin. Ultrasound*, **8**, 311–18

115. Varma, T. R., Taylor, H. and Bridges, C. (1979). Ultrasound assessment of fetal growth. *Br. J. Obstet. Gynaecol.*, **86**, 623–9

116. Campbell, S. (1970). Ultrasonic fetal cephalometry during the second trimester of pregnancy. *Br. J. Obstet. Gynaecol.*, **77**, 1057–62

117. Campbell, S. and Dewhurst, C. J. (1971). Diagnosis of the small-for-dates fetus by serial ultrasound cephalometry. *Lancet*, **2**, 1002–6

118. Seeds, J. W. (1984). Impaired fetal growth: ultrasonic evaluation and clinical management. *Obstet. Gynecol.*, **63**, 577–82

119. Rosendahl, H. and Kivinen, S. (1988). Routine ultrasound screening for early detection of small for gestational age fetuses. *Obstet. Gynecol.*, **71**, 518–21

120. Arias, F. (1977). The diagnosis and management of intauterine growth retardation. *Obstet. Gynecol.*, **49**, 293–8

121. Kurjak, A., Kirkinen, P. and Latin, U. (1980). Biometric and dynamic ultrasound assessment of small-for-dates infants: report of 260 cases. *Obstet. Gynecol.*, **56**, 281–4

122. Sabbagha, R., Hughey, M. and Depp, R. (1978). Growth adjusted sonographic age. A simplified method. *Obstet. Gynecol.*, **51**, 383–6

123. Macler, J., Rosenthal, C., Burgun, P. and Renaud, R. (1977). The interest of the echographic measurement of the transversal abdominal diameter in the poor intrauterine fetal growth. In Salvadori, B. and Bacchi-Modena, A. (eds.) *Poor Intrauterine Fetal Growth*, p.283–5. (Parma, Italy: Minerva Médica)

124. Jeanty, P., Coussaert, E. and Contraine, F. (1984). Normal growth of the abdominal perimeter. *Am. J. Perinatol.*, **1**, 129–35

125. Wittman, B. K., Robinson, H. P., Aitchison, T. and Fleming, J. E. *et al.* (1979). The value of diagnostic ultrasound as a screening test for intrauterine growth retardation. Comparison of nine parameters. *Am. J. Obstet. Gynecol.*, **134**, 30–5

126. O'Brien, G. and Queenan, J. J. (1981). Growth of the ultrasound fetal femur length during normal pregnancy. *Am. J. Obstet. Gynecol.*, **141**, 833–7

127. Hadlock, F. P., Deter, R. L., Harrist, R. B., Roecker, E. and Park, S. K. (1983). A date-independent predictor of intrauterine growth retardation: femur length/abdominal circumference ratio. *Am. J. Roentgenol.*, **141**, 979–84

128. Benson, C. B., Doubilet, P. M., Saltzman, D. H. and Jones, T. B. (1985). FL/AC ratio: poor predictor of intrauterine growth retardation. *Invest. Radiol.*, **20**, 727–30

129. Gohari, P., Berkowitz, R. L. and Hobbins, J. C. (1977). Prediction of intrauterine growth retardation by determination of total intrauterine growth. *Am. J. Obstet. Gynecol.*, **127**, 255–60

130. Geirsson, R. T., Patel, N. B. and Christie, A. D. (1985). Efficiency of intrauterine volume, fetal abdominal area and biparietal diameter measurements with ultrasound in screening for small-for-dates basis. *Br. J. Obstet. Gynaecol.*, **92**, 929–35

131. Geirsson, R. T., Patel, N. B. and Christie, A. D. (1985). Intrauterine volume, fetal abdominal area and biparietal diameter measurements with ultrasound in the prediction of small-for-dates babies in a high-risk obstetric population. *Br. J. Obstet. Gynaecol.*, **92**, 936–40

132. Kurjak, A. and Breyer, B. (1977). Estimation of fetal weight by ultrasonic abdominometry. *Am. J. Obstet. Gynecol.*, **125**, 962–5

133. Campbell, S., Wladimiroff, J. W. and Dewhurst, C. J. (1973). The antenatal measurement of fetal urine production. *Br. J. Obstet. Gynaecol.*, **80**, 680–6
134. Wladimiroff, J. and Campbell, S. (1974). Fetal urine production rates in normal and complicated pregnancy. *Lancet*, **1**, 151–4
135. Vintzileos, A. M., Campbell, W. A., Nochimson, D. J. and Weinbaum, P. J. (1987). The use and misuse of fetal biophysical profile. *Am. J. Obstet. Gynecol.*, **156**, 527–33
136. Vintzileos, A. M., Campbell, W. A., Feinstein, S. J., Lodeiro, J. G., Weinbaum, P. J. and Nochimson, D. J. (1987). The fetal biophysical profile in pregnancies with grade III placentas. *Am. J. Perinatol.*, **4**, 90–3
137. Ribbert, I. S. M., Snijders, R. J. M., Nicolaides, K. H. and Visser, G. H. A. (1990). Relationship of fetal biophysical profile and blood gas values at cordocentesis in severely growth retarded fetuses. *Am. J. Obstet. Gynecol.*, **163**, 569–71
138. Sival, D. A., Visser, G. H. A. and Preechtl, H. F. R. (1992). The effect of intrauterine growth retardation on the quality of general movements in the human fetus. *Early Hum. Dev.*, **28**, 119–32
139. Fisher, C. and Garret, W. (1976). Placental aging monitored by scale echography. *Am. J. Obstet. Gynecol.*, **124**, 483–8
140. Haney, A. F. and Trought, W. S. (1979). The sonolucent placenta in high risk obstetrics. *Obstet. Gynecol.*, **55**, 38–41
141. Catizone, F. A. (1981). Modelli ecografici di maturazione placentare. In Borruto, F. (ed.) *Ultrasonografia Ostetrica*. (Verona: Libreria Cortina)
142. Grannum, P. A. T., Berkowitz, R. L. and Hobbins, J. C. (1979). The ultrasonic changes in the maturing placenta and their relation to fetal pulmonic maturity. *Am. J. Obstet. Gynecol.*, **133**, 915–22
143. Kazzi, G. M., Gross, T. L., Sokil, R. J. and Kazzi, N. J. (1983). Detection of intrauterine growth retardation – a new use for sonographic placental grading. *Am. J. Obstet. Gynecol.*, **145**, 733–7
144. Flynn, A. M., Kelly, J. and O'Connor, M. (1979). Unstressed antepartum cardiotocography in the management of the foetus suspected of growth retardation. *Br. J. Obstet. Gynaecol.*, **86**, 106–10
145. Carrera, J. M. (1982). Intrauterine growth retardation. Ultrasonic and cardiotocographic assessments. In Borruto, F., Hansmann, M. and Wladimiroff, J. W. (eds.) *Fetal Ultrasonography*. (Chichester: John Wiley and Sons)
146. Pazos, R., Voulok, K., Aladjem, S., Lueck, J. and Anderson, C. (1982). Association of spontaneous fetal heart decelerations during antepartum nonstress testing and intrauterine growth retardation. *Am. J. Obstet. Gynecol.*, **144**, 574–7
147. Smith, C. V. and Phelan, J. P. (1988). Antepartum fetal heart rate testing of the small-for-gestational age fetus. *Semin. Perinatol.*, **12**, 52–6
148. Snijders, R. J. M., Ribbert, I. S. M., Visser, G. H. A. and Mulder, E. J. H. (1992). Numeric analysis of heart rate variation in intrauterine growth retarded fetuses. *Am. J. Obstet. Gynecol.*, **166**, 22–7
149. Bekedam, D. J., Visser, G. H. A., Mulder, E. J. H. and Poelmann Weejes, G. (1987). Heart rate variation and movement incidence in growth retarded fetuses: the significance of antenatal late heart rate deceleration. *Am. J. Obstet. Gynecol.*, **157**, 126–33
150. Visser, G. H. A., Sadovsky, G. and Nicolaides, K. H. (1990). Antepartum heart rate patterns in small-for-gestational age third trimester fetuses correlations with blood gas values obtained at cordocentesis. *Am. J. Obstet. Gynecol.*, **162**, 698–703
151. Henson, G. L., Dawes, G. S. and Redman, C. W. G. (1983). Antenatal fetal heart variability in relation to fetal acid–base status at caesarean section. *Br. J. Obstet. Gynaecol.*, **90**, 516–21
152. Bekedam, D. J. and Visser, G. H. A. (1985). Effects of hypoxemia events on breathing, body movements and heart rate variation. A study in growth retarded human fetuses. *Am. J. Obstet. Gynecol.*, **153**, 52–6
153. Slomka, C. V. and Phelan, J. P. (1981). Pregnancy outcome in the patient with a nonreactive nonstress test and a positive contraction stress test. *Am. J. Obstet. Gynecol.*, **139**, 11–15
154. Carrera, J. M., Alegre, M. and Torrents, M. (1987). La fluxometría Doppler transplancentaria en los estados hipertensivos del embarazo. In Stopelli, I. (ed.) *Gestosi 87*, pp. 89–94. (Rome: CIC Edizioni Internationali)
155. Reed, K. L., Anderson, C. F. and Shenker, L. (1987). Changes in intracardiac Doppler flow velocities in fetuses with absent umbilical artery diastolic flow. *Am. J. Obstet. Gynecol.*, **157**, 774–9
156. Burke, G., Stuart, B., Crowley, P., Scanaill, S. N. and Drumm, J. I. (1990). Intrauterine growth

retardation with normal umbilical artery blood flow a benign condition? *Br. Med. J.*, **300**, 1044–5

157. Ng, A. and Trudinger, B. (1992). The application of umbilical artery studies to complicated pregnancies. In Malcolm Pearce, J. (ed.) *Doppler Ultrasound in Perinatal Medicine*, pp.142–58 (Oxford: Oxford University Press)

158. Berkowitz, G. S., Mehalek, K. E., Chitkara, U., Rosenberg, J., Cogswell, C. and Berkowitz, R. L. (1988). Doppler umbilical velocimetry in prediction of adverse outcome in pregnancies at risk of intrauterine growth retardation. *Obstet. Gynecol.*, **71**, 742–6

159. Gaziano, E., Know, E., Wager, G. P., Bendel, R. P., Boyce, D. J. and Olson, J. (1988). The predictability of the small-for-gestational age infant by real time ultrasound derived measurements combined with pulsed Doppler umbilical artery velocimetry. *Am. J. Obstet. Gynecol.*, **158**, 1431–9

160. Chambers, S. E., Hoskins, P. R., Haddad, N. G., Johnstone, F. D., McDicken, W. N. and Muir, B. B. (1989). A comparison of fetal abdominal circumference measurements and Doppler ultrasound in the prediction of small-for-dates and fetal compromise. *Br. J. Obstet. Gynaecol.*, **96**, 803–8

161. Divon, M. Y., Girz, B. A., Bieblich, R. and Lauger, O. (1989). Clinical management of the fetus with markedly diminished umbilical artery end-diastolic flow. *Am. J. Obstet. Gynecol.*, **161**, 1523–7

162. Fleischer, A., Schulman, H., Farmakides, G., Bracero, L., Blattner, P. and Randolph, G. (1985). Umbilical artery velocity waveforms and intrauterine growth retardation. *Am. J. Obstet. Gynecol.*, **151**, 502–5

163. Laurin, J., Marsal, K., Persson, P. H. and Lingman, G. (1987). Ultrasound measurement of fetal blood in predicting fetal outcome. *Br. J. Obstet. Gynaecol.*, **94**, 940–8

164. Laurin, J., Lingman, G., Marsal, K. and Persson, P. H. (1987). Fetal blood flow in pregnancies complicated by intrauterine growth retardation. *Obstet. Gynecol.*, **69**, 895–902

165. Reuwer, P. J. H., Sijmons, E. A., Rietman, G. W., Van-Tiel, M. W. and Bruinse, H. W. (1987). Intrauterine growth retardation: prediction of perinatal distress by Doppler ultrasound. *Lancet*, **2**, 415–18

166. Dempster, J., Mieres, G. J., Patel, N. and Taylor, D. J. (1989). Umbilical artery velocity waveforms poor association with small-for-gestational age babies. *Br. J. Obstet. Gynaecol.*, **96**, 692–6

167. Lowery, C. L., Henso, B., Wan, I. and Brumfield, G. (1990). A comparison between umbilical velocimetry and standard antepartum surveillance in hospitalized high-risk patients. *Am. J. Obstet. Gynecol.*, **162**, 710–14

168. Maulik, D., Yarlagada, P., Younblood, J. P. and Ciston, P. (1990). The diagnostic efficacy of the umbilical arterial tool: a prospective blinded study. *Am. J. Obstet. Gynecol.*, **162**, 1518–25

169. Carrera, J. M., Mallafre, J., Torrents, M., Carreras, E., Salvador, M. J. and Alegre, M. (1990). Perfil biofísico progresivo. *Prog. Obstet. Ginecol.*, **33**, 89–104

170. Aickin, D. R., Smith, M. A. and Brown, J. B. (1974). Comparison between plasma and urinary oestrogen measurements in predicting fetal risk. *Aust. NZ J. Obstet. Gynecol.*, **14**, 59–76

171. Masson, G. M. (1973). Plasma oestriol in retarded intrauterine growth. *J. Obstet. Gynaecol. Br. Commonw.*, **80**, 423–8

172. Spellacy, W. N., Teoh, E. S., Buhi, W. C., Birk, S. A. and McCreary, S. A. (1971). Value of HCS in managing high-risk pregnancies. *Am. J. Obstet. Gynecol.*, **109**, 588–98

173. Letchworth, A. T. and Chard, T. (1972). HPL levels in preeclampsia. *J. Obstet. Gynaecol. Br. Commonw.*, **76**, 680–3

174. Rudolph, A. M. and Heymann, M. A. (1967). The circulation of the fetus '*in utero*'. Methods for studying distribution of blood flow, cardiac output and organ blood flow. *Circ. Res.*, **21**, 163–7

175. Reuss, M. L., Rudolph, A. M. and Heymann, M. A. (1981). Selective distribution of microspheres injected into the umbilical veins and inferior vena cava of fetal sheep. *Am. J. Obstet. Gynecol.*, **141**, 427–33

176. Behrman, R. E., Lees, M. H., Peterson, E. N., De Lannoy, C. W. and Seed, A. E. (1970). Distribution of the circulation in the normal and asphyxiated fetal primate. *Am. J. Obstet. Gynecol.*, **108**, 956–69

177. Morrow, R. J., Adamson, S. L., Bull, S. B. and Ritchie, J. W. K. (1990). Hypoxia acidemia, hyperviscosity and maternal hypertension do not affect the umbilical artery velocity waveforms in fetal sheep. *Am. J. Obstet. Gynecol.*, **163**, 1313–20

178. Trudinger, B. J. (1991). Doppler ultrasound study and fetal abnormality. In Drife, J. O. and Donnan, D. (eds.) *Antenatal Diagnosis of Fetal Abnormalities*, p. 113. (London: Springer-Verlag)

179. Gruenwald, P. (1975). The relation of deprivation to perinatal pathology and late sequels. In Gruenwald, P. (ed.) *The Placenta*. (Lancaster: Medical, Technical Publishing Co.)
180. Montenegro, C. A. B., Meirelles, J., Fonseca, A. L. A., Netto, H. C., Amin-Junior, J., Rezende-Filho, J. and Jacyntho, C. (1992). Cordocentèse et evaluation du bien-être foetal dans une population à très hant risque. *Rev. Fr. Gynecol. Obstet.*, **87**, 467–77
181. Giorlandino, C. A. and Vizzone, A. (1993). *Flussimetria Ostetrica Materna e Fetale*. (Rome: CIC Edizione Int.)
182. Morrow, R. J., Adamson, L., Richie, K. and Pearce, M. (1992). The pathophysiological basis of abnormal flow velocity waveforms. In Pearce, J. M. (ed.) *Doppler Ultrasound in Perinatal Medicine*. (Oxford: Oxford University Press)
183. De Haan, J. (1992). Fisipatología de los cambios en los índices de fluojo Doppler en la circulación fetal. In Carrera, J. M. (ed.) *Doppler en Obstetricia*. (Barcelona: Masson-Salvat)
184. Dawes, G. S., Duncan, S. L., Lewis, B. V., Merlet, C. L., Owen-Thomas, T. B. and Reeves, J. T. (1969). Cyanide stimulation of the systemic arterial chemoreceptors in foetal lambs. *J. Physiol.*, **201**, 1171–21
185. De Vore, G. R. (1988). Examination of the fetal heart in the fetus with intrauterine growth retardation using M-mode echocardiography. *Semin. Perinatol.*, **12**, 66–79
186. Lingman, G., Legarth, J., Rahman, F. and Stangenberg, M. (1991). Myocardial contracility in the anaemic human fetus. *Ultrasound Obstet. Gynecol.*, **1**, 266–8
187. Marsal, K., Lindblad, A., Lingman, G. and Eik-Nes, S. H. (1984). Blood flow in the fetal descending aorta: intrinsic factors affecting fetal blood flow i.e. fetal breathing movements and fetal cardiac arrhythmia. *Ultrasound Med. Biol.*, **10**, 339–48
188. Arabin, B., Bergmann, P. L. and Saling, E. (1987). Simultaneous assessment of blood flow velocity waveforms in uteroplacental vessels, the umbilical artery, the fetal aorta and the common carotid artery. *Fetal Therap.*, **2**, 17–26
189. Arabin, B., Siebert, M., Jimenez, E. and Saling, E. (1987). Obstetrical characteristic of a loss of end-diastolic velocities in the fetal aorta and/or umbilical artery using Doppler ultrasound. *Gynecol. Obstet. Invest.*, **25**, 173–80
190. Bilardo, C. M., Campbell, S. and Nicolaides, K. H. (1988). Mean blood velocity and flow impedance in the fetal descending thoracic aorta and common carotid artery in normal pregnancy. *Early Hum. Dev.*, **18**, 213–7
191. Gramellini, P., Folli, M. C., Raboni, S., Vadona, E. and Merialdi, A. (1992). Cerebral–umbilical Doppler ratio as a predictor of adverse perinatal outcome. *Obstet. Gynecol.*, **79**, 416–20
192. Indik, J. H., Chen, V. and Reed, K. L. (1991). Association of umbilical venous with inferior vena cava blood flow velocities. *Obstet. Gynecol.*, **77**, 551–7
193. Reed, K. L. (1992). Venous flow velocities in the fetus. In Jaffe, R. and Warson, S. L. (eds.) *Color Doppler Imaging in Obstetrics and Gynecology*, p. 179. (New York: McGraw-Hill)
194. Rizzo, G., Arduini, D. and Romanini, C. (1992). Inferior vena cava flow velocity waveforms in appropriate and small-for-gestational-age fetuses. *Am. J. Obstet. Gynecol.*, **166**, 1271–80
195. Van Uliet, M. A. T., Martin, C. B., Nijhuis, J. G. and Prechtl, H. F. R. (1985). Behavioural states in growth retarded human fetuses. *Early Hum. Dev.*, **12**, 183–98
196. Arduini, D., Rizzo, G., Romanini, C. and Mancuso, S. (1989). Are blood flow velocity waveforms related to umbilical cord acid–base status in the human fetus? *Gynecol. Obstet. Invest.*, **27**, 183–7
197. Bekedam, D. J., Mulder, E. J. H., Snijders, R. J. M. and Visser, G. H. A. (1991). The effects of a maternal hyperoxia on fetal breathing movements, body movements and heart rate variation in growth retarded fetuses. *Early Hum. Dev.*, **27**, 223–32
198. Arduini, D., Rizzo, G. and Romanini, C. (1992). Changes of pulsatility index from fetal vessels preceding the onset of late decelerations in growth-retarded fetuses. *Obstet. Gynecol.*, **79**, 605–10
199. Griffin, D. R., Bilardo, K., Diaz-Recasens, J., Pearce, J. M., Wilson, K. and Campbell, S. (1984). Doppler blood flow waveforms in the descending thoracic aorta of the human fetus. *Br. J. Obstet. Gynaecol.*, **91**, 997–1002
200. Phelan, J. P., Smith, C. V., Broussard, P. and Small, M. (1987). Amniotic fluid volume assessment with the four-quadrant technique at 36–42 weeks' gestation. *J. Reprod. Med.*, **32**, 540–2
201. Nicolaides, K. H., Bilardo, C. M., Soothill, P. W. and Campbell, S. (1987). Absence of end-diastolic frequencies in the umbilical artery: a sign of fetal hypoxia and acidosis. *Br. Med. J.*, **297**, 1026–7

202. Nicolaides, K. H., Bilardo, C. M. and Campbell, S. (1990). Prediction of fetal anaemia by measurement of mean blood velocity in the fetal aorta. *Am. J. Obstet. Gynecol.*, **162**, 209–12
203. Ferrazi, E., Pardi, G., Bauscaglia, M., Marconi, A. M., Gementi, B., Bellotti, M., Makowski, E. L. and Battaglia, F. C. (1988). The correlation of biochemical monitoring versus umbilical flow velocity measurements of the human fetus. *Am. J. Obstet. Gynecol.*, **159**, 1081–7
204. Tyrrell, S., Obais, A. H. and Lilford, R. J. (1989). Umbilical artery Doppler velocimetry as a predictor of fetal hypoxia and acidosis at birth. *Obstet. Gynecol.*, **74**, 332–7
205. Bilardo, C. M., Nicolaides, K. H. and Campbell, S. (1990). Doppler measurement of fetal and uteroplacental circulation: relationship with umbilical venous blood gases measured at cordocentesis. *Am. J. Obstet. Gynecol.*, **162**, 115–9
206. Vyas, S., Nicolaides, K. H., Bower, S. and Campbell, S. (1990). Middle cerebral artery flow velocity waveforms in fetal hypoxemia. *Br. J. Obstet. Gynaecol.*, **97**, 797–803
207. Marsal, K., Nicolaides, K. H., Kaminpetros, P. and Hackett, G. (1992). The clinical value of waveforms from the descending aorta. In Pearce, J. M. (ed.) *Doppler Ultrasound in Perinatal Medicine*. (Oxford: Oxford University Press)
208. Hackett, G. A., Campbell, S., Gamsu, H., Cohen-Overbeek, T. and Pearce, J. M. F. (1987). Doppler studies in the growth retarded fetus and prediction of neonatal necrotising enterocolitis, haemorrhage and neonatal morbidity. *Br. Med. J.*, **294**, 13–16
209. Myers, R. E., De Courtney-Myers, G. M. and Wagner, K. R. (1984). Effects of hypoxia on fetal brain. In Beard, R. W. and Nathanielsz, P. W. (eds.) *Fetal Physiology and Medicine*, p. 419. (London: Butterworth)
210. Richardson, B. S., Rurak, D., Patrick, I. E., Homan, J. and Carmichael, I. (1989). Cerebral oxidative metabolism during sustained hypoxaemia in fetal sheep. *J. Dev. Physiol.*, **2**, 37–43
211. Vyas, S. (1992). Pulsed Doppler examination of the normal human fetus. In Pearce, J. M. (ed.) *Doppler Ultrasound in Perinatal Medicine*. (Oxford: Oxford University Press)
212. Mari, G. and Wasserstrum, N. (1991). Flow velocity waveforms of the fetal circulation preceding fetal death in a case of lupus anticoagulant. *Am. J. Obstet. Gynecol.*, **164**, 776–8
213. Adams, R. D., Prod'hom, L. S. and Rabinowicz, T. H. (1977). Intrauterine brain death. *Acta Neuropathol.*, **40**, 419–9
214. Gaziano, E. P. and Freeman, D. W. (1977). Analysis of heart rate patterns preceding fetal death. *Obstet. Gynecol.*, **50**, 578–82
215. Van der Moer, P. E., Gerretsen, G. and Visser, G. H. A. (1985). Fixed fetal heart rate pattern after intrauterine accidental deceleration. *Obstet. Gynecol.*, **65**, 125–7
216. Nijhuis, J. G., Kruyt, N., Van Vijck, J. A. M. (1988). Fetal brain death. Two case reports. *Br. J. Obstet. Gynaecol.*, **85**, 197–200
217. Zimmer, E. Z., Jakobi, P., Goldstein, I. and Gutterman, E. (1992). Cardiotocographic and sonographic findings in two cases of antenatally diagnosed intrauterine fetal brain death. *Prenat. Diagn.*, **12**, 271–6
218. Ellis, W. G., Goetzman, B. W. and Lindenberg, J. A. (1988). Neuropathologic documentation of prenatal brain damage. *Am. J. Dis. Child.*, **142**, 858–66
219. Nwaesei, C. G., Pape, K. E., Martin, D. J., Becker, L. E. and Fitz, C. R. (1984). Periventricular infarction diagnosed by ultrasound: a postmortem correlation. *J. Pediatr.*, **105**, 106–10
220. Larroche, J. C. L., Droulle, P., Delezoide, A. L., Narey, F. and Nessmann, C. (1990). Brain damage in monozygous twins. *Biol. Neonat.*, **57**, 261–78
221. Visser, G. H. A. (1988). Abnormal antepartum fetal heart rate patterns and subsequent handicap. In Patel, N. (ed.) *Antenatal and Perinatal Causes of Handicap*, pp. 117–24. (London: Baillière's Clinical Obstetrics and Gynaecology)
222. Favre, R., Nissano, J. and Messer, G. (1991). Velocimetric sylvienne foetale. Critère de'extraction dans l'hypotrophic sévere. *J. Gynecol. Obstet. Biol. Reprod.*, **20**, 699–706

Computerized analysis of fetal heart rate in normal and growth-retarded fetuses

D. Arduini, G. Rizzo and C. Romanini

INTRODUCTION

Monitoring of fetal heart rate (FHR) is widely used in the monitoring of high-risk fetuses. However, its efficacy in improving perinatal outcome has been consistently questioned[1-3]. One major problem in assessing the diagnostic efficacy of this technique is the subjective nature of the evaluation, and several studies have shown poor intra-observer and inter-observer agreement[4-6]. Furthermore, fetal behavioral states greatly influence the characteristics of FHR patterns and they must be recognized and taken into account in the identification of fetal distress[7,8].

To reduce the problem, different automatic systems for analysis for FHR have been developed. However, limitations in the identification of the FHR baseline as well as lack of consideration of fetal behavior have recently been underlined in such systems.

In this chapter we describe a new computerized system (2CTG®, Hewlett Packard, Italy) that we developed for the fully automated and on-line analysis of FHR[9] as well as the changes in FHR occurring in normal fetuses and those with intrauterine growth retardation (IUGR).

DESCRIPTION OF THE SYSTEM

Hardware

FHR, uterine contractions and fetal movements were recorded by means of a commercially available fetal monitor (Hewlett Packard 8040A) equipped with a wide-range ultrasound transducer, a transabdominal tocodynamometer and a button activated by patients to identify fetal movements. The system of analysis was based on a 386 Personal Computer with an Intel 80386X processor running at 20 MHz (Hewlett Packard Vectra 386/20N). The configuration included 3 Mb of RAM and 50 Mb of hard disk. The operating system was MS-DOS 6.0 with MS-Windows 3.1 to provide an interface with the user including windows, icons, mouse and pointer.

The system employed priority interrupts every 100 ms from the central processor unit to address the fetal monitor via its RS232 port to acquire the current data on FHR (i.e. pulse interval), the autocorrelation function (i.e. quality of signal), the tocodynamometer value and fetal movements. The signals captured were displayed graphically in a dedicated window of the computer screen and stored on the hard disk. The quality of the signal was continuously evaluated and the percentage of signal loss of FHR, as determined by the autocorrelation function, was continuously provided on the computer screen.

Software

After the first 10 min of recording, the FHR baseline was fitted and accelerations, decelerations and FHR variability indices were calculated. Furthermore, uterine contractions were identified and analyzed. These parameters were reanalyzed every 5 min thereafter until the end of the recording. The procedures of analysis were the following:

Baseline determination

As the procedure described by Mantel and colleagues[10], resulting from a comparative trial, produced an algorithm better fitting the baseline, we followed this method for baseline determination. However, as this algorithm was originally described for off-line analysis taking 2 h, we implemented a real-time version. After 10 min of recording, the fetal heart pulse intervals were averaged over 2.5-s periods. A frequency distribution was obtained and the starting point was calculated on the basis of the first prominent peak near the high end of the frequency distribution, using a previously described algorithm[11]. The value of the starting point was then used as a guide for baseline calculation, based on a low pass filter with a time constant of 0.1/min and a trim function interacting in a five-run iterative process. Only the first 5 min of the resulting baseline was considered valid; the remainder was discarded. This selection was made in an attempt to minimize the border-effect errors that may result from the procedure of filtering used. After 5 more minutes (15 from the beginning of the acquisition), the computation window was shifted 5 min forward and the baseline was recalculated on the next 10 min using, as a starting point, the last valid value of the previously calculated baseline and similarly discarding at the end of the calculation the last 5 min. The procedure was repeated every 5 min until the recording stopped.

The selection of the 10-min window shifted every 5 min was the result of a compromise between theoretical considerations on the time constant of the low-pass filter (requiring a sufficiently long period of acquisition to have negligible border errors) and the clinical usefulness of frequent reanalysis of the data required.

Accelerations and decelerations

Accelerations and decelerations are defined as deviations from the baseline with a certain amplitude and duration. Accelerations were defined as periods longer than 15 s with an amplitude of > 15 bpm (large accelerations) or of > 10 bpm (small accelerations) above the baseline. A detection threshold of 5 bpm was used from the baseline for the determination of the duration to prevent small elevations of the baseline from being designated as accelerations. The detection of decelerations was performed similarly. Decelerations were considered as periods with an amplitude of > 20 bpm below the baseline and lasting for > 30 s, or as periods with an amplitude of > 10 bpm and lasting for > 60 s. For each deceleration the nadir, duration and area under the baseline was calculated and expressed. The temporal association with a uterine contraction (if present) was evaluated and the time interval between the onset of the contraction and the onset of the deceleration was recorded.

Analysis of FHR variability

Variability was calculated after exclusion of all the decelerations and large accelerations. For each minute the amplitude band-width around the baseline (delta) was then calculated as the difference between the maximum and minimum value of the FHR and expressed in beats per minute and milliseconds. Long-term variability was evaluated by means of the long-term irregularity index (LTI)[12]. Short-term variability was calculated every 60 s with two different indices: the short-term variation (STV) as the average of successive 2.5-s pulse interval differences (period-to-period variation)[13] and the interval index (II), calculated as the coefficient of variation (SD/mean) of the difference between averaged pulse intervals of consecutive 2.5-s periods[14].

Analysis of uterine contraction

The resulting tone (baseline of uterine activity) was calculated following the same method used for the FHR baseline. A contraction was defined as an increase from the resting tone lasting more than 30 s and exceeding a value of 25% from the basal value.

example of a FHR monitoring report is provided in Figure 2.

ASSESSMENT OF REPRODUCIBILITY

From the third-trimester high-risk patients attending our antepartum testing unit, we selected 34 FHR tracings lasting 25 min[6]. The FHR was recorded by means of a Hewlett Packard 8040a fetal monitor in a standard fashion and was simultaneously analyzed by the 2CTG computerized system. Tracings were independently assessed by ten experienced observers. All the experts were faculty members of the fetomaternal unit, unaware of the analysis of the computerized system. Clinical details of the patients were not provided, with the exception of gestational age. The experts were asked to define for each tracing the following variables:

(1) Baseline value categorized with values of 5 bpm;

(2) Delta expressed as the mean band-width around the baseline (expressed in beats per minute) over periods without accelerations or decelerations;

(3) Variability classified subjectively into four classes: normal, increased, reduced or silent;

(4) Accelerations defined as deviations from the baseline lasting for > 15 s and with an amplitude of > 15 bpm. The experts were asked to provide the total number of accelerations in the tracing and to draw an arrow on each acceleration identified; and

(5) Decelerations. Similarly to accelerations, the experts were asked to indicate the number and the position on the tracing of the decelerations. Additionally, each deceleration was defined as early, variable, late or unclassifiable.

Data obtained from the experts' analysis were tested for inter-observer variability by kappa-coefficient determination. For the FHR parameters showing an acceptable inter-observer variability (i.e. kappa > 0.40), a comparison with the computer interpretation was performed[16]. A

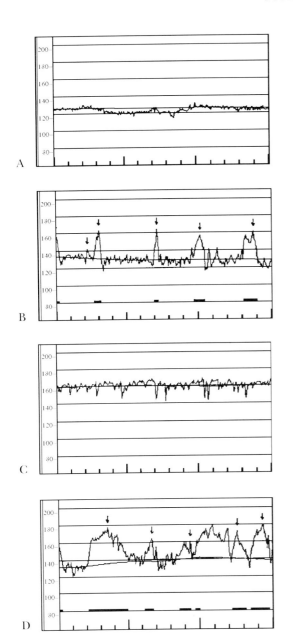

Figure 1 *Example of the four patterns of fetal heart rate defined according to Nijhuis[15] and automatically recognized by the system*

Identification of FHR patterns

At the end of the recording (off-line) the system reanalyzed the FHR data using a 3-min moving window shifted every 1 min. Following Nijhuis and associates[15], every 3-min period was classified into its pattern A–D. (Figure 1). An

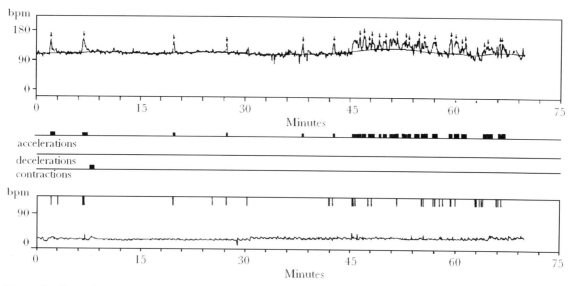

Figure 2 *Example of analysis of fetal heart rate, fetal movements and uterine activity of a normal fetus at 38 weeks by the computerized system*

conventional regression analysis was first performed between the mean value obtained for each parameter by the experts and by the computer. However, as correlation is not a measure of agreement, we also applied the procedure of Bland and Altman[17].

Accelerations and decelerations were present in 91% (31/34) and in 35% (12/34) of the tracings, respectively, as judged by at least of one expert or by the computer.

The agreement between experts was fair to good as judged by a kappa value of > 0.40 for the baseline determination (κ = 0.54), number of accelerations (κ = 0.42) and of decelerations (κ = 0.46). A poor agreement between experts (κ < 0.40) was shown for the delta value (κ = 0.27), variability (κ = 0.16) and classification of the type of accelerations (κ = 0.22) (Figure 3).

The relationship between the results of FHR analysis by the experts and by computer was calculated for the parameters showing acceptable inter-observer variability (i.e. baseline and number of accelerations and decelerations). A highly significant relationship was shown for all three parameters. The upper and lower limits of agreement for the FHR baseline were 5.14 bpm and –5.10 bpm, respectively (mean difference 0.02, SD 2.56). The upper and lower limits for

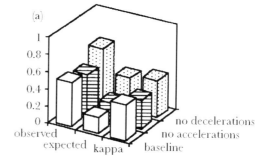
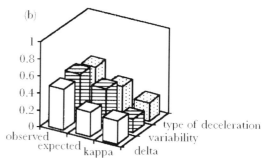

Figure 3 *Observed agreement, expected agreement by chance, and kappa value calculated from expert interpretations. Data are grouped for kappa values of > 0.40 (a) and < 0.40 (b) (from Arduini and colleagues[6], reproduced with permission of Springer-Verlag, New York)*

the number of accelerations were 1.06 and –0.98 (mean difference 0.04, SD 0.52) and 0.51 and

−0.65 and for the number of decelerations (mean difference −0.07, SD 0.29). All these limits are compatible with the clinical use of these parameters.

NORMAL RANGES DURING THE THIRD TRIMESTER

A total of 169 FHR recordings lasting more than 1 h cross-sectionally obtained at gestational ages from 31 to 42 weeks of gestation were selected to construct reference limits for gestation of the indices analyzed, taking into account the presence of different FHR patterns. After informed consent was acquired, these recordings were obtained from uncomplicated pregnancies of women recruited from our routine antenatal clinic and followed until delivery. Gestational age at delivery was 40.8 ± 1.67 weeks and birth weight was 3476 ± 342 g. None of the newborns showed complications.

A slight but significant decrease of the FHR baseline with gestation was found in the gestational period considered (constant = 161.54; slope = −0.63; residual SD = 8.93; $r = 0.161$; $p \leq 0.05$) associated with an increase in the number of large accelerations/h (constant = −6.57; slope = 0.58; residual SD = 7.42; $r = 0.177$; $p \leq 0.03$). The absolute number of small accelerations did not vary significantly with gestation ($r = 0.083$; mean = 5.89; SD = 3.44) while the ratio of small accelerations to the total number significantly decreased (constant = 72.72; slope = −1.18; residual SD = 17.16; $r = 0.156$; $p \leq 0.05$). No significant changes with gestation were found for the delta value expressed in bpm ($r = 0.052$; mean = 14.93; SD = 2.69), the delta value expressed in ms ($r = 0.035$; mean = 42.13; SD = 9.99), the LTI ($r = 0.078$; mean = 22.14; SD = 6.26), the STV ($r = 0.097$; mean = 7.69; SD = 2.25) and the II ($r = 0.083$; mean = 6.12; SD = 2.06).

FHR patterns A to D were recognized in 89.5% of the 3-min periods analyzed, while no specific patterns (unclassifiable patterns) were shown in the remaining periods. A slight but significant decrease of percentage of unclassifiable periods was shown with advancing gesta-

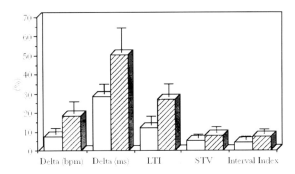

Figure 4 Differences of fetal heart rate (FHR) variability indices during FHR pattern A (white bars) and FHR pattern B (hatched bars). All differences were significant ($p \leq 0.001$). LTI, long-term irregularity index; STV, short-term variability

tion (constant = 34.68; slope = 0.73; residual SD = 4.12; $r = 0.123$; $p \leq 0.05$). The further analysis of FHR patterns was limited to patterns A and B, due to the low incidence of patterns C (3.7%) and D (5.2%). No significant changes were found in the gestational period considered in the incidence of FHR patterns A ($r = 0.123$; mean = 24.6%; SD 11.3%) and B ($r = 0.892$; mean = 56.0%; SD 21.4). The values of the indices of FHR variability are shown grouped according to FHR patterns A and B. Significantly lower values for all the parameters considered were found during FHR pattern A (Figure 4).

FHR INDICES IN IUGR

In order to assess the clinical efficacy of the newly constructed system in the identification of fetal acidosis, we considered 37 fetuses with IUGR in which FHR was recorded immediately before an elective Cesarean section due for maternal or fetal indications (Figure 5). Criteria of inclusion were the presence of Doppler signs of fetal blood-flow redistribution (i.e. ratio between umbilical artery and middle cerebral artery ≥ 95th centile of our reference limits for gestation[18], thus suggesting uteroplacental insufficiency as the more likely etiology) and the absence of structural or chromosomal abnormalities. At birth the umbilical cord was double-clamped and 1 ml of blood was withdrawn from the umbilical artery for pH determination. Acid-

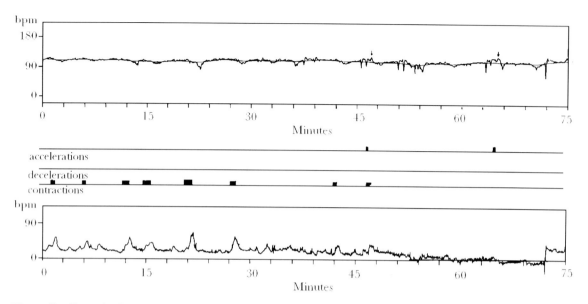

Figure 5 *Example of analysis of fetal heart rate in a fetus with intrauterine growth retardation at 33 weeks of gestation. Note the reduction of all the variability indices*

osis was considered in the presence of a value of < 7.210, corresponding to the lower 95% confidence limits of our reference values for umbilical artery pH obtained after a Cesarean section during the third trimester. The mean gestational age at birth was 33.9 ± 2.7 weeks and the mean birth weight 1245 ± 190 g. Acidosis was present in 15 cases (40.5%) while pH values above 7.210 were found in the remaining 22 newborns.

The number of large ($t = 3.56$; $p \leq 0.001$) as well as small decelerations ($t = 2.53$; $p \leq 0.05$) was significantly reduced in these fetuses when compared to the previously established reference limits. Similarly, delta values in beats per minute ($p \leq 0.01$) and in milliseconds ($p \leq 0.001$), LTI ($p \leq 0.01$), STV ($p \leq 0.05$) and II ($p \leq 0.05$) were significantly reduced with respect to normal fetuses. In 25 of the 37 fetuses with IUGR alternation between FHR patterns A and B was shown. Grouping together variability values for the respective FHR patterns allowed us to reach higher statistically significant difference for delta (bpm) ($p \leq 0.001$), LTI ($p \leq 0.001$), STV ($p \leq 0.01$) and II ($p \leq 0.01$). In Figure 5 the efficiency of the computerized indices in identifying acidosis are expressed in terms of specificity and sensitivity. Delta values

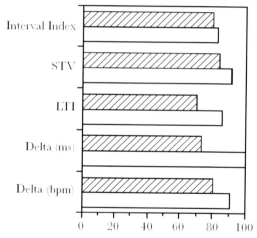

Figure 6 *Sensitivity (white bars) and specificity (hatched bars) of variability indices in predicting acidosis (i.e. umbilical artery pH < 7.210) at birth. STV, short-term variability; LTI, long-term irregularity index*

expressed in milliseconds showed the higher specificity (100%), since none of the fetuses with delta values within our reference limits for gestation showed acidosis at birth. Also, the STV showed higher sensitivity (91.6%) and all the cases except three with STV values below our reference limits showed acidosis at birth (Figure 6).

DISCUSSION

Our data show that the agreement between experts in the interpretation of FHR tracings is far from being optimal. This result is not surprising and confirms previous studies[4,5]. Of interest is the unacceptably low level of agreement obtained in the measurement of FHR band-width around the baseline, in FHR variability and in the classification of the type of decelerations, despite the importance usually attributed to these measurements, which are part of the more commonly used scoring systems[19-21]. This suggests a limited role for these parameters in the visual interpretation of FHR tracings, which may account for the discrepancies in the clinical management after the same tracings shown in previous experiences. On the other hand an acceptable level of agreement between experts was obtained for the determination of the baseline and of the number of accelerations and decelerations, suggesting that only these visual parameters should be used clinically and compared with different analytical techniques.

Comparison of baseline values and number of accelerations and decelerations between visual and computerized analysis is limited due to the nature of their definitions. Accelerations and decelerations are defined as deviations from the baseline, while the baseline itself is in fact an imaginary line corresponding to the mean level of the FHR in the absence of accelerations and decelerations. Because of the hypothetical nature of the baseline and its high interdependence on the definitions of accelerations and decelerations, there are no standards to verify the quality of the estimation.

The high r values found between the visual and computerized analysis of baseline and number of accelerations and decelerations suggest a close correlation between the two techniques. However, correlation does not provide a measure of agreement, and even a high coefficient of correlation may conceal a considerable lack of agreement[17]. We therefore applied a statistical method designed to compare two techniques when the true values are unknown[17]. This method is based on the calculation of the limits of agreement, which include more than 95% of the discrepancies between the measurements with two techniques of analysis for data normally distributed (as are those in this study). Provided that the variations in the measurements within the limits of agreement would not be clinically important, the two techniques may be used interchangeably. The limits of agreement established for the baseline (± 5 bpm), accelerations (± 1) and decelerations (± 0.5) are compatible with clinical purposes, suggesting that the computerized system may replace the visual analysis. In particular, the narrow limits found for decelerations must be pointed out, as their erroneous identification may be dangerous, inducing unnecessary obstetric interventions.

In this study we have shown the poor reproducibility of the visual interpretation of FHR variability based on the subjective estimation of the FHR variations around the baseline during periods without accelerations and decelerations. This implies a limited usefulness of this measure in clinical practice. Computerized analysis allows a numerical evaluation of FHR variability by applying mathematical formulas quantifying the short-term and long-term variations of FHR. The consistent recognition of the baseline and accelerations and decelerations performed by this computerized system supports the quality of the measurements of FHR variations. Similarly, the correct identification of decelerations allows an easy analysis with the computer of their morphology and latency from uterine contractions, resulting in a proper classification, which may overcome the disagreement found between the visual analyses of experts.

During the third trimester, changes in FHR variables occur. The slight decrease of the FHR baseline found in association with the increase in the absolute number and amplitude of FHR accelerations (as expressed by the ratio between the number of small accelerations and the total number) supports earlier reports showing that during the third trimester these parameters change with gestation[1,22]. On the other hand, the parameters describing FHR variability and the incidence of FHR patterns A and B remain unmodified during gestational age, considered to confirm previous observations[23,24].

Of interest are the profound differences of FHR variability values between FHR patterns A and B, with values that were highly significantly lower for all the indices calculated during FHR pattern A. This implies that the existence of FHR patterns should be considered in the evaluation of FHR variability, as values normal for FHR pattern A may be abnormal for FHR pattern B. Moreover, if the FHR variability is considered as a mean value over a fixed period of recording, the relative incidence of FHR pattern A on this time interval should be taken into account, as a high incidence of FHR pattern A would result in lower mean values of FHR variability indices. This concept has recently been validated by Mantel and co-workers[8] by showing that during fetal quiet sleep (corresponding to FHR pattern A) the FHR variability in 11 out of 16 healthy fetuses resulted in questionable or abnormal values when compared to normal reference limits. The importance of recognizing FHR patterns before evaluating FHR variability must therefore be pointed out.

In fetuses with IUGR all the variability indices are reduced and these differences are particularly evident when data are grouped according to FHR patterns. Of interest is that in the presence of normal delta values, acidosis was never shown at birth, while in the presence of abnormal STV values, acidosis was almost constantly present. If these data are confirmed on a larger population, it might be suggested that FHR indices may be used to give guidance on the time of delivery in fetuses with IUGR.

In conclusion, the computerized system developed for FHR analysis provides an estimation of the baseline and an identification of accelerations and decelerations that are interchangeable with the interpretation of experts. Furthermore, the reliable assessment of these parameters allows the performance of an objective and numerical analysis of FHR variability that may be useful in the monitoring of fetuses with IUGR. These measurements may improve the validity of conventional interpretation of FHR monitoring, by providing numerical indices that seem to be related to fetal acid–base status.

References

1. Lumley, J., Lester, A., Anderson, I., Renou, P. and Wood, C. (1983). A randomized trial of weekly cardiotocography in high risk obstetrics patients. *Br. J. Obstet. Gynaecol.*, **90**, 1018–26
2. Schneider, E. P., Hutson, J. M. and Petrie, R. H. (1988). An assessment of the first decade's experience with antepartum fetal heart rate testing. *Am. J. Perinatol.*, **5**, 134–41
3. Arduini, D. and Rizzo, G. (1993). New trends in fetal heart rate monitoring. *J. Matern. Fetal Invest.*, **3**, 153
4. Trimbos, J. B. and Keirse, M. J. N. C. (1978). Observer variability in assessment of antepartum cardiotocograms. *Br. J. Obstet. Gynecol.*, **85**, 900–6
5. Schneider, E., Schulman, H., Farmakides, G. and Paksima, S. (1991). Comparison of the interpretation of antepartum fetal heart rate tracings between a computer program and experts. *J. Matern. Fetal Invest.*, **1**, 205–8
6. Arduini, D., Rizzo, G., Giannini, F., Garzetti, G. G. and Romanini, C. (1993). Computerized analysis of fetal heart rate. II Comparison with the interpretation of experts. *J. Matern. Fetal Invest.*, **3**, 165–9
7. Visser, G. H. A., Goodman, J. D. S., Levine, D. H. and Dawes, G. S. (1982). Diurnal and other cyclic variations in human fetal heart rate near term. *Am. J. Obstet. Gynecol.*, **142**, 535–44
8. Mantel, R., Van Geijn, H. P., Ververs, I. A. P. and Copray, F. J. A. (1992). Automated analysis of near term antepartum fetal heart rate in relation to fetal behavioral states: the Sonicaid system 8000. *Am. J. Obstet. Gynecol.*, **165**, 57–65
9. Arduini, D., Rizzo, G., Piana, G., Bonalumi, A., Brambilla, P. and Romanini, C. (1993). Computerized analysis of fetal heart rate. I Description of the system (2CTG). *J. Matern. Fetal Invest.*, **3**, 159–64
10. Mantel, R., Van Geijn, H. P., Caron, F. J. M., Swartijes, J. M., van Worden, E. E. and Jongsma, H. W. (1990). Computer analysis of antepartum fetal heart rate: 1. Baseline determination. *Int. J. Biomed. Comput.*, **25**, 261–72

11. Dawes, G. S., Redman, C. W. G., Smith, J. H. (1985). Improvements in the registration and analysis of fetal heart rate records at the bedside. *Br. J. Obstet. Gynaecol.*, **92**, 317–25
12. De Haan, J. V., Bemmel, J. H. V., Versteeg, B., Veth, A. F. L., Stolte, F. L., Janssens, L. A. M. and Eskes, T. K. A. (1971). Quantitative evaluation of fetal heart rate patterns. I Processing methods. *Eur. J. Obstet. Gynecol.*, **3**, 95–102
13. Dalton, K. S., Dawes, G. S. and Patrick, J. E. (1977). Diurnal, respiratory and other rhythms of fetal heart rate in lambs. *Am. J. Obstet. Gynecol.*, **127**, 414–24
14. Yeh, S. S., Forsythe, A. and Hon, E. A. (1973). Quantification of fetal heart beat to beat interval differences. *Obstet. Gynecol.*, **41**, 355–63
15. Nijhuis, J. G., Prechtl, H. F. R., Martin, C. B. Jr and Bots, R. S. G. M. (1982). Are there behavioural states in the human fetus? *Early Hum. Dev.*, **6**, 177–95
16. Landis, J. R. and Koch, J. J. (1979). The measurement of observer agreement for categorical data. *Biometrics*, **33**, 159–74
17. Bland, J. M. and Altman, D. G. (1986). Statistical methods for assessing agreement between two methods of clinical measurement. *Lancet*, **1**, 307–10
18. Arduini, D. and Rizzo, G. (1992). Prediction of fetal outcome in small for gestational age fetuses: comparison of Doppler measurements obtained from different vessels. *J. Perinat. Med.*, **20**, 29–38
19. Fisher, W. M., Stude, I. and Brandt, H. (1976). Ein vorschlag zur beurteilung des antepartalen kardiotokocogramms. *Z. Geburtshilfe Perinatol.*, **180**, 117–23
20. Hammacher, K. (1978). *Einfuhrung in die Cardiotokographie.* Hewlett Packard's Editions No. 5953–1109
21. Flynn, A. M., Kelly, J. and O'Conor, M. (1979). Unstressed antepartum cardiotocography in the management of fetuses suspected of growth retardation. *Br. J. Obstet. Gynaecol.*, **89**, 106–10
22. Wheeler, T. and Murrils, A. (1975). Patterns of fetal heart rate during normal pregnancy. *Br. J. Obstet. Gynaecol.*, **85**, 18–24
23. Arduini, D., Rizzo, G., Giorlandino, C., Valensise, H., Dell' Acqua, S. and Romanini, C. (1986). The development of fetal behavioural states: a longitudinal study. *Prenat. Diagn.*, **6**, 117–24
24. Dawes, G. S. (1991). Computerised analysis of fetal heart rate. *Eur. J. Obstet. Gynecol. Reprod. Biol.*, **42**, S5–8

Fetal hemodynamics in growth retardation

G. Rizzo, D. Arduini and C. Romanini

INTRODUCTION

Fetuses with abnormally low intrauterine growth greatly contribute to perinatal mortality and morbidity. The smallness of a fetus can be secondary to various multiple etiologies, including chromosomal aberrations, structural abnormalities, constitutionally low growth potentialities or so-called uteroplacental insufficiency[1]. One of the main challenges of the management of these fetuses is to identify and properly monitor those in which the growth retardation is secondary to uteroplacental insufficiency, as these fetuses have an increased risk of developing perinatal mortality and morbidity[2,3]. Fetuses that are small secondary to constitutional factors do not show any significant increase in perinatal complications[4], while the prognosis of fetuses with chromosomal and structural abnormalities is related to the severity of the underlying disease[1]. In this chapter we therefore restrict our interest to fetuses in which the intrauterine growth retardation (IUGR) is secondary to uteroplacental insufficiency.

Much of the understanding and present knowledge of this phenomenon is derived from animal research and pathological studies of the human placenta or uterine biopsies. Furthermore, the advent of pulsed and color Doppler ultrasonography has allowed us to obtain non-invasive hemodynamic measurements from several vascular beds of the uterine, placental and fetal circulation in humans. Thus it has been possible to improve our understanding of the pathophysiology of the fetal circulation in IUGR.

After a brief summary of the pathophysiology of uteroplacental insufficiency in this chapter we describe the hemodynamic modification in IUGR detectable by Doppler ultrasonography and consider the potential clinical role of this technique in the management of these fetuses.

PATHOPHYSIOLOGY

The underlying pathophysiology of uteroplacental insufficiency is a reduction in the supply of nutrients provided from the mother to the fetus through the placenta. In normal pregnancies the blood supply to the uterus increases markedly from 50 ml/min in early pregnancy to approximately 500 ml/min at term[5]. It has been clearly demonstrated that fetal growth is directly related to the normal incremental increases in uterine blood flow through pregnancy[6] and that, in cases of prolonged reduction of uterine blood, fetal growth is slowed[7]. Systemic events occurring during pregnancy, such as the expansion in maternal blood volume and the rise of cardiac output, have a partial role in this increase of uterine blood flow, but its main origin may be found in local factors causing the decrease of uterine vascular resistance.

In normal early pregnancy the trophoblastic cells invade the placental bed and migrate through the spiral arteries of the uterine circulation. The invading trophoblast destroys the elastic lamina and replaces the smooth-muscle cells of the vascular wall of the spiral arteries. This transformation, completed by 20 weeks of gestation, leads to the formation of a system of low vascular resistance in which relatively large arteries pump blood directly to the placental intervillous space[8]. Failure or impairment of trophoblast invasion does not allow the fall of uterine vascular resistance and impairs the maternal–fetal exchange of nutrients and oxygen, thus leading to IUGR and/or maternal hypertension[9].

Moreover, IUGR might also occur in the presence of a normal uterine blood supply associated with an abnormal placental function. The difficulties in studying placental function have limited our present knowledge. However, it has been shown that the number of small muscular arteries in the tertiary stem villi is reduced in fetuses with IUGR, thus resulting in an impaired supply of oxygen and nutrients from the mother to the fetus. There has been debate as to whether this reduction is secondary to a developmental arrest of placental angiogenesis[10], or to an obliterative process of small muscular arteries[11]; however, it is possible that both phenomena might occur.

The decrease of uterine blood flow and/or placental exchange capability leads to a reduced supply to the fetus of oxygen, glucose and essential nutrients[12-14]. This limitation of substrates causes concomitant circulatory responses.

Umbilical venous blood flow that passes through the ductus venosus increases, whereas the passage to the liver decreases, thus improving the impaired concentration of oxygen and nutrients in the inferior vena cava and consequently in the heart[15]. Concomitantly there is a change of arterial vascular resistance in the fetal circulation with vasodilatation at the level of the brain and myocardium, and a constriction at the level of the muscles and viscera[16]. Consequently, a redistribution of cardiac output occurs (the so-called 'brain-sparing effect') in favor of the priority organs (i.e. the brain and heart) with a reduction of flow to the other organs that are less essential for the immediate survival of the fetus, and a consequent impairment of their growth. The persistence or the worsening of this condition of nutritional deprivation leads to a progressive deterioration of fetal conditions with further hemodynamic changes, mainly characterized by a reduction of cardiac output and an impairment of cardiac function[17]. Further modifications include abnormalities in fetal motor behavior and heart-rate patterns[18]. Finally, if the fetus is not delivered in due course, fetal death will occur.

HEMODYNAMIC MODIFICATIONS

Since the earlier signs of fetal impairment secondary to reduced nutrient and oxygen supply are adaptive circulatory responses, Doppler ultrasound provides a unique tool to examine these changes non-invasively. In particular, the combined use of color and pulsed Doppler techniques in obstetrics has greatly enhanced the possibilities of studying IUGR[19].

Uterine circulation

Velocity waveforms from uterine vessels can be recorded at different levels, and transvaginal color Doppler ultrasonography has allowed us to visualize, even in early pregnancy, the main uterine arteries, arcuate arteries, radial arteries and the flows near the trophoblastic area representing spiral arteries[20,21]. The small dimensions of the uterine vessels and the difficulties of obtaining a low angle of insonation have limited the analysis of blood-flow velocity waveforms mainly to qualitative angle-independent indices considered directly related to vascular resistance such as the S/D ratio (systolic velocity/diastolic velocity) or resistance index (RI = (systolic velocity − diastolic velocity)/systolic velocity). Attempts to record absolute uterine blood flow have recently been performed with the aid of color Doppler[22]. Their reproducibility and clinical significance still remain to be defined.

In normal pregnancy a progressive decrease of Doppler-measured vascular resistance is present at the level of both uterine arteries and the branches thereof[20,21,23]. There are no particular advantages in obtaining recordings from the peripheral areas of uterine circulation and the main uterine artery is the most commonly analyzed vessel[23]. This choice is based on two factors. The first is the higher reproducibility of the recordings due to the easier identification of this vessel when compared to a single arcuate or spiral artery. Furthermore, as the indices measured reflect the vascular resistance of the downstream circulation, the main uterine artery provides information on the whole uterine circulation, while an arcuate or spiral artery provides information only on a limited vascular area that may differ from the general situation.

In normal pregnancies the S/D or RI values significantly decrease with advancing gestation until 24 to 26 weeks, when a plateau is reached[23]. In the absence of this physiological decrease, a higher incidence of hypertensive diseases and/or IUGR has been widely documented[23–26]. On the other hand, as previously described, several IUGR fetuses present normal uterine artery waveforms, despite severe compromise of the maternal–fetal exchange of substrates because of a pathological disease limited to the fetal side of the uteroplacental circulation.

Umbilical artery

Similarly to the uterine circulation, velocity waveforms from the umbilical artery are usually analyzed by angle-independent indices, mainly the S/D ratio or pulsatility index (PI = (systolic velocity – diastolic velocity)/mean velocity). The latter index is preferred by several authors, as it allows the evaluation of the waveforms even in the absence of end-diastolic flow. Normal pregnancies show a progressive decrease of S/D and PI values, mainly due to an increase of the end-diastolic velocities[27]. End-diastolic velocities are physiologically absent in the first trimester, whereas they are always present from 16 weeks of gestation onwards[28]. These changes in Doppler indices are considered an expression of the physiological decrease of placental resistance (i.e. progressive opening and merging of small muscular arteries in the tertiary stem villi).

In fetuses with IUGR there is an increase of these indices secondary to the decrease, absence or reversal of end-diastolic flow. The changes in these waveform patterns are thought to be indicative of increased placental resistance. However, other explanations, such as an increase in blood viscosity or a reduction in arterial blood pressure, have not been excluded. There is no report of whether the abnormalities in the umbilical artery occur earlier than, simultaneously with, or later than, those in fetal vessels. As already described, despite the common denominator of a reduced supply of nutrients, IUGR has multiple etiologies, which may involve the placenta primarily, with an early increase of its vascular resistance. On the other hand, different causes (e.g. impaired uterine circulation) might primarily induce the brain-sparing phenomenon with a consequent reduction of the blood supply to the placenta, and secondary obliterative and degenerative phenomena leading to increased vascular resistance.

The absent or reversed end-diastolic flows are strongly associated with an abnormal course of pregnancy and a higher incidence of perinatal complications, when compared to fetuses with IUGR of similar severity but characterized by the presence of end-diastolic flow[29].

Fetal descending aorta

Velocity waveforms from the fetal descending aorta are usually recorded at the lower thoracic level, keeping the angle of insonation of the Doppler beam below 45°. Diastolic velocities are always present during the second and third trimester of normal pregnancy and the PI remains constant through gestation[27]. Flow velocity waveforms in the descending aorta represent the summation of flows to the kidneys, other abdominal organs, femoral arteries and the placenta. The absence of modifications of the PI during pregnancy suggests that despite the decrease of placental and renal resistances (see below) with advancing gestation, aortic resistances remain constant, implying a concomitant increase of vascular resistances in other areas, such as the extremities.

Moreover, fetuses with IUGR show an increase of PI with reduction, absence or reversal of diastolic velocities[3]. The absence of end-diastolic velocities, suggestive of profound vascular changes causing a severe reduction of flow to splanchnic organs, has been associated with a higher incidence of neonatal complications, particularly necrotizing enterocolitis, when compared with matched controls with the presence of end-diastolic flow[3].

Fetal renal artery

Color Doppler allows the identification, in a longitudinal view of the fetal abdomen, of the fetal renal artery, from its origin as a lateral branch of the abdominal aorta to the hilum of the kidney[27]. Diastolic velocities are physiologically absent until 34 weeks, and the PI significantly decreases with advancing gestation[27,30]. If it is assumed that arterial pressure remains constant through gestation, then fetal renal perfusion increases. This may offer an explanation for the increase of fetal urine production that occurs with advancing gestation.

Fetuses with IUGR show higher PI values from the renal artery and this increase is proportional to the severity of fetal hypoxemia[30]. Furthermore, the abnormalities of the renal artery PI are inversely related to the volume of amniotic fluid[31]. This suggests that the PI from the renal artery can be considered a good marker of renal perfusion and may be used to monitor the fetal adapting response to hypoxemia.

Fetal cerebral circulation

With the color Doppler technique it is possible to investigate the main cerebral arteries from 8 weeks onwards[32]. In healthy fetuses the vascular resistances remain constant during the second and early third trimester of pregnancy, whereas they significantly decrease during the late third trimester[27]. The PI is significantly higher in the middle cerebral artery than in the internal carotid artery or in the anterior and posterior cerebral arteries. It is therefore important to know exactly which cerebral vessel is sampled during a Doppler examination, as a PI value might be normal for the internal carotid artery but abnormal for the middle cerebral artery[33]. The use of color Doppler has greatly improved the identification of the cerebral vessels, thus limiting the possibility of sampling errors.

The middle cerebral artery is usually considered the vessel of choice in the evaluation of the fetal cerebral circulation, as it is possible to obtain velocity waveforms with an angle of insonation near $0°$ and with a high reproducibility. However, the physiological differences between the cerebral vessels still remain to be clarified.

In fetuses with IUGR, the PI from cerebral arteries decreases and these changes are secondary to a vasomotor response (vasodilatation) occurring during the brain-sparing phenomenon. Comparison between cerebral PI and the measurement of umbilical pO_2, CO_2, pH and O_2 content obtained by cordocentesis or at birth has shown significant correlations between these parameters[34,35]. However, these correlations do not appear to be sufficiently strong to use the cerebral Doppler indices in clinical practice to quantify the compromise of fetal acid–base status and to take decisions on the time of delivery. Nevertheless, a satisfying relationship has been found between the existence of significantly decreased fetal cerebral resistances and the development in the newborn of post-asphyxial encephalopathy, thus suggesting an important prognostic role for cerebral Doppler velocimetry[36].

Fetal cardiac flows

Secondary to the brain-sparing effect, selective changes in cardiac afterload occur in fetuses with IUGR (i.e. decreased left-ventricle afterload, due to the cerebral vasodilatation and increased right-ventricle afterload, due to the systemic vasoconstriction). Furthermore, hypoxemia might impair myocardial contractility while the polycythemia usually present[12] might alter blood viscosity and therefore preload. As a consequence, fetuses with IUGR show impaired ventricular filling properties[37,38], lower peak velocities in the aorta and pulmonary arteries[39,40], increased aortic and decreased pulmonary time to peak velocity (TPV)[41] and a relative increase of left cardiac output (LCO) associated with decreased right cardiac output (RCO)[40,42]. These hemodynamic intracardiac changes are compatible with a preferential shift of cardiac output in favor of the left ventricle, leading to improved perfusion to the brain. Thus, the supply of substrate and oxygen can be maintained at near-normal levels despite any absolute reduction of placental transfer.

Fetal venous blood flow

The fetal supply of oxygen and nutrients depends on blood returning to the heart from the placenta via the umbilical vein, ductus venosus and inferior vena cava. In the human fetus the inferior vena cava blood flow has a triphasic pulsatile pattern[43]. The first forward wave begins to increase with atrial relaxation, reaches a peak during ventricular systole and then falls to reach a nadir at the end of ventricular systole. The second forward wave occurs during early diastole, while the third wave, characterized by a reverse flow, is present in late diastole with atrial contraction. In healthy fetuses a significant decrease of reverse flow during atrial contraction is present with advancing gestation[43]. As the amount of reverse flow is proportional to the pressure gradient present between the right atrium and the right ventricle at the end of diastole, these changes are considered to be related both to the improvement of ventricular compliance and to the reduction of right-ventricular afterload, due to the fall of placental resistances occurring with gestation.

In fetuses with IUGR an increase of reverse flow during atrial contraction might be present in the most severely compromised fetuses[43]. As a consequence of these venous abnormal flow patterns, the return of blood from the placenta to the heart is impaired, thus further reducing the supply of oxygen and nutrients.

Concomitant changes are present in the ductus venosus of fetuses with IUGR, where the velocity during atrial contraction is significantly reduced or reversed[44]. Umbilical venous blood flow is usually continuous. However, in the presence of a relevant amount of reverse flow during atrial contraction in the inferior vena cava, pulsations with heart rate occur in umbilical venous flows. In normal pregnancies these pulsations occur only before the 12th week of gestation and they are secondary to the stiffness of the ventricles present at this gestational age, causing a high percentage of reverse flow in the inferior vena cava[45]. Later in gestation the presence of pulsations in the umbilical vein indicates severe cardiac compromise and has a significance similar to that of increased reverse flow in the inferior vena cava. Particularly in fetuses with IUGR, the presence of pulsations in the umbilical vein is associated with a five-fold increase in perinatal mortality when compared to such fetuses with continuous umbilical flow[46].

HEMODYNAMIC CHANGES OCCURRING IN DETERIORATING FETUSES WITH IUGR

Fetuses with IUGR are usually delivered on the basis of either the results of other biophysical tests, such as fetal heart rate monitoring and a biophysical profile, or uncontrollable co-existing maternal diseases (e.g. pre-eclampsia). The time interval elapsing between the first Doppler abnormalities in the umbilical or fetal circulation (i.e. brain-sparing effect) and delivery is usually wide and, according to published data, may range from 1 to 9 weeks[47,48].

The knowledge of the temporal hemodynamic sequence occurring in fetuses with IUGR after the establishment of the brain-sparing phenomenon has important clinical implications. In fact, recent studies have reported that fetuses with IUGR, acidotic during intrauterine life, or exhibiting antepartum abnormal heart-rate tracings, showed a poor neurological development at 2 years[49,50]. This has led some authors to suggest that fetuses with IUGR should be delivered before the onset of abnormal fetal heart-rate patterns (suggestive of fetal acidemia) in order to avoid the consequence on the brain of prolonged malnutrition[51]. Moreover, gestational age should be taken into account, as the anticipation of the time of delivery may increase the risk of prematurity-related neonatal complications. Randomized controlled studies are required to clarify this issue.

At present, irrespective of the program of management for the timing of delivery of these fetuses, the knowledge of the progressive hemodynamic changes in deteriorating fetuses with IUGR may help to clarify their natural history and to predict the time interval left before the onset of abnormal heart-rate patterns.

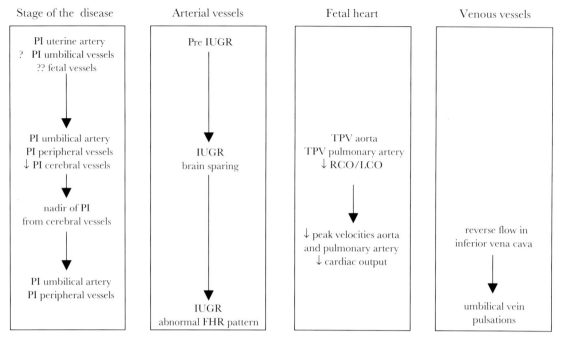

Figure 1 Suggested pathophysiological steps and corresponding hemodynamic changes in different vascular compartments occurring in chronically deteriorating intrauterine growth retardation (IUGR). PI, pulsatility index; TPV, time to peak velocity; RCO, right cardiac output; LCO, left cardiac output; FHR, fetal heart rate

Serial studies on fetuses with IUGR followed from the diagnosis to the onset of late decelerations of the heart rate have allowed the partial clarification of the hemodynamic changes occurring in different placental and fetal areas. A theoretical scheme for the temporal sequence of Doppler changes secondary to uteroplacental insufficiency is shown in Figure 1.

Doppler studies on the umbilical artery, fetal descending thoracic aorta and fetal renal artery have shown that after the establishment of the brain-sparing phenomenon, further modifications of the PI occur and are characterized by a slight increase in the first stage of the disease followed by a rapid increase at the last stage of the disease[52] (Figure 2). After the establishment of the brain-sparing effect, further changes occur in the cerebral circulation, as assessed by the PI in the middle cerebral artery or internal carotid artery, but the trend of these changes differs from that described for the umbilical artery and fetal peripheral vessels[52]. In particular, the decrease of the PI is progressive in the first stage of the disease and reaches a nadir at least 2 weeks before the onset of abnormal patterns of fetal heart rate (Figure 3). Furthermore, it has been shown that a few hours before fetal death, there is a loss of cerebral vasodilatation, despite the persistence of high resistances in peripheral vessels[53,54]. These terminal changes are consistent with data obtained in animal models[55].

At intracardiac level, the TPV and the ratio between the outputs of the right and left ventricles remain stable during repeated recordings in deteriorating fetuses with IUGR[40]. This implies that there are no other significant changes in outflow resistances and cardiac output redistribution after the establishment of the brain-sparing mechanism. However, in deteriorating fetuses with IUGR, peak velocities and cardiac output decline progressively, rather than showing the expected rise with gestation[40] (Figure 4). The physiological significance of these longitudinal changes is subject to several interpretations. However, as they are closely followed by the onset of abnormal heart-rate patterns, one might speculate that the terminal fall in cardiac

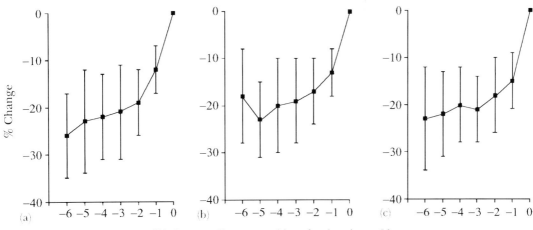

Figure 2 Longitudinal changes of pulsatility index from (a) the umbilical artery, (b) the descending aorta, and (c) the renal artery in deteriorating intrauterine growth retardation. Data are expressed as mean percentage changes (± 1 SD) from the values obtained at the last recording (time 0) close to the onset of antepartum late decelerations of the heart rate. Reproduced with permission from The American College of Obstetricians and Gynecologists[52]

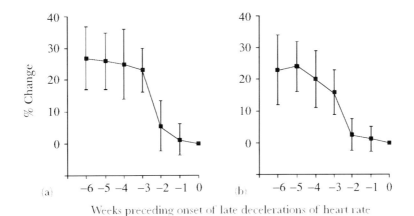

Figure 3 Longitudinal changes of pulsatility index from (a) the internal carotid artery and (b) the middle cerebral artery. Data are expressed as mean percentage changes (± 1 SD) from the values obtained at the last recording (time 0) close to the onset of antepartum late decelerations of the heart rate. Reproduced with permission from The American College of Obstetricians and Gynecologists[52]

output may reflect a decompensation of a normally protective mechanism responsible for the brain-sparing effect. According to this model, the fetal heart adapts to placental insufficiency in a manner which helps to maximize the brain supply of substrate and oxygen. With progressive deterioration of fetal conditions, this protective mechanism is overwhelmed by the fall of cardiac output, and fetal distress occurs.

Concomitantly, the percentage of reverse flow in the inferior vena cava increases[13] (Figure 5), the peak velocity occurs during atrial contraction in the ductus venosus[44], and pulsations occur in the umbilical vein[18]. These findings are

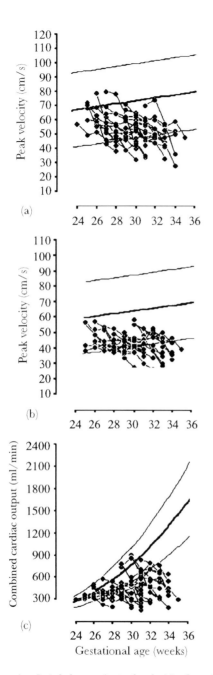

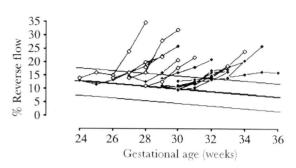

Figure 5 *Serial changes in percentage reverse flow in inferior vena cava obtained in chronically deteriorating intrauterine growth retardation. Filled symbols indicate fetuses with absent end-diastolic flow in the umbilical artery. Reproduced with permission from Rizzo and colleagues*[45]

compatible with the fall of cardiac output previously described. All these changes are the expression of the same phenomenon, namely cardiac decompensation, which impairs both the filling and the output of the heart.

CONCLUSION

Fetuses with IUGR show evident modifications of Doppler parameters in the uteroplacental and fetal circulation. The examination of the fetal circulation by Doppler techniques is providing evidence of some of the mechanisms of adaptation and decompensation of the fetus in response to uteroplacental insufficiency. At present the condition of fetuses with IUGR can quite accurately be assessed by sequential studies of Doppler waveforms from different vascular areas. There are, however, still many uncertainties concerning the relationships between the Doppler changes and the metabolic situation of the fetus and therefore on the optimal timing of delivery to prevent an intrauterine injury. Controlled trials on earlier versus later delivery of fetuses at similar gestational ages are required to clarify this issue.

Figure 4 *Serial changes in peak velocities from (a) aorta and (b) pulmonary valve and (c) combined cardiac output obtained in chronically deteriorating intrauterine growth retardation. Reproduced with permission from Rizzo and colleagues*[40]

References

1. Lin, C. C. and Evans, M. I. (1984). *Intrauterine Growth Retardation. Pathophysiology and Clinical Management.* (New York: McGraw-Hill)
2. Dobson, P. C., Abell, D. A. and Beisher, N. A. (1981). Mortality and morbidity of fetal growth retardation. *Aust. NZ J. Obstet. Gynaecol.*, **21**, 69–72
3. Hackett, G. A., Campbell, S., Gamsu, H., Cohen-Overbeek, T. and Pearce, J. M. F. (1987). Doppler studies in the growth retarded fetus and prediction of neonatal necrotising enterocolitis, haemorrhage, and neonatal morbidity. *Br. Med. J.*, **294**, 13–18
4. Burke, G., Stuart, B., Crowley, P., Scanail, S. N. and Drumm, J. (1990). Is intrauterine growth retardation with normal umbilical blood flow a benign condition? *Br. Med. J.*, **300**, 1044–5
5. Blechner, J. N., Stenger, V. G. and Prystowsky, H. (1974). Uterine blood flow in women at term. *Am. J. Obstet. Gynecol.*, **120**, 633–8
6. Creasy, R. K., Barret, C. T., De Swiet, M., Kahanpaa, K. V. and Rudolph, A. M. (1972). Experimental growth retardation in the sheep. *Am. J. Obstet. Gynecol.*, **112**, 566–73
7. Gu, W., Jones, C. T. and Parer, J. T. (1985). Metabolic and cardiovascular effects on fetal sheep of sustained reduction of uterine blood flow. *J. Physiol.*, **368**, 109–21
8. Brosens, I., Robertson, W. B. and Dixon, H. G. (1967). The physiological response of the vessels of the placental bed to normal pregnancy. *J. Pathol. Bacteriol.*, **93**, 569–79
9. Sheppard, B. L. and Bonnar, J. (1981). An ultrastructural study of uteroplacental spiral arteries in hypertensive and normotensive pregnancy and fetal growth retardation. *Br. J. Obstet. Gynaecol.*, **88**, 695–705
10. Giles, W. B., Trudinger, B. J., Baird, P. J. and Cook, C. M. (1985). Fetal umbilical artery flow velocity waveforms and placental resistance: pathological correlation. *Br. J. Obstet. Gynaecol.*, **92**, 31–6
11. Bracero, L. A., Beneck, D., Kirshenbaum, N., Peiffer, M., Stalter, P. and Schlman, H. (1989). Doppler velocimetry and placental disease. *Am. J. Obstet. Gynecol.*, **161**, 388–93
12. Soothill, P. W., Nicholaides, K. H. and Campbell, S. (1987). Prenatal asphyxia, hyperlactemia and erythroblastosis in growth retarded fetuses. *Br. Med. J.*, **294**, 1051–3
13. Economides, D. L., Nicolaides, K. H. and Campbell, S. (1987). Blood glucose and oxygen tension in small for gestational age fetuses. *Am. J. Obstet. Gynecol.*, **160**, 385–9
14. Cetin, I., Corbetta, C., Sereni, L. P., Marconi, A. M., Bozzetti, P. and Pardi, G. (1990). Umbilical amino acid concentrations in normal and growth retarded fetuses sampled *in utero* by cordocentesis. *Am. J. Obstet. Gynecol.*, **162**, 253–61
15. Rudolph, A. M. (1985). Distribution and regulation of blood flow in the fetal and neonatal lamb. *Circ. Res.*, **57**, 811–21
16. Peeters, L. L. H., Sheldon, R. F., Jones, M. D., Makowsky, E. I. and Meschia, G. (1979). Blood flow to fetal organ as a function of arterial oxygen content. *Am. J. Obstet. Gynecol.*, **135**, 637–46
17. Creasy, R. K., De Swiet, M., Kahanpaa, K. V., Young, W. P. and Rudolph, A. M. (1973). Pathophysiological changes in the foetal lamb with growth retardation. In Comline, R. S., Croos, K. W., Dawes, G. S. and Nathanielz, P. W. (eds.) *Foetal and Neonatal Physiology*, pp. 398–402. (London: Cambridge University Press)
18. Visser, G. H. A. and Bekedam, D. J. (1990). Serial observations on adaptation in the human fetus. In Dawes, G. S., Borruto, F., Zacutti, A. and Zacutti, A. Jr (eds.) *Fetal Autonomy and Adaptation*, pp. 67–80 (Chichester: Wiley)
19. Arduini, D., Rizzo, G., Boccolini, M. R., Romanini, C. and Mancuso, S. (1990). Functional assessment of utero-placental and fetal circulations by means of color doppler ultrasonography. *J. Ultrasound Med.*, **9**, 249–53
20. Alfirevic, Z. and Kurjak, A. (1990). Transvaginal colour Doppler ultrasound in normal and abnormal early pregnancy. *J. Perinat. Med.*, **18**, 173–80
21. Arduini, D., Rizzo, G. and Romanini, C. (1991). Doppler ultrasonography in early pregnancy does not predict adverse pregnancy outcome. *Ultrasound Obstet. Gynecol.*, **1**, 180–5
22. Thaler, I., Manor, D., Itskovitz, J., Rottem, S., Levit, N., Timor Tritsch, I. and Brandes, J. M. (1990). Changes in uterine blood flow during human pregnancy. *Am. J. Obstet. Gynecol.*, **162**, 121–5
23. Schulman, H., Fleisher, A., Farmakides, G., Bracero, L., Rochelson, B. and Grunfeld, L. (1986). Development of uterine artery compliance in pregnancy as detected by ultrasound. *Am. J. Obstet. Gynecol.*, **155**, 1031–6
24. Trudinger, B. J., Giles, W. B. and Cook, C. M. (1985). Uteroplacental blood flow velocity time waveforms in normal and complicated pregnancies. *Br. J. Obstet. Gynaecol.*, **92**, 39–45
25. Campbell, S., Pearce, J. M. F., Hackett, G., Cohen-Overbeek, T. E. and Hernandez, C. (1986). Qualitative assessment of uteroplacental

blood flow: early screening test for high-risk pregnancies. *Obstet. Gynecol.*, **68**, 649–53
26. Arduini, D., Rizzo, G., Romanini, C. and Mancuso, S. (1987). Utero-placental blood flow velocity waveforms as predictors of pregnancy-induced hypertension. *Eur. J. Obstet. Gynecol. Reprod. Biol.*, **26**, 335–41
27. Arduini, D. and Rizzo, G. (1990). Normal values of pulsatility index from fetal vessels: a cross sectional study on 1556 healthy fetuses. *J. Perinat. Med.*, **18**, 165–72
28. Arduini, D. and Rizzo, G. (1991). Umbilical artery velocity waveforms in early pregnancy: a transvaginal color Doppler study. *J. Clin. Ultrasound*, **19**, 335–9
29. Rochelson, B., Schulman, H., Farmakides, J., Bracero, L., Ducey, J., Fleisher, A., Penny, B. and Winter, D. (1987). The significance of absent end diastolic velocity in umbilical artery velocity waveforms. *Am. J. Obstet. Gynecol.*, **156**, 1213–7
30. Vyas, S., Nicolaides, K. H. and Campbell, S. (1989). Renal flow-velocity waveforms in normal and hypoxemic fetuses. *Am. J. Obstet. Gynecol.*, **161**, 168–72
31. Arduini, D. and Rizzo, G. (1991). Fetal renal artery velocity waveforms and amniotic fluid volume in growth-retarded and post-term fetuses. *Obstet. Gynecol.*, **77**, 370–4
32. Kurjak, A., Predanic, M., Kupesic-Urek, S., Funduk-Kurjak, B., Demarin, V. and Salihagic, A. (1992). Transvaginal color Doppler study of middle cerebral artery blood flow in early normal and abnormal pregnancy. *Ultrasound Obstet. Gynecol.*, **2**, 424–8
33. Mari, G., Moise, K. J., Deter, R. L., Kirshon, B., Carpenter, R. J. and Hutha, J. C. (1989). Doppler assessment of the pulsatility index in the cerebral circulation of the human fetus. *Am. J. Obstet. Gynecol.*, **160**, 698–703
34. Bilardo, C. M., Nicolaides, K. H. and Campbell, S. (1990). Doppler measurement of fetal and uteroplacental circulation: relationship with umbilical venous blood gases measured at cordocentesis. *Am. J. Obstet. Gynecol.*, **162**, 115–21
35. Arduini, D., Rizzo, G., Romanini, C. and Mancuso, S. (1989). Are blood flow velocity waveforms related to umbilical cord acid–base status in the human fetus? *Gynecol. Obstet. Inv.*, **27**, 183–7
36. Rizzo, G., Luciano, R. Arduini, D., Rizzo, C., Tortorolo, G., Romanini, C. and Mancuso, S. (1989). Prenatal cerebral Doppler ultrasonography and neonatal neurological outcome. *J. Ultrasound Med.*, **8**, 237–40
37. Rizzo, G., Arduini, D., Romanini, C. and Mancuso, S. (1988). Doppler echocardiographic assessment of atrioventricular velocity waveforms in normal and small for gestational age fetuses. *Br. J. Obstet. Gynaecol.*, **95**, 65–9
38. Reed, K. L., Anderson, C. F. and Shenker, L. (1987). Changes in intracardiac Doppler blood flow velocities in fetuses with absent umbilical artery diastolic flow. *Am. J. Obstet. Gynecol.*, **157**, 774–9
39. Groenenberg, I. A. L., Wladimiroff, J. W. and Hop, W. C. J. (1989). Fetal cardiac and peripheral arterial flow velocity waveforms in intrauterine growth retardation. *Circulation*, **80**, 1711–7
40. Rizzo, G. and Arduini, D. (1991). Fetal cardiac function in intrauterine growth retardation. *Am. J. Obstet. Gynecol.*, **165**, 876–82
41. Rizzo, G., Arduini, D., Romanini, C. and Mancuso, S. (1990). Doppler echocardiographic evaluation of time to peak velocity in the aorta and pulmonary artery of small for gestational age fetuses. *Br. J. Obstet. Gynaecol.*, **97**, 603–7
42. Al-Ghazali, W., Chita, S. K., Chapman, M. G. and Allan, L. D. (1989). Evidence of redistribution of cardiac output in asymmetrical growth retardation. *Br. J. Obstet. Gynaecol.*, **96**, 697–704
43. Rizzo, G., Arduini, G. and Romanini, C. (1992). Inferior vena cava flow velocity waveforms in appropriate and small for gestational age fetuses. *Am. J. Obstet. Gynecol.*, **166**, 1271–80
44. Rizzo, G., Pietropolli, A., Bufalino, L. M., Soldano, S., Arduini, D. and Romanini, C. (1993). Ductus venosus systolic to atrial peak velocities ratio in appropriate and small for gestational age fetuses. *J. Matern. Fetal. Inv.*, **3**, 198
45. Rizzo, G., Arduini, D. and Romanini, C. (1992). Pulsations in umbilical vein: a physiological finding in early pregnancy. *Am. J. Obstet. Gynecol.*, **167**, 675–7
46. Indick, J. H., Chen, V. and Reed, K. L. (1991). Association of umbilical venous with inferior vena cava blood flow velocities. *Obstet. Gynecol.*, **77**, 551–7
47. Bekedam, D. J., Visser, G. H. A., van der Zee, A. G. J., Snijders, R. and Poelmann-Weesjes, G. (1990). Abnormal umbilical artery waveform patterns in growth retarded fetuses: relationship to antepartum late heart rate decelerations and outcome. *Early Hum. Dev.*, **24**, 79–90
48. Arduini, D., Rizzo, G. and Romanini, C. (1993). The development of abnormal heart rate patterns after absent end diastolic velocity in umbilical artery: analysis of risk factors. *Am. J. Obstet. Gynecol.*, **168**, 43–9
49. Soothill, P. W., Ajayi, R. A., Campbell, S., Ross, E. M., Candy, D. C. A., Snijders, R. M. and Nicolaides, K. H. (1992). Relationship between acidemia at cordocentesis and subsequent neurodevelopment. *Ultrasound Obstet. Gynecol.*, **2**, 80–4

50. Todds, A. L., Trudinger, B. J., Cole, M. J. and Cooney, G. H. (1992). Antenatal tests of fetal welfare and development at age 2 years. *Am. J. Obstet. Gynecol.*, **167**, 66–71
51. Visser, G. H. A., Stitger, R. H. and Bruinse, H. W. (1991). Management of the growth-retarded fetus. *Eur. J. Obstet. Gynecol. Repr. Biol.*, **42**, S73–8
52. Arduini, D., Rizzo, G. and Romanini, C. (1992). Changes of pulsatility index from fetal vessels preceding the onset of late decelerations in growth retarded fetuses. *Obstet. Gynecol.*, **79**, 605–10
53. Mari, G. and Wasserstrum, N. (1991). Flow velocity waveforms of the fetal circulation preceding fetal death in a case of lupus anticoagulant. *Am. J. Obstet. Gynecol.*, **164**, 776–8
54. Rizzo, G., Capponi, A., Pietropolli, A., Cacciatore, C., Arduini, D. and Romanini, C. (1994). Cardiac and extra-cardiac flow changes preceding intrauterine fetal death. *Ultrasound Obstet. Gynecol.*, **4**, in press
55. Richardson, B. S., Rurak, D., Patrick, J. E., Homan, J. and Charmichael, L. (1989). Cerebral oxidative metabolism during sustained hypoxemia in fetal sheep. *J. Dev. Physiol.*, **11**, 37–43

Advances in neonatology   26

M. Levene

INTRODUCTION

In the era of neonatal intensive care the mortality rate of infants born extremely prematurely has fallen year on year. In 1994 the survival rate for infants born at gestational ages 24–25 weeks is in the order of 50% in many centers. These impressive statistics beg at least two important questions. First, what is the outcome of babies surviving of this gestational age?, and second what has been the cause of this reduction in mortality? This chapter reviews some of the recent advances in neonatal care that have contributed to the reduction in mortality, in particular the widespread introduction of exogenous surfactant therapy. The role of perinatal infection in neonatal death is another important area that has shown a promising response with new hyperimmune intravenous immunoglobulin treatment, and this is reviewed. It is now recognized that early feeding in the first week of life with appropriate milks makes a significant difference to cognitive ability in preschool children, and recent advances in this field are discussed.

OUTCOME FOLLOWING NEONATAL INTENSIVE CARE

If the success of neonatal intensive care is measured by the survival rate of babies, then the results of this complicated form of therapy have clearly dramatically improved over the last 30 years. If outcome of surviving babies is considered, then it becomes more difficult to argue convincingly that results are improving. It is very difficult to compare studies reporting outcome of very premature infants with each other, because of differences in study designs, definition of outcome and comparability of groups. The term 'handicap' is commonly used to describe babies who have an adverse outcome, but this may be misleading unless it is carefully defined. The World Health Organization has defined outcome[1] in terms of impairment (a defect in the structure or function of an organ or sense), disability (the result of an impairment, which restricts the child's ability to perform an activity in a manner that is considered normal) and a handicap (the result of an impairment or disability, which leads to a social or cultural disadvantage for the individual child).

A recent overview[2] of 111 studies describing the outcome of infants with very low birth weight (birth weight ≤ 1.5 kg) reported the incidence of disability in these children. The median number of children they considered as being 'disabled' (defined as severe or moderate disabilities or handicaps) was reported to be 25% (confidence interval [CI] 20.9–30.0). Another recent study[3] defined a major handicap as cerebral palsy, mental retardation, severe retinopathy of prematurity or neurosensory hearing impairment. They found 83 of 462 (18%) babies with extremely low birth weight (birth weight ≤ 1000 g) to have a 'major handicap'. Msall and associates[4] reported major impairments in 25% of infants with extremely low birth weight surviving to a mean age of 5 years. If cerebral palsy alone is taken as an indicator of bad outcome, then this is likely significantly to underestimate the risks of neonatal intensive care. Escobar and colleagues[2], in a meta-analysis of published data, reported the overall median prevalence of cerebral palsy to be 7.7% (CI 5.3–9.0), and there were no differences when babies below 1000 g were compared with babies of birth weight 1000–1500 g. There does not appear to have been any reduction in the incidence of cerebral palsy since the 1960s[2], although there was a reduction in median incidence of disabilities in 1960–77 compared with the period 1978–86[2].

A review of recent studies[5] has indicated that even the group of prematurely born babies who survived and were thought to be 'normal' may have important functional disabilities. These children had no 'hard' neurological deficits but underachieved at school for a number of measurable reasons. When prematurely born babies reached 5 years of age or more, and were compared with control children of the same age, and as far as possible were matched for socioeconomic class, there were significant differences in personal and social proficiency, receptive and expressive language, problem solving, academic achievement and measures of motor performance. The prematurely born babies at school age had more learning problems, were twice as likely to have repeated grades at school and had a three-fold increase in the rate of attention deficit disorder with hyperactivity.

These studies focus attention on the assumption that the outcome of neonatal intensive care is good. The results reviewed above do not support this contention. There are many possible reasons for this apparently poor outcome, but research in recent years has highlighted some important innovations in neonatal intensive care that may reduce some of these disabilities.

SURFACTANT THERAPY

Respiratory distress syndrome (RDS) and its complications are the commonest cause of death in prematurely born infants. The cause of RDS is surfactant deficiency. Surfactant, a complicated phospholipid, is produced from type II pneumatocytes, which are present in the fetal lung from the end of the first trimester. Its physiological action lies in its ability to form a thin molecular monolayer in the luminal alveolus, which has the effect of lowering the surface tension. The major component of surfactant is lecithin or dipalmitoylphosphatidyl choline (DPPC), with lesser amounts of other phospholipids. Since Avery and Mead[6] first described the association between RDS and surfactant deficiency, there has been considerable interest in the preparation and testing of surfactant-like preparations given to the baby exogenously. These substances are liquid and are injected directly into the endotracheal tube.

There are two main types of exogenous surfactant, their classification being based on their origin: synthetic and natural. The main synthetic surfactant preparation is Exosurf®, which is a protein-free compound comprising mainly DPPC with an alcohol (hexadecanol) and a spreading agent (tyloxapol). A second synthetic agent, artificial lung expanding compound (ALEC), is much less widely used in clinical practice.

A number of natural surfactant compounds (Survanta, Curosurf, Alveofact, Surfactant TA) have gained widespread clinical use. They are produced commercially by lung lavage from either pigs or calves. Human natural surfactant is no longer used, due to the risk of viral contamination.

Exogenous surfactant is the most carefully and widely evaluated 'drug' to be used in neonatal medicine. To date, over 10 000 babies have been enroled in randomized controlled studies. Unfortunately, evaluating the overall efficacy of these studies has proved difficult, because of different study designs, varying dosage regimens from study to study and different preparation of surfactant in use. Despite these confounding factors, a number of generalizations can be made. There is now little doubt that exogenous surfactant (of any type) reduces neonatal mortality by up to 40%. Meta-analysis has shown that there is a marked fall in inspired oxygen concentration and a significant reduction in the incidence of pneumothorax compared with control babies not given the substance[7]. These results appear to be independent of the type and timing of the administration of the surfactant.

The therapeutic use of surfactant has been evaluated as very early treatment at, or immediately after, resuscitation (prophylactic use) and treatment when the baby shows signs of acute respiratory distress syndrome (rescue treatment). Prophylactic use has concentrated on giving the surfactant to high-risk premature infants (usually of ≤ 30 weeks' gestation) either at the time of the first breath or after a short period of resuscitation. These studies have shown that the initial dose of surfactant needs to be followed by at least one further dose in the next 12–24 h to maintain reduction of levels of inspired oxygen. Rescue therapy has also been shown to reduce inspired oxygen concentration, although the rate at which the oxygen requirement can be dropped depends on the type of surfactant given; natural surfactant appears to have a considerably more rapid action than synthetic.

The use of exogenous surfactant does not appear to have a significant benefit in reducing the risk of chronic lung disease or of reducing the risk of intracranial hemorrhage. Early fears that surfactant therapy increased the risk of patent ductus arteriosus do not seem to have been borne out.

There is little doubt that exogenous surfactant represents a major advance in the management of premature babies with RDS. Preliminary evidence suggests that it is also of value in the most immature infants of < 26 weeks' gestation. Unfortunately, approximately 30% of babies treated with either artificial or natural surfactants are oxygen-dependent at 28 days[8], and further studies must be constructed to assess the combined or sequential role of surfactant and corticosteroids to reduce chronic lung disease in these babies. There are unresolved questions as to which is the best type of surfactant to use, and whether it should be given prophylactically or as a rescue therapy. The evidence to date is that the earlier the substance is used, the better the results will be. The cost–benefit argument must also be considered for this expensive form of treatment, and there can be little doubt that the most effective and cheapest way of reducing the incidence and severity of RDS in cases at risk is to use antenatal steroids.

INFECTION

After congenital malformations and lung disease, infection is the commonest cause of death in prematurely born neonates. The very immature baby is particularly prone to infection for two main reasons: first, the immune system is functionally compromised, due to immaturity, and second, there is a failure in the passive transfer of immunoglobulins from mother to fetus.

The fetal immune system is largely mediated through lymphocytes, of which there are two types, T cells and B cells. T cells derive from the fetal bone marrow and migrate to the thymus. On stimulation by an antigen, they transform into one of a number of different types of lymphocyte, and lymphokines are produced, which amplify the immune response. In addition, opsonins, such as complement and fibronectin, are necessary for phagocytic ingestion, to complete the bacterial process. Opsonic activity is impaired in the premature neonate.

B lymphocytes, when stimulated, transform into plasma cells and produce immunoglobulin. IgM is the first type to be produced at 15 weeks, followed by IgG at 20 weeks. Endogenous levels of fetal immunoglobulins remain very low at birth, but in the final trimester, there is an increasing infusion of maternal IgG, a relatively small molecule that crosses the placenta. This gives the neonate effective passive immunity at birth, but the levels decay by 3 months.

In view of the low levels of IgG in prematurely born infants, various attempts have been made to enhance the neonatal immune response by administration of immunoglobulins, but the results of these studies remain inconclusive. Immunoglobulins have been administered in two regimens, prophylaxis and rescue.

Intravenous immunoglobulin (IVIg) has been given to groups of susceptible premature infants without signs of infection, to reduce the risk of septicemia and meningitis. Weisman and colleagues[9] have critically evaluated the results of five published controlled randomized trials and concluded that in only one study of prophylactic IVIg was there an impressive reduction in infection in the group treated compared with controls[10].

Four further clinical trials (only two of which were blind) have evaluated the role of IVIg as adjunct to therapy in infants suspected of having severe infection. Comparison between these studies is difficult, due to the small numbers of patients and varying dosage of immunoglobulins, but overall there appears to be a three-fold increase in the ratio of the relative-risk of death in those babies not treated with IVIg compared with IVIg in addition to a standard antibiotic and supportive regimen[9].

Group B β-hemolytic streptococcus (GBS) is a particularly virulent and dangerous perinatal pathogen that causes early infection, which is often severe and rapidly fatal. Although IVIg may have an important effect in reducing mortality in infants who are suspected of having GBS infection, recent work using GBS hyperimmune IVIg suggests that this may be of additional benefit[11].

Reducing mortality due to infection, particularly due to perinatal pathogens, may occur as the result of routine surveillance of women in premature labor, very early antigen diagnosis in the neonatal period, and adjunct therapy such as IVIg. Immunoglobulins with specific activity against particular perinatal pathogens appear to be a promising way forward.

THE SIGNIFICANCE OF ENTERAL FEEDS AND SUBSEQUENT OUTCOME

The extremely premature baby must rapidly adapt to a non-placental source of nutrients, but functional immaturity of the brain (inability to suck), bowel (impaired activity of disaccharidase enzymes) and kidneys (sodium leak) all conspire to make enteral feeding more difficult and potentially harmful. For these reasons parenteral intravenous nutrition has been widely used in very immature infants. Recent studies have suggested that rather than having a negative effect on the infant's well-being, appropriate enteral feeding may give the baby a significant advantage in terms of early growth, and intelligence in early childhood. Milk feeding of the very immature infant may be the preferred method for sustaining appropriate nutrition.

If milk feeding is considered possible, then there is a choice of milks available, natural or formula. Human milk does not have a constant composition; its nutritional constitution varies with the gestation at which the mother delivers, and the duration of breast feeding. Breast milk for premature babies may derive from the baby's own mother, and the composition is significantly different from that of the milk of mothers who deliver at full-term. If the mother of a premature baby cannot, or does not wish to, breast feed her infant, the only natural alternative is to provide breast milk from a woman who has established lactation and who will donate milk at the end of feeding her own baby (hindmilk) or drip-milk from the non-suckling breast. Unfortunately, the nutritional status of these types of milk is even less appropriate for premature infants than is that of other types of mature breast milk.

Formula feeds can be divided into preterm artificial formula and term artificial formula. The nutritional constitution of these milks vary in number of important ways. Preterm formulae typically have a higher concentration of protein, sodium, other electrolytes and vitamins, with a higher energy density compared with standard formula.

Lucas and colleagues[12,13] have undertaken a number of controlled studies evaluating the effects of various types of milk on premature babies' growth and development. In a comparison of term versus preterm artificial formula, there were clear advantages to the babies who had been fed preterm formula[12]. They gained weight and their head size grew significantly more rapidly than a control group fed term formula. At 18 months, the infants fed on the preterm formula showed marked improvement in their developmental outcomes[12].

In a comparative study of preterm formula compared with mature breast milk, premature infants grew more rapidly in the preterm formula group than the breast milk group[13]. There has been only one randomized study of banked term breast milk versus banked preterm breast milk in prematurely born infants[14]. The group of babies given preterm formula grew better and had a significantly shorter period of time to regain birth weight than the term breast-milk group.

The most interesting and clinically important question is: do babies grow and develop better if they are initially fed on a preterm formula rather than their own mother's breast milk? For obvious ethical reasons, it will prove very difficult to undertake such a study, but current understanding indicates that mothers who deliver prematurely should be encouraged to express milk to feed their own babies, but if this is not possible, then they should be given a preterm formula from as early as they are able to tolerate enteral feeds. If the baby's growth is poor on its own mother's milk, then this should be supplemented with preterm formula.

References

1. World Health Organization (1980). *International Classification of Impairments, Disabilities, and Handicaps*, p.207 (Geneva: World Health Organization)
2. Escobar, G. J., Littenberg, B. and Petitti, D. B. (1991). Outcome among surviving very low birthweight infants: a meta-analysis. *Arch. Dis. Child.*, **66**, 204–11
3. Teplin, S. W., Burchinal, M., Johnson-Martin, N., Humphry, R. A. and Kraybill, E. N. (1991). Neurodevelopmental, health, and growth status at age 6 years of children with birth weights less than 1001 grams. *J. Pediatr.*, **118**, 768–7
4. Msall, M. E., Buch, G. M., Rogers, B. L., Merke, D., Catanzaro, N. L. and Zorn, W. A. (1991). Risk factors for major neurodevelopmental impairments and need for special education resources in extremely premature infants. *J. Pediatr.*, **119**, 606–14
5. Levene, M. I. (1992). The impact of intensive neonatal care on the frequency of mental and motor handicap. *Curr. Opin. Neurol. Neurosurg.*, **5**, 333–8
6. Avery, M. E. and Mead, J. (1959). Surface properties in relation to atelectasis and hyaline membrane disease. *Am. J. Dis. Child.*, **97**, 517–23
7. Soll, R. F., and McQueen, M. (1992). Respiratory distress syndrome. In Sinclair, J. C. and Bracken, M. B. (eds.) *Effective Care of the Newborn Infant*, pp. 325–58. (Oxford: Oxford University Press)
8. Halliday, H. L., Tarnow-Mordi, W. O. and Patterson, C. C. (1993). Multicentre randomised trial comparing high and low dose surfactant regimens for the treatment of respiratory distress syndrome (the Curosurf 4 trial). *Arch. Dis. Child.*, **69**, 276–80
9. Weisman, L. E., Cruess, D. F., Fischer, G. W. (1993). Standard versus hyperimmune intravenous immunoglobulin in preventing or treating neonatal bacterial infections. *Clin. Perinatol.*, **20**, 211–24
10. Baker, C. J. (1989). Multicenter trial of intravenous immunoglobulin to prevent late-onset infection in preterm infants: preliminary results. *Pediatr. Res.*, **25**, 275A
11. Weisman, L. E., Wilson, S. R. and Roberts, D. (1990). Group B streptococcal hyperimmune intravenous immunoglobulin in suspected neonatal sepsis. *Pediatr. Res.*, **27**, 278A
12. Lucas, A., Morley, R., Cole, T., Gore, S. M., Lucas, P. J., Crowle, P., Pearse, R., Boon, A. and Powell, R. (1990). Early diet in preterm babies and developmental status at 18 months. *Lancet*, **335**, 1477–81
13. Lucas, A., Gore, S. M. and Cole, T. J. (1984). Multicentre trial on feeding low birthweight infants: effects of diet on early growth. *Arch. Dis. Child.*, **59**, 722–30
14. Gross, S. J. (1983). Growth and biochemical response of preterm infants fed human milk or modified infant formula. *N. Engl. J. Med.*, **308**, 237–41

Amniotic fluid analysis

27

C. P. O'Reilly-Green and M. Y. Divon

RATIONALE FOR AMNIOTIC FLUID ANALYSIS

Amniotic fluid analysis is undertaken because amniotic fluid is a dynamic product of fetal, placental and maternal metabolism. Consequently, study of the physiology and pathophysiology of amniotic fluid can give insight into the normal and abnormal interactions of these three components of an ongoing pregnancy.

A great many aspects of amniotic fluid have been analyzed. Much of this analysis has occurred in an effort to elicit the physiology of amniotic fluid and the systems responsible for its formation. Many such analyses have, in recent years, taken the form of assays for various endocrine, paracrine and autocrine hormones, cytokines and substances of unknown function on a number of readily available body fluids, including amniotic fluid.

Some of these studies have failed to control for gestational age and maternal characteristics, or have proposed no hypothetical mechanism of function. Such analyses[1–10] must be considered preliminary and in need of further exploration.

However, a number of studies have been directed at answering specific questions, with appropriate formulation of hypotheses. These studies have increased our ability to understand both normal and abnormal processes of pregnancy that involve amniotic fluid. Some of these analytical methods are limited to specific research laboratories, while others have come into widespread common and commercial use. It can be expected that those specialized tests with consistent and predictive results will, in the future, become widely available, and this is the rationale for discussing these tests here.

PHYSIOLOGY OF AMNIOTIC FLUID COMPOSITION AND DYNAMICS

The dynamics and physiology of amniotic fluid vary continuously over gestation and during parturition. Consequently, amniotic fluid analysis varies over gestation, with different objectives and possibilities in the first, second and third trimesters and during parturition.

Hertig and Rock[11] noted amniotic fluid first distending the amniotic cavity between the seventh and ninth days of gestation. Brace[12] suggested that amniotic fluid initially has the character of a transudate, with an electrolyte composition and osmolality similar to fetal and maternal blood. Seeds[13] suggested that, since the active transport of solutes but not water has been demonstrated in tissues, the accumulation of water in the amniotic cavity must occur passively following osmotic or pressure gradients. Consequently, there must be small transplacental chemical gradients responsible for this early accumulation of fluids. Alternatively, some mechanism for forming a hypotonic fluid, such as that found in kidneys and sweat glands, must exist in the embryo or amnion.

Indeed, recent studies comparing amniotic fluid and extraembryonic celomic fluid with maternal serum, and with each other, suggest significant differences when sampled between 5 and 13 weeks' gestation[14,15]. Many solutes are in lower concentration in amniotic fluid than in maternal serum, while significant differences exist between amniotic fluid and extraembryonic fluid as well, in spite of their separation only by the amnion. For example, lower concentrations of protein, potassium, sodium, and creatinine were found in amniotic fluid and extraembryonic celom than in maternal serum between 5 and 13 weeks of gestation[15]

(Tables 1 and 2). Moreover, levels of sodium, potassium and bicarbonate were higher in amniotic fluid than in the extraembryonic celom, while levels of chloride, urea, bilirubin, protein, albumin, glucose, creatinine, calcium and phosphate were lower in amniotic fluid than in extraembryonic celomic fluid between 8 and 12 weeks of gestation[14] (Table 3). Human chorionic gonadotropin (hCG) was lower in amniotic fluid and higher in exocelomic fluid than in maternal serum[15,16] (Tables 1, 2 and 4). Erythropoietin was lower in amniotic fluid than in extraembryonic celomic fluid or maternal serum[17]. These differences cannot be accounted for by diffusion equilibrium across a passive membrane, and suggest that mechanisms exist for the formation of a hypotonic amniotic fluid even before fetal urination makes a significant contribution.

Fetal urine begins to contribute to amniotic fluid at around 10 to 11 weeks[18], the amount rising steadily throughout gestation. Fetal swallowing also begins at around 8 to 11 weeks[19], so that the dynamic flux of amniotic fluid from these sources begins early and rises steadily.

Fluid is also produced in the fetal respiratory tree. It is uncertain how much of this becomes added to amniotic fluid and how much is swallowed without exiting the mouth. For example, after esophageal occlusion, amniotic fluid volume increased nearly three-fold[20], whereas urine flow did not change, suggesting that the usual function of the fetal gastrointestinal tract is to remove amniotic fluid, along with respiratory-tract secretions. However, the presence of lamellar bodies and pulmonary surfactant lipids in amniotic fluid during the second half of gestation indicates that there is some contribution of respiratory secretions to amniotic fluid.

Nasal and buccal mucosa and glands also produce copious secretions during fetal life and similarly may contribute to amniotic fluid.

Fetal skin is probably a major source of amniotic fluid during the first half of pregnancy, since the amount of fluid is proportional to body surface area up till around 24 weeks, and the skin is permeable to water. After that time, the skin becomes keratinized and so much less permeable to water, although preterm infants clearly have a greater tendency toward water loss through the skin than full-term infants.

Transport of water may occur across the amnion and chorion as well as across fetal vessels that traverse them. It is estimated that at term, urine production is 500 ml per day, lung fluid entry into amniotic fluid is 200 ml per day, and swallowing accounts for the removal of only 400 ml per day[12]. Thus it is estimated that at least 300 ml per day leaves the amniotic cavity across the membranes late in gestation. Recently, an intramembranous pathway has been demonstrated. Utilizing esophageal occlusion and urinary drainage[21], it was suggested that water is absorbed from the amniotic fluid through the intramembranous pathway into the fetal circulation at a rate of 1.25% of the total amniotic fluid volume per hour, or 240 ml per day, in the term ovine fetus. The oral–nasal membranes are not likely to be the major route of absorption in these experiments, because arginine vasopressin injected into amniotic fluid had immediate fetal systemic effects[22], while injection of the same dose into a glove covering the fetal head had no measureable effects.

The net transfer of water across membranes can be accomplished through an osmotic gradient. An osmotic gradient develops during pregnancy, due to the formation of increasingly hypotonic amniotic fluid, reflecting chiefly the contribution of an increasingly hypotonic urine[23] (see Figure 1). The composition of amniotic fluid changes from that of a transudate of plasma to a much more hypotonic solution, providing an osmotic drive for the flow of amni-

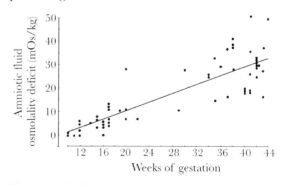

Figure 1 *Difference in osmolality between maternal serum and amniotic fluid with advancing pregnancy. (From Reference 23)*

Table 1 Comparison of maternal serum and amniotic fluid composition in 17 matched samples. (From Reference 15). NS, not significant; hCG, human chorionic gonadotropin

	Maternal serum	Amniotic fluid	p
Urea (mmol/l)	6.8	7.2	NS
Protein (g/l)	71.3	0.2	< 0.001
Potassium (mmol/l)	4.0	3.5	< 0.05
Sodium (mmol/l)	135.7	127.1	< 0.05
Creatinine (µmol/l)	49.1	27.7	< 0.001
hCG (IU/l)	74 568	1 052	< 0.001
α-Fetoprotein (kIU/l)	2.9	27 096	< 0.001

Table 2 Comparison of maternal serum and exocelomic fluid composition in 25 matched samples. (From Reference 15). NS, not significant; hCG, human chorionic gonadotropin

	Maternal serum	Exocelomic fluid	p
Urea (mmol/l)	7.2	8.3	NS
Protein (g/l)	71.3	3.5	< 0.001
Potassium (mmol/l)	4.1	3.8	< 0.005
Sodium (mmol/l)	135.9	130.9	< 0.001
Creatinine (µmol/l)	50.1	43.6	< 0.01
hCG (IU/l)	67 630	174 001	< 0.001
α-Fetoprotein (kIU/l)	1.4	21 816	< 0.001

Table 3 Comparison of amniotic fluid composition with exocelomic fluid composition in pregnancies between 5 and 13 weeks of gestation. (From Reference 15)

	Amniotic fluid	Exocelomic fluid	p
Urea (mmol/l)	3.3	3.9	0.02
Protein (g/l)	1.0	5.4	< 0.0001
Potassium (mmol/l)	4.0	3.9	0.004
Sodium (mmol/l)	141.2	138.1	< 0.0001
Creatinine (µmol/l)	37.1	72.3	< 0.0001
Chloride (mmol/l)	97.4	110.1	< 0.0001
Bicarbonate (mmol/l)	34.2	20.9	< 0.0001
Calcium (mmol/l)	1.4	2.7	< 0.0001
Phosphate (mmol/l)	1.1	2.7	< 0.0001
Bilirubin (µmol/l)	0.6	3.4	< 0.0001
Albumin (g/l)	0.5	4.6	< 0.0001
Glucose (mmol/l)	3.2	3.7	0.02
Osmolality (mOsm/kg)	273.6	270.6	NS

Table 4 Comparison of exocelomic fluid composition in 12 pregnancies between 5 and 8 weeks and in 13 pregnancies between 9 and 12 weeks of gestation. (From Reference 15). NS, not significant; hCG, human chorionic gonadotropin

	Exocelomic fluid		p
	5–8 weeks	9–12 weeks	
Urea (mmol/l)	9.7	7.1	< 0.005
Protein (g/l)	3.1	3.9	< 0.05
Potassium (mmol/l)	3.9	3.6	NS
Sodium (mmol/l)	133.4	128.8	NS
Creatinine (µmol/l)	45.1	40.6	NS
hCG (IU/l)	259 358	120 375	< 0.001
α-Fetoprotein (kIU/l)	19 999	14 392	NS

otic fluid across the fetal membranes. It is the change in composition of fetal urine as well as the increased contribution of fetal urine to amniotic fluid relative to skin that causes the progressive change in amniotic fluid composition. As early as 24 weeks, fetal kidneys are reabsorbing sodium, potassium and chloride to produce urine that is hypotonic[24,25]. In the second trimester, pH and bicarbonate are significantly lower in amniotic fluid than in fetal umbilical arterial or venous blood or in maternal venous blood[26], and this difference is most likely due to substances contributing to base deficit, such as sulfate and phosphate excreted by the kidneys.

Amniotic fluid volume rises during pregnancy[27] (see Figure 2). Amniotic fluid pressure also rises during pregnancy[28], peaking in midgestation, and is not apparently related to intrauterine volume. Amniotic fluid volume at term remains between 500 and 2000 ml, unless some unusual disturbance leads to oligohydramnios or polyhydramnios. Turnover of amniotic fluid is rapid. Indeed, studies with deuterium tracer techniques[29] indicated that the water in amniotic fluid is replaced every 2.9 h. It is uncertain what mechanism regulates the maintenance of amniotic fluid volume within these limits. Amniotic fluid volume increases in response to maternal hydration with hypotonic fluid[30–32], in conjunction with a decrease in fetal plasma osmolality and increased fetal urination. Fetal hydration with large volumes of isotonic fluid[33] or hypertonic saline solution[34] also leads to increases in fetal urination and amniotic fluid volume, but not to fetal hydrops, because fluid infused also crosses the placenta and enters the maternal circulation, with a high filtration coefficient. Diuretic infusion into the fetus causes a dose-dependent increase in fetal arterial pressure[35]. Apparently, the subsequent increases in fetal urination and amniotic fluid volume are mediated through these increases in fetal arterial pressure.

METHODS OF CLINICAL AMNIOTIC FLUID ANALYSIS

Study of amniotic fluid in normal and abnormal conditions has revealed that components of amniotic fluid are altered in a number of pregnancy abnormalities. This has formed the basis for devising diagnostic tests for confirmation and for following the progress of abnormal conditions in pregnancy (see Table 5).

In clinical settings, it is parsimonious to utilize a non-invasive method in preference to an invasive method to answer specific questions. This chapter will consider both approaches.

Table 5 *Conditions amenable to amniotic fluid analysis*

Karyotypic abnormality
Genetic abnormality
Oligohydramnios
Polyhydramnios
Structural abnormality
Hemolytic anemia
Diabetes
Multiple gestation
Preterm labor
Infection
Rupture of membranes
Pulmonary hypoplasia
Prematurity
Growth retardation
Postmaturity
Hypoxemia or acidosis
Hemorrhage
Embolism
Meconium passage
Drug levels

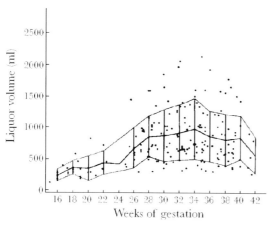

Figure 2 *Amniotic fluid volumes in normal pregnancies by the para-aminohippurate method. (From Reference 27)*

Non-invasive methods

Non-invasive methods of amniotic fluid analysis at present are divided into those that utilize some energy source to define the physical characteristics of the fluid when access is limited by the abdominal wall, closed cervix and intact membranes, and those in the limited situation of physical, biochemical and microbial analysis of fluid obtained vaginally with rupture of membranes.

Physical examination

An experienced practitioner can sometimes gain an estimate of the quantity of amniotic fluid by palpation of the abdomen[36]. This is enhanced when the abdominal wall is thin, and is impeded by central obesity. Fundal height is a typical semi-quantitative adjunct to the clinical assessment of fluid volume. Decreased fundal height leads to a suspicion of oligohydramnios, intrauterine growth retardation (IUGR), or both. Increased fundal height leads to a suspicion of polyhydramnios, macrosomia, or both. As a consequence, the practitioner can formulate a hypothesis regarding the presence of abnormal quantities of amniotic fluid, either oligohydramnios or polyhydramnios. Detection of these abnormalities is the simplest goal of amniotic fluid analysis.

The significance of abnormal quantities of amniotic fluid lies in anecdotal observations of fetal outcome in association with the observation of abnormalities of fluid volume during labor when membranes are ruptured. Thus, abnormal quantities of amniotic fluid have been associated with antepartum, intrapartum and neonatal demise and morbidity. It has been the objective of individuals developing methods of amniotic fluid analysis to convert these anecdotal observations into systematic observations that can be reproduced and utilized to predict and then avoid perinatal death and morbidity.

X-ray

Amniotic fluid is translucent to X-rays. Radiographs were used early to gather indirect evidence of amniotic fluid quantity. Thus, radiographs or fluoroscopy showing a fetus compressed and immobile were compatible with decreased fluid, and those showing the fetus lying in a large radiolucent oval were compatible with excess fluid. As the dangers of fluoroscopic exposure became better known, such analyses were replaced with newer methods imparting less energy to the fetus.

Computerized tomography

Similar indirect conclusions about amniotic fluid volume can be drawn from images generated by computed tomography (CT) equipment. However, such a use for CT has not become popular, partly because the radiation associated with CT is not thought warranted, and because the problem of fetal movement obscuring interpretation has yet to be solved. An estimate of amniotic fluid volume can be obtained in the course of performing CT pelvimetry for evaluation of breech presentation for vaginal delivery[37,38], but is not the main objective of this evaluation.

Magnetic resonance imaging

Magnetic resonance imaging (MRI) has also not become a popular method of analyzing amniotic fluid. MRI has the theoretical advantage of the absence of ionizing radiation, although the problem of movement is even less ready to be solved in this modality. Nevertheless, anticipated improvements in this technology, combined with its ability to generate an image in three axes (see Figures 3 and 4) and potentially in a three-dimensional display, may make MRI the imaging modality of the future.

Nuclear medicine

Radionuclides have not been utilized in the analysis of amniotic fluid, due to worries about potential teratogenicity and carcinogenicity for the fetus. In addition, imaging systems have the same difficulties dealing with fetal movement as do CT and MRI.

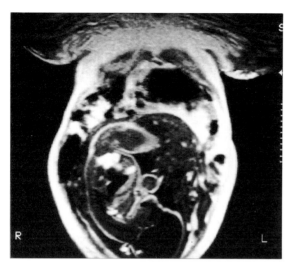

Figure 3 *Magnetic resonance image of 36-week pregnancy showing fetus in sagittal section at level of ductus arteriosus, surrounded by amniotic fluid. (Courtesy of Dr Allah Rosenblit, Department of Radiology, Montefiore Medical Center)*

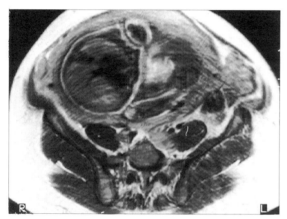

Figure 4 *Magnetic resonance image of 36-week pregnancy showing fetus in transverse section at level of four-chamber view of the heart, with surrounding amniotic fluid obscured by motion artefact. (Courtesy of Dr Allah Rosenblit, Department of Radiology, Montefiore Medical Center)*

Sonography

Since ultrasonic energy delivered with the power proven useful for imaging has not been shown to be theoretically or practically harmful to the fetus, this imaging modality has gained huge popularity in non-invasive amniotic fluid analysis. While the images have a disadvantage in resolution with current technology compared with CT and MRI, there is a considerable advantage gained since the advent of real-time imaging technology, analogous to the advantage of fluoroscopy over conventional radiographs. Thus, fluid can be imaged instantaneously, eliminating artifact due to fetal movement. Nevertheless, the older B-mode technology allowed imaging of the entire uterus in two dimensions, which is no longer possible with linear, curvilinear or sector arrays. Thus, B-mode lent itself to calculation of a figure for total intrauterine volume and total uterine volume, which were among the first semi-quantitative approaches to analyzing amniotic fluid volume with ultrasound[39,40].

Imaging fluid with ultrasound is based on the principle that fluid has virtually complete through-sound-transmission and forms a sharp acoustic interface with tissue. Thus, on sonographic images, amniotic fluid appears dark in contrast to bright tissue echoes and is well demarcated, except when it underlies structures with significant acoustic shadowing or scattering, such as bone, uterine leiomyomata or a thick maternal pannus. Thus in some patients, and in some fetal positions, portions of amniotic fluid are poorly visualized, leading to errors in the estimation of fluid volume. In addition, the measurements possible for amniotic fluid pockets are crude in comparison with the complicated geometric shapes of those pockets, leading to further error.

Subjective amniotic fluid volume Crowley[41] described qualitative assessment of amniotic fluid volume based on an intuitive integration by the sonographic examiner of all the images of amniotic fluid pockets seen in the vicinity of the fetal limbs, a kind of real-time Gestalt, comparable to the total intrauterine volume. Perinatal morbidity was greater in post-date patients if fluid was considered reduced or absent. Manning and associates[42] combined subjective estimates of amniotic fluid volume with a semi-quantitative measure. Oligohydramnios was diagnosed if there was no pocket of amniotic fluid greater than 1 cm in depth and a distinct impression of crowding. Of 31 fetuses, 26 (84%) meeting these criteria were growth retarded. Hill and colleagues[43] found the incidence of oligohydramnios in a prospectively screened, unselected population over 27 weeks to be 0.43% using these criteria. If a subjective decrease in amniotic fluid volume for gestational age were used, instead of the semiquantitative criteria, the sensitivity and specificity were 50% and 100% respectively, in detecting IUGR. Benson and co-workers[44] recommended adding blood pressure and estimated fetal weight to subjective amniotic fluid volume, in a Bayesian approach to improve the prediction of IUGR. Similarly, polyhydramnios has been assessed using subjective criteria. Damato and colleagues[45] recently reported a series of patients with polyhydramnios determined subjectively by the sonographic examiner, and the association with anomalies increased in relation to the impression of the severity of the polyhydramnios.

1-cm Pocket Subjective methods, although claimed to be quite accurate, have given way to various semi-quantitative measures thought to reflect amniotic fluid volume. Manning's description of the biophysical profile (BPP) utilized a maximal pocket depth found in two perpendicular planes throughout the uterus of less than 1 cm to define oligohydramnios[42], and correlated this with fetal and neonatal outcome. He found a maximal pocket of 1 cm or less correlated with poor outcome regardless of the status of the dynamic parameters of the BPP, which can be influenced by behavioral state[46]. Other reports[47–52] on oligohydramnios utilized this 1-cm-pocket definition.

2-cm Pocket Chamberlain and associates[53] showed that outcome was intermediate for individuals with a maximal pocket between 1 and 2 cm and good for individuals with a pocket greater than 2 cm. Lin and co-workers[54] utilized a 2-cm pocket in defining oligohydramnios in association with IUGR. Oligohydramnios developed a mean of 2 weeks after IUGR was suspected on the basis of an abdominal circumference less than the 10th centile.

3-cm Pocket Crowley and associates[55] revised their definition of oligohydramnios to include a maximal pocket 3 cm or less. This definition was utilized by Bochner and colleagues[56] and Cruz and colleagues[57] in evaluating the morbidity associated with oligohydramnios, and is widely used in Europe. Recently, Fischer and co-workers[58], using receiver-operating characteristic curve (ROCC) analysis, showed that a 2.7-cm or smaller pocket was optimal for predicting abnormal perinatal outcome (see below).

8-cm Pocket Chamberlain and associates[53] found a maximal pocket greater than 8 cm in only 3.2% of referred high-risk patients and used this as a definition of excessive fluid on sonographic imaging.

Four-quadrant sum of pockets Rutherford and colleagues[59] correlated a summation of four standardized measurements of maximal pocket size in the four abdominal quadrants, termed the amniotic fluid index (AFI), with various measures of fetal outcome. Outcome was worse when the AFI summed less than 5.1 cm, intermediate when it lay between 5.1 and 8 cm, and good between 8.1 and 18 cm. Over 18 cm was a rare finding, and was associated with increased Cesarean delivery rate. Carlson and co-workers[60] found an AFI of 24 cm or more to be associated with serious fetal structural defects

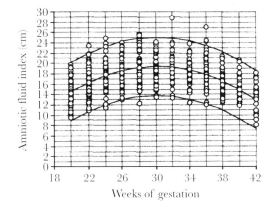

Figure 5 *Range of amniotic fluid index in two groups of women followed longitudinally throughout pregnancy at 4 week intervals, with superimposed curve of the mean ± 2 standard deviations. (From Reference 62)*

and/or death. Moore and Cayle[61] analyzed the AFI of 791 referred patients with normal outcomes to generate a table of normal values. These data were generated cross-sectionally from single measurements in women referred for antepartum testing or sonography. An AFI of 6.2 cm was at the 2.5th centile and an AFI of 5.5 cm was at the 1.0st centile in term patients (5.6 cm was at the 1.0th centile in post-term patients). Recently, Nwosu and associates[62] described the AFI in 105 normal women divided into two equal groups, and followed longitudinally throughout pregnancy (see Figure 5). Superposition of Nwosu's reference range on Moore's dataset shows the mean and lower limit of AFI were raised in comparison with Moore's data in Nwosu's group of normal women followed longitudinally (see Figure 6).

Cord- or limb-containing pockets There has been some controversy over whether to include pockets containing umbilical cord in the AFI. Rutherford and colleagues[59] ignored 'brief appearances of cord or extremity' but excluded parts of fluid pockets containing an 'aggregation of either one' in their definition. Subsequently, Moore and Cayle[61] included only pockets completely clear of cord or extremities. Sadovsky[63], utilizing Rutherford's definition of AFI, assessed the outcome of women with an AFI no greater than 5 cm, who also had an additional cord-containing pocket larger than 5 cm. Perinatal risk in these women was lower than in women with a smaller cord-containing pocket. Sadovsky speculated that the need for intervention might be reduced if a cord-containing pocket larger than 5 cm were present.

Comparison of maximal vertical pocket with AFI
Youssef and colleagues[64] found that the AFI improved the sensitivity and positive predictive value of the BPP. However, doubt remains whether maximum vertical pocket (MVP) or AFI is the best sonographic predictor of amniotic fluid volume. A number of authors have compared the AFI with the MVP[58,65–69]. Moore[65] showed a correlation of 0.51 between AFI and MVP. Hoskins and associates[69] reported no accurate correlation, but did not report the R-value. Fischer and co-workers[58] compared AFI and MVP utilizing ROCC analysis. The curve for MVP had a much more ideal characteristic than the flattened curve for AFI. The maximum utility of MVP occurred at a cut-off volume of 2.7 cm. The sensitivity of MVP at this cut-off volume (using fetal outcome as a substitute for the 'gold standard' of clinical oligohydramnios), was 50% and the specificity was 87.9%, somewhat better than they found for an AFI cut-off value of 5 cm.

Three studies compared AFI with MVP using dye dilution studies. Dildy and colleagues[66] found large percentage errors for both measures. Croom and associates[67] found the AFI slightly better in reflecting dye-determined amniotic fluid volume. Magann and associates[68] found the two moderately accurate in identifying normal fluid and hydramnios, but not in identifying oligohydramnios. Magann's group also described a two-diameter pocket obtained as the product of the vertical and horizontal measurements of the largest pocket of amniotic fluid. This proved superior to AFI in detecting oligohydramnios. The optimal two-diameter pocket cut-off was found to be 15 cm^2 by ROCC analysis utilizing dye-dilution studies as the gold standard for amniotic fluid volume. Recently,

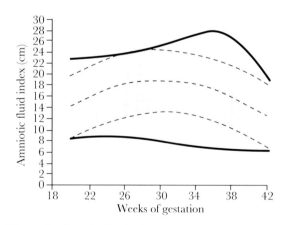

Figure 6 *Longitudinal reference range of amniotic fluid index (AFI) in normal patients (from reference 62 - shaded area) superimposed on the cross-sectional reference range in normal referred patients (from reference 61 – open area). Heavy lines[61], mean ± 2 SD; thin, dashed lines[62], mean ± 2 SD*

Chauhan and associates[70] and Ross[71] pointed out that selecting the ROCC of one test as superior to another was inappropriate without statistical analysis showing the two curves were not different by chance alone. Thus, the conclusions[58,68] regarding superiority of one method over another may not be valid, since this statistical analysis is not presented.

Correlation of AFI with clinical oligohydramnios
Absent from any of these studies were attempts to correlate sonographic measurements with the actual quantity of fluid observed at rupture of membranes. As noted by Druzin and Adams[72], this finding is consistent with oligohydramnios and subsequent meconium staining, as well as with increased perinatal morbidity. Recently, we have generated a ROCC for AFI, comparing it with oligohydramnios as perceived by the patient's care-giver at the time of rupture of membranes (Figure 7). The sensitivity and specificity of a 5-cm or smaller pocket in predicting oligohydramnios were 63% and 86%, respectively. The utility of these functions was maximized at an AFI cut-off of 6.5 cm, but with sensitivity and specificity of only 75% and 78%, respectively, the AFI proved to be less than an ideal test in predicting amniotic fluid volume at delivery.

The three-dye dilution studies corroborated this finding. Dildy and associates[66] found an error of 7% (± SD 38.7%) comparing AFI with dye dilution results, with a 95% confidence interval of −53.9% to 88.7%. Croom and colleagues[67] found a correlation coefficient of 0.753 for AFI compared with dye-determined amniotic fluid volume. Magann and associates[68] found a sensitivity for an AFI of 5 cm in predicting oligohydramnios (less than 500 ml) of 6.7% and a specificity of 100%. For predicting polyhydramnios (over 1500 ml) with an AFI over 18 cm, the specificity and sensitivity were 83.3% and 85.3%, respectively. The two-dimensional pocket performed slightly better in predicting oligohydramnios (60% and 84%, respectively), but not as well with polyhydramnios (50% and 97%, respectively).

Variability in AFI measurement Moore and Cayle[61] found a 5.0 mm ± 1.2 mm intraobserver error, and a 9.7 mm ± 0.7 mm interobserver error in the measurement of AFI. Bruner and associates[73] found that the coefficient of variation for amniotic fluid index measurements varied from 10.8% within examiners to 15.4% between examiners. Nwosu and co-workers[62] found the intraobserver error for AFI measurements done twice at one sitting, separated by 15 min, by a single observer to be 8% in either direction. Wax and co-workers[74] found that three discrete episodes of fetal movement changed the AFI by 1.5 cm with a single observer and 2.5 cm with a blinded second observer, and that these changes could be accounted for simply on the basis of interobserver and intraobserver variation.

Clinical outcome after normal or low AFI
Hoskins and associates[75] evaluated a subset of antepartum-tested patients with severe decelerations and an amniotic fluid index less than 5 cm. These patients had significantly increased rates of neonatal acidosis and low Apgar scores. AFI was part of the antepartum evaluation in

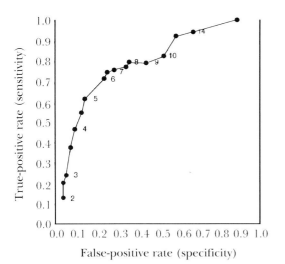

Figure 7 *Receiver operating characteristic curve of amniotic fluid index (AFI) as a diagnostic test for the clinical outcome of oligohydramnios as perceived by the patient's care-giver at the time of rupture of membranes. Numbers to the right of points forming the line correspond to the cut-off value for AFI at that point*

16 191 women at Los Angeles County/University of Southern California Medical Center Women's Hospital, reported by Grubb[76]. 8038 women were tested only because of post-dates. The fetal death rate with AFI over 5.0 cm and a reactive non-stress test (NST), or BPP of 8, was 1.12 per 1000. She also reported that when an AFI less then 2.0 cm was associated with antepartum fetal heart rate (FHR) decelerations, indices of perinatal morbidity, including Cesarean section for fetal distress, meconium passage and 1-min Apgar score less than 7, were increased. All patients were delivered who had an AFI less than 5.1 cm. However, Lagrew and colleagues[78] followed 107 patients with AFI less than 5.1 cm for 4 to 7 days, and found a reversion to low-normal or normal values in 41% of these patients. Although they raised the question whether intervention for AFI less than 5.1 was appropriate, their study was not designed to answer this question directly. Nevertheless, they recommended evaluation for delivery in term and post-term patients with AFI less than 5.1 cm. Petrikovsky and co-workers[79] found that fetal acoustic stimulation increased the percentage of time a fetus spent in swallowing. Of fetuses with borderline AFI, 41% developed oligohydramnios following acoustic stimulation, and two developed persistent variable decelerations requiring operative intervention. Zimmer and associates[80] found vibro-acoustic stimulation caused the fetus to empty its bladder, which could potentially lead to an increase in AFI. Pearce and McFarland[81] found amniotic fluid determinations combined with umbilical artery Doppler waveforms an adequate method of monitoring post-date patients. However, others have found Doppler studies less useful in the evaluation of post-date patients and rely instead on the model developed at USC based on NST and AFI.

Dynamics of amniotic fluid volume The dynamics of amniotic fluid have been followed with ultrasound. Weinbaum and colleagues[82] and Clement and colleagues[83] noted the abrupt development of oligohydramnios in post-date patients over the course of 24 h. Trimmer and associates[51] compared the dynamics of bladder filling in post-term patients with and without oligohydramnios by the 1-cm pocket criterion and found fewer bladder cycles, a longer bladder filling time and decreased fetal urine production in post-term patients with oligohydramnios. Arduini and Rizzo[84] found an inverse linear relationship between AFI and renal artery pulsatility index (PI) normalized for gestational age. Growth-retarded fetuses showed a higher PI than controls, and the difference was increased as amniotic fluid declined. However, post-term fetuses showed no significant correlation between amniotic fluid volume and renal artery PI. Marks and Divon[85] demonstrated a decline in AFI with increasing gestational age in post-date patients followed with serial semi-weekly testing. However, there was considerable scatter about this trend line. Lagrew and colleagues[78] followed up 7393 patients within 4 days and found a 2.6% chance of developing oligohydramnios in patients at 41 or more weeks' gestation who had initial AFI between 8 and 15 cm, and a 5% chance if the previous AFI was 5 to 8 cm, i.e. in the low-normal range.

Intrapartum screening for amniotic fluid volume
When AFI was used as a screening test for unselected or normal patients intrapartum, Sarno and co-workers[86] found an AFI of 5 cm or less was a risk factor for perinatal morbidity. Teoh and associates[87] also found measurement of amniotic fluid volume in early labor a useful admission test. However, when Sarno[88] evaluated fetal heart-rate decelerations after acoustic stimulation in the latent phase of labor, he found that the AFI played an insignificant role in the genesis of the decelerations. The physiological mechanism of variable decelerations can either be on the basis of cord compression or head compression[89]. The latter may have dominated Sarno's study, resulting in poor predictive value for AFI, since only the former type of decelerations are likely to be produced on the basis of low amniotic fluid volume.

The distribution of amniotic fluid at the onset of labor is apparently related to perinatal outcome. Myles and Strassner[90] found a worse perinatal outcome when the sum of the two upper pockets of fluid was greater than the sum of the two lower pockets, when the AFI was measured on admission for labor.

Saunders and co-workers screened 101 women about to undergo induction of labor[91] and found marked oligohydramnios in five of seven women delivered by emergency Cesarean section early in the first stage of labor for significant abnormality of the fetal heart-rate trace. These seven women had fetuses with small abdominal circumference. If amniotic fluid was normal, small or average-sized babies tended to be born spontaneously, while large babies had a greater risk of operative delivery. Robson and associates[92] compared women with an AFI of 6.5 cm or more after rupture of membranes to women with an AFI less than 6.2 cm. Women in the latter group had a higher incidence of fetal heart-rate abnormalities in the first stage of labor, meconium at delivery, and operative delivery for fetal distress. Crawford and co-workers found screening for oligohydramnios useful in deciding whether patients with gastroschisis could undergo vaginal delivery[93].

Multiple gestation and amniotic fluid volume
Normal values for sonographic amniotic fluid volume have not been reported in twins. However, generally some variation of the largest pocket of amniotic fluid is used, ideally with visualization of a membrane separating the two pockets. The extremes of amniotic fluid volume abnormality are seen in the 'stuck-twin' phenomenon. Frequently the membrane cannot be visualized or is seen tightly adherent to one twin that remains relatively fixed to the uterine wall in one position, even with changes in maternal position. The other twin may demonstrate polyhydramnios. This situation may be missed, unless a meticulous search for the membrane is made. Its absence must be connected to a suspicion of oligohydramnios in one twin, the stuck twin, and rigorous attempts must be made to demonstrate fetal movement away from the uterine wall. If this cannot be demonstrated, one must conclude that severe oligohydramnios is present, and the twins must be evaluated for possible delivery. Recently, the role of amniocentesis in managing this problem has been investigated[94,95], as discussed below.

Particulate analysis in amniotic fluid Attempts have been made to assess sonographically the presence of vernix caseosa and meconium as particulates in amniotic fluid. However, the two cannot be reliably distinguished by sonography. Homogeneous echogenic amniotic fluid is also not correlated with meconium staining at delivery[96].

Use of amniotic fluid volume in monitoring polyhydramnios Polyhydramnios is associated with fetal anomalies, and leads to preterm labor and preterm premature rupture of the membranes (PROM). It should be suspected if size is greater than dates, the uterus feels distended and the fetus is poorly felt or very mobile on palpation. A sonogram showing a single pocket of amniotic fluid greater than 8 cm or an AFI of 24 cm or more is indicative of probable polyhydramnios. Twins can develop polyhydramnios in association with the twin–twin transfusion syndrome discussed above.

Polyhydramnios is associated with immune hydrops and warrants re-examination of the Coombs test on maternal blood for previously undetected isoimmunization. Polyhydramnios has been associated with diabetes[97,98]. However, in a recent paper, Girz and associates[99] were unable to confirm this association in a controlled study, although there was an association between birth weight and AFI. Similarly, in a recent sonographic series of 130 patients with polyhydramnios[45], only five had diabetes and each of these had an additional fetal anomaly explaining the polyhydramnios. The improved control of diabetes and detection of anomalies may account for the lower incidence of polyhydramnios among diabetics suggested by these studies in comparison with older series.

Anomalies associated with polyhydramnios include those affecting the central nervous system, the skeleton, the gastrointestinal tract, the respiratory tract and the genitourinary tract[45].

The syndrome of non-immune hydrops is also associated with polyhydramnios. Thus, confirmation of polyhydramnios ultrasonographically should prompt the search for other anomalies. Should these be found, the risk of a chromosomal anomaly may be as high as 27%[60]. Even when the anatomical survey is normal and glucose screening and antibody screening are normal, the risk of chromosomal abnormality was as high as 3.2% in an unselected population[100]. This incidence is much higher than the incidence of chromosomal abnormality found in women over the age of 35, for whom genetic screening is recommended. Consequently, a recommendation for study of fetal karyotype is warranted in all cases of polyhydramnios, if the same criteria are applied.

One modality of treatment for polyhydramnios is the use of prostaglandin synthetase inhibitors, such as indomethacin[101,102]. The mechanism is uncertain, but fetal urinary flow is known to decrease. Moise and associates[103] have followed patients on indomethacin therapy with serial echocardiograms, because of the risk of reversible ductal closure. Serial measurements of amniotic fluid volume are necessary as well, to follow fetal renal function and determine an end-point of therapy. Besinger and colleagues[104] found pulmonary hypertension in several newborns treated with indomethacin for a prolonged period of time. Because of the complexity of treatment and attendant complications, the use of indomethacin therapy should be considered only for the symptomatic patient.

Vaginal collection after spontaneous rupture of membranes

Amniotic fluid obtained after spontaneous rupture of membranes (SROM) may be assessed directly with a variety of biochemical tests, including those that confirm its identity. These tests are of particular value when the membranes rupture without associated labor. This is referred to as PROM, since it is most usual for membranes to rupture in the course and as a consequence of labor. Sonographic assessment continues to have value.

Amniotic fluid volume If the rupture is observed, its volume may be estimated by an experienced clinician as normal, increased, decreased or absent. Increased amniotic fluid suggests polyhydramnios, including the differential diagnoses of diabetes, gastrointestinal obstruction, neurological abnormality and trisomy, among others[105]. Decreased amniotic fluid suggests oligohydramnios, including the differential diagnoses of urinary tract obstruction, occult prior rupture of membranes, acute or chronic oliguria due to uteroplacental insufficiency, absent kidneys and trisomy, among others[106].

Visual inspection Visual inspection can lead to a number of hypotheses regarding pathological processes in the fetus. Amniotic fluid can be observed qualitatively as clear, vernix-bearing, meconium-stained, cloudy, purulent, foul-smelling, bloody, brown or yellow. The presence of vernix signifies a fetus likely to have lung maturity and not to be post-date. Meconium staining signifies a fetus late in gestation, passing meconium physiologically, or earlier in gestation, passing meconium in response to some vagal stimulus, such as hypoxia. Cloudy fluid may contain bacteria, yeast, white blood cells, or mucus. Purulent fluid contains the infectious elements in greater quantity and may or may not be foul-smelling from some particular product of bacterial metabolism or necrosis. Bloody fluid should suggest possible abruption, or marginal placental separation, if it is not the typical blood-tinged mucus of the bloody show seen at the onset of labor. Brown fluid may contain oxidized breakdown products of old blood or meconium and should bring to mind abruption and fetal hypoxia. Yellow fluid may contain excess amounts of fetal bilirubin from hemolytic disease such as Rh(D) sensitization or of maternal bilirubin from hepatitis or biliary obstruction.

Meconium

Meconium may be gauged as grade III, or thick or spreadable; grade II, or moderate or opaque with particulate meconium; or grade I, or thin or light or greenish-tinged but translucent. The amniotic fluid may be centrifuged to separate the particulate phase from fluid and the amount of particulates quantitated in an analogy with the hematocrit measurement. With meconium, this would be the 'meconium-crit'[107]. The grade or thickness of meconium relates to the degree of associated oligohydramnios. It is probably the intermittent hypoxia and pulmonary vascular hyperplasia associated with oligohydramnios that gives the more ominous prognosis to thick meconium than the chemical or mechanical properties of meconium itself, according to Katz and Bowes[108].

Hematocrit
If the sample is grossly bloody, an hematocrit can estimate the amount of blood present. An abruption should immediately be suspected and preparations should be made for transfusion, monitoring of maternal vital signs, fetal heart-rate monitoring, blood studies for disseminated intravascular coagulation, and most likely delivery.

Ferning The vaginally collected pool can be observed for ferning, a typical microscopic pattern seen when amniotic fluid dries on a slide[109]. Ferning should be evaluated only if a sample is obtained from an obvious vaginal pool, since cervical mucus and semen also produce a ferning pattern on drying that can be indistinguishable from that seen with amniotic fluid. Rosemond and colleagues[110] found that blood may inhibit ferning and give a false-negative test.

Cell content It is not possible reliably to discern infection of amniotic fluid when collected vaginally because the vagina typically contains large numbers of white blood cells and bacteria identical to those expected from chorioamnionitis. However, as noted above, continuous emergence of purulent, foul-smelling amniotic fluid in quantity sufficient to wash the vagina out should prompt investigation for chorioamnionitis. Cell content is seldom analyzed on a vaginal specimen, because of the problem of contamination with vaginal elements noted above.

pH The pH can also be measured on a vaginal pool. Typically the vagina has a pH of less than 5, while amniotic fluid has a pH greater than 7, that is, close to the physiological pH of 7.4 seen in tissue. Urine, however, if infected with urea-splitting organisms, can have a pH greater than 7, and the differential diagnosis for ruptured membranes late in pregnancy typically includes the involuntary passage of urine, which can appear as a vaginal pool. Bloody show also may give a false-positive test, as blood has an alkaline pH.

Phospholipids The vaginal pool, if determined by these simple tests to be amniotic fluid, can be sent for analysis for fetal lung maturity if it is in question. A number of tests have been designed to look for the evidence of fetal lung function in amniotic fluid. This is because the fetal respiratory tract contributes to the significantly to the volume of amniotic fluid. Lamellar bodies and phospholipid components of pulmonary surfactant can be found in amniotic fluid. In fact, the rescue of preterm fetuses from respiratory distress syndrome is performed using surfactant recovered from bovine amniotic fluid. The physiology[111] and immunogenic structure[112] of human surfactant obtained from amniotic fluid is being analyzed. Human lung surfactant protein D cDNA has been cloned[113] and will become valuable in the study of surfactant pathophysiology in prematurity.

A variety of tests that reflect fetal lung maturity have been developed over the past years, the most common being measurement of the lecithin/sphingomyelin (L/S) ratio[114] and analysis for the presence of phosphatidyl glycerol. An L/S ratio of 2.5 or larger in the non-diabetic patient, and the presence of phosphatidyl glycerol in the diabetic, are predictive of fetal lung maturity. Newer tests promise both speed and accuracy relative to these standards[115–123].

An immature L/S ratio may be associated with congenital hypothyroidism[124]. Analysis of

L/S ratios and saturated phosphatidylcholine levels in fetuses exposed *in utero* to maternal cigarette smoke demonstrated earlier lung maturity than non-exposed fetuses, occurring by an abnormal developmental process that may contribute to decreased lung function and the increased respiratory illness seen in these infants[125].

Use of amniotic fluid volume in evaluation of PROM
A normal amniotic fluid volume (AFV) cannot rule out PROM, nor does a low AFI confirm PROM. However, measurement of AFV has been useful in establishing the prognosis in PROM. Vintzileos and associates[126] have shown that a normal AFV in PROM is associated with a longer latent period and less perinatal morbidity and mortality, including fewer Cesarean sections and better Apgar scores. A low AFV is more likely to be associated with chorioamnionitis[126,127]. A low AFV had sensitivity and specificity for predicting amnionitis and neonatal infection similar to that of the Gram stain and amniotic fluid culture in preterm PROM[128]. However, abnormalities of the daily non-stress test identified clinically significant lower fluid volumes among patients with low amniotic fluid volume after rupture of membranes[129]. Fetal weight estimates are frequently difficult in the presence of oligohydramnios, as the boundary of the abdominal circumference is difficult to visualize. However, Toohey and co-workers[130] found estimated fetal weight calculations in patients with preterm PROM as accurate as those in patients in preterm labor with normal amniotic fluid volume. Clinical judgement is required to balance the risk of premature delivery with the risk of subclinical chorioamnionitis presented by an asymptomatic patient with a decreased AFV.

Preterm PROM and pulmonary hypoplasia Pulmonary hypoplasia is thought to be associated with oligohydramnios at a time of active lung differentiation, particularly at gestational ages of less than 24 weeks. However, Thibeault and colleagues131 have shown that prolonged PROM may be associated with pulmonary hypoplasia in as little as 6 days, and with little or no deformation, at gestational ages of less than or equal to 34 weeks. Sonographically determined amniotic fluid volume was the most predictive parameter for pulmonary hypoplasia[132]. Outcome was better in preterm PROM without oligohydramnios[133]. Serial thoracic abdominal circumference ratios predicted pulmonary hypoplasia, and persistent oligohydramnios was associated with lethal pulmonary hypoplasia in six fetuses, and pulmonary complications in the remaining two[134]. However, recently, regression analysis has suggested that gestational age at onset of rupture of membranes has a significant effect on development of pulmonary hypoplasia, while duration of PROM and degree of oligohydramnios do not[135]. It is interesting that hypertensive patients exposed to angiotensin-converting enzyme inhibitors in the second and third trimesters developed oligohydramnios, but their fetuses survived, apparently without pulmonary hypoplasia[136], if dialysis was instituted at birth.

In an experimental model, chronic pharyngeal drainage did not impair lung development in fetal sheep[137]. This model mimicked low amniotic fluid pressure at the level of the upper airway in the presence of normal amniotic fluid volume, thus arguing against an effect of lowered airway pressure in the development of oligohydramnios. In another experimental model, it was found that lung maturation was normal only in the presence of both intact kidneys and amniotic fluid[138]. Lung growth and structural maturity were dissociated in the presence of structurally damaged kidneys. When amniotic fluid was normal, growth was normal but maturation was impaired. Amniotic fluid activity of N-acetyl-β-D-glucosaminidase was elevated in the presence of kidney damage[139] and may serve as an assay of renal impairment. It is uncertain what role renal abnormalities play in the development of pulmonary hypoplasia associated with preterm PROM, or what causes some patients to develop oligohydramnios with preterm PROM while others maintain minimally reduced or normal amniotic fluid volumes. Finally, it is uncertain what causes some patients with preterm PROM to regain amniotic fluid and stop leaking, apparently 'resealing' the membranes[140].

Culture Culture of vaginally collected amniotic fluid is likely to yield cervical, vaginal or rectal organisms, and may not reflect the presence of intra-amniotic organisms. Some vaginal organisms are nevertheless considered pathogenic. Prophylactic therapy to prevent ascending Group B streptococcal infection is still controversial[141–144]. It is of interest that cultures for Group B streptococci (GBS) are more likely to be falsely negative after rupture of membranes[145]. This supports the recommendations of Boyer and Gotoff[146] that effective prevention of GBS disease requires universal culturing at 28 weeks, prior to the onset of preterm labor or PROM.

Invasive methods

Amnioscopy/fetoscopy/embryoscopy

Amnioscopy (visual inspection of the amniotic cavity through an endoscope) has waned in popularity until recently. It has been used to assess amniotic fluid for the presence of meconium and to allow access to the fetus for intrauterine transfusions and skin biopsies. A form of amnioscope is used commonly after membrane rupture to sample fetal scalp blood. More recently, Cullen and associates[147] and Reece and colleagues[148] have explored the use of fetoscopy and embryoscopy, using a vascular endoscope to puncture the chorion and observe the embryo or fetus and surrounding amniotic fluid through the intact amnion. One disturbing result of these investigations was the observation of petechiae covering the skin of fetuses immediately following first-trimester chorionic villus sampling[149].

Amniocentesis

Amniocentesis involves puncture of the amniotic membrane and removal of amniotic fluid for analysis, or instillation into the amniotic cavity of substances that are subsequently analyzed.

Today, amniocentesis is almost universally performed with real-time sonographic guidance of the needle into an appropriate pocket of amniotic fluid. With the precision of this method, it is possible to obtain samples of fluid from pockets as small as 1 cm. The maternal risks of amniocentesis are, rarely, significant infection or blood loss. Occasionally, fetal loss is experienced, due to infection or rupture of membranes at a pre-viable stage. Fetal loss is typically quoted as 0.5%, but is probably much less than this, particularly when amniocentesis is performed in the third trimester.

Dye dilution The instillation of dye into the amniotic cavity can have a number of purposes. In the past, amniography, or the infusion of radio-opaque substances into the amniotic cavity, followed by radiography or fluoroscopy, was used to assess anomalies of fluid, placenta or fetus. Sutter and co-workers[150] used such an approach to confirm monoamnionic twinning. Methylene blue is now avoided, because of its association with methemoglobinemia and hemolysis in the fetus[151]. Indigo carmine can be infused in a search for occult rupture of membranes, shown by the vaginal appearance of the dye. Caution must be exercised by looking for the emergence of the dye within 15 min, and in high concentration, as the dye is rapidly passed transplacentally and appears in maternal urine and vaginal transudates. This dye can also be infused as a marker for a sac previously entered in attempts to sample each sac of a multiple gestation. If dye is observed on fluid withdrawal at a subsequent puncture, it signifies that this sac has been sampled previously. Dye can also be infused into the amniotic cavity, mixed with the amniotic fluid by maternal position change, and withdrawn again in dilute form, to assess the volume of amniotic fluid. This is not performed routinely, but forms the basis for many research studies of amniotic fluid dynamics[27,152].

Karyotype and genotype Fetal squamous cells are found suspended in amniotic fluid and will grow in tissue-culture medium if not frozen. This forms the basis for karyotypic analysis of amniotic fluid, which can be performed as early as 11 weeks and is useful up to 10 to 14 days prior to delivery (the time it takes for the analysis), in helping plan the mode of and support needed for delivery[153]. If performed before 22 weeks, it can form the basis of a decision on abortion for genetic reasons. In addition, the information is useful to pediatricians, obstetricians, parents and their counselors at any time during pregnancy. A karyotype is useful in the presence of unexplained growth retardation[154]. Newer methods, such as fluorescence *in situ* hybridization (FISH) can rapidly identify specific karyotypic abnormalities in uncultured cells[155], similar in principle to fetal sex determination by looking for the Barr body and the 'Y-body'[156].

Fetal DNA obtained from cultured amniocytes can be used for DNA hybridization studies to identify carriers of a variety of abnormal genetic material that leads to a variety of genetic diseases such as cystic fibrosis[157,158] and Duchenne muscular dystrophy[159].

Recently, DNA repair measurements in trophoblasts and amniotic cells has allowed prenatal diagnosis of a rare lethal autosomal recessive disease involving defective repair[160]. The abnormal products of numerous inheritable enzymatic blocks can be assayed in amniotic fluid, thus leading to a genetic diagnosis[161–167]. One interesting application of this approach involves congenital adrenal hyperplasia, an autosomal recessive enzymatic defect. Therapy to prevent masculinization of female fetuses with this disease must begin by 7 weeks, too early for accurate genetic diagnosis. Thus, in pregnancies at risk, 7 out of 8 mothers must be treated unnecessarily until the fetal sex can be determined, and 3 out of 4 mothers must be treated unnecessarily even if the sex can be determined unequivocally. The treatment has significant maternal side-effects[168]. Door and Sippell[169] interrupted dexamethasone treatment for 5 days before second-trimester amniocentesis and then measured steroid levels in amniotic fluid. Prenatal diagnosis was possible for both the salt-wasting and simple virilizing forms of congenital adrenal hyperplasia, thus allowing discontinuation of therapy in unaffected pregnancies. Congenital lipoid adrenal hyperplasia, the rarest form of congenital adrenal hyperplasia, has now also been diagnosed prenatally[170].

This information can be used for counseling, planning and decision making, as regard the current pregnancy and future fertility.

Phospholipid Considerations are identical to those noted under the discussion of the analysis of the vaginal pool (see above).

Cells and particulates As noted above, on the contents of the vaginal pool, a variety of simple and widely used tests are available to assess the physical and chemical properties of amniotic fluid. These are seldom used on specimens obtained at amniocentesis, except for cellular analysis. This includes a Wright's stain for leukocytes and a Gram stain for bacteria, which will be discussed below, under infection.

The presence of meconium is an important and worrisome finding at amniocentesis. Romero and colleagues[171] have recently shown that meconium-stained amniotic fluid removed at amniocentesis in the setting of preterm labor has a 33% chance of a positive culture, compared with 11% if the fluid was clear. Altshuler and associates[172] have found meconium-induced umbilical-cord vascular necrosis and ulceration in association with poor neonatal outcome. On the other hand, in post-date patients, meconium passage may be physiologic. This explains why Knox and co-workers[173] found that induction of labor for meconium detected at amniocentesis in prolonged pregnancy did not improve perinatal outcome in comparison with a program of non-intervention, unless the contraction stress test was positive.

The detection of old or unusually large amounts of blood that cannot be accounted for as iatrogenic in origin is also disturbing, suggesting infarction or abruption either remotely or recently, depending on the state of decomposition of the blood. This finding warrants careful sonographic survey of fetal and placental anat-

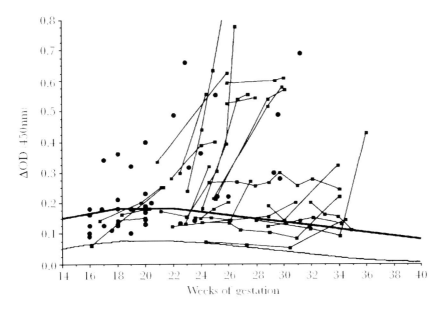

Figure 8 *Amniotic fluid change in optical density (OD) (single circles) and serial (squares) values in fetuses at risk of dying; lower line represents mean values of Rh-negative, unaffected fetuses; upper line represents demarcation of intrauterine-death risk. (Fom Reference 175)*

omy and intensive fetal surveillance if no indication for delivery is found.

Bilirubin Amniocentesis is widely used to assess the amniotic fluid content of fetal urinary bilirubin. The change in optical density observed at a frequency of 450 nm contributed by bilirubin (ΔOD_{450}) is recorded on the Liley curve. Increases in amniotic fluid ΔOD_{450} reflect increasing severity of fetal hemolysis in fetal isoimmune hemolytic disease. Spinnato and co-workers[174] recently examined six methods for assessing amniotic fluid bilirubin. They found the chloroform-extraction method accurately predicted fetal status in 111 samples from 37 patients, while lesser degrees of accuracy were observed with the other five methods.

Recently, Queenan and colleagues[175] (see Figure 8) studied ΔOD_{450} from 14 to 40 weeks in unaffected and affected fetuses. Rather than showing the linear extrapolation of Liley prior to 28 weeks, the normal values of ΔOD_{450} followed a curve that increased steadily until 22 to 26 weeks before decreasing to term. The authors proposed replacement of the extrapolated por-

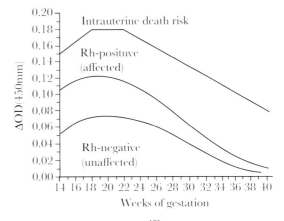

Figure 9 *Queenan's curve[175]: amniotic fluid management zones for change in optical density (OD)*

tions of the Liley curve with a new series of curves that reflect these findings (see Figure 9). Serious complications are unlikely when amniotic fluid ΔOD_{450} values fall in the lower zone or the lower side of the mid-zone of the Liley curve[176]. When bilirubin values fall in the upper mid-zone or upper zone, cordocentesis is warranted. Isoimmunization to Rh(D) antigen is less common now, with the widespread use of

Rh(D) immunoglobulin. Consequently, other blood-group isoimmunization is becoming relatively more common and may have different characteristics in amniotic fluid analysis. For example, Kell isoimmunization can be followed with amniotic fluid bilirubin[177]. It may be as severe as Rh(D) hemolytic disease. However, in one recent series[178], the applicability of the Liley curve for management of patients with Kell isoimmunization has been disputed.

A new approach to the prediction of fetal Rh(D) hemolytic disease involves the analysis of fetal Rh genotype by the amplification by the polymerase chain reaction of fetal Rh(D) gene DNA from amniocytes obtained by amniocentesis[179].

Glucose Another fetal metabolite found in amniotic fluid is glucose. This is elevated in the presence of maternal diabetes and decreased in fetal infection (see below).

Inherited metabolic disorders In recent years, amniotic fluid has been analyzed for the presence of various fetal metabolites excreted in fetal urine and associated with a variety of fetal diseases not amenable to DNA analysis, as noted above under karyotype and genotype.

Growth factors A variety of growth factors have been isolated and characterized over the past several decades[180]. These include insulin, insulin-like growth factors, fibroblast growth factors, hematopoietic colony-stimulating growth factors and epidermal growth factors. These are present in a variety of tissues and biological fluids, including amniotic fluid.

The physiology of insulin-like growth factors (IGF) is currently under investigation in a number of research laboratories. Two species, IGF-I and IGF-II, have been characterized and produced as pure species using recombinant DNA techniques. Current investigations involve characterizing the proteins which bind IGF-I and -II in various biological fluids[181–189].

Amniotic fluid is particularly rich in IGF-binding protein-1. This protein can inhibit DNA synthesis stimulated by IGF-I. In amniotic fluid obtained at second-trimester amniocentesis, elevated levels of IGF-binding protein-1 were found more commonly in women whose fetuses developed growth retardation in the third trimester[190]. In another study[191], cord serum was analyzed for IGF-I, IGF-II, IGF-binding protein-1 and insulin C-peptide at various gestational ages. IGF-I levels were decreased by 40% in small-for-gestational-age newborns, and increased by 28% in large-for-gestational-age newborns, in the absence of diabetes. IGF-I levels correlated best with birth weight. IGF-II concentrations were six- to ten-fold higher than those of IGF-I, and 8 to 10% higher in newborns that were large than in those that were average or small for gestational age. Cord serum C-peptide concentrations were 28% and 34% higher in newborns that were large than in those that were average or small for gestational age respectively. IGF-binding protein-1 levels were increased in preterm average- and in term small-for-gestational-age newborns, compared with term newborns that were average for gestational age. IGF-binding protein-1 showed negative correlation with birth weight.

The function of IGFs and their binding proteins in amniotic fluid or maternal or fetal tissues is not fully elucidated, but the role of this system in fetal growth may have important implications. For example, the regulation of IGF may relate to macrosomia. The importance of this is underscored by the recently reported follow-up of offspring of diabetic mothers to 8 years of age[192]. At birth, 50% were greater than the 90th centile for weight. Although weight was similar to that of the general population by 12 months, the relative weight increased dramatically after 5 years and by 8 years of age, half had weights classified as obese. This obesity correlated with maternal pre-pregnant weight, and independently with amniotic-fluid level of insulin at 32–38 weeks. Since this study was initiated, the role of IGFs as growth regulators *in utero* has begun to be elucidated. Their role in the development of macrosomia and IUGR may soon be explained[193].

Colony stimulating factor-1 (CSF-1) may regulate placental development[194]. It has been detected in human pregnancy in serum, endometrium, placenta, chorion, amnion, and amniotic fluid. The placental source of CSF-1 varies with trimester as the villous circulation matures. This strongly supports a role for CSF-1 in the regulation of placental function by autocrine and/or paracrine mechanisms.

Epidermal growth factor has been isolated and produced in pure form using recombinant technology. It has been injected into amniotic fluid and shown to increase the cytoplasmic volume fraction of lamellar bodies and to elevate the percentage of phosphatidyl glycerol in lung phospholipids[195].

Recently, scarless wound healing has been demonstrated in mammalian fetuses[196,197]. The underlying mechanisms that regulate fetal wound repair are currently not well understood. An altered supply or activity of growth factors may be instrumental. Open wounds do not contract in some species, possibly due to the presence of an inhibitor of wound contraction in amniotic fluid. In other species, wounds do contract, and in sheep this is under the influence of a protein factor found in amniotic fluid. Fetal antigens isolated from amniotic fluid play a role in the healing of adult wounds[198].

α-Fetoprotein α-Fetoprotein is the major serum protein found in fetal blood during early gestation. It is normally found in only tiny amounts in amniotic fluid, from transudation across fetal vessels and placental membranes or fetal skin, or excreted in fetal urine after the majority is reabsorbed in the distal tubules. Consequently, elevated amounts of α-fetoprotein in amniotic fluid signify either some compromise in the integrity of the fetal vascular–dermal barrier, or abnormal kidney function, such as Finnish nephrosis. Many neural tube defects present such a compromise in the dermal–vascular barrier through the meningocele sac, the exposed anencephalic cranium or an encephalocele. Amniotic fluid analysis for elevated α-fetoprotein thus allows detection of neural tube defects as well as a number of other anomalies. Most of these can be visualized sonographically. Amniotic fluid acetylcholinesterase is also elevated in most cases of neural tube defects, since this enzyme is abundant in cerebrospinal fluid. It is also routinely measured along with α-fetoprotein when neural tube defects are suspected.

Measurement of maternal serum α-fetoprotein has become a routine screening test for neural tube defects. When it is inappropriately elevated, analysis for amniotic fluid α-fetoprotein[199,200] and acetylcholinesterase[201] is indicated, as is a sonographic scan targeted for anomalies. Since α-fetoprotein levels in amniotic fluid and extraembryonic celomic fluid follow distinctly different curves of physiological variation during the first trimester[202], it is important to identify the site of first-trimester amniocentesis accurately. In addition to neural tube defects, numerous other anomalies such as omphalocele and gastroschisis are associated with elevated values. Acetylcholinesterase has been used to differentiate between neural tube defects and other anomalies when sonography is inconclusive because of its high concentration in the central nervous system. However, there have been false-positives reported. It may be possible to differentiate neural tube defects from these other anomalies more accurately now with the addition of butyrylcholinesterase analysis in amniotic fluid to rule out a false-positive acetylcholinesterase[200]. Isoelectric focusing of amniotic fluid α-fetoprotein may improve the diagnosis of neural tube defect[203]. Finnish nephrosis should be considered with marked elevations of amniotic fluid of α-fetoprotein and normal acetylcholinesterase[204]. Maternal serum α-fetoprotein levels have been reported to be increased in two patients with congenital hypothyroidism. However, Haddow and colleagues[205] with comment by Cuckle and associates found no general association in reviews of 35 pregnancies affected by congenital hypothyroidism. They concluded it was premature to recommend measuring amniotic-fluid thyroid-stimulating hormone in cases of elevated maternal serum α-fetoprotein.

Folic acid supplementation has been recommended in the prevention of neural-tube defects based on epidemiologic and experimental studies. The mechanism is uncertain. Recently, maternal blood, amniotic fluid and fetal blood folate and vitamin B_{12} levels have been measured in normal pregnancies and eight affected by neural tube defects[206] and no difference was found. This supports the hypothesis that other mechanisms for formation of neural tube defects exist.

Maternal serum α-fetoprotein measurement is now also used as a screen for trisomy 21. The sensitivity has been improved by use of the triple screen, to include unconjugated estriol and hCG. Recently[207], amniotic fluid levels of unconjugated estriol, total estriol, and dehydroepiandrosterone sulfate (DHEAS) have been measured. The amniotic fluid levels of these in affected pregnancies were low, while hCG level was high, suggesting that the abnormal maternal serum levels of unconjugated estriol and hCG in affected pregnancies are due mainly to abnormal fetal–placental synthesis rather than abnormal fetal–maternal transfer.

Amniocentesis and polyhydramnios Amniocentesis to remove excess amniotic fluid has not met with much success, due to the rapid reaccumulation of fluid, since turnover of amniotic fluid is so dynamic (see above). Nevertheless, Mahoney[94] and Urig and associates[95] recently reported some success treating twin–twin transfusion syndrome with amniocentesis, although not without complications. Amniocentesis should be reserved for symptomatic patients only.

Amniotic fluid embolism Because of the reported 50% maternal mortality associated with amniotic fluid embolism[208–210], attempts have been made to identify the component(s) of amniotic fluid responsible for this severe complication of pregnancy. Since subsequent pregnancy in survivors can be normal, Clark[208] concluded that amniotic fluid embolism involves chemically abnormal fluid rather than an abnormal maternal response to chemically normal fluid. In a pregnant-goat model, Hankins and co workers[211] found transient left-ventricular dysfunction accompanied by an acute increase in extravascular lung water and dysoxia only when amniotic fluid containing meconium was infused. There was a pressor effect with all other amniotic fluid infusions, including amniotic fluid that had been filtered and boiled, but no other effect on cardiac function. A monoclonal antibody to an unusual oligosaccharide structure of mucin, characteristic of amniotic fluid and meconium, has been used to detect amniotic fluid embolism in women with a clinical picture suggesting its presence[212]. It is unclear whether this is a causative agent or simply a marker for the presence of amniotic fluid.

Amniotic fluid contains a poorly characterized potent initiator of coagulation[213], which increases with gestational age. Amniotic fluid also contains protein-C-inhibitor antigenic activity[214]. Since absence of protein-C leads to abnormal coagulation, its inhibitor could also play a role in abnormal coagulation. Epithelium-derived fluids, including amniotic fluid, also contain a factor VII-dependent procoagulant activity[215]. Amniotic epithelium stains prominently for plasminogen and plasminogen activators[216], but not for inhibitors of plasminogen activators, while chorionic trophoblast and decidua do stain heavily for the inhibitors. Amniotic fluid contains high inhibitor concentrations measured by immunoreactivity, but low biologic activity. The regulation of this system is thus also likely to involve still another element, an inhibitor of the inhibitor. The malfunction of such a delicately regulated fibrinolytic system in the amniotic fluid and adjoining tissues could well release components into the maternal circulation responsible for the disseminated intravascular coagulation seen in amniotic fluid embolism.

Indicators of amniotic fluid infection Numerous rapid diagnostic tests have been developed to detect microbial invasion of the amniotic cavity.

Culture and other specific tests: Amniotic fluid can be cultured for the presence of aerobic and anaerobic bacteria, such as *Listeria*, GBS, *E. coli* and *Bacteroides*, among others, and viruses, notably cytomegalovirus and rubella[217,218]. The treponeme causing syphilis cannot be cultured. However, Wendel and associates[219] reported seeing treponemes on dark-field examination of amniotic fluid from pregnancies complicated by congenital syphilis. Fetal blood sampling was positive for syphilis by testing for monoclonal anti-treponemal antibody and rabbit infectivity. The flow velocity ratios of the uterine and umbilical arteries in these pregnancies showed markedly increased placental vascular resistance[220]. Chlamydia has been demonstrated in amniotic fluid using amplification of specific DNA sequences by the polymerase chain using amplification of specific DNA sequences by the polymerase chain reaction technique[221], although culture is more widely available. Two of nine women with positive cervicovaginal chlamydial DNA identification also had this finding in amniotic fluid, compared with none of 22 women with negative cervicovaginal DNA analysis. Human immunodeficiency virus (HIV) infection of the fetus has been identified antenatally[222]. Thirteen seropositive women underwent amniocentesis and fetal blood sampling. Antibody to HIV was found in maternal serum, amniotic fluid and fetal serum. However, p24 antigen was found in the serum of only three of 13 fetuses and probably represents active fetal infection.

A positive culture is used as the 'gold standard' for the presence of amniotic fluid infection. Chorioamnionitis is the maternal clinical syndrome of fever, leukocytosis and sometimes bacteremia that occurs when bacterial invasion of the amniotic cavity, membranes or adjacent tissue results in clinically evident maternal disease[223]. It is becoming evident that culture-proven amniotic fluid infection occurs in other syndromes, such as preterm labor and premature rupture of membranes, without clinical evidence of chorioamnionitis. Harger and associates[224] found no positive amniotic fluid cultures in 38 asymptomatic afebrile women with normal leukocyte counts in preterm labor with intact membranes between 27 and 32 weeks, testing for bacteria, fungi, *Mycoplasma hominis*, *Ureaplasma urealyticum*, *Chlamydia trachomatis*, and viruses. Watts and colleagues[224] found positive cultures in 20% of such women. The frequency was inversely related to gestational age. Of positive cultures of amniotic fluid facultative and anaerobic organisms in the research laboratory, 40% were negative in the clinical laboratory. The clinical characteristics and leukocyte count did not differ between women with positive and negative cultures. Women with positive cultures delivered a median of 1 day after enrolment, while women with negative cultures delivered a median of 29 days later. Romero and co-workers[226] found positive amniotic fluid cultures in 38% of women admitted with preterm labor and intact membranes delivered within 48 h of amniocentesis. Inflammatory lesions of the placenta had a strong association with positive amniotic fluid cultures. Gauthier and Meyer[227] found amniocentesis specimens yielded positive cultures in 48% of women with preterm premature rupture of membranes and no clinical evidence of infection. Romero and associates[228] found amniocentesis specimens yielded positive cultures in 34% of women with term premature rupture of the membranes. In this study, of those with a positive culture, 33% went on to develop postpartum endometritis compared with 0% of those with a negative culture. Poka and Lampe[229] commented that this risk was increased in the face of both a positive amniotic fluid culture and Cesarean section. Romero and colleagues[230] also found 52% of women with apparent incompetent cervix and intact membranes admitted between 14 and 24 weeks of gestation had positive amniotic fluid cultures. If cultures were negative, nine of 16 women who had cerclage went on to deliver after 34 weeks, while patients who underwent cerclage in the presence of a positive culture had rupture of membranes, clinical chorioamnionitis or pregnancy loss. A rabbit model also confirms that inoculation of a pregnant uterine horn with bacteria results in preterm delivery compared with inoculation of a saline solution[231]. Finally, Romero and associates[232] reported eradication of culture-proven intra-amniotic infection with *Ureaplasma urealyticum* with 6 days of maternal intravenous erythromycin, ampicillin, gentamicin and clindamycin at 24 weeks, with continuation of the pregnancy for 22 days.

Amniotic fluid esterase: Bacterial esterases are present in infected amniotic fluid[233,234]. Therefore the presence of bacterial esterase activity can predict amniotic fluid infection. However, uninfected amniotic fluid also has some esterase activity, and esterases of differing origin respond differently when tested with a variety of esterase inhibitors. The specificity and sensitivity of this method will improve as these assays are further explored. Interestingly, amniotic fluid at term stimulated the production of fibroblast collagenase and other proteases[235], while preterm amniotic fluid failed to do so. Whether this stimulation is a property of term amniotic fluid or a result of undetected microbial invasion near term remains to be elucidated. The production of collagenase could weaken the membranes and contribute to premature rupture of membranes.

Amniotic fluid glucose: Amniotic fluid glucose levels are significantly lower in amniotic fluid in the presence of culture-proven intra-amniotic infection in the setting of preterm labor or premature rupture of membranes. The sensitiity and specificity of this test has been described[236–239] and is discussed at greater length below. In infected amniotic fluid, the level of glucose declines from baseline values at 37°C or even at 22°C, but remains unchanged in frozen samples[240]. However, the glucose level does not decline in amniotic fluid stored at room temperature or even at 37°C in the absence of infection. This is the expected result of bacterial metabolism and probably explains the correlation of low values with infection.

Amniotic-fluid white blood-cell count: Romero and colleagues[241] found positive amniotic-fluid cultures in 13% of a group of women with preterm labor and intact membranes. Amniotic-fluid white blood-cell count was significantly higher (320 cells/mm^3) in patients with a positive culture compared with patients with negative cultures (6/mm^3). Moreover, 88% of patients with a negative culture and a white blood-cell count in amniotic fluid greater than 50 cells/mm^3 had a spontaneous preterm delivery.

Mediators of inflammation: Amniotic fluid can be examined for mediators of inflammation. Besides leukocytes and bacteria, various paracrine and autocrine substances are known to be associated with inflammation and can be found in the amniotic fluid of patients with preterm premature rupture of membranes, preterm labor and chorioamnionitis. The assays for these substances are difficult and limited at present to research laboratories, but will come into increasing use in future years in clinical settings in attempts to define and correct the causes of preterm labor.

Interleukins: Leukoattractants are cytokines that attract white blood cells. In a leukotaxis bioassay, the detection of amniotic fluid leukoattractants was a better predictor of histological chorioamnionitis in patients with idiopathic preterm labor than were microbiologic tests[242]. In patients with detectable leukoattractants, tocolysis failed significantly more often (93%) than in patients without them (7%). Hillier and associates[243] found increased levels of amniotic-fluid cytokines in women in preterm labor who delivered at or before 34 weeks, compared with women in preterm labor who delivered later. These included interleukin-6 (IL-6), interleukin-1α (IL-1α), interleukin-1β (IL-1β) and prostaglandin E$_2$. In fluid from which bacteria were isolated, all these cytokines were elevated, as was tumor necrosis factor-α (TNF-α), and all were associated with histological chorioamnionitis among women who delivered within one week of the amniocentesis. Amniotic-fluid level of IL-6 at a cut-off of 600 pg/ml or greater had a specificity of 100% and a sensitivity of 89% for identification of intrauterine infection in women with preterm labor and intact membranes[244]. IL-6 was present at levels of less than 714 pg/ml in amniotic fluid of women not in labor, but elevated in the amniotic fluid of some women in term labor. Opsjøn and colleagues[245] sampled IL-1, IL-6 and TNF-α throughout normal pregnancy in celomic fluid and amniotic fluid. Little was found in the first trimester. IL-6 appeared in second-trimester amniotic fluid. TNF was present at term. All increased with the onset of labor. Therefore, these cytokines may play a role in the onset of labor. Austgulen and associates[246] compared levels of IL-1, IL-6 and TNF with levels of the soluble receptors for TNF in amniotic fluid of women in spontaneous labor at term and in the maternal and newborn urine.

Although soluble receptors for TNF were elevated in amniotic fluid compared with maternal or fetal urine, there was no significant correlation with levels of the cytokines. Therefore, the receptor proteins are probably produced by intrauterine tissues, but may not have a role in regulation of these cytokines during labor. Romero and co-workers[217] found neutrophil attractant/activating peptide-1/interleukin-8 elevated in amniotic fluid from women with preterm labor and intact membranes who had proven microbial invasion of the amniotic cavity. It was also elevated in the amniotic fluid from women with sterile amniotic fluid and preterm labor who delivered preterm compared with women who responded to tocolysis and delivered at term. Finally, it was elevated in the amniotic fluid of women at term in active labor. It was absent from the amniotic fluid of most women in mid-trimester and women at term, not in labor.

Endothelins: Endothelins are cytokines originally isolated from endothelial tissue. The level of endothelin-1 rises in amniotic fluid during pregnancy[248–250], and is present in much higher concentrations in amniotic fluid than in maternal or fetal plasma. Endothelin-1 is secreted by avascular human amnion tissue and by amnion cells maintained in primary monolayer culture[251]. Endothelin-1 mRNA is expressed in amnion cells in response to factors found in amniotic fluid, including epidermal growth factor, IL-1 and TNF. Endothelin levels are increased in amniotic fluid of women with spontaneous preterm labor, more so if intraamniotic infection is present[252]. It is known that endothelin-1 increases cytoplasmic calcium ion concentration in the target cell[248]. Thus, that endothelin may play a role in the initiation of parturition by triggering the production of prostaglandins in fetal membranes through a calcium-dependent mechanism.

Tumor necrosis factor: In a study of intrauterine growth retardation, Heyborne and associates[253] showed that TNF-α had been elevated in amniotic fluid obtained at mid-trimester from fetuses who were small for gestational age at birth. TNF-α was not elevated in amniotic fluid of the controls who gave birth to a term baby that was average for gestational age. Bacterial lipopolysaccharide (LPS) can induce fetal resorption in mice[254]. In an infection-mediated model of early pregnancy loss, injection of LPS was associated with the appearance of TNF-α in the amniotic fluid, suggesting that it is a mediator of fetal resorption. In a rabbit model of intrauterine infection, levels of amniotic fluid TNF-α, IL-1α and IL-1β rose as early as four hours after inoculation in some animals and by 12 to 16 hours in all animals[255]. Levels of amniotic fluid prostaglandin E_2 (PGE_2) and prostaglandin $F_{2\alpha}$ ($PGF2\alpha$) also rose, and levels correlated significantly with time from intracervical inoculation. Romero and co-workers[256] showed that amniotic fluid from women in the second and third trimesters who were not in labor did not contain TNF. Among women in preterm labor, 92% of those with a positive amniotic fluid culture had detectable TNF in the amniotic fluid, whereas only 10% of those with a negative culture had detectable TNF. Histopathological chorioamnionitis was found in placentas of all women with positive amniotic fluid cultures, and TNF was found in the amniotic fluid of 12 out of 13. Among women in active labor at term, 25% had TNF detectable in amniotic fluid. TNF was detectable among 47% of those with a positive amniotic-fluid culture and only 20% of those with a negative culture. TNF was also elevated in the presence of preterm premature rupture of membranes. Leukemia inhibitory factor has many biological actions that parallel those of IL-1, IL-6 and TNF-α[257]. It has been found in moderately elevated concentration in the amniotic fluid of a woman with chorioamnionitis but in low concentration in the amniotic fluid of women in labor.

Prostaglandins: In a sheep model, partial occlusion of the uterine circulation led to an increase in PGF metabolites in amniotic fluid[258], suggesting that hypoxemia as well as infection can serve as a stimulus for prostaglandin release. This may explain why preterm labor develops in some small-for-gestational-age fetuses who are experiencing chronic intrauterine hypoxia, and underscores the need for individualizing tocolytic therapy. Fetal membranes obtained after labor released PGE_2 and $PGF_{2\alpha}$ into a buffer solution[259]. Amniotic fluid obtained before labor caused a 3- to 5-fold increase in PGE_2 secretion from the amnion, but a relative decrease in the release of PGE_2 and $PGF_{2\alpha}$ from chorion, while release of arachidonic acid from both sides was increased. This argues for some as yet uncharacterized paracrine effect.

Romero and colleagues[260], in a study of spontaneous rupture of membranes at term, found increases in amniotic fluid concentrations of PGE_2, $PGF_{2\alpha}$, and thromboxane B_2, but not 6-keto-prostaglandin $F_{1\alpha}$. Early labor in these patients was associated with a significant increase in all these eicosanoids, whether the women had microbial invasion of the amniotic cavity or sterile fluid. This is in distinct contrast to findings in women with preterm labor, in whom absence of microbial invasion of amniotic fluid was also associated with absence of significant increase in amniotic fluid prostaglandins. This argues for a different mechanism of prostaglandin production induced by rupture of membranes at term compared with that induced by microbial invasion with intact membranes in preterm labor.

MacDonald and Casey[261] sampled amniotic fluid transabdominally at term before labor, and from the upper compartment of the uterine cavity during labor, and by needle aspiration of the forebag during labor. There was no increase in amniotic-fluid prostaglandins in the upper compartment during early labor compared with those present before labor began. At 3 to 5 cm dilatation there was an increase in amniotic-fluid prostaglandins in the upper compartment. This increase was less than the increase found in the forebag at 3 to 5 cm dilatation. Prostaglandins did not increase further in the upper uterine cavity from this point, but the concentration of prostaglandins in the forebag continued to increase during labor, as a function of cervical dilatation, until delivery.

These findings suggest that production of prostaglandins by amniotic membranes is not a cause of labor, but rather is a result of labor, particularly the exposure of the forebag to trauma as it stretches and comes in contact with vaginal microbes during labor. Nevertheless, these findings do not conclusively prove this point. As Carsten and Miller[262] pointed out, prostaglandins are involved in uterine contraction even in the absence of fetal membranes, so that anti-prostaglandins are effective in ablating menstrual cramping. Anti-prostaglandins are effective in quietening uterine contractions due to preterm labor, which is unlikely if the prostaglandins are an effect of labor rather than a cause. It may be that the decidual production of prostaglandin is most important, or that the rises in the upper compartment are sufficient to produce labor, while those in the lower compartment are caused not only by labor but also by the mechanisms proposed.

In cows, labor may be initiated by a single injection of flumethasone[263]. Observations on myometrial activity were divided into four periods, the first one prior to injection and then three periods characterized by different patterns of activity following injection. During period 3, contractures nearly disappeared, and $PGF_{2\alpha}$ in amniotic fluid was not significantly changed compared with previous periods, while maternal plasma $PGF_{2\alpha}$ was significantly higher and progesterone was significantly lower than before. Finally, in period 4, a pattern of labor contractions gradually emerged accompanied by a further decline in progesterone and rise in $PGF_{2\alpha}$ in maternal plasma.

Cytokine inhibitors and immunosuppressive factors: IL-1 receptor antagonist inhibits the effects of IL-1 by blocking its receptors. IL-1 receptor antagonist was present in amniotic fluid of women at mid-trimester, at term with and without labor and in preterm labor, and in concentrations higher than in any other biological fluid studied so far[264]. However, IL-1 receptor antagonist was not increased by the presence of infection or preterm labor in spite of dramatically increased levels of IL-1α and IL-1β in the same fluids. IL-1 receptor antagonist reduced production of PGE_2 stimulated by IL-1β in amnion and chorion in a dose-dependent manner, but did not by itself cause release of PGE_2 from these tissues. It has been concluded tentatively that exogenous cytokine antagonists may be of value in the treatment of preterm labor.

Transforming growth factor-beta 2 (TGF-β2) is an inhibitor of cytokine-induced prostaglandin synthesis, such as that caused by IL-1α and TNF-α. Recently it has been shown that a combination of TNF-α and IL-1α can provoke preterm parturition in the rabbit, and that TGF-β2 can prevent the cytokine-induced increase in preterm delivery[265]. Fluids from immunologically privileged sites such as amniotic fluid, the aqueous humor of the anterior chamber of the eye, and cerebrospinal fluid can induce a deviant form of systemic immunity which is characterized by a selective inability to display antigen-specific delayed hypersensitivity[266]. TGF-β2 can induce this form of altered immunity in naive macrophages, and is found in amniotic fluid as well as these other fluids. The relationship between these two actions of TGF-β2 has yet to be elucidated.

Amniotic fluid has immunosuppressive effects that can prolong the survival of renal allografts in rats[267]. In concanavalin A-stimulated lymphocytes, amniotic fluid suppressed interferon and IL-2 production but did not suppress IL-3 or IL-6 production or IL-2 receptor expression.

Gravidin is a phospholipase inhibitor previously characterized as a component of amniotic fluid[268]. Recently, gravidin was shown to be identical to the secretory component of IgA[268,269]. The concentration of free secretory component in amniotic fluid rises during gestation to reach levels found in other external secretions. The relationship between this structural component of secretory immunoglobulin and its capacity to affect the prostaglandin cascade through phospholipase inhibition is not known.

Amnion and amniotic fluid contain membrane-attack-complex inhibitory protein[270]. This may be important in protecting the fetus from maternal complement *in utero*.

Prolactin is known to inhibit prostaglandin production. Recently, Kinoshita and colleagues[271] showed a decline in the amniotic fluid levels of prolactin with time during labor. Prolactin levels in decidua also declined during labor, compared with those before labor.

Factors of uncertain function: Fetal fibronectin is found in amniotic fluid after rupture of membranes[272], and can be used as a biochemical test of membrane rupture. Recently, Lockwood and associates[273] showed that fetal fibronectin could be found in cervicovaginal secretions of some patients with apparently intact membranes and preterm labor. Its presence served as a predictor of actual preterm delivery. Whether fibronectin is a cause or consequence of factors leading to preterm delivery is uncertain.

Relaxin is present in maternal blood at ten times the concentration found in amniotic fluid and follows different kinetics with time during the pregnancy[274]. Relaxin is absent from fetal blood samples. Thus, the source of relaxin in amniotic fluid may be the decidua rather than the maternal circulation.

Corticotropin releasing hormone (CRH)-binding protein appears in the amniotic fluid after 15 weeks' gestation and in umbilical-cord plasma after 24 weeks[275]. The saturation during the third trimester was similar to that in neonates and adults. However, the saturation of this protein decreased at 40 weeks of pregnancy, indicating a decline in free CRH, which may play a role in initiating labor. Adrenocorticotropic hormone (ACTH) and its byproducts α-melanocyte stimulating hormone and β-endorphin rise in amniotic fluid during labor[276]. In pregnancies complicated by pre-eclampsia, the rise of β-endorphin was much higher, confirming its role as a marker of fetal distress and pituitary response.

Catechol estrogens in amniotic fluid rise progressively during pregnancy[277]. Moreover, levels were significantly higher in spontaneous labor at term than during Cesarean section at term in patients not in labor. This supports a role for catechol estrogens in initiating labor, possibly through stimulating effects on prostaglandin synthesis. Nocturnal uterine activity in Rhesus macaques was not related to maternal arterial or amniotic fluid catecholamine concentrations[278].

Steroid hormones can now be analyzed in amniotic fluid by high-performance liquid chromatography[279]. Stress steroids were lower in amniotic fluid of mid-trimester fetuses during fetoscopy with pre-medication than during amniocentesis without sedation[280].

Inhibin present in the serum of women during pregnancy is virtually undetectable 24 h after delivery[281]. It is also found in amniotic fluid, retroplacental serum and placental extract and cord serum. The levels of immunoreactive inhibin were much higher in the placental specimens than in maternal or fetal serum or in amniotic fluid, suggesting the placenta as the site of origin.

Comparisons of rapid diagnostic tests: Gauthier and Meyer[227] found a leukocyte esterase activity of 1+ or 2+ and an amniotic-fluid glucose concentration of 16 mg/dl or less significantly more sensitive than Gram stain in detecting positive amniotic fluid cultures among women with preterm PROM (73%, 68% and 41%, respectively). Gauthier and associates[282] did not find the biophysical profile useful in predicting results of culture of fluid obtained at amniocentesis, although women with positive cultures had significantly lower overall scores as well as lower individual test scores. Coultrip and Grossman[283] studied predictive indices of four tests for a positive amniotic fluid culture and for clinical infection in women with either preterm labor or preterm premature rupture of the membranes, and generated ROCC for each test. Low glucose level had the greatest sensitivity for predicting either outcome. In patients with preterm labor, Gram stain provided the greatest positive predictive value. Combining Gram stain with intraamniotic glucose did not improve the sensitivity of a low glucose test or the positive predictive value of Gram stain. The leukocyte esterase assay and *Limulus* amebocyte lysate assays were both found to be insensitive indicators of intra-amniotic infection. Watts and colleagues[225] found elevated levels of C-reactive protein and a positive amniotic fluid Gram stain the two most sensitive and specific methods to predict positive amniotic-fluid cultures in women with preterm labor and intact membranes. Romero and co-workers[241] compared amniotic fluid white blood-cell (WBC) count with Gram stain in a similar group of patients. They found the WBC count had a higher sensitivity (80%) in detecting patients with a positive culture compared with Gram stain (48%), but a lower specificity (88% vs. 99%). Thus, they found Gram stain had a high false-negative rate compared with WBC count, and a lower false-positive rate in the prediction of positive culture results. As noted above, however, WBC count had a lower false-positive rate in the prediction of preterm delivery. Therefore, there may be inflammatory stimuli resulting in preterm delivery that are not detected by current culture methods. These may or may not be infectious agents. Romero and colleagues[284] also compared IL-6, Gram stain, WBC count and glucose as diagnostic tests in the detection of microbial invasion of the amniotic cavity and in prediction of preterm delivery and neonatal complications in patients with preterm labor and intact membranes. Amniotic-fluid IL-6 was shown to have a more ideal ROCC than amniotic-fluid glucose or WBC in the prediction of amniotic fluid infection. Even when IL-6 was falsely positive for prediction of amniotic fluid infection, 100% still had preterm delivery and 92% had histological chorioamnionitis. Unfortunately, a multi-center randomized trial of a bactericidal and a bacteriostatic antibiotic in the prevention of preterm delivery in the setting of preterm labor with intact membranes has been unable to show a difference in the outcome of preterm labor[285]. It may be that once infection is detectable, the outcome cannot be reversed. In the face of preterm premature rupture of membranes, none of these diagnostic tests predicts amniotic fluid cultures as well as they do if membranes are intact[286]. However, IL-6 still appears to be the best test by ROCC analysis, although none of these curves have been compared using appropriate statistical techniques[70,71].

Drugs in amniotic fluid It is possible to study fetal excretion of drugs utilizing amniocentesis. Hallak and associates[287] studied amniotic fluid magnesium levels in relation to maternal and fetal magnesium levels in women receiving magnesium sulfate to quieten uterine contractions during cordocentesis, and compared them with those in controls who had not received magnesium. Magnesium rose in fetal serum obtained 1 h after infusion but had not yet appeared in amniotic fluid. When mothers had received magnesium 3 h before, magnesium levels were lower in fetal serum compared with the previous group, and amniotic fluid magnesium levels had risen. This correlates with postnatal studies of neonates whose mothers received magnesium.

Fetal cocaine exposure can be detected in amniotic fluid[288,289]. In a guinea pig model, cocaine accumulated in amniotic fluid at 3 to 4 times plasma concentrations and the *in vitro* half-life in amniotic fluid was 30 times the half-life in plasma *in vivo*. Thus amniotic fluid may serve as a reservoir for prolonged fetal exposure to cocaine.

Transplacental passage of vancomycin[290] and cefuroxime[291] have been studied in chorioamnionitis.

Artificial rupture of membranes

A variety of assessments may be made at the time of artificial rupture of membranes (AROM). Typical are qualitative and semi-quantitative amniotic fluid assessments. These are performed in a fashion identical to that noted under observed SROM. Tests analogous to those performed on specimens obtained after SROM, noted above, may be performed, but in practice are seldom used. If no fluid is observed at AROM, this is consistent with oligohydramnios[72].

Amnioinfusion

Amnioinfusion is the infusion of physiological solutions into the amniotic cavity for the purpose of increasing or augmenting amniotic fluid. This may be monitored sonographically with the amniotic fluid index. Amnioinfusion was derived from the practice of infusing small amounts of fluid through the commonly used fluid column intrauterine pressure catheters into the amniotic cavity to maintain patency of the catheter. Some of the current uses of amnioinfusion include the infusion of a physiological solution into the amniotic cavity in the presence of thick meconium to prevent aspiration[292], in the presence of oligohydramnios[293], to prevent or relieve decelerations from cord occlusions[294], and in women attempting vaginal birth after Cesarean section[295]. The practice remains controversial[296,297]. One complication of amnioinfusion is the acute development of iatrogenic polyhydramnios[298]. Serial monitoring of fundal height, maternal girth, amniotic fluid index and intrauterine pressure[299,300] can help avoid this complication.

One recent development is the use of amnioinfusion to define fetal anatomy and to attempt to prevent pulmonary hypoplasia from the oligohydramnios sequence. Several attempts have been made in recent years to infuse a physiological solution into an amniotic cavity where oligohydramnios apparently exists, either from fetal anatomic problems or from preterm premature rupture of membranes[301,302]. Antibiotics have been added to the infusate to prevent infection[303].

SUMMARY

Amniotic fluid is a readily available biological fluid produced by the fetus and its surrounding membranes. Consequently, it has been studied extensively in relation to normal and abnormal fetal physiology. Management of a variety of fetal conditions is aided through multiple modalities of amniotic fluid analysis.

References

1. Itoh, H., Sagawa, N., Hasegawa, M., Okagaki, A., Inamori, K., Ihara, Y., Mori Ogawa, Y., Suga, S., Mukoyama, M. et al. (1993). Brain natriuretic peptide is present in the human amniotic fluid and is secreted from amnion cells. *J. Clin. Endocrinol. Metab.*, **76**, 907–11
2. Shipley, C. F. III and Nelson, G. H. (1993). Prenatal diagnosis of a placental cyst: comparison of postnatal biochemical analyses of cyst fluid, amniotic fluid, cord serum, and maternal serum. *Am. J. Obstet. Gynecol.*, **168**, 211–13
3. Vernof, K. K., Benirschke, K., Kephart, G. M., Wasmoen, T. L. and Gleich, G. J. (1992). Maternal floor infarction: relationship to X cells, major basic protein, and adverse perinatal outcome. *Am. J. Obstet. Gynecol.*, **167**, 1355–63
4. Fraser, M., Carter, A. M., Challis, J. R. and McDonald, T. J. (1992). Gastrin releasing peptide immunoreactivity is present in ovine amniotic fluid and fetal and maternal circulations. MRC Group in Fetal and Neonatal Health and Development. *Endocrinology*, **131**, 2033–5
5. Wu, S., Polk, D., Wong, S., Reviczky, A., Vu, R. and Fisher, D. A. (1992). Thyroxine sulfate is a major thyroid hormone metabolite and a potential intermediate in the monodeiodination pathway in fetal sheep. *Endocrinology*, **131**, 1751–6
6. Morita, I., Kawamoto, M. and Yoshida, H. (1992). Difference in the concentration of tryptophan metabolites between maternal and umbilical foetal blood. *J. Chromatogr.*, **576**, 334–9
7. Chopra, I. J., Wu, S. Y., Teco, G. N. and Santini, F. (1992). A radioimmunossay for measurement of 3,5,3′-triiodothyronine sulfate: studies in thyroidal and nonthyroidal diseases, pregnancy, and neonatal life. *J. Clin. Endocrinol. Metab.*, **75**, 189–94
8. Shinagawa, T., Do, Y. S., Baxter, J. and Hsueh, W. A. (1992). Purification and characterization of human truncated prorenin. *Biochemistry*, **31**, 2758–64
9. Schwonzen, M., Schmits, R., Baldus, S. E., Vierbuchen, M., Hanisch, F. G., Pfreundschuh, M., Diehl, V., Bara, J. and Uhlenbruck, G. (1992). Monoclonal antibody FW6 generated against a mucin-carbohydrate of human amniotic fluid recognizes a colonic tumour-associated epitope. *Br. J. Cancer*, **65**, 559–65
10. Hanisch, F. G. and Peter-Katalinic, J. (1992). Structural studies on fetal mucins from human amniotic fluid. Core typing of short-chain O-linked glycans. *Eur. J. Biochem.*, **205**, 527–35
11. Hertig, A. T. and Rock, J. (1945). Two human ova in the previllous stage, having a developmental age of about 7 and 9 days respectively. *Contrib. Embryol.*, **31**, 65
12. Gilbert, N. M. and Brace, R. A. (1993). Amniotic fluid volume and normal flows to and from the amniotic cavity. *Semin. Perinatol.*, **17**,150–7
13. Seeds, A. E. (1980). Current concepts of amniotic fluid dynamics. *Am. J. Obstet. Gynecol.*, **138**, 575
14. Campbell, J., Wathen, N., Macintosh, M., Cass, P., Chard, T. and Mainwaring Burton, R. (1992). Biochemical composition of amniotic fluid and extraembryonic coelomic fluid in the first trimester of pregnancy. *Br. J. Obstet. Gynaecol.*, **99**, 563–5
15. Jauniaux, E., Jurkovic, D., Gulbis, B., Gervy, C., Ooms, H. A. and Campbell, S. (1991). Biochemical composition of exocoelomic fluid in early human pregnancy. *Obstet. Gynecol.*, **78**, 1124–8
16. Iles, R. K., Wathen, N. C., Campbell, D. J. and Chard, T. (1992). Human chorionic gonadotrophin and subunit composition of maternal serum and coelomic and amniotic fluids in the first trimester of pregnancy. *J. Endocrinol.*, **135**, 563–9
17. Campbell, J., Wathen, N., Lewis, M., Fingerova, H. and Chard, T. (1992). Erythroprotein levels in amniotic fluid and extraembryonic coelomic fluid in the first trimester of pregnancy. *Br. J. Obstet. Gynaecol.*, **99**, 974–6
18. Engle, W. D. (1986). Development of fetal and neonatal renal function. *Semin. Perinatol.*, **10**, 113–24
19. Pritchard, J. A. (1965). Deglutition by normal and ancencephalic fetuses. *Obstet. Gynecol.*, **25**, 289
20. Fujino, Y., Agnew, C. L., Schreyer, P., Ervin, M. G., Sherman, D. J. and Ross, M. G. (1991). Amniotic fluid volume response to esophageal occlusion in fetal sheep. *Am. J. Obstet. Gynecol.*, **165**, 1620–6
21. Jang, P. R. and Brace, R. A. (1992). Amniotic fluid composition changes during urine drainage and tracheoesophageal occlusion

in fetal sheep. *Am. J. Obstet. Gynecol.*, **167**, 1732–41
22. Gilbert, W. M., Cheung, C. Y. and Brace, R. A. (1991). Oral-nasal membranes are not the major route for fetal absorption of amniotic fluid arginine vasopressin. *Am. J. Obstet. Gynecol.*, **165**, 1614–20
23. Gillibrand, P. N. (1969). Changes in the electrolytes, urea, and osmolality of the amniotic fluid with advancing pregnancy. *J. Obstet. Gynaecol. Br. Commonw.*, **76**, 898–905
24. Mandelbaum, B. and Evans, T. N. (1969). Life in the amniotic fluid. *Am. J. Obstet. Gynecol.*, **104**, 365–77
25. Adzick, N. S. and Harrison, M. R. (1992). The fetus at surgery. In Reece, E. A., Hobbins, J. C., Mahoney, M. J. and Petrie, R. H. (eds.) *Medicine of the Fetus and Mother*, pp. 791–9. (Philadelphia: J. B. Lippincott)
26. Economides, D. L., Johnson, P. and MacKenzie, I. Z. (1992). Does amniotic fluid analysis reflect acid–base balance in fetal blood? *Am. J. Obstet. Gynecol.*, **166**, 970–3
27. Queenan, J. T., Thompson, W., Whitfield, C. R. and Shah, S. I. (1972). Amniotic fluid volumes in normal pregnancy. *Am. J. Obstet. Gynecol.*, **114**, 34–8
28. Fisk, N. M., Ronderos-Dumit, D., Tannirandorn, Y., Nicolini, U., Talbert, D. and Rodeck, C. H. (1992). Normal amniotic pressure throughout gestation. *Br. J. Obstet. Gynaecol.*, **99**, 18–22
29. Vosburgh, G. H., Flexner, L. B., Cowie, D. B., Hellman, L. M., Proctor, N. K. and Wilde, W. S. (1948). The rate of renewal in woman of the water and sodium of the amniotic fluid as determined by tracer techniques. *Am. J. Obstet. Gynecol.*, **56**, 1156–9
30. Kilpatrick, S. J. and Safford, K. L. (1993). Maternal hydration increases amniotic fluid index in women with normal amniotic fluid. *Obstet. Gynecol.*, **81**, 49–52
31. Powers, D. R. and Brace, R. A. (1991). Fetal cardiovascular and fluid responses to maternal volume loading with lactated Ringer's or hypotonic solution. *Am. J. Obstet. Gynecol.*, **165**, 1504–15
32. Kilpatrick, S. J., Safford, K. L., Pomeroy, T., Hoedt, L., Scheerer, L. and Laros, R. K. (1991). Maternal hydration increases amniotic fluid index. *Obstet. Gynecol.*, **78**, 1098–102
33. Brace, R. A. and Moore, T. R. (1991). Transplacental, amniotic, urinary, and fetal fluid dynamics during very-large-volume fetal intravenous infusions. *Am. J. Obstet. Gynecol.*, **164**, 907–16
34. Powell, T. L. and Brace, R. A. (1991). Fetal fluid responses to long-term 5 M NaCl infusion: where does all the salt go? *Am. J. Physiol.*, **261**, R412–9
35. Kelly, T. F., Moore, T. R. and Brace, R. A. (1993). Hemodynamic and fluid responses to furosemide infusion in the ovine fetus. *Am. J. Obstet. Gynecol.*, **168**, 260–8
36. Rankin, S. (1989). Disorders of the pregnancy. In Bennett, V. R. and Brown, L. K. (eds.) *Myles Textbook for Midwives*, pp. 306–16. (New York: Churchill Livingstone)
37. Christian, S. S., Brady, K., Read, J. A. and Kopelman, J. N. (1990). Vaginal breech delivery: a five-year prospective evaluation of a protocol using computed tomographic pelvimetry. *Am. J. Obstet. Gynecol.*, **163**, 848–55
38. Gimovsky, M. L., Willard, K., Neglio, M., Howard, T. and Zerne, S. (1985). X-ray pelvimetry in a breech protocol: a comparison of digital radiography and conventional methods. *Am. J. Obstet. Gynecol.*, **153**, 887–8
39. Gohari, P., Berkowitz, R. L. and Hobbins, J. C. (1979). Prediction of intrauterine growth retardation by determination of total intrauterine volume. *Am. J. Obstet. Gynecol.*, **127**, 225–60
40. Kurz, A. B., Kurz, R. J., Rifkin, M. D., Pasto, M. E., Cole-Beuglet, C., Wapner, R. J., Tsatalis, J. and Goldberg, B. B. (1984). Total uterine volume: a new graph and its clinical implications. *J. Ultrasound Med.*, **3**, 299–308
41. Crowley, P. (1980). Non-quantitative estimation of amniotic fluid volume in suspected prolonged pregnancy. *J. Perinat. Med.*, **8**, 249–51
42. Manning, F. A., Platt, L. D. and Sipos, L. (1980). Antepartum fetal evaluation: development of a fetal biophysical profile. *Am. J. Obstet. Gynecol.*, **136**, 787–95
43. Hill, L. M., Breckle, R., Wolfgram, K. R. and O'Brien, P. C. (1983). Oligohydramnios: ultrasonically detected incidence and subsequent fetal outcome. *Am. J. Obstet. Gynecol.*, **147**, 407–10
44. Benson, C. B., Boswell, S. B., Brown, D. L., Saltzman, D. H. and Doubilet, P. M. (1988). Improved prediction of intrauterine growth retardation with use of multiple parameters. *Radiology*, **168**, 7–12
45. Damato, N., Filly, R. A., Goldstein, R. B., Callen, P. W., Goldberg, J. and Golbus, M. (1993). Frequency of fetal anomalies in sonographi-

cally detected polyhydramnios. *J. Ultrasound Med.*, **12**, 11–15

46. Pillai, M. and James, D. (1990). The importance of the behavioural state in biophysical assessment of the term human fetus. *Br. J. Obstet. Gynaecol.*, **97**, 1130–4

47. Phelan, J. P., Platt, L. D., Yeh, S., Broussard, P. and Paul, R. H. (1985). The role of ultrasound assessment of amniotic fluid in the management of the postdate pregnancy. *Am. J. Obstet. Gynecol.*, **151**, 304–8

48. Bastide, A., Manning, F., Harman, C., Lange, I. and Morrison, I. (1986). Ultrasound evaluation of amniotic fluid: outcome of pregnancies with severe oligohydramnios. *Am. J. Obstet. Gynecol.*, **154**, 895–900

49. Dyer, S N., Burton, B. K. and Nelson, L. H. (1987). Elevated maternal serum alpha-fetoprotein levels and oligohydramnios: poor prognosis for pregnancy outcome. *Am. J. Obstet. Gynecol.*, **157**, 336–9

50. Small, M. L., Phelan, J. P., Smith, C. V. and Paul, R. H. (1987). An active management approach to the postdate fetus with a reactive nonstress test and fetal heart rate decelerations. *Obstet. Gynecol.*, **70**, 636–40

51. Trimmer, K. J., Leveno, K. J., Peters, M. T. and Kelly, M. A. (1990). Observations on the cause of oligohydramnios in prolonged pregnancy. *Am. J. Obstet. Gynecol.*, **163**, 1900–3

52. Shenker, L., Reed, K. L., Anderson, C. F. and Borjon, N. A. (1991). Significance of oligohydramnios complicating pregnancy. *Am. J. Obstet. Gynecol.*, **164**, 1597–600

53. Chamberlain, P. F., Manning, F. A., Morrison, I., Harman, C. R. and Lange, I. R. (1984). I. The relationship of marginal and decreased amniotic fluid volumes to perinatal outcome. *Am. J. Obstet. Gynecol.*, **150**, 245–9

54. Lin, C.-C., Sheikh, Z. and Lopata, R. (1990). The association between oligohydramnios and intrauterine growth retardation. *Obstet. Gynecol.*, **76**, 1100–4

55. Crowley, P., O'Herlihey, C. and Boylan, P. (1984). The value of ultrasound measurement of amniotic fluid volume on the management of prolonged pregnancies. *Br. J. Obstet. Gynaecol.*, **91**, 444–8

56. Bochner, C. J., Medearis, A. L., Davis, J., Oakes, G. K., Hobel, C. J. and Wade, M. E. (1987). Antepartum predictors of fetal distress in postterm pregnancy. *Am. J. Obstet. Gynecol.*, **157**, 353–8

57. Cruz, A. C., Frentzen, B. H., Gomez, K. J., Allen, G. and Tyson-Thomas, M. (1988). Continuous-wave Doppler ultrasound and decreased amniotic fluid in pregnant women with intact or ruptured membranes. *Am. J. Obstet. Gynecol.*, **159**, 708

58. Fischer, R. L., McDonnell, M., Bianculli, K. W., Perry, R. L., Hediger, M. L. and Scholl, T. O. (1993). Amniotic fluid volume estimation in the postdate pregnancy: a comparison of techniques. *Obstet. Gynecol.*, **81**, 698–704

59. Rutherford, S. E., Phelan, J. P., Smith, C. V. and Jacobs, N. (1987). The four-quadrant assessment of amniotic fluid volume: an adjunct to antepartum fetal heart rate testing. *Obstet. Gynecol.*, **70**, 353–6

60. Carlson, D. E., Platt, L. D., Medearis, A. L. and Horenstein, J. (1990). Quantifiable polyhydramnios: diagnosis and management. *Obstet. Gynecol.*, **75**, 989–93

61. Moore, T. R. and Cayle, J. E. (1990). The amniotic fluid index in normal human pregnancy. *Am. J. Obstet. Gynecol.*, **162**, 1168–73

62. Nwosu, E. C., Welch, C. R., Manasse, P. R. and Walkinshaw, S. A. (1993). Longitudinal assessment of amniotic fluid index. *Br. J. Obstet. Gynaecol.*, **100**, 816–19

63. Sadovsky, Y., Christensen, M. W., Scheerer, L. and Crombleholme, W. R. (1992). Cord-containing amniotic fluid pocket: a useful measurement in the management of oligohydramnios. *Obstet. Gynecol.*, **80**, 775–7

64. Youssef, A. A., Abdulla, S. A., Sayed, E. H., Salem, H. T., Abdelalim, A. M. and Devoe, L. D. (1993). Superiority of amniotic fluid index over amniotic pocket fluid measurement for predicting bad fetal outcome. *South. Med. J.*, **86**, 426–9

65. Moore, T. R. (1990). Superiority of the four-quadrant sum over the single-deepest-pocket technique in ultrasonographic identification of abnormal amniotic fluid volumes. *Am. J. Obstet. Gynecol.*, **163**, 762–7

66. Dildy, G. A. III, Lira, N., Moise, K. J. Jr, Riddle, G. D. and Deter, R. L. (1992). Amniotic fluid volume assessment: comparison of ultrasonographic estimates versus direct measurements with a dye-dilution technique in human pregnancy. *Am. J. Obstet. Gynecol.*, **167**, 986–94

67. Croom, C. S., Banias, B. B., Ramos-Santos, E., Devoe, L. D., Bezhadian, A. and Hiett, A. (1992). Do semiquantitative amniotic fluid indexes reflect actual volume? *Am. J. Obstet. Gynecol.*, **167**, 995–9

68. Magann, E. F., Nolan, T. E., Hess, L. W., Martin, R. W., Whitworth, N. S. and Morrison, J. C. (1992). Measurement of amniotic fluid volume: accuracy of ultrasonography techniques. *Am. J. Obstet. Gynecol.*, **167**, 1533–7
69. Hoskins, I. A., McGovern, P. G., Ordorica, S. A., Freiden, F. J. and Young, B. K. (1992). Amniotic fluid index: correlation with amniotic fluid volume. *Am. J. Perinatol.*, **9**, 315–18
70. Chauhan, S. P., Magann, E. F. and Morrison, J. C. (1993). Amniotic fluid volume estimation in the postdate pregnancy: a comparison of techniques. *Obstet. Gynecol.*, **82**, 635–6
71. Ross, M. G. (1993). Amniotic fluid volume determination. *Am. J. Obstet. Gynecol.*, **169**, 435–7
72. Druzin, M. L. and Adams, D. M. (1990). Significance of observing no fluid at amniotomy. *Am. J. Obstet. Gynecol.*, **162**, 1006–7
73. Bruner, J. P., Reed, G. W., Sarno, A. P. Jr, Harrington, R. A. and Goodman, M. A. (1993). Intraobserver and interobserver variability of the amniotic fluid index. *Am. J. Obstet. Gynecol.*, **168**, 1309–13
74. Wax, J. R., Costigan, K., Callan, N. A., Gegor, C. and Johnson, T. R. (1993). Effect of fetal movement on amniotic fluid index. *AM. J. Obstet. Gynecol.*, **168**, 188–9
75. Hoskins, I. A., Frieden, F. J. and Young, B. K. (1991). Variable decelerations in reactive nonstress tests with decreased amniotic fluid index predict fetal compromise. *Am. J. Obstet. Gynecol.*, **165**, 1094–8
76. Grubb, D. K., Rabello, Y. A. and Paul, R. H. (1992). Post-term pregnancy: fetal death rate with antepartum surveillance. *Obstet. Gynecol.*, **79**, 1024–6
77. Grubb, D. K. and Paul, R. H. (1992). Amniotic fluid index and prolonged antepartum fetal heart rate decelerations. *Obstet. Gynecol.*, **79**, 558–60
78. Lagrew, D. C., Pircon, R. A., Nageotte, M., Freeman, R. K. and Dorchester, W. (1992). How frequently should the amniotic fluid index be repeated? *Am. J. Obstet. Gynecol.*, **167**, 1129–33
79. Petrikovsky, B. M., Schifrin, B. and Diana, L. (1993). The effect of fetal acoustic stimulation on fetal swallowing and amniotic fluid index. *Obstet. Gynecol.*, **81**, 548–50
80. Zimmer, E. Z., Chao, C. R., Guy, G. P., Marks, F. and Fifer, W. P. (1993). Vibroacoustic stimulation evokes human fetal micturition. *Obstet. Gynecol.*, **81**, 178–79
81. Pearce, J. M. and McParland, P. J. (1991). A comparison of Doppler flow velocity waveforms, amniotic fluid columns, and the nonstress test as a means of monitoring postdates pregnancies. *Obstet. Gynecol.*, **77**, 204–8
82. Weinbaum, P. J., Vintzileos, A. M., Campbell, W. A., Leidy, A. M. and Nochimson, D. (1986). Acute development of oligohydramnios in a pregnancy complicated by chronic hypertension and superimposed preeclampsia. *Am. J. Perinatol.*, **3**, 47
83. Clement, D., Schifrin, B. S. and Kates, R. B. (1987). Acute oligohydramnios in postdate pregnancy. *Am. J. Obstet. Gynecol.*, **157**, 884
84. Arduini, D. and Rizzo, G. (1991). Fetal renal artery velocity waveforms and amniotic fluid volume in growth-retarded and post-term fetuses. *Obstet. Gynecol.*, **77**, 370–3
85. Marks, A. D. and Divon, M. Y. (1992). Longitudinal study of the amniotic fluid index in post-dates pregnancy. *Obstet. Gynecol.*, **79**, 229–33
86. Sarno, A. P., Ahn, M. O., Brar, H. S., Phelan, J. P. and Platt, L. D. (1989). Intrapartum doppler velocimetry, amniotic fluid volume, and fetal heart rate as predictors of subsequent fetal distress. *Am. J. Obstet. Gynecol.*, **161**, 1508
87. Teoh, T. G., Gleeson, R. P. and Darling, M. R. (1992). Measurement of amniotic fluid volume in early labour is a useful admission test. *Br. J. Obstet. Gynaecol.*, **99**, 859–60
88. Sarno, A. P. (1991). The significance of amniotic fluid volume during intrapartum fetal acoustic stimulation. *Am. J. Obstet. Gynecol.*, **164**, 1100–1
89. Ball, R. H. and Parer, J. T. (1992). The physiologic mechanisms of variable decelerations. *Am. J. Obstet. Gynecol.*, **166**, 1683–8
90. Myles, T. D. and Strassner, H. T. (1992). Four-quadrant assessment of volume: distribution's role in predicting fetal outcome. *Obstet. Gynecol.*, **80**, 769–74
91. Saunders, N., Amis, S. and Marsh, M. (1992). The prognostic value of fetal ultrasonography before induction of labour. *Br. J. Obstet. Gynaecol.*, **99**, 303–6
92. Robson, S. C., Crawford, R. A., Spencer, J. A. and Lee, A. (1992). Intrapartum amniotic fluid index and its relationship to fetal distress. *Am. J. Obstet. Gynecol.*, **166**, 78–82
93. Crawford, R. A., Ryan, G., Wright, V. M. and Rodeck, C. H. (1992). The importance of serial biophysical assessment of fetal wellbeing in gastroschisis. *Br. J. Obstet. Gynaecol.*, **99**, 899–902

94. Mahony, B. S., Petty, C. N., Nyberg, D. A., Luthy, D. A., Hickok, D. E. and Hirsch, J. H. (1990). The 'stuck twin' phenomenon: ultrasonographic findings, pregnancy outcome, and management with serial amniocenteses. *Am. J. Obstet. Gynecol.*, **163**, 1513–22

95. Urig, M. A., Clewell, W. H. and Elliott, J. P. (1990). Twin–twin transfusion syndrome. *Am. J. Obstet. Gynecol.*, **163**, 1522–6

96. Sherer, D. M., Abramowicz, J. S., Smith, S. A. and Woods, J. R. Jr (1991). Sonographically homogeneous echogenic amniotic fluid in detecting meconium-stained amniotic fluid. *Obstet. Gynecol.*, **78**, 819–22

97. Jacoby, H. E. and Charles, D. (1966). Clinical conditions associated with hydramnios. *Am. J. Obstet. Gynecol.*, **94**, 910–19

98. Queenan, J. T. and Gadow, E. C. (1970). Polyhydramnios: chronic versus acute. *Am. J. Obstet. Gynecol.*, **108**, 349–55

99. Girz, B. A., Divon, M. Y., Papajohn, M. and Merkatz, I. R. (1992). Amniotic fluid volume in diabetic pregnancy. *J. Matern. Fetal Invest.*, **1**, 237–40

100. Brady, K., Polzin, W. J., Kopelman, J. N. and Read, J. A. (1992). Risk of chromosomal abnormalities in patients with idiopathic polyhydramnios. *Obstet. Gynecol.*, **79**, 234–8

101. Cabrol, D., Landesman, R., Muller, J., Uzan, M., Sureau, C. and Saxena, B. B. (1987). Treatment of polyhydramnios with prostaglandin synthetase inhibitor (indomethacin). *Am. J. Obstet. Gynecol.*, **157**, 422–6

102. Kirshon, B., Mari, G. and Moise, K. J. (1990). Indomethacin therapy in the treatment of symptomatic polyhydramnios. *Obstet. Gynecol.*, **75**, 202–5

103. Moise, K. J., Huhta, J. C., Sharif, D. S., Ou, C-N., Kirshon, B., Wasserstrum, N. and Cano, L. (1988). Indomethacin in the treatment of premature labor: effects on the fetal ductus arteriosus. *N. Engl. J. Med.*, **319**, 327–31

104. Besinger, R. E., Niebyl, J. R., Keyes, W. G. and Johnson, T. R. (1991). Randomized comparative trial of indomethacin and ritodrine for the long-term treatment of preterm labor. *Am. J. Obstet. Gynecol.*, **164**, 981–6

105. Cardwell, M. S. (1987). Polyhydramnios: a review. *Obstet. Gynecol. Surv.*, **42**, 612–17

106. Peipert, J. F. and Donnenfeld, A. E. (1991). Oligohydramnios: a review. *Obstet. Gynecol. Surv.*, **46**, 325–39

107. Weitzner, J. S., Strassner, H. T., Rawlins, R. G., Mack, S. R. and Anderson, R. A. (1990). Objective assessment of meconium content of amniotic fluid. *Obstet. Gynecol.*, **76**, 1143–4

108. Katz, V. L. and Bowes, W. A. (1992). Meconium aspiration syndrome: reflections on a murky subject. *Am. J. Obstet. Gynecol.*, **166**, 171–83

109. Benett, S. L., Cullen, J. B. H., Sherer, D. M. and Woods, J. R. (1993). The ferning and nitrazine tests of amniotic fluid between 12 and 41 weeks' gestation. *Am. J. Perinatol.*, **10**, 101–4

110. Rosemond, R. L., Lombardi, S. J. and Boehm, F. H. (1990). Ferning of amniotic fluid contaminated with blood. *Obstet. Gynecol.*, **75**, 338–401

111. Gorree, G. C., Egberts, J., Bakker, G. C., Beintema, A. and Top, M. A. (1991). Development of a human lung surfactant, derived from extracted amniotic fluid. *Biochim. Biophys. Acta*, **1086**, 209–16

112. Strayer, D. S., Hallman, M. and Merritt, T. A. (1991). Immunogenicity of surfactant. I. Human alveolar surfactant. *Clin. Exp. Immunol.*, **83**, 35–40

113. Lu, J., Willis, A. C. and Reid, K. B. (1992). Purification, characterization and cDNA cloning of human lung surfactant protein D. *Biochem. J.*, **284**, 795–802

114. Harper, M. D. and Lorentz, W. B. Jr. (1993). Immature lecithin/sphingomyelin ratios and neonatal respiratory course. *Am. J. Obstet. Gynecol.*, **168**, 495–8

115. Ashwood, E. R., Palmer, S. E., Taylor, J. S. and Pingree, S. S. (1993). Lamellar body counts for rapid fetal lung maturity testing. *Obstet. Gynecol.*, **81**, 619–24

116. Herbert, W. N., Chapman, J. F. and Schnoor, M. M. (1993). Role of the TDx FLM assay in fetal lung maturity. *Am. J. Obstet. Gynecol.*, **168**, 808–12

117. Ashwood, E. R., Palmer, S. E. and Lenke, R. R. (1992). Rapid fetal lung maturity testing: commercial versus NBD-phosphatidylcholine assay. *Obstet. Gynecol.*, **80**, 1048–53

118. Chen, C., Roby, P. V., Weiss, N. S., Wilson, J. A., Benedetti, T. J. and Tait, J. F. (1992). Clinical evaluation of the NBD-PC fluorescence polarization assay for prediction of fetal lung maturity. *Obstet. Gynecol.*, **80**, 688–92

119. Sbarra, A. J., Chaudhury, A., Cetrulo, C. L., Mittendorf, R., Shakr, C., Kennison, R., Jones, J. and Kennedy, J. Jr. (1991). A rapid visual test for predicting fetal lung maturity. *Am. J. Obstet. Gynecol.*, **165**, 1351–3

120. Steinfeld, J. D., Samuels, P., Bulley, M. A., Cohen, A. W., Goodman, D. B. and Senior,

M. B. (1992). The utility of the TDx test in the assessment of fetal lung maturity. *Obstet. Gynecol.*, **79**, 460–4
121. Bowie, L. J., Shammo, J., Dohnal, J. C., Farrell, E. and Vye, M. V. (1991). Lamellar body number density and the prediction of respiratory distress. *Am. J. Clin. Pathol.*, **95**, 781–6
122. Pearlman, E. S., Baiocchi, J. M., Lease, J. A., Gilbert, J. and Cooper, J. H. (1991). Utility of a rapid lamellar body count in the assessment of fetal maturity. *Am. J. Clin. Pathol.*, **95**, 778–80
123. Guidozzi, F. and Gobetz, L. (1991). The tap test — a rapid bedside indicator of fetal lung maturity. *Br. J. Obstet. Gynaecol.*, **98**, 479–81
124. Cohen, G. R., Thorp, J., Yeast, J. D., Meyer, B. A., O'Kell, R. and Macy, C. (1991). A markedly immature lecithin–sphingomyelin ratio at term and congenital hypothyroidism (letter). *Am. J. Dis. Child.*, **145**, 1227–8
125. Liberman, E., Torday, J., Barbieri, R., Cohen, A., Van Nunakis, H. and Weiss, S. T. (1992). Association of intrauterine cigarette smoke exposure with indices of fetal lung maturation. *Obstet. Gynecol.*, **79**, 564–70
126. Vintzileos, A. M., Campbell, W. A., Nochimson, D. J. and Weinbaum, P. J. (1985). Degree of oligohydramnios and pregnancy outcome in patients with premature rupture of the membranes. *Obstet. Gynecol.*, **66**, 162–7
127. Gonik, B., Bottoms, S. F. and Cotton, D. B. (1985). Amniotic fluid volume as a risk factor in preterm premature rupture of the membranes. *Obstet. Gynecol.*, **65**, 456–9
128. Vintzileos, A. M., Campbell, W. A., Nochimson, D. J., Weinbaum, P. J., Escoto, D. T. and Mirochnick, M. H. (1986). Qualitative amniotic fluid volume versus amniocentesis in predicting infection in preterm premature rupture of the membranes. *Obstet. Gynecol.*, **67**, 579–83
129. Harding, J. A., Jackson, D. M., Lewis, D. F., Major, C. A., Nageotte, M. P. and Asrat, T. (1991). Correlation of amniotic fluid index and nonstress test in patients with preterm premature rupture of membranes. *Am. J. Obstet. Gynecol.*, **165**, 1088–94
130. Toohey, J. S., Lewis, D. F., Harding, J. A., Crade, M., Asrat, T., Major, C. A., Garite, T. J. and Porto, M. (1991). Does amniotic fluid index affect the accuracy of estimated fetal weight in premature rupture of membranes? *Am. J. Obstet. Gynecol.*, **165**, 1060–2
131. Thibeault, D. W., Beatty, E. C., Hall, R. T., Bowen, S. K. and O'Neill, D. H. (1985). Neonatal pulmonary hypoplasia with premature rupture of fetal membranes and oligohydramnios. *J. Pediatr.*, **107**, 273–7
132. Kilbride, H. W., Thibeault, D. W., Yeast, J., Maulik, D. and Grundy, J. (1988). Amniotic fluid volume from ultrasound assessment is the most predictive parameter for pulmonary hypoplasia (PH) following premature rupture of membranes (PROM). *Pediatr. Res.*, **22**, 512A
133. Van Reempts, P., Kegelaers, B., Van Dam, K. and Van Overmeire, B. (1993). Neonatal outcome after very prolonged and premature rupture of membranes. *Am. J. Perinatol.*, **10**, 288
134. D'Alton, M., Mercer, B., Riddick, E. and Dudley, D. (1992). Serial thoracic versus abdominal circumference ratios for the prediction of pulmonary hypoplasia in premature rupture of the membranes remote from term. *Am. J. Obstet. Gynecol.*, **166**, 658–83
135. Rotschild, A., Ling, E. W., Puterman, M. L. and Farquharson, D. (1990). Neonatal outcome after prolonged preterm rupture of the membranes. *Am. J. Obstet. Gynecol.*, **162**, 46
136. Piper, J. M., Ray, W. A. and Rosa, F. W. (1992). Pregnancy outcome following exposure to angiotensin-converting enzyme inhibitors. *Obstet. Gynecol.*, **80**, 429–32
137. Fisk, N. M., Parkes, M. J., Moore, P. G., Hanson, M. A., Wigglesworth, J. and Rodeck, C. H. (1992). Mimicking low amniotic pressure by chronic pharyngeal drainage does not impair lung development in fetal sheep. *Am. J. Obstet. Gynecol.*, **166**, 991–6
138. Peters, C. A., Reid, L. M., Docimo, S., Luetic, T., Carr, M., Retik, A. B. and Mandell, (1991). The role of the kidney in lung growth and maturation in the setting of obstructive uropathy and oligohydramnios. *J. Urol.*, **146**, 597–600
139. Ring, E., Hofmann, H., Erwa, W., Riccabona, M., Zobel, G. and Hausler, M. (1991). Amniotic fluid N-acetyl-beta-D-glucosaminidase activity and renal abnormalities. *Arch. Dis. Child.*, **66**, 1147–9
140. Johnson, J. W. C., Egerman, R. S. and Moorhead, J. (1990). Cases with ruptured membranes that 'reseal'. *Am. J. Obstet. Gynecol.*, **163**, 1024–32
141. Silver, H. M., Gibbs, R. S., Gray, B. M. and Dilon, H. C. (1990). Risk factors for perinatal group B streptococcal disease after amniotic fluid colonization. *Am. J. Obstet. Gynecol.*, **163**, 19–25
142. Matorras, R., Garcia-Perea, A., Usandizaga, J. A. and Omenaca, F. (1991). Group B streptococ-

cal disease (letter; comment). *Am. J. Obstet. Gynecol.*, **164**, 1152–3

143. American Academy of Pediatrics. Committee on Infectious Diseases and Committee on Fetus and Newborn. (1992). Guidelines for prevention of group B streptococci (GBS) infection by chemoprophylaxis. *Pediatrics*, **90**, 775–8

144. Larson, J. and Dooley, S. (1993). Group B streptococcal infections: an obstetrical viewpoint. *Pediatrics*, **91**, 148

145. Henderson, C. E., Egre, H., Turk, R., Aning, V., Szilagyi, G. and Divon, M. Y. (1993). Amniorrhexis lowers the incidence of positive cultures for group B streptococci. *Am. J. Obstet. Gynecol.*, **168**, 624–5

146. Boyer, K. M. and Gotoff, S. P. (1986). Prevention of early-onset neonatal group B streptococcal disease with selective intrapartum chemoprophylaxis. *N. Engl. J. Med.*, **314**, 1665–9

147. Cullen, M. T., Reece, E. A., Whetham, J. and Hobbins, J. C. (1990). Embryoscopy: description of a new technique. *Am. J. Obstet. Gynecol.*, **162**, 82–6

148. Reece, E. A., Whetham, J., Rothmensch, S. and Wiznitzer, A. (1993). Gaining access to the embryonic-fetal circulation via first-trimester endoscopy: a step into the future. *Obstet. Gynecol.*, **82**, 876–9

149. Quintero, R. A., Romero, R., Mahoney, M. J., Vecchio, M., Holden, J. and Hobbins, J. C. (1992). Fetal haemorrhagic lesions after chorionic villous sampling. *Lancet*, **339**, 193

150. Sutter, J., Arab, H. and Manning, F. A. (1986). Monoamnaiotic twins: antenatal diagnosis and management. *Am. J. Obstet. Gynecol.*, **155**, 836–7

151. Briggs, G. G., Freeman, R. K. and Yaffe, S. J. (1990). *Drugs in Pregnancy and Lactation*, 3rd edn., pp. 288–9. (Baltimore: Williams and Wilkins)

152. Vorherr, H. (1975). Placental insufficiency in relation to postterm pregnancy and fetal postmaturity. *Am. J. Obstet. Gynecol.*, **123**, 67–103

153. D'Alton, M. E. and DeCherney, A. H. (1993). Prenatal diagnosis. *N. Engl. J. Med.*, **328**, 114–20

154. Snijders, R. J., Sherrod, C., Gosden, C. M. and Nicolaides, K. H. (1993). Fetal growth retardation: associated malformations and chromosomal abnormalities. *Am. J. Obstet. Gynecol.*, **168**, 547–55

155. Bryndorf, T., Christensen, B., Philip, J., Hansen, W., Yokobata, K., Bui, N. and Gaiser, C. (1992). New rapid test for prenatal detection of trisomy 21 (Down's syndrome): preliminary report. *Br. Med. J.*, **304**, 1536–9

156. Cervenka, J., Gorlin, R. J. and Bendel, R. P. (1971). Prenatal sex determination. Detection of 'Y body'. *Obstet. Gynecol.*, **37**, 912–5

157. Hitzeroth, H. W., Petersen, E. M., Herbert, J. and Denter, M. (1991). Preventing cystic fibrosis in the RSA. *S. Afr. Med. J.*, **80**, 92–8

158. Elias, S., Arnas, G. J. and Simpson, J. L. (1991). Carrier screening for cystic fibrosis: implications for obstetric and gynecologic practice. *Am. J. Obstet. Gynecol.*, **164**, 1077–83

159. Simard, L. R., Gingras, F. and Labuda, D. (1991). Direct analysis of amniotic fluid cells by multiplex PCR provides rapid prenatal diagnosis for Duchenne muscular dystrophy. *Nucleic Acids Res.*, **19**, 2501

160. Sarasin, A., Blanchet-Bardon, C., Renault, G., Lehmann, A., Arlett, C. and Dumez, Y. (1992). Prenatal diagnosis in a subset of trichothiodystrophy patients defective in DNA repair. *Br. J. Dermatol.*, **127**, 485–91

161. Hyland, K., Surtees, R. A., Rodeck, C. and Clayton, P. T. (1992). Aromatic L-amino acid decarboxylase deficiency: clinical features, diagnosis, and treatment of a new inborn error of neurotransmitter amine synthesis. *Neurology*, **42**, 1980–8

162. Lieberman, J. (1991). A CF-lectin factor in amniotic fluid from pregnancies at risk for cystic fibrosis. *Am. J. Med. Sci.*, **302**, 142–4

163. Chitayat, D., Meagher-Villemure, K., Mamer, O. A., O'Gorman, A., Hoar, D. I., Silver, K. and Scriver, C. R. (1992). Brain dysgenesis and congenital intracerebral calcification associated with 3-hydroxyisobutyric aciduria. *J. Pediatr.*, **121**, 86–9

164. Barratt, T. M., Kasidas, G. P., Murdoch, I. and Rose, G. A. (1991). Urinary oxalate and glycolate excretion and plasma oxalate concentration. *Arch. Dis. Child.*, **66**, 501–3

165. Shoemaker, J. D. and Elliott, W. H. (1991). Automated screening of urine samples for carbohydrates, organic and amino acids after treatment with urease. *J. Chromatogr.*, **562**, 125–38

166. Kaartinen, V. and Mononen, I. (1990). Assay of aspartylglycosylaminase by high-performance liquid chromatography. *Anal Biochem.*, **190**, 98–101

167. Wiley, D. M., Szabo, I., Maguire, M. H., Finley, B. E. and Bennett, T. L. (1990). Measurement of hypoxanthine and xanthine in late-gestation human amniotic fluid by reversed-phase high-performance liquid chromatography with photodiode-array detection. *J. Chromatogr.*, **533**, 73–86

168. Pang, S., Clark, A. T., Freeman, L. C., Dolan, L. M., Immken, L., Mueller, O. T., Stiff, D. and Shulman, D. I. (1992). Maternal side effects of prenatal dexamethasone therapy for fetal congenital adrenal hyperplasia. *J. Clin. Endocrinol. Metab.*, **75**, 249–53

169. Dorr, H. G. and Sippell, W. G. (1993). Prenatal dexamethasone treatment in pregnancies at risk for congenital adrenal hyperplasia due to 21-hydroxylase deficiency: effect on midgestational amniotic fluid steroid levels. *J. Clin. Endocrinol. Metab.*, **76**, 117–20

170. Izumi, H., Saito, N., Ichiki, S., Makino, Y., Yukitake, K. and Kaneoka, T. (1993). Prenatal diagnosis of congenital lipoid adrenal hyperplasia. *Obstet. Gynecol.*, **81**, 839–41

171. Romero, R., Hanaoka, S., Mazor, M., Athanassiadis, A. P., Callahan, R., Hsu, Y. C., Avila, C., Nores, J. and Jiminez, C. (1991). Meconium-stained amniotic fluid: a risk factor for microbial invasion of the amniotic cavity. *Am. J. Obstet. Gynecol.*, **164**, 859–62

172. Altshuler, G., Arizawa, M. and Molnar-Nadasdy, G. (1992). Meconium-induced umbilical cord vascular necrosis and ulceration: a potential link between the placenta and poor pregnancy outcome. *Obstet. Gynecol.*, **79**, 760–6

173. Knox, G. E., Huddleston, J. F., Flowers, C. E., Eubanks, A. and Sutliff, G. (1979). Management of prolonged pregnancy: results of a prospective randomizedf trial. *Am. J. Obstet. Gynecol.*, **134**, 376–84

174. Spinnato, J. A., Ralston, K. K., Greenwell, E. R., Marcell, C. A. and Spinnato, J. A. III (1991). Amniotic fluid bilirubin and fetal hemolytic disease. *Am. J. Obstet. Gynecol.*, **165**, 1030–5

175. Queenan, J. T., Tomai, T. P., Ural, S. H. and King, J. C. (1993). Deviation in amniotic fluid optical density at a wavelength of 450 nm in Rh-immunized pregnancies from 14 to 40 weeks' gestation: a proposal for clinical management. *Am. J. Obstet. Gynecol.*, **168**, 1370–6

176. Steyn, D. W., Pattinson, R. C. and Odendaal, H. J. (1992). Amniocentesis — still important in the management of severe rhesus incompatibility. *S. Afr. Med. J.*, **82**, 321–4

177. Bowman, J. M., Pollack, J. M., Manning, F. A., Harman, C. R. and Menticoglou, S. (1992). Maternal Kell blood group alloimmunization. *Obstet. Gynecol.*, **79**, 239–44

178. Leggat, H. M., Gibson, J. M., Barron, S. L. and Reid, M. M. (1991). Anti-Kell in pregnancy. *Br. J. Obstet. Gynaecol.*, **98**, 162–5

179. Bennett, P. R., Le Van Kim, C., Colin, Y., Warwick, R. M., Chérif-Zahar, B., Fisk, N. M. and Cartron, J.-P. (1993). Prenatal determination of fetal RhD type by DNA amplification. *N. Engl. J. Med.*, **329**, 607–10

180. Miyazawa, K. (1992). Role of epidermal growth factor in obstetrics and gynecology. *Obstet. Gynecol.*, **79**, 1032–40

181. Kubota, T., Kamada, S., Taguchi, M. and Aso, T. (1992). Determination of insulin-like growth factor-2 in feto-maternal circulation during human pregnancy. *Acta Endocrinol. (Copenh.)*, **127**, 359–65

182. Oh, Y., Muller, H. L., Lee, D. Y., Fielder, P. J. and Rosenfeld, R. G. (1993). Characterization of the affinities of insulin-like growth factor (IGF)-binding proteins 1–4 for IGF-I, IGF-II, IGF-I/insulin hybrid, and IGF-I analogs. *Endocrinology*, **132**, 1337–44

183. Gargosky, S. E., Pham, H. M., Wilson, K. F., Liu, F., Guidice, L. C. and Rosenfeld, R. G. (1992). Measurement and characterization of insulin-like growth factor binding protein-3 in human biological fluids: discrepancies between radioimmunoassay and ligand blotting. *Endocrinology*, **131**, 3051–60

184. Baxter, R. C. and Saunders, H. (1992). Radioimmunoassay of insulin-like growth factor-binding protein-6 in human serum and other body fluids. *J. Endocrinol.*, **134**, 133–9

185. Roghani, M., Lassarre, C., Zapf, J., Povoa, G. and Binoux, M. (1991). Two insulin-like growth factor (IGF)-binding proteins are responsible for the selectiuve affinity for IGF-II of cerebrospinal fluid binding proteins. *J. Clin. Endocrinol. Metab.*, **73**, 658–66

186. Liu, L., Brinkman, A., Blat, C. and Harel, L. (1991). IGFBP-1, an insulin like growth factor binding protein, is a cell growth inhibitor. *Biochem. Biophys. Res. Commun.*, **1174**, 673–9

187. Wang, H. S., Perry, L. A., Kanisius, J., Iles, R. K., Holly, J. M. and Chard, T. (1991). Purification and assay of insulin-like growth factor-binding protein-1: measurement of circulating levels throughout pregnancy. *J. Endocrinol.*, **128**, 161–8

188. Gargosky, S. E., Walton, P. E., Wallace, J. C. and Ballard, F. J. (1990). Characterization of insulin-like growth factor-binding proteins in rat serum, lymph, cerebrospinal and amniotic fluids, and in media conditioned by liver, bone and muscle cells. *J. Endocrinol.*, **127**, 391–400

189. Wang, J. F., Fraher, L. J. and Hill, D. J. (1990). Characterization of insulin-like growth factor-

binding protein in ovine amniotic fluid. *J. Endocrinol.*, **127**, 325–33
190. Hakala-Ala-Pietila, T. H., Koistinen, R. A., Salonen, R. K. and Seppala, M. T. (1993). Elevated second-trimester amniotic fluid concentration of insulin-like growth factor binding protein-1 in fetal growth retardation. *Am. J. Obstet. Gynecol.*, **169**, 35–9
191. Verhaeghe, J., Van Bree, R., Van Herck, E., Laureys, J., Bouillon, R. and Van Assche, F. A. (1993). C-peptide, insulin-like growth factors I and II, and insulin-like growth factor binding protein-1 in umbilical cord serum: correlations with birth weight. *Am. J. Obstet. Gynecol.*, **169**, 89–97
192. Silverman, B. L., Rizzo, T., Green, O. C., Cho, N. H., Winter, R. J., Ogata, E. S., Richards, G. E. and Metzger, B. E. (1991). Long-term prospective evaluation of offspring of diabetic mothers. *Diabetes*, **40**, 121–5
193. Heffner, L. J., Bromley, B. S. and Copeland, K. C. (1992). Secretion of prolactin and insulin like growth factor I by decidual explant cultures from pregnancies complicated by intrauterine growth retardation. *Am. J. Obstet. Gynecol.*, **167**, 1431–6
194. Daiter, E., Pampfer, S., Yeung, Y. G., Barad, D., Stanley, E. R. and Pollard, J. W. (1992). Expression of colony-stimulating factor-1 in the human uterus and placenta. *J. Clin. Endocrinol. Metab.*, **74**, 850–8
195. Plopper, C. G., St. George, J. A., Read, L. C., Nishio, S. J., Weir, A. J., Edwards, L., Tarantal, A. F., Pinkerton, K. E., Merritt, T. A., Whitsett, J. A. *et al.* (1992). Acceleration of alveolar type II cell differentiation in fetal rhesus monkey lung by administration of EGF. *Am. J. Physiol.*, **262**, L313–21
196. Rittenburg, T., Longaker, M. T., Adzick, N. S. and Ehrlich, H. P. (1991). Sheep amniotic fluid has a protein factor which stimulates human fibroblast populated collagen lattice contraction. *J. Cell Physiol.*, **149**, 444–50
197. Mast, B. A., Diegelmann, R. F., Krummel, T. M. and Cohen, I. K. (1992). Scarless wound healing in the mammalian fetus. *Surg. Gynecol. Obstet.*, **174**, 441–51
198. Rasmussen, H. B., Teisner, B., Andersen, J. A., Yde-Anderson, E. and Leigh, I. (1992). Foetal antigen 2 (FA2) in relation to wound healing and fibroblast proliferation. *Br. J. Dermatol.*, **126**, 148–53
199. Wathen, N. C., Campbell, D. J., Kitau, M. J. and Chard, T. (1993). Alpha-fetoprotein levels in amniotic fluid from 8 to 18 weeks of pregnancy. *Br. J. Obstet. Gynaecol.*, **100**, 380–2
200. Fogarty, P. P. (1992). Early amniocentesis: alpha-fetoprotein levels in amniotic fluid, extraembronic coelomic fluid and maternal serum between 8 and 13 weeks (letter). *Br. J. Obstet. Gynaecol.*, **99**, 530
201. Loft, A. G., Mortensen, V., Hangaard, J. and Nargaard-Pedersen, B. (1991). Ratio of immunochemically determined amniotic fluid acetylcholinesterase to butyrylcholinesterase in the differential diagnosis of fetal abnormalities. *Br. J. Obstet. Gynaecol.*, **98**, 52–6
202. Wathen, N. C., Cass, P. L., Campbell, D. J., Kitau, M. J. and Chard, T. (1991). Early amniocentesis: alpha-fetoprotein levels in amniotic fluid, extraembryonic coelomic fluid and maternal serum between 8 and 13 weeks. *Br. J. Obstet. Gynaecol.*, **98**, 866–70
203. Wiechen, K., Plendl, H. and Grote, W. (1991). Isoelectric focusing of amniotic fluid alpha-fetoprotein to improve diagnosis of neural tube defects (letter). *Lancet*, **337**, 674
204. Hogge, W. A., Hogge, J. S., Schnatterly, P., Sun, C. J. and Blitzer, M. G. (1992). Congenital nephrosis: detection of index case through maternal serum alpha-fetoprotein. *Am. J. Obstet. Gynecol.*, **167**, 1330–3
205. Haddow, J. E., Knight, G. J., Palomaki, G. E. and Johnson, A. M. (1991). Maternal serum alpha-fetoprotein in congenital hypothyroidism (letter; comment). *Lancet*, **337**, 922
206. Economides, D. L., Ferguson, J., Mackenzie, I. Z., Darley, J., Ware, I. I. and Holmes-Siedle, M. (1992). Folate and vitamin B12 concentrations in maternal and fetal blood, and amniotic fluid in second trimester pregnancies complicated by neural tube defects. *Br. J. Obstet. Gynaecol.*, **99**, 23–5
207. Cuckle, H. S., Wald, N. J., Densem, J. W., Canick, J. and Abell, K. B. (1991). Second trimester amniotic fluid oestriol, dehydroepiandrosterone sulphate, and human chorionic gonaodtrophin levels in Down's syndrome. *Br. J. Obstet. Gynaecol.*, **98**, 1160–2
208. Clark, S. L. (1992). Successful pregnancy outcomes after amniotic fluid embolism. *Am. J. Obstet. Gynecol.*, **167**, 511–2
209. Kool, M. J. (1991). Successful treatment of postpartum shock caused by amniotic fluid embolism with cardiopulmonary bypass and pulmonary artery thromboembolectomy (letter). *Am. J. Obstet. Gynecol.*, **164**, 701–2

210. Hardin, L., Fox, L. S. and O'Quinn, A. G. (1991). Amniotic fluid embolism. *South. Med. J.*, **84**, 1046–8
211. Hankins, G. D., Snyder, R. R., Clark, S. L., Schwartz, L., Patterson, W. R. and Butzin, C. A. (1993). Acute hemodynamic and respiratory effects of amniotic fluid embolism in the pregnant goat model. *Am. J. Obstet. Gynecol.*, **168**, 1113–29; Discussion, 1129–30
212. Kobayashi, H., Ohi, H. and Terao, T. (1993). A simple, noninvasive, sensitive method for diagnosis of amniotic fluid embolism by monoclonal antibody TKH-2 that recognizes NeuAc alpha 2-6GalNAc. *Am. J. Obstet. Gynecol.*, **168**, 848–53
213. Lockwood, C. J., Bach, R., Guha, A., Zhou, X. D., Miller, W. A. and Nemerson, Y. (1991). Amniotic fluid contains tissue factor, a potent initiator of coagulation. *Am. J. Obstet. Gynecol.*, **165**, 1335–41
214. España, F., Gilabert, J., Estellés, A., Romeu, A., Aznar, J. and Cabo, A. (1991). Functionally active protein C inhibitor/plasminogen activator inhibitor-2 (PCI/PAI-3) is secreted in seminal vesicles, occurs at high concentrations in human seminal plasma and complexes with prostate-specific antigen. *Thromb. Res.*, **64**, 309–20
215. O'Brodovich, H., Berry, L., D'Costa, M., Burrows, R. and Andrew, M. (1991). Influence of fetal pulmonary epithelium on thrombin activity. *Am. J. Physiol.*, **261**, L262–70
216. Watanabe, T., Araki, M., Mimuro, J., Tamada, T. and Sakata, Y. (1993). Fibrinolytic components in fetal membranes and amniotic fluid. *Am. J. Obstet. Gynecol.*, **68**, 1283–9
217. Lamy, M. E., Mulongo, K. N., Gadisseux, J. F., Lyon, G., Gaudy, V. and Van Lierde, M. (1992). Prenatal diagnosis of fetal cytomegalovirus infection. *Am. J. Obstet. Gynecol.*, **166**, 91–4
218. Skvorc-Ranko, R., Lavoie, H., St-Denis, P., Villeneuve, R., Gagnon, M., Chicoine, R., Boucher, M., Guimond, J. and Dontigny, Y. (1991). Intrauterine diagnosis of cytomegalovirus and rubella infections by amniocentesis. *Can. Med. Assoc. J.*, **145**, 649–54
219. Wendel, G. D. Jr, Sanchez, P. J., Peters, M. T., Harstad, T. W., Potter, L. L. and Norgard, M. V. (1991). Identification of *Treponema pallidum* in amniotic fluid and fetal blood from pregnancies complicated by congenital syphilis. *Obstet. Gynecol.*, **78**, 890–5
220. Lucas, M. J., Theriot, S. K. and Wendel, G. D. Jr (1991). Doppler systolic-diastolic ratios in pregnancies complicated by syphilis. *Obstet. Gynecol.*, **77**, 217–22
221. Pao, C. C., Kao, S. M., Wang, H. C. and Lee, C. C. (1991). Intraamniotic detection of *Chlamydia trachomatis* deoxyribonucleic acid sequences by polymerase chain reaction. *Am. J. Obstet. Gynecol.*, **164**, 1295–9
222. Viscarello, R. R., Cullen, M. T., DeGennaro, N. J. and Hobbins, J. C. (1992). Fetal blood sampling in human-immunodeficiency-virus-seropositive women before elective midtrimester termination of pregnancy. *Am. J. Obstet. Gynecol.*, **167**, 1075–9
223. Gibbs, R. S. and Duff, P. (1991). Progress in pathogenesis and management of clinical intraamniotic infection. *Am. J. Obstet. Gynecol.*, **164**, 1317–26
224. Harger, J. H., Meyer, M. P., Amortegui, A., Macpherson, T. A., Kaplain, L. and Mueller-Heubach, E. (1991). Low incidence of positive amnionic fluid cultures in preterm labor at 27–32 weeks in the absence of clinical evidence of chorioamnionitis. *Obstet. Gynecol.*, **77**, 228–34
225. Watts, D. H., Krohn, M. A., Hillier, S. L. and Eschenbach, D. A. (1992). The association of occult amniotic fluid infection with gestational age and neonatal outcome among women in preterm labor. *Obstet. Gynecol.*, **79**, 351–7
226. Romero, R., Salafia, C. M., Athanassiadis, A. P., Hanaoka, S., Mazor, M., Sepulveda, W. and Bracken, M. B. (1992). The relationship between acute inflammatory lesions of the preterm placenta and amniotic fluid microbiology. *Am. J. Obstet. Gynecol.*, **166**, 1382–8
227. Gauthier, D. W. and Meyer, W. J. (1992). Comparison of gram stain, leukocyte esterase activity, and amniotic fluid glucose concentration in predicting amniotic fluid culture results in preterm premature rupture of membranes. *Am. J. Obstet. Gynecol.*, **167**, 1092–5
228. Romero, R., Mazor, M., Morrotti, R., Avila, C., Oyarzun, E., Insunza, A., Parra, M., Behnke, E., Montiel, F. and Cassell, G. H. (1992). Infection and labor. VII. Microbial invasion of the amniotic cavity in spontaneous rupture of membranes at term. *Am. J. Obstet. Gynecol.*, **166**, 129–33
229. Poka, R. and Lampe, L. (1993). Microinvasion of the amniotic cavity increases the risk of post-cesarean section endometritis (letter). *Am. J. Obstet. Gynecol.*, **168**, 275–6
230. Romero, R., Gonzalez, R., Sepulveda, W., Brandt, F., Ramirez, M., Sorokin, Y., Mazor, M., Treadwell, M. C. and Cotton, D. B. (1992). In-

fection and labor. VII. Microbial invasion of the amniotic cavity in patients with suspected cervical incompetence: prevalence and clinical significance. *Am. J. Obstet. Gynecol.*, **167**, 1086–91

231. Dombroski, R. A., Woodard, D. S., Harper, M. J. and Gibbs, R. S. (1991). A rabbit model for bacteria-induced preterm pregnancy loss. *Am. J. Obstet. Gynecol.*, **163**, 1938–43

232. Romero, R., Hagay, Z., Nores, J., Sepulveda, W. and Mazor, M. (1992). Eradication of *Ureaplasma urealyticum* from the amniotic fluid with transplacental antibiotic treatment. *Am. J. Obstet. Gynecol.*, **166**, 618–20

233. Hoskins, I. A., Katz, J., Kadner, S. S., Young, B. K. and Finlay, T. (1992). Use of esterase inhibitors and zone electrophoresis to define bacterial esterases in amniotic fluid. *Am. J. Obstet. Gynecol.*, **167**, 1579–82

234. Hoskins, I. A., Katz, J., Frieden, F. J., Ordorica, S. A. and Young, B. K. (1990). *In vitro* inhibition of esterase activity in amniotic fluid: comparison with bacterial cultures. *Am. J. Obstet. Gynecol.*, **163**, 1944–7

235. Vadillo-Ortega, F., González-Avila, G., Villanueva-Diaz, C., Bañales, J. L., Selman-Lama, M., Alvarado-Durán, A. (1991). Human amniotic fluid modulation of collagenase production in cultured fibroblasts. A model of fetal membrane rupture. *Am. J. Obstet. Gynecol.*, **164**, 664–8

236. Gauthier, D. W., Meyer, W. J. and Bieniarz, A. (1991). Correlation of amniotic fluid glucose concentration and intraamniotic infection in patients with preterm labor or premature rupture of membranes. *Am. J. Obstet. Gynecol.*, **165**, 1105–10

237. Kiltz, R. J., Burke, M. S. and Porreco, R. P. (1991). Amniotic fluid glucose concentration as a marker for intra-amniotic infection. *Obstet. Gynecol.*, **78**, 619–22

238. Kirshon, B., Rosenfeld, B., Mari, G. and Belfort, M. (1991). Amniotic fluid glucose and intraamniotic infection. *Am. J. Obstet. Gynecol.*, **164**, 818–20

239. Gonen, R. (1992). Amniotic fluid glucose and intraamniotic infection: sensitivity, specificity, and predictive values (letter). *Am. J. Obstet. Gynecol.*, **166**, 1863–4

240. Meyer, W. J. and Gauthier, D. W. (1992). Effect of time and storage temperature on amniotic fluid glucose concentrations. *Obstet. Gynecol.*, **80**, 1017–9

241. Romero, R., Quintero, R., Nores, J., Avila, C., Mazor, M., Hanaoka, S., Hagay, Z., Merchant, L. and Hobbins, J. C. (1991). Amniotic fluid white blood cell count: a rapid and simple test to diagnose microbial invasion of the amniotic cavity and predict preterm delivery. *Am. J. Obstet. Gynecol.*, **165**, 821–30

242. Cherouny, P. H., Pankuch, G. A., Botti, J. J. and Appelbaum, P. C. (1992). The presence of fluid leukoattractants accurately identifies histologic chorioamnionitis and predicts tocolytic efficacy in patients with idiopathic preterm labor. *Am. J. Obstet. Gynecol.*, **167**, 683–8

243. Hillier, S. L., Witkin, S. S., Krohn, M. A., Watts, D. H., Kiviat, N. B. and Eschenbach, D. A. (1993). The relationship of amniotic fluid cytokines and preterm delivery, amniotic fluid infection, histologic chorioamnionitis, and chorioamnion infection. *Obstet. Gynecol.*, **81**, 941–8

244. Greig, P. C., Ernest, J. M., Teot, L., Erikson, M. and Talley, R. (1993). Amniotic fluid interleukin-6 levels correlate with histologic chorioamnionitis and amniotic fluid cultures in patients in premature labor with intact membranes. *Am. J. Obstet. Gynecol.*, **169**, 1035–44

245. Opsjøn, S.-L., Wathen, N. C., Tingulstad, S., Wiedswang, G., Sundan, A., Waage, A. and Austgulen, R. (1993). Tumor necrosis factor, interleukin-1 and interleukin-6 in normal human pregnancy. *Am. J. Obstet. Gynecol.*, **169**, 397–404

246. Austgulen, R., Johnson, H., Kjøllesdal, A. M., Liabakk, N. B. and Espevik, T. (1993). Soluble receptors for tumor necrosis factor: occurrence in association with normal delivery at term. *Obstet. Gynecol.*, **82**, 343

247. Romero, R., Ceska, M., Avila, C., Mazor, M., Behnke, E. and Lindley, I. (1991). Neutrophil attractant/activating peptide-1/interleukin-8 in term and preterm parturition. *Am. J. Obstet. Gynecol.*, **165**, 813–20

248. Hasegawa, M., Sagawa, N., Ihara, Y., Okagawi, A., Li, X. M., Inamori, M., Itoh, H., Mori, T., Saito, Y., Shirakami, G. *et al.* (1991). Concentrations of endothelin-1 in human amniotic fluid at various stages of pregnancy. *J. Cardiovasc. Pharmacol.*, **17** (Suppl. 7), S440–2

249. Chou, J., Wang, Y. N., Chang, D., Chang, J. K., Avila, C. and Romero, R. (1991). Big endothelin in plasma and amniotic fluid. *J. Cardiovasc. Pharmacol.*, **7** (Suppl. 7), S430–3

250. Iwata, I., Takagim T., Yamaji, K. and Tanizawa, O. (1991). Increase in the concentration of immunoreactive endothelin in human pregnancy. *J. Endocrinol.*, **129**, 301–7

251. Casey, M. L., Word, R. A. and MacDonald, P. C. (1991). Endothelin-1 gene expression and regulation of endothelin mRNA and protein biosynthesis in avascular human amnion. Potential source of amniotic fluid endothelin. *J. Biol. Chem.*, **266**, 5762–8
252. Romero, R., Avila, C., Edwin, S. S. and Mitchell, M. D. (1992). Endothelin-1,2 levels are increased in the amniotic fluid of women with preterm labor and microbial invasion of the amniotic cavity. *Am. J. Obstet. Gynecol.*, **166**, 95–9
253. Heyborne, K. D., Witkin, S. S. and McGregor, J. A. (1992). Tumor necrosis factor-alpha in midtrimester amniotic fluid is associated with impaired intrauterine fetal growth. *Am. J. Obstet. Gynecol.*, **167**, 920–5
254. Gendron, R. L., Nestel, F. P., Lapp, W. S. and Baines, M. G. (1990). Lipopolysaccharide-induced fetal resorption in mice is associated with the intrauterine production of tumor necrosis factor-alpha. *J. Reprod. Fertil.*, **90**, 395–402
255. McDuffie, R. S. Jr, Sherman, M. P. and Gibbs, R. S. (1992). Amniotic fluid tumor necrosis factor-alpha and interleukin-1 in a rabbit model of bacterially induced preterm pregnancy loss. *Am. J. Obstet. Gynecol.*, **167**, 1583–8
256. Romero, R., Mazor, M., Sepulveda, W., Avila, C., Copeland, D. and Williams, J. (1992). Tumor necrosis factor in preterm and term labor. *Am. J. Obstet. Gynecol.*, **166**, 1576–87
257. Waring, P., Wycherley, K., Cary, D., Nicola, N. and Metcalf, D. (1992). Leukemia inhibitory factor levels are elevated in septic shock and various inflammatory body fluids. *J. Clin. Invest.*, **90**, 2031–7
258. Valenzuela, G. J., Norburg, M. and Ducsay, C. A. (1992). Acute intrauterine hypoxia increases amniotic fluid prostaglandin F metabolites in the pregnant sheep. *Am. J. Obstet. Gynecol.*, **167**, 1459–64
259. Collins, P. L., Goldfien, A. and Roberts, J. M. (1992). Exposure of human amnion to amniotic fluid obtained before labor causes a decrease in chorion/decidual prostaglandin release. *J. Clin. Endocrinol. Metab.*, **74**, 1198–205
260. Romero, R., Baumann, P., Gomez, R., Salafia, C., Rittenhouse, L., Barberio, D., Behnke, E., Cotton, D. B. and Mitchell, M. D. (1993). The relationship between spontaneous rupture of membranes, labor, and microbial invasion of the amniotic cavity and amniotic fluid concentrations of prostaglandins and thromboxane B2 in term pregnancy. *Am. J. Obstet. Gynecol.*, **168**, 1654–64
261. MacDonald, P. C. and Casey, M. L. (1993). The accumulation of prostaglandins (PG) in amniotic fluid is an aftereffect of labor and not indicative of a role for PGE2 or PGF2 alpha in the initiation of human parturition. *J. Clin. Endocrinol. Metab.*, **76**, 1332–9
262. Carsten, M. E. and Miller, J. D. (1987). A new look at uterine muscle contraction. *Am. J. Obstet. Gynecol.*, **157**, 1303–15
263. Janszen, B. P., Bnign, H., Van der Weyden, G. C., Bevers, M. M., Dieleman, S. J. and Taverne, M. A. (1990). Flumethason-induced calving is preceded by a period of myometrial inhibition during luteolysis. *Biol. Reprod.*, **43**, 466–71
264. Romero, R., Sepulveda, W., Mazor, M., Brandt, F., Cotton, D. B., Dinarello, C. A. and Mitchell, M. D. (1992). The natural interleukin-1 receptor antagonist in term and preterm parturition. *Am. J. Obstet. Gynecol.*, **167**, 863–72
265. Bry, K. and Hallman, M. (1993). Transforming growth factor-beta 2 prevent preterm delivery induced by interleukin-1 alpha and tumor necrosis factor-alpha in the rabbit. *Am. J. Obstet. Gynecol.*, **168**, 1318–22
266. Wilbanks, G. A. and Steilein, J. W. (1992). Fluids from immune privileged sites endow macrophages with the capacity to induce antigen-specific immune deviation via a mechanism involving transforming growth factor-beta. *Eur. J. Immunol.*, **22**, 1031–6
267. Yoshimura, N., Matsui, S., Hamashima, T., Lee, C. J., Ohsaka, Y., Hirakawa, K. and Oka, T. (1991). Prolongation of renal allograft survivalk in the rat treated with amniotic fluid. *Transplantation*, **52**, 540–5
268. Wilson, T. and Christie, D. L. (1991). Gravidin, an endogenous inhibitor of phospholipase A2 activity, is a secretory component of IgA. *Biochem. Biophys. Res. Commun.*, **176**, 447–52
269. Cleveland, M. G., Bakos, M. A., Pyron, D. L., Rajaraman, S. and Goldblum, R. M. (1991). Characterization of secretory component in amniotic fluid. Identification of new forms of secretory IgA. *J. Immunol.*, **147**, 181–8
270. Rooney, I. A. and Morgan, B. P. (1992). Characterization of the membrane attack complex inhibitory protein CD59 antigen on human amniotic cells and in amniotic fluid. *Immunology*, **76**, 541–7
271. Kinoshita, T., Taketani, Y. and Mizuno, M. (1991). A decline in prolactin levels in amniotic fluid and decidua at term pregnancy after the initation of labour. *J. Endocrinol.*, **130**, 151–3

272. Eriksen, N. L., Parisi, V. M., Daoust, S., Flamm, B., Garite, T. J. and Cox, S. M. (1992). Fetal fibronectin: a method for detecting the presence of amniotic fluid. *Obstet. Gynecol.*, **80**, 451–4

273. Lockwood, C. J., Senyei, A. E., Dische, M. R., Casal, D., Shah, K. D., Thung, S. N., Jones, L., Deligdisch, L. and Garite, T. J. (1991). Fetal fibronectin in cervical and vaginal secretions as a predictor of preterm delivery. *N. Engl. J. Med.*, **325**, 669–74

274. Johnson, M. R., Abbas, A., Nicolaides, K. H. and Lightman, S. L. (1992). Distribution of relaxin between human maternal and fetal circulations and amniotic fluid. *J. Endocrinol.*, **134**, 313–7

275. Suda, T., Iwashita, M., Sumitomo, T., Nakano, Y., Tozawa, F. and Demura, H. (1991). Presence of CRH-binding protein in amniotic fluid and in umbilical cord plasma. *Acta Endocrinol (Copenh.)*, **125**, 165–9

276. Mauri, A., Serri, F., Caminiti, F., Mancuso, S., Fratta, W., Gessa, G. L. and Argiolas, A. (1990). Correlation between amniotic levels of alpha-MSH, ACTH and beta-endorphin in late gestation and labour in normal and complicated pregnancies. *Acta Endocrinol. (Copenh.)*, **123**, 637–42

277. Biswas, A., Chaudhury, A., Chattoraj, S. C. and Dale, S. L. (1991). Do catechol estrogens participate in the initiation of labor? *Am. J. Obstet. Gynecol.*, **165**, 984–7

278. McNutt, C. M. and Ducsay, C. A. (1991). Catecholamines and uterine activity rhythms in the pregnant rhesus macaque. *Biol. Reprod.*, **45**, 373–9

279. Noma, J., Hayashi, N. and Sekiba, K. (1991). Automated direct high-performance liquid chromatographic assay for esterol, estriol, cortisone and cortisol in serum and amniotic fluid. *J. Chromatogr.*, **568**, 35–44

280. Partsch, C. J., Sippell, W. G., MacKenzie, I. Z. and Aynsley-Green, A. (1991). The steroid hormonal milieu of the undisturbed human fetus and mother at 16–20 weeks' gestation. *J. Clin. Endocrinol. Metab.*, **73**, 9969–74

281. Qu, J. and Thomas, K. (1992). Changes in bioactive and immunoactive inhibin levels around human labor. *J. Clin. Endocrinol. Metab.*, **74**, 1290–5

282. Gauthier, D. W., Meyer, W. J. and Bieniarz, A. (1992). Biophysical profile as a predictor of amniotic fluid culture results. *Obstet. Gynecol.*, **80**, 102–5

283. Coultrip, L. L. and Grossman, J. H. (1992). Evaluation of rapid diagnostic tests in the detection of microbial invasion of the amniotic cavity. *Am. J. Obstet. Gynecol.*, **167**, 1231–42

284. Romero, R., Yoon, B. H., Mazor, M., Gomez, R., Diamond, M. P., Kenney, J. S., Ramirez, M., Fidel, P. L., Sorokin, Y., Cotton, D. and Sehgal, P. (1993). The diagnostic and prognostic value of amniotic fluid white blood cell count, glucose, interleukin-6, and Gram stain in patients with preterm labor and intact membranes. *Am. J. Obstet. Gynecol.*, **169**, 805

285. Romero, R., Sibai, B., Caritis, S., Paul, R., Depp, R., Rosen, M., Klebanoff, M., Sabo, V., Evans, J., Thom, E., Cefalo, R. and McNellis, D. (1993). Antibiotic treatment of preterm labor with intact membranes: a multicenter, randomized, double-blinded, placebo-controlled trial. *Am. J. Obstet. Gynecol.*, **169**, 764

286. Romero, R., Yoon, B. H., Mazor, M., Gomez, R., Gonzalez, R., Diamond, M. P., Baumann, P., Araneda, H., Kenney, J. S., Cotton, D. and Sehgal, P. (1993). A comparative study of the diagnostic performance of amniotic fluid glucose, white blood cell count, interleukin-6, and Gram stain in the detection of microbial invasion in patients with preterm premature rupture of membranes. *Am. J. Obstet. Gynecol.*, **169**, 839–51

287. Hallak, M., Berry, S. M., Madincea, F., Romero, R., Evans, M. I. and Cotton, D. B. (1993). Fetal serum and amniotic fluid magnesium concentrations with maternal treatment. *Obstet. Gynecol.*, **81**, 185–8

288. Jain, L., Meyer, W., Moore, C., Tebbett, I., Gauthier, D. and Vidyasagar, D. (1993). Detection of fetal cocaine exposure by analysis of amniotic fluid. *Obstet. Gynecol.*, **81**, 787–90

289. Sandberg, J. A. and Olsen, G. D. (1992). Cocaine and metabolite concentrations in the fetal guinea pig after chronic maternal cocaine administration. *J. Pharmacol. Exp. Ther.*, **260**, 587–91

290. Bourget, P., Fernandez, H., Delouis, C. and Ribou, F. (1991). Transplacental passage of vancomycin during the second trimester of pregnancy. *Obstet. Gynecol.*, **78**, 908–11

291. De Leeuw, J. W., Roumen, F. J., Bouckaert, P. X., Cremers, H. M. and Vree, T. B. (1993). Achievement of therapeutic concentrations of cefuroxime in early preterm gestations with premature rupture of the membranes. *Obstet. Gynecol.*, **81**, 255–60

292. Sadovxky, Y., Amon, E., Bade, M. E. and Petrie, R. H. (1989). Prophylactic amnioinfusion

during labor complicated by meconium: a preliminary report. *Am. J. Obstet. Gynecol.*, **161**, 613–17

293. Schrimmer, D. B., Macri, C. J. and Paul, R. H. (1991). Prophylactic amnioinfusion as a treatment for oligohydramnios in laboring patients: a prospective, randomized trial. *Am. J. Obstet. Gynecol.*, **165**, 972–5
294. Miyazaki, F. S. and Nevarez, F. (1985). Saline amnioinfusion for relief of repetitive variable decelerations: a prospective randomized study. *Am. J. Obstet. Gynecol.*, **153**, 301–6
295. Strong, T. H., Vega, J. S., O'Shaughnessy, M. J. et al. (1992). Amnioinfusion among women attempting vaginal birth after cesarean delivery. *Obstet. Gynecol.*, **79**, 673–4
296. Chauhan, S. P. (1991). Questions about prophylactic intrapartum amnioinfusion (letter; comment). *Am. J. Obstet. Gynecol.*, **164**, 1365–6
297. Chauhan, S. P. and Morrison, J. C. (1993). Questions on prophylactic amnioinfusion as a treatment for oligohydramnios (letter). *Am. J. Obstet. Gynecol.*, **168**, 1006–7
298. Sorenson, T., Sobeck, J. and Benedetti, T. (1991). Intrauterine pressure in acute iatrogenic hydramnios. *Obstet. Gynecol.*, **78**, 917–19
299. Arulkumaran, S., Yang, M., Tien, C. Y. and Ratnan, S. S. (1991). Reliability of intrauterine pressure measurements. *Obstet. Gynecol.*, **78**, 800–2
300. Miyazuki, F. S. (1991). The effect of amnioinfusion on uterine pressure and activity (letter). *Am. J. Obstet. Gynecol.*, **165**, 1898–9
301. Fisk, N. M., Ronderos-Dumit, D., Soliani, A., Nicolini, U., Vaughan, J. and Rodeck, C. H. (1991). Diagnostic and therapeutic transabdominal amnioinfusion in oligohydramnios. *Obstet. Gynecol.*, **78**, 270–8
302. Imanaka, M., Ogita, S. and Sugawa, T. (1989). Saline solution amnioinfusion for oligohydramnios after premature rupture of membranes: a preliminary report. *Am. J. Obstet. Gynecol.*, **161**, 102–6
303. Ogita, S., Imanaka, M., Matsumoto, M., Oka, T. and Sugawa, T. (1988). Transcervical amnioinfusion of antibiotics: a basic study of managing premature rupture of membranes. *Am. J. Obstet. Gynecol.*, **158**, 23–7

Prenatal diagnosis of skin disease

S. Brenner, A. Kurjak, D. Jurković, T. Kobayasi, R. E. Brandsen, H. Matz and U. Marton

The purpose of prenatal diagnosis is the detection or exclusion of a hereditary disease or congenital defect *in utero*[1]. Most prenatal diagnosis nowadays relies upon the cytogenetic or biochemical analysis of cultured amniotic fluid cells, fetal blood samples or placental tissue, and molecular biology. It is well known that chromosomal abnormalities are associated with multiple congenital abnormalities, high mortality and morbidity rates, and a poor long-term prognosis. Amniocentesis and ultrasonography, or ultrasound, are established methods, while fetoscopy and fetal blood and skin sampling are newer techniques, and chorionic villus sampling is the most recent development.

Prenatal diagnosis of genetic disease with major cutaneous manifestations is still largely limited to the detection of morphological or immunohistochemical abnormalities in fetal skin biopsies[1]. Amniotic fluid and its cells are used for diagnosing a variety of metabolic diseases with skin involvement. Direct analysis of fetal skin cells obtained by fetoscopy or ultrasonically guided biopsy is the only method for the proper prenatal diagnosis of some conditions[2,3].

FETAL SKIN BIOPSY

This procedure, which can be performed with the aid of a fetoscope or ultrasound scanners, consists of percutaneously inserting a biopsy forceps under continuous ultrasound guidance. Fetal skin sampling is performed optimally at 17–20 weeks' gestation[4].

Fetal skin biopsy has been used to diagnose a variety of diseases associated with characteristic or specific histological or ultrastructural changes. For example, epidermolysis bullosa of the junctional and dystrophic types is diagnosed at 15–18 weeks of gestation by finding a split in the dermo–epidermal junction on light microscopy; the precise level of cleavage is then determined by electron microscopy. Bullous ichthyosiform erythroderma, can be diagnosed at 20 weeks by detection of epidermal vacuolation and abnormal cellular inclusions[1], or, more specifically, highly characteristic tonofilament clumps in both fetal epidermal and amniotic fluid cells.

Certain inherited skin disorders that can be diagnosed or excluded by fetal skin biopsy include disorders of keratinization such as epidermolytic hyperkeratosis, lamellar ichthyosis, harlequin ichthyosis and Sjögren–Larsson syndrome; blistering disorders such as epidermolysis bullosa; pigmentary disorder such as oculocutaneous albinism; and other conditions such as Ehlers–Danlos syndrome type VI, and anhidrotic ectodermal dysplasia.

The risks associated with fetal skin sampling, apart from spontaneous abortion, include leakage of amniotic fluid per vagina, infection, prematurity, hemorrhage from injury to the anterior abdominal wall, uterus or placenta, fetal and maternal injuries, difficulty in interpreting the morphological and immunohistochemical features (this varies with the experience of the obstetrician and microscopist), artifact caused by the biopsy procedure and by processing the very small fetal skin samples, and scarring, which is rarely severe.

Zagreb experience

At the Ultrasonic Institute, University of Zagreb, 20 fetal skin biopsies have been performed under continuous ultrasound guidance since

1985. A TRU-CUT needle, 15 cm long and 1.7 mm in outer diameter is used. With the available high-resolution ultrasound equipment (Aloka 680 with sector transducer 3.5 MHz), the needle can be visualized easily within the uterus and directed toward virtually any anatomic area of the fetal skin. Thirty minutes before commencing the procedure, 10 mg of diazepam and 30 mg pentazocin are administered intravenously for maternal sedation; diazepam is used because it crosses the placenta and reduces fetal activity. The procedure is performed between 20 and 24 weeks of gestation with full aseptic technique. A preliminary ultrasound examination is needed to confirm gestational age by biometry, localize the position of placenta (especially the insertion of the cord), exclude multiple gestation, to confirm fetal viability and to determine the position of the fetus.

The biopsy needle is inserted transabdominally into the amniotic cavity under continuous guidance and placed against a stationary part of the fetus (usually the gluteal region), preselected depending on the suspected disorder. The point of insertion of the umbilical cord and the face, neck and genital regions should be avoided. During the procedure the open and closed needle tip echos are followed on the ultrasound screen, enabling safe placement of the needle on the fetal surface. We usually obtain multiple specimens (4–6) in a short period of time and, if necessary, more than one anatomic site can be sampled. The skin samples obtained are typically 1–2 mm in diameter and are full thickness. They may be placed in sterile saline or directly into culture medium. The tissue is refrigerated if electron and light microscopy are to be performed. The tissue specimens are sufficient to allow evaluation of the structure of the dermis, epidermis, dermo-epidermal junction, and epidermal appendages and to perform certain biochemical assays. Analysis of most of the skin specimens obtained from our 20 cases have been performed in the electron microscopy laboratory at Department of Dermatoloty, Rigshopital, Coopenhagen, Denmark by Professor T. Kobayasi.

Four pregnancies in which the fetus was affected by epidermolysis bullosa letalis, and four with the dystrophic type of epidermolysis bullosa were terminated by instillation of prostaglandins into the amniotic fluid. At autopsy the skin biopsy site was easily recognized. In cases where histological analysis revealed normal skin without cleavage in the dermo–epidermal junction, pregnancy has been allowed to continue, resulting in the birth of normal term infants with no cosmetic or functional injuries in the region from which samples had been obtained. According to data published in the literature, and in our own experience, ultrasonically guided fetal skin sampling is a safe and simple method with a minimal rate of maternal and fetal injuries[5–8].

The advantages of this method over fetoscopy include the greater field of view of the fetus, the opportunity to select specific sites to be biopsied (avoiding above mentioned regions), and the ability to sample a range of body regions. Despite problems such as procedures performed relatively late in pregnancy, misinterpretation because of artifacts and regional variability in expression of some disorders, transabdominal skin biopsy under continuous ultrasonic monitoring is a successful diagnostic technique with an undoubtedly promising future for the prenatal diagnosis of hereditary epidermal disorders.

Enzymatic assay

This form of biochemical analysis may be used as an adjunct or alternative to morphological analysis of fetal tissue for prenatal diagnosis. Cultured fibroblasts derived from a 20-week aborted fetus with recessive dystrophic epidermolysis bullosa were found to express an abnormally high level of immunoreactive collagenase, consistent with that seen in patients with the disease.

Determination of keratins and fillagrin in fetal skin samples

Keratins are proteins that form intermediate filaments (tonofilament) and are found in all epithelial cells. There are 19 different keratins, and each layer of the epidermis contains its

Table 1 *Fetal skin development. (From Reference 6)*

	14–16 weeks	19–20 weeks
Hypodermis	+	+
Nerves/vessels	+	+
Dermis		
appendages	± sebaceous gland − apocrine glands − eccrine glands (body) hair germs, hair pegs, few bulbous hair pegs	+ sebaceous gland + apocrine glands + eccrine glands hair germs, fewer hair pegs, mostly bulbous hair pegs
collagen organization	Types I, III, IV, V + papillary + recticular	same + papillary + recticular
elastin	+ microfibrils − elastin	+ microfibrils + elastin
Dermo-epidermal junction	+ anchoring filaments + anchoring fibrils + hemidesmosomes + bullous pemphigoid, type IV collagen, laminin, and antigens	+ anchoring filaments + anchoring fibrils + hemidesmosomes + bullous pemphigoid, type IV collagen, laminin, and antigens
Epidermis periderm cell layers	single or multiple blebs basal 2–3 intermediate periderm	regressing basal 3–4 intermediate periderm
keratinization	parts of nail, hair follicle, palms, and soles	interfollicular epidermis of scalp increasing amount in nail follicles, palms, and soles
pigment production immigrant cells	premelanin and melanin Langerhans	melanin Langerhans Merkel

Table 2 *Keratins and fillagrin – localization and time of appearance in fetal skin. (From References 29, 75, 76)*

Keratin type	Molecular weight (kD)	Localization	Time of appearance (weeks of gestation)
1	67	suprabasal layer	
10	56.5	suprabasal layer	9–11 weeks
5	58	basal layer	
14	50	basal layer	< 9 weeks
8	52	periderm	
19	40	periderm	< 9 weeks, disappear
18	45	periderm	after 24 weeks
6	48	suprabasal	13 weeks
16	56	layers of palms and soles	term
Fillagrin	37	follicles interfollicular	15 weeks 24 weeks

specific type. Some, such as 40 kD keratin, are found only in embryonic and not in adult skin. Fillagrin is a protein that aggregates with keratin filaments and probably functions as a keratin matrix protein in the cornified cells of the epidermis. Profillagrin, the precursor of fillagrin, is synthesized in the stratum spinosum, where it is associated with the keratohyalin granules. When the cells reach the stratum corneum, the profillagrin is converted to fillagrin. Because of its specificity for the stratum spinosum and stratum corneum, fillagrin is often cited as a marker for epidermal differentiation (Tables 1 and 2).

The different keratins and fillagrin can be detected with monoclonal and polyclonal antibodies. Keratins with molecular weights of 40, 45 and 52 kD are found in the early embryonic stage in the periderm; they gradually disappear as keratinization proceeds and cannot be found after 24 weeks of gestation. Keratins 5 and 14 (molecular weights 50 kD and 58 kD, respectively) can be found in the embryonic basal layer and are also typical of the adult basal layer. Keratins 1 and 10 (molecular weights 56.5 kD and 67 kD, respectively) begin to appear in the fetal skin at 9–11 weeks of gestation, and their appearance histologically parallels the formation of the intermediate cell layer. In adults these keratins can be found in the suprabasal layers, and they are considered to be specific to keratinized epithelia. The onset of their expression in fetal skin heralds the time of stratification. At 12–14 weeks, as the hair follicles start to cornify, there is a dramatic increase in the expression of keratins 1 and 10. At 15 weeks the cells in the hair follicles start to cornify and fillagrin appears. In the interfollicullar epidermis, keratinization and the simultaneous appearance of fillagrin occur at about 24 weeks[9]. The skin of the palms and soles expresses keratins 6 and 16 (molecular weights 48 kD and 56 kD). These have been called they hyperproliferative keratins because they are found in the skin of patients with several hyperproliferative skin diseases, such as psoriasis and seborrheic dermatitis[10]. By 14–16 weeks all the keratins and fillagrin are present in the fetal skin. This finding has relevance for amniocentesis, which is performed at this time for prenatal diagnosis[11].

In genodermatoses such as epidermolytic hyperkeratosis, the diagnosis can be made on the basis of clumping of the keratin filament bundles in the cells of the spinous layer, and cytolysis of spinous and granular cells. This can be detected by ultrastructural study of fetal skin biopsies taken at 19–20 weeks. Some authors have also investigated the amniotic fluid cells for these features, since 25% of amniotic fluid cells are derived from fetal epithelia[10,11]. The finding of keratin filament aggregations in the amniotic fluid cells of affected fetuses led Holbrook and co-workers[10] to suggest that the diagnosis could be made one month earlier, at 14–16 weeks, by amniocentesis. Other authors, however, obtained false-negative results and concluded that the lack of tonofibrillar aggregations in amniotic fluid cells precludes a safe exclusion of the disorder[12].

In an attempt to provide an even earlier prenatal diagnosis of genodermatoses, chorionic villi samples obtained at 8–12 weeks were examined ultrastructurally. Chorionic villi were, however, found to have only a few of the characteristics of differentiated skin, rendering them inappropriate for such prenatal diagnosis[13].

The determination of keratins and fillagrin in fetal skin samples may be useful in establishing the diagnosis of genetic disorders of keratinization.

PRENATAL DIAGNOSIS OF DISEASES AND DISORDERS OF THE SKIN

Ichthyoses

The ichthyoses are a group of keratinization disorders that can be subdivided into four major forms and a group of rare associated syndromes. The major forms are ichthyosis vulgaris, X-linked ichthyosis, epidermolytic hyperkeratosis, and autosomal recessive ichthyosis, which can be subdivided into lamellar ichthyosis and congenital ichthyosiform erythroderma[14]. Ichthyosis vulgaris is inherited in an autosomal dominant manner and is common, with an incidence of 1 : 300. The disease appears a few months to one year after birth with adherent scales, especially on the extensor surfaces. It is not present at birth and therefore cannot be diagnosed prenatally.

X-linked ichthyosis

The incidence of X-linked ichthyosis is about 1 : 6000 men. The disease is not usually present at birth but develops in the first months of life with small brown, adherent scales on the extensor surfaces of the extremities, on the flexor surfaces and on the trunk. This finding differentiates it clinically from ichthyosis vulgaris, in which the trunk and flexural areas are usually spared. Characteristically the sides of the neck are involved, giving the child an unwashed look. The face, scalp, palms, soles and mucosa are spared. The condition is ameliorated by warm humid weather, and does not improve with age.

The histological picture shows hyperkeratosis with a normal or slightly thickened granular layer. This finding differentiates X-linked ichthyosis from ichthyosis vulgaris, in which the granular layer is absent or thinned[14]. Associated findings consist of corneal opacities, which can be found in adult female carriers and patients and do not affect vision. Cryptorchidism is present in approximately 25% of patients, and the incidence of testicular cancer exceeds that of the normal population[15].

The defect in X-linked ichthyosis is the congenital absence of steroid (aryl) sulfatase, an enzyme associated with the microsomal fraction of liver, placenta, adrenal cortex, brain and skin. Steroid sulfatase removes the sulfate moiety from sulfated steroid hormones and cholesterol sulfate. Dehydroepiandrosterone sulfate (DHA-S), which is produced by the fetal adrenal glands, is the main estrogen precursor. In the absence of aryl sulfatase C, DHA-S cannot be hydrolyzed: estrogen levels in maternal blood and urine are low, and levels of sulfated estrogen precursors are high. Absence of placental aryl sulfatase causes delay in the onset and progress of labor and Cesarean section is often necessary. Due to the absence of estrogen stimulation of lactalbumin, breast feeding fails to be established[16]. Aryl sulfatase breaks down cholesterol sulfate in the granular layer of the skin: in the absence of the enzyme cholesterol sulfate accumulates in the stratum corneum, causing the skin to scale. Serum levels of cholesterol sulfate are also elevated, expressed by a rise in the LDL fraction, which contains about 70% of the total cholesterol sulfate in plasma.

Prenatal diagnosis can be made by measuring estrogen levels in maternal urine at 16 weeks of gestation. The diagnosis can be confirmed by measuring steroid sulfatase activity in cultured amniocytes, fibroblasts and leukocytes[15,16].

Epidermolytic hyperkeratosis

Also called bullous icthyosiform erythroderma (BIE), this very rare disease (1 : 300 000) is transmitted as an autosomal dominant trait. It presents at birth as erythroderma, blistering and erosions of the skin; large areas denuded of skin make these infants prone to secondary infection and sepsis.

Hyperkeratosis develops only in the first year of life, after the erythema and bullae subside. The scales are thick, brown and verrucous and have a preference for flexural areas. Because of bacterial colonization, these children have a foul body odor. The face may be involved, but usually only mildly. The palms and soles show hyperkeratosis that may be severe. Mucous membranes and hair are spared. Nails may be dystrophic. There are no systemic or associated manifestations, but the perinatal morbidity and mortality are high because of sepsis and loss of fluid and electrolytes. At birth, differential diagnosis includes epidermolysis bullosa and staphylococcal scalded skin syndrome. BIE tends to improve with age.

In ichthyosis vulgaris and X-linked ichthyosis, the scaling results from delayed shedding of the epidermal cells. In BIE and lamellar ichthyosis, the scaling results from increased epidermal turnover rate. Normally, the cell transit time from the basal layer to stratum corneum is about 2 weeks. In BIE and lamellar ichthyosis this time is reduced to 4 days. The histologic picture of BIE is characteristic: the granular layer is markedly thickened and the cells of the middle and upper portions of the stratum malpighii show pronounced vacuolization. The edematous cells may separate from one another, forming intra-epidermal bullae and the keratohyaline granules in the granular layer are increased in number and irregular in shape.

Electron microscopy shows excessive production and clumping of tonofilaments and keratohyaline granules. The desmosomes, which are the connection between two keratinocytes, are normal but their association with the tonofilaments is disturbed, and therefore blistering can occur[14].

Prenatal diagnosis of this disease can be made by fetal skin biopsy at 19 or 20 weeks. Keratinization normally starts at about 15 weeks in the hair follicles and by 24 weeks over the rest of the skin. Precocious keratinization before 24 weeks and clumping of the tonofilaments make the diagnosis of epidermolytic hyperkeratosis likely. Eady and colleagues[11] suggest the diagnosis might even by suspected on finding clumping of tonofilaments in amniotic fluid cells, thus saving fetal skin biopsy. However, according to Arnold and Anton Lamprecht[14], the lack of tonofibrillar aggregations in amnion fluid cells does not allow a safe exclusion of the disorder.

Autosomal recessive ichthyosis

Lever[14] subdivides recessive ichthyosis into two types: lamellar ichthyosis and the less severe congenital ichthyosiform erythroderma (CIE). Both diseases are rare with an incidence of approximately 1 : 300 000. The child is born encased in a collodion membrane that sheds after 10–14 days, leaving erythema and scaling of the entire skin, including scalp, face, palms and soles. The tight skin around the eyes and mouth causes ectropion and eclabion. The babies are often born premature and suffer from temperature instability due to erythroderma. They are also exposed to water loss and bacterial invasion through deep cracks in the skin.

Lamellar ichthyosis is more severe than CIE, with severe ectropion and thick plate-like scales and a progressive course. Keratotic plugging of the sweat ducts causes a decrease in normal sweating, resulting in hyperpyrexia in warm weather or during exercise. The histologic picture is non-specific. There is thickening of the stratum corneum with focal parakeratosis in CIE, whereas the hyperkeratosis in lamellar ichthyosis is more marked and parakeratosis is absent. The lipid content of the scales shows elevated levels of *n*-alkanes in CIE and normal levels in lamellar ichthyosis[17].

Prenatal diagnosis of recessive ichthyosis can be made by fetal skin biopsy at 19–21 weeks, with the diagnosis likely when precocious keratinization and hyperkeratosis are found. However, differentiation and keratinization of the epidermis vary in different anatomical regions at any one point in time, complicating the sampling for diagnosis. Keratinization starts in the hair follicles at about 15 weeks and in the interfollicular skin at about 24 weeks. The skin of the scalp, face, palms and soles differentiates ahead of the trunk. It is therefore advisable to obtain skin biopsies from a few areas, including the scalp, to optimize the chances of diagnosing the disorder[17].

Rare syndromes associated with ichthyosis

Harlequin fetus

In this extremely rare condition, children are born with hard, thick whitish-yellow skin with deep red fissures. Ectropion and eclabion results from the extremely tight skin, the nose is depressed and underdeveloped, and there are flexion contractures of the extremities. The condition is thought to be the result of mutations associated with a heterogeneous group of disorders with autosomal recessive inheritance patterns[13]. Less than 100 cases have been described in the world literature[18].

Most infants die within 2 weeks of birth due to infection, loss of fluids and electrolytes, and mechanical restriction of respiration and feeding. The histopathology of the skin shows massive hyperkeratosis, the stratum corneum being 20–30 times thicker than the stratum malpighii. Droplets of neutral fat can be seen throughout the cornified cells with fat stains. Sometimes papillomatosis or parakeratosis is seen[14,19].

Prenatal diagnosis can be made by fetal skin biopsy at 20–21 weeks, when the skin shows the characteristically hyperkeratotic stratum corneum in the interfollicular epidermis. The amniotic fluid contains well-matured keratinocytes and is yellow and turbid in color. This finding is probably not unique to harlequin ichthyosis and is common to other severe forms of ichthyosis[20]. The condition can also be diagnosed by ultrasonic scan in the early third trimester[21,22], when the sonographic signs leading to the diagnosis of harlequin fetus are widely opened mouth, hypoplastic nose with evident apertures corresponding to the nostrils, large ectropion, lack of fetal breathing movements, edematous-like limbs and intrauterine membranes[22]. It remains to be seen whether diagnosis by ultrasound scan alone can be made early enough to offer therapeutic possibilities.

Sjögren–Larsson syndrome

Only some 200 cases of this autosomal recessive inherited disease have been reported[18]. The clinical features consist of a triad of mental retardation, ichthyosis and spastic paraparesis of the extremities.

The skin disease is usually present at birth as erythroderma or scaling and hyperkeratosis. By the age of 2 years spasticity becomes apparent, usually accompanied by speech deficits and seizures. In about 50% of affected children a characteristic retinopathy develops, showing 'glistening dots' on the retinal macula. Other occasionally reported features of this syndrome are enamel hypoplasia, skeletal anomalies and hypertelorism.

Sjören–Larsson syndrome is associated with an inborn error of lipid metabolism. Deficient activity of the enzyme fatty alcohol oxidoreductase (FAO) can be demonstrated in fibroblasts, leukocytes, keratinocytes and jejunal enterocytes[19,23]. This enzyme converts fatty alcohol into fatty acid and its activity is also somewhat reduced in obligate carriers of the disease.

Prenatal diagnosis can be made on fetal skin biopsy, as described by Kousseff and colleagues[24]. In their patient a biopsy taken in the 23rd week showed orthokeratotic thickening of the keratin layer, and a prominent granular layer with prominent keratohyalin granules. Electron microscopy demonstrated concentric laminated membranous structures in the stratum corneum, which appeared to be keratinosomes (also called Odland bodies). These structures are usually found in the stratum spinosum and granulosum but not in the stratum corneum.

Measurement of alcohol dehydrogenase activity in fetal cells would be a rapid and precise test for prenatal diagnosis of Sjögren–Larsson syndrome, and this subject needs further study[25].

Refsum's disease

This very rare autosomal recessively inherited disease, also called heredopathia atactica polyneuritiformis, is caused by a deficiency of the enzyme phytanic acid oxidase, a mitochondrial enzyme that initiates the catabolism of phytanic acid[25].

The onset of the syndrome may be in early childhood or as late as the 4th or 5th decade. The symptoms are primarily neurologic, consisting of peripheral neuropathy, cerebellar ataxia and night blindness due to retinitis pigmentosa. The skin exhibits a mild ichthyosis that clinically resembles ichthyosis vulgaris. The histologic picture differs from that of ichthyosis vulgaris, showing hyperkeratosis with hypergranulosis and vacuoles in the basal and suprabasal cells of the epidermis that stain with lipid stains[14]. Refsum's disease is treatable with dietary restriction of phytanic acid, although the damage to nerve fibers is irreversible. Prenatal diagnosis has been made by measuring phytanic acid oxidase activity in cultured amniotic cells sampled in the 18th week of pregnancy[26].

Chondrodysplasia punctata syndrome

This disorder is usually divided into an autosomal recessive inherited rhizomelic type, and the non-rhizomelic type, also called Conradi–Hunermann syndrome, which can be dominantly inherited or X-linked. The common symptom of these disorders is chondrodysplasia punctata, which is visible on X-rays as stippling of the epiphyses[19]. Congenital ichthyosiform erythroderma occurs in about 30% of patients, showing a whorled pattern.

The rhizomelic type is the most severe, with dwarfism, shortened proximal extremities, saddle nose and cataracts. Most patients die in the first year of life due to respiratory failure. Prenatal diagnosis relies largely on sonographic examination which shows the shortened limbs and the depressed nose. Attempts to confirm the diagnosis by fetal skin biopsy at 22 weeks of menstrual age failed when the biopsies showed normal skin and the ultrasound showed the fetus was affected[27]; the authors concluded that this genodermatosis cannot be diagnosed prenatally on the basis of disturbance of keratinization detected on fetal biopsies.

Epidermolysis bullosa

The term epidermolysis bullosa (EB) describes a group of inherited diseases characterized by bullous lesions that appear spontaneously or after minor trauma. The disorder is quite rare, with an estimated incidence of 1 in 50 000 births[28]. According to inheritance, clinical, histological and ultrastructural features, 16 different types can be distinguished[29]. Lever[14] recognizes three main groups, defined by the level of separation on electron microscopy: epidermal (epidermolytic), junctional (within the lamina lucida), and dermal (sublamina densa). The clinical features, histology, ultrastructural changes and possibilities for prenatal diagnosis will be discussed for each group.

Epidermolytic epidermolysis bullosa EB simplex, the generalized type (Koebner type), is inherited in an autosomal dominant fashion. The bullae may be present at birth, but generally develop within the first year of life on areas of local trauma. Because the bullae are located intraepidermally, they do not leave scars after healing. The mucosa can be mildly affected. Nails, hair and teeth develop normally, although the nails may be temporarily shed. The condition worsens with hot weather, improves with age, and patients have a normal life span[29].

Localized EB simplex (Weber–Cockayne type) is an autosomal dominant inherited variant in which the bullae are localized to the hands and feet. Blistering does not usually occur until childhood or adolescence. The condition is associated with hyperhydrosis and hyperkeratosis of the palms and soles. This is probably the most common and the least debilitating form of epidermolysis bullosa[29]. Hair, teeth, nails and mucosa are unaffected.

EB simplex herpetiformis (Dowling–Meara type) is inherited in an autosomal dominant fashion. The disease is present at birth or early infancy with herpetiform blistering on the hands and feet but also on the proximal extremities and the trunk. In contrast to the other forms of EB simplex, the blistering in this variant occurs spontaneously without prior trauma. Because of the severe blistering, the disease is sometimes difficult to distinguish from the junctional or dystrophic types of EB. The oral mucosa is frequently involved and nail dystrophy may occur. Although the lesions heal without scarring, transient milia formation is characteristic. The symptoms tend to improve with age, but palmoplantar hyperkeratosis frequently develops.

Histopathology of all three epidermal types of EB[12] shows cytolysis of the lower portion of the basal cells, resulting in intraepidermal blistering[12]. Ultrastructurally, the Dowling-Meara type differs from the other EB simplex types by clumping of filaments of keratins 15 and 4 in the basal and suprabasal layers.

There are no reports in the literature of prenatal diagnosis of the generalized (Koebner) and localized (Weber–Cockayne) types of EB simplex types, and it is questionable whether their severity warrants prenatal diagnosis.

EB herpetiformis (Dowling–Meara type) can cause severe blistering at birth, associated with increased perinatal mortality, and therefore justifies prenatal diagnosis. This disease was successfully diagnosed prenatally by Holbrook and colleagues[30] in 1992 from a fetal skin biopsy obtained at 20 weeks of gestation in a mother with two affected children, one of whom had died at 1 month of age. Light microscopy of the biopsy showed separation of the epidermis from the dermis, leaving only small epidermal fragments attached to the dermo-epidermal junction. Electron microscopy showed the plane of cleavage to be within the basal layer of the epidermis. Keratin filament aggregates, characteristic of EB Dowling–Meara type in adult patients, were evident in the attached remnants of basal cells and in the basal and intermediate layer cells of the separated epidermal sheets of the fetal skin biopsy. The fetus was aborted and post-mortem examination of the skin confirmed the prenatal diagnosis.

Junctional epidermolysis bullosa The junctional variants of epidermolysis bullosa are characterized by autosomal recessive inheritance and separation at the dermo-epidermal junction at the level of the lamina lucida. At least three different variants have been described, one of which is lethal in 50% of patients in the first few months of life. The other types show the same ultrastructural features but are less extensive and non-lethal. In the lethal or Herlitz variant, the blisters are present at birth or appear soon after, mainly on the buttocks, trunk and scalp. They heal without scarring or milia formation but can leave atrophy[29].

Multiple non-cutaneous epithelia can be involved, most notably the eye, oral cavity, esophagus and tracheobronchial tree[31]. The teeth show defective enamel formation and are dysplastic. Because of the involvement of the digestive tract, feeding difficulties and malnutrition are common. The infants suffer from severe anemia and growth retardation. Early death may result from fluid loss and sepsis. Light microscopy shows a subepidermal separation with an intact basal membrane zone[14]. Electron microscopy reveals structural and numerically abnormal hemidesmosomes, structures that are normally found between the plasma membrane of the basal cells and the underlying basal lamina, and represent the anchoring points between dermis and epidermis[32].

Hemidesmosomes first appear at 12 weeks of gestational age, and by the time fetal skin biopsy is performed (18–20 weeks), they have acquired the normal ultrastructural morphology[28], enabling diagnosis of junctional EB. Two recently developed monoclonal antibodies, GB3 and 19-DEJ-1[33,34], are used in the prenatal diagnosis. The GB3 monoclonal antibody is directed against five polypeptides in the lamina lucida that can be detected in fetal skin as early as 7.5 weeks[33]. This antigen is absent or weakly expressed in patients affected with junctional EB, but was found in about 50% of those with non-Herlitz junctional EB.

Fine and coworkers[34] developed the monoclonal antibody 19-DEJ-1, which detects an antigen that bears a close relationship to the hemidesmosomes, is detectable in normal fetal skin as early as 81 days, and is absent in all variants of junctional EB[34]. Thus, the diagnosis can be made by immunohistochemical staining of fetal skin biopsy taken at 18–20 weeks.

Dermolytic epidermolysis bullosa The dermolytic variants of epidermolysis bullosa are also called dystrophic because the blisters heal with scarring. They are inherited in an autosomal dominant or recessive fashion. Dominant EB dystrophica (Cockayne–Touraine type) is the less severe disease, and has its onset in infancy or early childhood with blistering mainly on the extremities, which heal with milia formation and scarring. The scars may be hypertrophic, and hypertrophic nails are commonly seen. There is little or no involvement of the hair and teeth, and the mucosa is usually not affected. The general healthy of these patients is not affected and physical development is normal. The disease tends to improve with age. A unique variant is the albopapuloid form (Pasini variant), in which small ivory-white perifollicular papules appear, usually later in childhood.

The recessive form of dystrophic EB is a severe disease when generalized (Hallopeau–Siemens type). There is widespread blistering either at birth or shortly thereafter and the blisters leave extensive scarring and milia, with deformities and contractures of the extremities. The so-called 'mitten' deformity of the hands is characteristic, and is caused by fusion of the skin

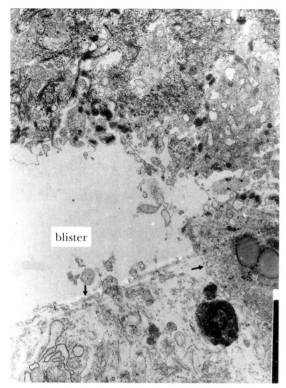 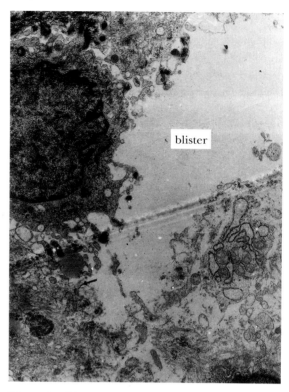

Figure 1 *Electron micrograph showing histogical findings of epidermolysis bullosa. In the dermo-epidermal junction, basal lamina (arrows) can be seen with irregular shape and thickness; it is partially interrupted or disappears completely*

Figure 2 *Electron micrograph showing histogical findings of epidermolysis bullosa. Blister roof is composed of basal keratinocytes seen with or without junctional structures. Separation of the epidermis (suprabasal) is seen over the area of dermo-epidermal separation*

of the fingers due to recurrent blistering[29]. There is severe involvement of the mucous membranes, resulting in malnutrition, anemia and growth retardation. Esophageal strictures lead to aspiration pneumonia. Involvement of the eyes causes corneal ulceration and scarring. Ectropion and lacrimal duct obstruction may occur. The ears may be affected, resulting in recurrent otitis and strictures of the external auditory canal. Hoarseness may result from laryngeal involvement and the teeth are malformed and susceptible to severe caries. Death may occur in infancy due to sepsis, fluid loss or amyloidosis caused by recurrent infections. Surviving patients are at risk for developing squamous cell carcinoma in scarred areas of skin, oropharynx, esophagus, stomach and upper bronchial tree. These tumors behave aggressively and two-thirds of these patients die of metastasis[29].

Light microscopy of skin of patients with dystrophic EB (dominant and recessive) shows separation of the epidermis from the dermis below the basal membrane zone[16]. Electron microscopy of recessive dystrophic EB shows complete absence of the anchoring fibrils. In the dominant and localized forms, structurally normal anchoring fibrils are present but their number is reduced[14] (Figures 1 and 2).

Direct immunofluorescence after labeling of the skin with the monoclonal antibody KF-1 shows a complete absence of the corresponding antigen in recessive dystrophic EB, and weak fluorescence in dominant dystrophic EB. The KF-1 antibody identifies a non-collagenous constituent of the lamina densa of the basement membrane zone of the skin[35]. In the normal fetus this is expressed by week 16[36].

The monoclonal antibody LH 7:2 is directed against a 37 kD protein in the epidermal basement membrane and can be found in normal fetal skin at 10 weeks[37], but is absent or markedly reduced in recessive dystrophic EB. Fibroblasts of patients with recessive dystrophic EB produce increased amounts of collagenase, resulting in lysis of the collagen fibrils and blistering[38].

Prenatal diagnosis of the dystrophic EB variants is made by fetal skin biopsy at 18–20 weeks of gestational age. Electron microscopic examination shows absent or reduced numbers of anchoring fibrils in recessive and dominant dystrophic EB, respectively.

Immunohistochemical staining with monoclonal antibodies KF 1 and LH 7:2 can be used in the prenatal diagnosis of recessive dystrophic EB, but this is not sufficiently reliable in the diagnosis of dominant dystrophic EB[36]. Bauer and co-workers[39] cultured fetal fibroblasts obtained at 20 weeks from a fetus at risk for recessive dystrophic EB, and found collagenase production greater than that of control fibroblast cultures, thereby establishing the diagnosis of recessive dystrophic EB[39].

CONGENITAL ECTODERMAL DEFECTS

Ectodermal dysplasias

The ectodermal dysplasias are a heterogeneous group of genodermatoses characterized by numerous anomalies of the epidermis and its appendages. They result from faulty development of the ectodermal structures during embryogenesis[40].

Anhidrotic (hypohydrotic) ectodermal dysplasia (Christ–Siemens–Touraine syndrome)

This in an X-linked recessive condition in which the main defects are anhydrosis or hypohydrosis, hypotrichosis and total or partial anodontia. In the more complete forms the appearance of the patients is distinctive, with characteristic facies. These patients may also suffer from onychodysplasia, decreased pigmentation of hair and eyes, atopic dermatitis, and palmoplanar hyperkeratosis[40].

Histopathology shows thin and flattened epidermis, absent or poorly developed eccrine sweat glands, and a reduced number of hair follicles and sebaceous glands. Dermal connective tissue usually appears grossly normal, but collagen and elastic fibers may be fragmented or sparse. In some cases mucous glands are absent from the upper respiratory tract and bronchi. Salivary glands display inflammatory changes and ectasia of ducts. The cell-mediated immune response may be depressed and serum IgE level elevated, as in atopic states. There can be a paucity of amniotic fluid at birth[41].

Little treatment can be offered except advice concerning restriction of physical exertion, choice of suitable occupation and avoidance of warm climates. Psychological support and special schooling may be needed.

Two prenatal diagnostic methods have been carried out:

(1) Direct histological analysis of fetal skin taken from various regions by fetoscopy in the late second trimester (20th week of gestation). Light and electron microscopy demonstrate lack of skin appendages, including hair follicles, sebaceous glands and sweat glands. The lack of pilosebaceous follicles can be used as a diagnostic criterion, since these structures are fully developed in normal fetuses of 20 weeks while sweat glands do not begin to develop until weeks 20–24[42].

(2) Indirect prenatal diagnosis by linkage analysis, using restriction fragment length polymorphisms on closely linked marker loci, from a DNA sample obtained by a chorionic villus biopsy at 9 weeks' gestation[43].

Ectrodactyly – ectodermal dysplasia and cleft lip and/or cleft palate (EEC)

EEC is a rare autosomal dominant syndrome comprising ectrodactyly (split hand and foot), ectodermal dysplasia (hypoplastic nails, sparse hair, eyelashes and eyebrows, albinoid changes of skin and hair), nasolacrimal duct obstruction, and clefting of the lip and palate[44]. Not all the defects are present in every patient, but the most constant finding is ectodermal dysplasia. Ultrasound will show cleft lip and palate after the 16th week of gestation[43].

Aplasia cutis congenita

This congenital defect of the skin has a predilection for the midline of the vertex of the scalp. A small bleb in fetal life may develop into a coin-sized absence of skin and subcutaneous tissue, rarely penetrating into the cranium. In another rare condition, multiple symmetrical defects occur on the skin, generally on the lower extremities. There is a tendency for these aplasias to heal spontaneously[45].

Aplasia cutis congenita belongs to the disorders in which midtrimester (16 weeks) amniotic fluids exhibit elevated concentrations of α-fetoprotein and presence of acetylcholinesterase. This disorder should be considered part of the differential diagnosis of these amniotic fluid findings. Ultrasound examination produces normal results throughout the pregnancy[45,46].

PIGMENTARY DISORDERS

Albinism

In oculocutaneous albinism there is a partial or complete failure of melanin production in the skin, hair and eyes. Tyrosinase-negative and tyrosinase-positive oculocutaneous albinism are autosomal recessive disorders caused by mutations in the tyrosinase gene[47]. Tyrosinase-negative albinism is characterized by hair bulbs which, after incubation with tyrosine, fail to darken due to complete absence of the enzyme responsible for converting tyrosine into melanin. The hair bulbs do darken in the more common tyrosinase-positive albinism, but the enzyme is reduced or its appearance delayed. In tyrosinase-negative albinism, most of the melanosomes are stage I and stage II, with no melanization, while stage III melanosomes may be present in tyrosinase-positive albinism[48].

In tyrosinase-negative albinism, the skin is pink in color, the hair is white and the patients show a prominent red light reflex in the eye. In the tyrosinase-positive type some pigment is formed, and with increasing age is to be found in the iris, skin and hair. Both types of patients have photophobia, and may have a characteristic facial expression. Almost all patients have horizontal or rotatory nystagmus, visual disturbances due to optic nerve defects, and develop various malignant skin tumors[55].

Prenatal diagnosis consists of histochemistry and electron microscopy of samples of scalp hair taken by fetoscopy at 16–20 weeks of pregnancy, which demonstrate the stage of development of melanosomes. The degree of melanization varies in the tyrosinase-positive form and is less easy to establish. Diagnosis of the tyrosinase-negative form is based on absence of stage IV melanosomes in the melanocytes. This method is technically difficult[48].

In another procedure, skin samples taken by fetoscopy guided by ultrasonography from the upper trunk of the fetus at 19–20 weeks of gestation are examined by electron microscopy for melanocytes containing stage I and II, but not stage III and IV melanosomes. Observation of only stage I and II melanosomes after incubation with L-dopa confirms the lack of tyrosinase activity in these fetal melanocytes. The electron microscopic dopa reaction test on a fetal skin biopsy specimen is safe and practical[48].

Chediak–Higashi syndrome

Chediak–Higashi syndrome is an autosomal recessive disorder characterized by partial albinism with fair skin, pale retina, and translucent irides[50]. The hair is light blond or silvery grey, and there is photophobia with nystagmus. As well as the cutaneous manifestation there is a severe immune deficiency. Affected children are highly susceptible to bacterial and viral infection and intractable respiratory and cutaneous infections that usually cause death before the age of 10. Longer survival is possible, but later the lymph nodes, spleen and liver become enlarged and a malignant lymphoma frequently develops. Histopathological examination shows abnormal cytoskeleton and lysosome formation leading to giant cytoplasmic granules in all cells containing lysosomes: leukocytes, skin melanocytes and hair bulb melanocytes.

Bone marrow transplantation can cure Chediak–Higashi disease

Prenatal diagnosis is justified for families at risk, especially in the absence of a suitable HLA-identical bone marrow donor[49]. Prenatal diagnosis is made by a morphological approach only, since the immune deficiency is too subtle to be diagnosed *in utero*. Fetal blood and fetal hair are obtained by fetoscopy in the 21st week of gestation. Light microscopy of the fetal hair shaft shows pigmentation abnormalities, and the giant, irregular melanin granules are easily detected. Diagnosis is confirmed by examination of polymorphonuclear leukocytes, which gives evidence of the typical giant granules on both light and electron microscopy[50].

Griscelli syndrome

Griscelli syndrome is an autosomal recessive disorder characterized by partial albinism and immune deficiency. The pigmentary deletion is characterized by large clumps of pigment in the hair shaft and accumulation of melanosomes in melanocytes. The immune deficiency consists of both T and B cell effector dysfunction. Polymorphonuclear cells are normal, both morphologically and functionally. The disease has a poor prognosis and most children die within the first decade of life from infection or the lymphoma-like accelerated phase[50].

Prenatal diagnosis can be made at 21 weeks of gestation based on light microscopic examination of hair taken by fetoscopy. The immune deficiency cannot be detected before birth[50].

IMMUNE DISORDERS

Wiskott–Aldrich syndrome

The clinical manifestations of this rare X-linked recessive disorder are chronic eczematous dermatitis, increased susceptibility to recurrent infections, thrombocytopenic purpura with hepatosplenomegaly, and an increased incidence of lymphoreticular malignancy. There is a low level of IgM, low or normal level of IgG, elevated levels of IgA and IgE, thrombocytopenia, and a decrease in the quantity and activity of T cells. Death occurs by age 6 from infection or bleeding. Treatment includes platelet transfusions, antibiotics, immune globulin, splenectomy and allogeneic marrow transplantation[51].

Prenatal diagnosis requires fetal blood sampling in the 20th week of pregnancy and measurement of fetal platelet size and number. Alternatively chorionic villus samples obtained in the 9th week can be used for DNA analysis, based on the known location of the responsible gene on the X-chromosome[52].

CHROMOSOME INSTABILITY SYNDROMES

Ataxia telangiectasia

Ataxia telangiectasia is an autosomal recessive disease. There is extensive genetic heterogeneity of the disease, and five different complementation groups have been described. Clinically, it is characterized by cerebellar ataxia, oculocutaneous telangiectasia, and abnormal development of ovaries and testicles. Thymus development is deficient, leading to humoral and cellular immunodeficiency and an increased predisposition to cancer, predominantly lymphoreticular. Heterozygous carriers exhibit an excess risk of cancer, especially breast cancer[53]. There is an increased plasma level of α-fetoprotein[54]. The primary defect is unknown. Patients with ataxia telangiectasia exhibit a high level of spontaneous chromosome aberations with hypersensitivity to γ-radiation and radiomimetic chemicals at the chromosomal and cellular levels. Severe pulmonary infection and progressive bronchiectasis occur in most patients. Predominantly lymphorecticular malignancies are the most common cause of death.

Two prenatal diagnostic methods are described:

(1) Amniocentesis at 16 weeks of gestation with analysis of amniotic fluid samples for chromosome instability and biochemical abnormalities[54].
(2) Cytogenetic approach using chorionic villi sampling in the first trimester of pregnancy (9 weeks' gestation). Levels of spontaneous and induced (γ-radiation) chromosome breakage are measured 9 days after sampling[55].

Xeroderma pigmentosum

Xeroderma pigmentosum refers to a group of autosomal recessively inherited conditions characterized by hypersensitivity of the skin to sunlight. The regions most often affected are the sun-exposed areas such as the face, neck, hands and arms. Skin changes consist of ephelidies, lentigenes, telangiectases, keratoses, papillomas, carcinoma and melanoma. There can be variable neurological abnormalities, such as low intelligence, areflexia, impaired hearing and abnormal speech. Malignancy can occur in sites other than the skin. The effects of the disease on the eyes include photophobia, lacrimation, keratitis and tumors of the lids that can cause loss of vision. Xeroderma pigmentosum can be associated with congenital ichthyosis, porphyria and lupus erythematosus.

Pathogenesis consists of an altered reaction of the epidermis to light. The main biochemical defect is a failure to repair UV-induced DNA damage because of a deficiency of DNA endonuclease. Treatment consists of avoidance of sunlight, removal of tumor and symptomatic treatment. Prognosis varies from no serious trouble to death early in adulthood from metastasis of malignant tumors[56].

Amniocentesis is performed at 17 weeks of pregnancy, the amniotic fluids cells are cultivated, and the rate of excision repair of UV-induced pyrimidine dimers of the DNA measured[57].

Cockayne's syndrome

This rare autosomal recessive disorder is characterized by dwarfism, optic atropy, deafness and mental retardation. The dermatologic features are photodermatitis resulting in hyperpigmentation and scarring. Other changes are microcephaly, a facial appearance resembling Mickey Mouse, severe flexion contractures, retardation of growth and retinitis pigmentosa with optic atrophy. There is impaired colony forming ability and decreased DNA and RNA synthesis after ultraviolet exposure in fibroblasts, lymphoblastoid cell lines and cultured amniotic fluid cells[53,58]. Prognosis consists of progressive neurologic disturbance with shortened lifespan. There is no increased susceptibility to carcinogenesis.

Prenatal diagnosis is performed on amniotic cells cultured *in vitro* following amniocentesis at 16–17 weeks of gestation. Anomalies in DNA and RNA synthesis characteristic of Cockayne's syndrome can be detected after irradiating cultured amniotic cells with UV light. There is increased sensitivity to the lethal effect of UV[59].

Fanconi's anemia

Fanconi's anemia is an autosomal recessive disorder characterized by widespread brown skin, hyperpigmentation, petechiae, microcephaly, genital hypoplasia, generalized hyper-reflexia, internal strabismus, normal intelligence and absence of the thumbs. There is severe hypoplastic anemia and thrombocytopenia, and renal malformations and endocrine abnormalities are frequently found. These patients usually die at an early age from hemorrhage, infection or leukemia. There is an increased incidence of leukemia, hepatocellular carcinoma and squamous cell carcinoma in patients who survive to adulthood[59,60]. The specific molecular defects in Fanconi's anemia are not known. Cultured cells from these patients show increased transformation by oncogenic viruses, marked hypersensitivity to agents that produce interstrand cross-links in DNA, such as mitomycin C, nitrogen mustard and psoralen plus UVA light, no hypersensitivity to X-rays, ultraviolet light and chemical agents that mimic these agents, increased cell killing and chromosome aberrations. Lower than normal levels of nicotinamide adenine dinucleotide (NAD), a coenzyme possibly associated with DNA ligase activity in the repair system, have been reported in these cells[60].

Two methods of prenatal diagnosis have been described.

(1) Quantitation of chromosome breakage in cultured amniotic fluid cells obtained by amniocentesis in the 16th week of gestation.

(2) Analysis of chromosomal breakage in cells from chorionic villi at 9 weeks of gestation and cultured in diepoxy-butane (DEB) medium, which induces chromosomal breakage[61].

METABOLIC DISORDERS

Menke's syndrome

This congenital disturbance of the copper metabolism is an X-linked recessively inherited disorder characterized by increased copper accumulation in multiple cell types in the body and in culture combined with extremely low serum copper and ceruloplasmin levels[62]. The syndrome consists of severe neurologic involvement, abnormal arteries (fragmentation and reduplication of the internal elastic lamina of the arteries), and sparse thin hair with pili torti[63].

Two methods of prenatal diagnosis have been described:

(1) In the second trimester, by copper incorporation into cultured amniotic fluid cells. Copper incorporation into amniotic fluid cells from affected male fetuses is negatively correlated with gestational age. After the 18th week of gestation the risk of misclassification is significant[62].

(2) Direct copper measurement in chorionic villi in the first trimester (10th week of gestation). Affected males accumulate excessive amounts of copper in their tissues, mainly in the trophoblast cells. The high proportion of this cell type in chorionic villi should make them useful for prenatal diagnosis of Menke's disease[62].

Fabry's disease

Fabry's disease is an X-linked recessive storage disease caused by a deficiency of one or more lysosomal hydrolases. The lack of α-galactosidase-A activity causes an accumulation of glycosphingolipids (ceramide trihexoside) in the lysosomes of many cell types, particularly endothelial cells, fibroblasts and pericytes of the dermis, in the heart, in the kidneys, and in the autonomic nervous system. Clinical symptoms include edema of ankles, paralysis, extreme pain, hypohydrosis, high blood pressure, angiokeratoma of the skin, abnormal vascular structures in the conjunctiva and retina. Heterozygotes exhibit a milder form of the same disorders. Treatment is symptomatic only[64]. Cardiac disease and renal insufficiency cause death, usually in the 5th decade.

Prenatal diagnosis can be made by quantitative measurements of α-galactosidase-A in cultured amniotic fluid cells, or by chorionic villi biopsy, which can be performed earlier[65].

Erythropoietic porphyria (Gunther's disease or congenital photosensitive porphyria)

This autosomal recessively inherited disorder is caused by deficiency of uroporphyrinogen III cosynthetase, an enzyme necessary in the synthesis of heme. Clinical manifestations include photosensitivity, splenomegaly, hemolytic anemia, red urine in early infancy and erythrodontia. Vesicles and subepidermal bullae develop on light-exposed skin areas and heal with scarring and hyperpigmentation. This phenomenon, together with hypertrichosis of the cheeks, profuse eyebrows and long eyelashes, prompted the terms 'monkey face' or 'werewolf'. Cicatricial alopecia of the scalp may develop. Other chronic findings are increased fragility of the skin, photophobia, irregular hyper- and hypopigmentation, keratoconjunctivitis, ectropion and symblepharon. Treatment consists of strict avoidance of sunlight and, sometimes, splenectomy[64].

Prenatal diagnosis is made by measuring uroporphyrinogen III cosynthetase activity in cultured amniotic fluid cells obtained after 17 weeks in a pregnancy at risk for congenital erythropoietic porphyria[66]. The activity of the uroporphyrinogen III cosynthetase in this disease is much lower (25–40%) than normal.

INHERITED CONNECTIVE TISSUE DISORDERS

Ehlers–Danlos syndrome (EDS)

EDS is a group of autosomal dominant disorders of collagen metabolism, with at least 10 syndromes identified to date. It is characterized by fragility of the skin and blood vessels, hyperelasticity of the skin and hypermobility of the joints. The essential defect is a quantitative deficiency of collagen[50]. This may result from mutations in collagen genes, type I collagen (EDS type VII), or type III collagen (EDS type IV, the most severe form). The individual has thin or translucent skin through which the underlying venous pattern is noticeable. Arterial fragility is manifested by easy bruisability and arterial rupture, which is one of the major causes of morbidity and mortality. Other complications include rupture of the colon and rupture of the uterus during pregnancy.

Chorionic villus biopsy is the procedure of choice for prenatal diagnosis of EDS, because the defects responsible for this syndrome are limited to analysis by molecular genetic techniques or to biochemical analysis of type I collagen (EDS type VII) or type III collagen (EDS type IV) produced by cultured cells. EDS can also be diagnosed by linkage analysis and/or detection of a known mutation in families with these dominantly inherited disorders on a chorionic villus biopsy. Molecular genetic analysis using DNA derived from amniocentesis has also been described[67].

OTHER DISORDERS

Trichothiodystrophy

Trichothiodystrophy (TTD) is an autosomal recessive disorder characterized by brittle hair with reduced sulfur content, and mental and physical retardation. The hair is dry and sparse and the hair shafts break easily[68]. Various syndrome complexes are associated with TTD, including brittle hair–intellectual impairment–decreased fertility–short stature (BIDS), ichthyosis and BIDS (IBIDS), and photosensitivity and IBIDS (PIBIDS).

TTD patients die at an early age and no treatment has been proposed, making prenatal diagnosis important. Lehmann[69], analyzing cellular responses to UV, found a remarkable heterogeneity among fibroblasts isolated from different patients. Approximately 70% of cell strains showed defective DNA repair[70], and in general, this correlated with photosensitivity[68]. Prenatal diagnosis of TTD can be performed at about 14 weeks of gestation in families at risk by measuring the level of unscheduled DNA synthesis (UDS) after UV irradiation of trophoblast cells obtained from chorionic villi in the 9th week and cultured for 4 weeks. This procedure is limited to the 70% of TTD families in which the disorder is known to be associated with defective DNA repair.

This early detection allows confirmation of the results either by measurement of UDS in cells from amniotic fluid at 16–18 weeks' gestation, or by fetal hair biopsy at 20 weeks' gestation. The hair biopsy is an absolute confirmation of the diagnosis since the hair structure abnormality is characteristic of TTD.

Acid lipase deficiency: Wolman's disease

Wolman's disease is the infantile form of acid lipase deficiency, which causes accumulation of triglycerides and cholesterol esters in lysosomes. Onset of this autosomal recessive inherited disease occurs between 0 and 3 months, and is characterized by mental retardation, liver or spleen enlargement, adrenal calcification, anemia, vomiting and poor growth. There are no skeletal or ophthalmic manifestations[71].

Prenatal diagnosis was made in the past by enzyme analysis of amniotic fluid cells cultured after amniocentesis in the second trimester. Today, Wolman's disease can be diagnosed in the first trimester of pregnancy (10th week) by the direct demonstration of acid lipase deficiency in chorionic villi. The diagnosis is confirmed by studies on cultured chorionic villi cells and fetal skin fibroblasts. The na 633 0.(-40-) ashow olesterol oleate should be used in the prenatal diagnosis[72].

References

1. Eady, R. A. J. (1992). Prenatal diagnosis of skin disease. In: *Textbook of Dermatology*, 5th edn. pp. 373–80. (London: Blackwell Scientific)
2. Hoewell, D. H., Loeffler, F. E. and Coleman, D. V. (1983). Assessment of transcervical aspiration technique for chorion villus sampling in the first trimester of pregnancy. *Br. J. Obstet. Gynecol.*, **39**, 394–7
3. Rodeck, C. H. and Nicolaides, K. H. (1983). Invasive procedures in obstetrics. *Clin. Obstet. Gynecol.*, **10**, 515–39
4. Beharev, V. A., Aivazyan, A. A., Karetnikova, N. A., Mordovtser, V. N. and Yantovsky, Y. R. (1990). Fetal skin biopsy in prenatal diagnosis of some genodermatoses. *Prenat. Diagn.*, **10**, 1–12
5. Kurjak, A., Relja, Z., Zergollern-Cupak, L., Jurkovic, D. and Miric, D. (1993). Ultrasonically guided prenatal diagnostic procedures – benefits and risks. *J. Maternal Fetal Invest.*, **3**, 25–8
6. Elias, S. (1993). Fetal skin sampling for prenatal diagnosis of heritable skin disease. In Chervenak, F. A., Isaacon, G. C. and Campbell, S. (eds.) *Ultrasound in Obstetrics and Gynecology*. pp. 1259–65. (Boston, Toronto, London: Little Brown)
7. Kurjak, A., Alfirevic, Z. and Jurkovic, D. (1987). Ultrasonically guided fetal tissue biopsy. *Acta Obstet. Gynecol. Scand.*, **66**, 523–7
8. Jurkovic, D. and Kurjak, A. (1989). Prenatal diagnosis of epidermyolisis bullosa hereditaria by ultrasonically guided fetal skin biopsy. *Lijec Vjesn*, **111**, 60–3
9. Dale, B. A. and Holbrook, K. A. (1987). Developmental expression of human epidermal keratins and fillagrin. *Curr. Topics Dev. Biol.*, **22**, 127–51
10. Holbrook, K. A., Dales, B. A., Sybett, V. P. and Sagebiel, R. W. (1983). Epidermolytic hyperkeratosis: ultrastructure and biochemistry of skin and amniotic fluid cells from two affected fetuses and a newborn infant. *J. Invest. Dermatol.*, **80**, 222–7
11. Eady, R. A. J., Gunner, G. B., Lamba Caibone, C. D., Bricarelli, F. O., Gosden, G. M. and Rodech, C. H. (1986). Prenatal diagnosis of bullous ichthyosiform erythroderma: detection of tonofilament clumps in fetal epidermal and amniotic fluid cells. *J. Med. Genet.*, **23**, 46–51
12. Arnold, M. L. and Anton-Lamprecht, I. (1987). Prenatal diagnosis of epidermal disorders. *Curr. Probl. Dermatol.*, **16**, 120–8
13. Hausser, I. and Anton-Lamprecht, I. (1988). Ultrastructure of first trimester chorionic villi with regard to the prenatal diagnosis of genodermatoses. *Prenatal Diagn.*, **8**, 511–24
14. Lever, W. F. and Schaumburg-Lever, G. (1990). *Histopathology of the Skin*, 7th edn. (Philadelphia: J.B. Lippincott Company)
15. Shwayder, T. and Ott, F. (1991). All about ichthyosis. *Pediatr. Clin. N. Am.*, **38**, 835–57
16. Honour, J. W. Goolamali, S. K. and Taylor, N. F. (1985). Prenatal diagnosis and variable presentation of recessive x-linked ichthyosis. *Br. J. Dermatol.*, **112**, 423–30
17. Holbrook, K. A., Dale, B. A., Williams, M., Perry, T. B., Hoff, M. S., Hamilton, E. F., Fisher, C. and Senikas, V. (1988). The expression of congenital ichthyosiform erythroderma in second trimester fetuses of the same family: morphologic and biochemical studies. *J. Invest. Dermatol.*, **91**, 521–31
18. Buxhan, M., Goodkin, P. E., Fahrenbach, W. H. and Dimond, R.L. (1979). Harlequin ichthyosis with epidermal lipid abnormality. *Arch. Dermatol.*, **115**, 189
19. Williams, M. L. and Elias, P. M. (1987). Genetically transmitted, generalized disorders of cornification. The ichthyoses. *Dermatol. Clin.*, **5**, 155–78
20. Suzumori, K. and Kanzaki, T. (1991). Prenatal diagnosis of harlequin ichthyosis by fetal skin biopsy; report of 2 cases. *Prenatal Diagn.*, **11**, 451–7

21. Mihalko, M., Lindfors, K. K., Grix, A. W., Brant, W. E. and McGahan, J. P. (1989). Prenatal sonographic diagnosis of harlequin ichthyosis. *Am. J. Radiol.*, **153**, 827–8
22. Meizer, I. (1992). Prenatal ultrasonic features in a rare case of congenital ichthyosis (harlequin fetus). *J. Clin. Ultrasound*, **20**, 132–4
23. Judge, M. R., Lake, B. D., Smith, V. V., Besley, G. T. N. and Harper, J. I. (1990). Depletion of alcohol (Hexanol). Dehydrogenase activity in the epidermis and jejunal mucosa in Sjögren–Larsson syndrome. *J. Invest. Dermatol.*, **95**, 632–4
24. Kousseff, B. G., Matsuoka, L. Y., Stenn, K. S., Hobbins, J. C., Mahoney, M. J. and Hashimoto, K. (1982). Prenatal diagnosis of Sjögren–Larsson syndrome. *J. Pediatr.*, **101**, 998–1000
25. Poulos, A., Pollard, A. C., Mitchell, J. D., Wise, G. and Mortimer, G. (1984). Patterns of Refsum's disease. *Arch. Dis. Childhood*, **59**, 222–9
26. Poll-The, B. T., Poulos, A., Sharp, P., Boue, J., Ogier, H., Odievre, M. and Saudubray, J. M. (1985). Antenatal diagnosis of infantile Refsum's disease. *Clin. Genet.*, **27**, 524–6
27. Arnold, M. L. and Anton-Lamprecht, I. (1985). Problems in prenatal diagnosis of the ichthyosis congenita group. *Hum. Genet.*, **71**, 301–11
28. Gedde-Dahl, T. (1981). Sixteen types of epidermolysis bullosa. *Acta Dermato-Venereol.*, **Suppl 95**: 74–87
29. Tabas, M., Gibbons, S. and Bauer, E. A. (1987). The mechanobullous diseases. *Dermatol. Clin.*, **5**, 123–36
30. Holbrook, K. A., Wapner, R., Jackson, L. and Zaen, N. (1992). Diagnosis and prenatal diagnosis of epidermolysis bullosa herpetiformis (Dowling–Meara) in a mother, two affected children and an affected fetus. *Prenatal Diagn.*, **12**, 725–39
31. Smith, L. T., Miller, A. W., Kirz, D. A., Elias, S., Brumbaugh, S. and Holbrook, K. A. (1992). Separation of non-cutaneous epithelia in a fetus diagnosed *in utero* with junctional epidermolysis bullosa. *Pediatr. Res.*, **31**, 561–6
32. Rodeck, C. H., Eady, R. A. J. and Gosden, C. M. (1980). Prenatal diagnosis of epidermolysis bullosa letalis. *Lancet*, **1**, 949–52
33. Heagerty, A. H. M., Eady, R. A. J., Kennedy, A. R., Nicolaides, K. H., Rodeck, C. H., Hsi, B. L. and Ortonne, J. P. (1987). Rapid prenatal diagnosis of epidermolysis bullosa letalis using GB3 monoclonal antibody. *Br. J. Dermatol.*, **117**, 271–5
34. Fine, J. D., Holbrook, K. A., Elias, S., Anton-Lamprecht, I. and Rauskolb, R. (1990). Applicability of Ig DEJ-I monoclonal antibody for the prenatal diagnosis or exclusion of junctional epidermolysis bullosa. *Prenatal Diagn.*, **10**, 219–29
35. Fine, J. D., Breathnach, S. M., Hinter, H. and Katz, S. I. (1984). KF-I monoclonal antibody defines a specific basement membrane antigen defect in dystrophic forms of epidermolysis bullosa. *J. Invest. Dermatol.*, **82**, 35–38
36. Fine, J. D., Eady, R. A. J., Levy, M. L., Fielding Heitmancik, J., Courtney, K. B., Carpenter, R. J., Holbrook, K. A. and Hawkins, H. K. (1988). Prenatal diagnosis of dominant and recessive dystrophic epidermolysis bullosa: application and limitations in the use of KF-I and LH 7:2 monoclonal antibodies and immunofluorescence mapping technique. *J. Invest. Dermatol.*, **91**, 456–71
37. Heagerty, A. H. M., Kennedy, A. R., Gunner, D. B. and Eady, R. A. J. (1986). Rapid prenatal diagnosis and exclusion of epidermolysis bullosa using novel antibody probes. *J. Invest. Dermatol.*, **86** 603–5
38. Valle, K. J. and Bauer, E. A. (1980). Enhanced biosynthesis of human skin collagenase in fibroblast cultures from recessive dystrophic epidermolysis bullosa. *J. Clin. Invest.*, **66**, 176–87
39. Bauer, E. A., Ludman, M. D., Goldberg, J. D., Berkowitz, R. L. and Holbrook, K. A. (1986). Antenatal diagnosis of recessive dystrophic epidermolysis bullosa – collagenase expression in cultured fibroblasts as a biochemical marker. *J. Invest. Dermatol.*, **87**, 597–601
40. Arnold, M. L., Rauskolb, R., Anton-Lamprecht, I., Schinzel, A. and Schmid, W. (1984). Prenatal diagnosis of anhidrotic ectodermal dysplasia. *Prenatal Diagn.*, **4**, 85–98
41. Harper, J. (1992). *Genetics and Genodermatoses.* In: *Textbook of Dermatology*, 5th edn. pp. 305–372, (London: Blackwell Scientific Publications)
42. Gilgenkrantz, S., Blanchet-Bardon, C., Nazzaro, V., Formiga, I., Mujica, P. and Alembik, Y. (1989). Hypohidrotic ectodermal dysplasia. *Hum. Genet.*, **81**, 120–2
43. Zonana, J., Schinzel, A., Upadhyaya, M., Thomas, N. S. T., Anton-Lamprecht, I. and Harper, P. S. (1990). Prenatal diagnosis of X-linked hypohidrotic ectodermal dysplasia by linkage analysis. *Am. J. Med. Genet.*, **35**, 132–5
44. Anneren, G., Andersson, T., Lindgren, P. G. and Kjartansson, S. (1991). Ectrodactyly–etodermal dysplasia–clefting syndrome (EEC): the clinical variation and prenatal diagnosis. *Clin. Genet.*, **40**, 257–62
45. Bick, D. P., Balkite, E. A., Baumgarten, A., Hobbins, J. C. and Mahoney, M. J. (1987). The association of congenital skin disorders with acetylcholinesterase in amniotic fluid. *Prenatal Diagn.*, **7**, 543–9
46. Shah, Y. G. and Moodley, S. (1992). Report of a case with aplasia cutis congenita, elevated amniotic fluid alpha-fetoprotein and positive acetylcholinesterase band. *Am. J. Perinatol.*, **9**, 411–3
47. Taylor, W. O. G. (1987). Prenatal diagnosis in albinism. *Lancet*, **1**, 1307–8

48. Shimizu, H., Ishiko, A., Kikuchi, A., Akiyama, M., Suzumori, K. and Nishikava, I. (1992). Prenatal diagnosis of tyrosinase-negative oculocutaneous albinism. *Lancet*, **340**, 739–40
49. Bleechen, S. S., Ebling, F. J. G. and Champion, R. H. (1992). Disorders of Skin Colour. In Champion R. H., Burton, J. I. and Ebling, F. J. G. (eds.) *Textbook of Dermatology*, 5th edn. pp. 1561–622.(London: Blackwell Scientific Publications)
50. Durandy, A., Brelon-Gorius, J. Guy-Grand, D., Dumez, L. and Grisicelli, I. (1993) Prenatal diagnosis of syndromes associating albinism and immune deficiencies (Chediak–Higashi syndrome and variant). *Prenatal Diagn.*, **13**, 13–20
51. Atopic dermatitis, eczema, non-infectious immunodeficiency disorders. (1990). In *Andrews' Diseases of the Skin*, 8th edn. pp. 68–88. (Philadelphia: Saunders)
52. Schwartz, M., Mibashan, R. S., Nicolaides, K. H., Millar, D. S. and Jenkins, E. (1989). First trimester diagnosis of Wiskott–Aldrich syndrome by DNA markers. *Lancet*, **2**, 1405
53. Some genodermatoses. (1990). In: *Andrews' Diseases of the Skin*, 8th edn. pp. 637–81. (Philadelphial: Saunders)
54. Jaspers, N. G. J., Van Der Kraan, M., Linssen, P. C. M. L., Macek, M., Seemanova, E. and Kleijer, W. J. (1990). First trimester prenatal diagnosis of the Nijmegen breakage syndrome and ataxia telengiectasia using an assay of radioresistant DNA synthesis. *Prenatal Diagn.*, **10**, 667–74
55. Lierena, J., Murer-Orlando, M., McGuire, M., Zahed, L., Sheridan, R.J., Berry, A. C. and Bobrow, M. (1989). Spontaneous and induced chromosome breakage in chorionic villus samples: a cytogenetic approach to first trimester prenatal diagnosis of ataxia telengiectasia syndrome. *J. Med. Genet.*, **26**, 174–8
56. Dermatoses due to physical factors (1990). In: *Andrews' Diseases of the Skin*, 8th edn. pp. 22–50. (Philadelphia: Saunders)
57. Halley, D. J. J., Keiyzer, W., Jaspers, N. G. J., Niemeijer, M. I., Kliejer, W. J., Bove, J., Bove, A. and Bootsma, D. (1979). Prenatal diagnosis of xeroderma pigmentosum (Group C). Using assays of unscheduled DNA synthesis and postreplication repair. *Clin. Genet.*, **16**, 137–46
58. Lehmann, A. R. (1985). Prenatal diagnosis of Cockayne's syndrome. *Lancet*, **1**, 486–8
59. Sugita, T., Ikenaga, M. and Suehara, N. (1982). Prenatal diagnosis of Cockayne syndrome using assay of colony-forming ability in ultraviolet light irradiated cells. *Clin. Genet.*, **22**, 137–42
60. Lambert, W. C. (1987). Genetic disease associated with DNA and chromosomal instability. *Dermatol. Clin.*, **5**, 85–108
61. Auerbach, A. D., Min, Z., Ghosh, R., Pergament, E., Verlinsky, Y., Nicolas, H. and Bove, J. (1986). Clastogen-induced chromosomal breakage as a marker for first trimester prenatal diagnosis of Faconi anemia. *Hum. Genet.*, **73**, 86–8
62. Tonnesen, T., Horn, N., Sonergaard, F., Jensen, O. A., Gerdes, A. M., Girard, S. and Damsgaard, I. (1987). Experience with first trimester prenatal diagnosis of Menkes' disease. *Prenatal Diagn.*, **7**, 497–509
63. Burton, J. L. (1992). Disorders of connective tissue. In *Textbook of Dermatology*, 5th edn. pp. 1763–826. (London: Blackwell Scientific Publications)
64. Errors of metabolism. (1990). In *Andrew's Diseases of the Skin*, 8th edn. pp. 599–636. (Philadelphia: Saunders)
65. Hasholt, L., Wandall, A. and Sorensen, S. A. (1989). Fabry's disease. *Clin. Genet.*, **36**, 335–6
66. Deybach, J. C. H., Grandchamp, B., Grelier, M., Nordmann, Y., Bove, J. and Berranger, P. (1980). Prenatal exclusion of congenital erythropoietic prophyria (Gunther's disease) in a fetus at risk. *Hum. Genet.*, **53**, 217–21
67. Cohn, D. H. and Byers, P. H. (1990). Clinical screening for collagen defects in connective tissue diseases. *Clin. Perinatol.*, **17**, 793–809
68. Sarasin, A., Blanchet-Bardon, C., Renault, G., Lehmann, A., Arlett, L. and Dumez, Y. (1992). Prenatal diagnosis in a subset of trichothiodystrophy patients defective in DNA repair. *Br. J. Dermatol.*, **127**, 485–91
69. Lehmann, A. R., Arlett, C. F., Broughton, C. C., (1988). Trichothiodystrophy, a human DNA repair disorder with heterogeneity in the cellular response to UV light. *Cancer Res.*, **48**, 6090–6
70. Dawber, R. P. R., Ebling, F. J. G. and Waynarowska, F. T. (1992). Disorders of the hair. In Champion, R. H., Burton, J. I. and Ebling, I. J. G. (eds.) *Textbook of Dermatology*, 5th edn. pp. 2533–638 (London: Blackwell Scientific Publications)
71. Beaudet, A. L. (1991). Lysosomal storage diseases. In *Harrison's Principles of Internal Medicine*, 12th edn. pp. 1845–53. (New York: McGraw-Hill)
72. Van Diggelen, O. P., Von Koskull, H., Ammala, P., Vredeveldt, G. T. M., Janse, H. C. and Klieijer, W. J. (1988). First trimester diagnosis of Wolman's disease. *Prenatal Diagn.*, **8**, 661–3

Section 4

Doppler ultrasound

The prenatal assessment of fetal hypoxia

S. Campbell, K. Harrington and C. Lees

INTRODUCTION

Color Doppler/duplex machines have enabled a more detailed examination of the fetal circulation, allowing a greater knowledge of the physiological changes in the fetus during pregnancy. Interestingly, this provides an insight into how the fetus adapts when there is impaired placental transfer, in particular when it is deprived of oxygen and other substrates *in utero*. When this information is combined with that derived from cordocentesis, we can build an accurate picture of the fetal response to hypoxemia. This intelligence helps us to recognize the 'at risk' fetus, and allows us to determine with greater accuracy the progression of the disease processes. Fetal Doppler ultrasound also has the potential for being able to identify the optimum time for delivery of the compromised fetus.

Although actual measurement of volume flow changes in an organ would be ideal, the current methods for determining volume flow *in vivo* are too inaccurate, due to the poor resolution of color Doppler or B-mode in determining the size of vessel walls. Consequently, we rely on indices of resistance (e.g. the resistance index, RI, or the pulsatility index, PI), derived from the flow velocity waveform (FVW) and absolute blood velocity changes (e.g. time-averaged velocity TAV), to give us information on changes in the hemodynamics of a particular organ. The FVW can also be assessed qualitatively, by noting the absence or presence of end-diastolic frequencies, or by the presence or absence or early diastolic notching. Both methods of analysis represent the interaction between the forward compression wave, due to cardiac systole, and the peripheral resistance arresting flow.

PHYSIOLOGICAL CHANGES IN FETAL CIRCULATION DURING PREGNANCY

Doppler studies of the umbilical artery provide information on perfusion of the fetoplacental circulation, and Doppler studies of the fetus itself are valuable in observing the hemodynamic response of the fetus to an altered environment, in particular hypoxia. The FVW from the umbilical arteries can easily be obtained using continuous-wave or pulsed-wave Doppler ultrasound[1]. They have a saw-tooth appearance of arterial flow in one direction and continuous umbilical venous blood flow in the other (Figure 1). The resistance indices of the umbilical artery FVW gradually decrease with gestation, and a positive end-diastolic frequency is usually present by 15 weeks' gestation. This decrease in resistance is secondary to the increase in the number of tertiary stem villi of the placenta, and in addition to fetal cardiac output[2].

The introduction of pulsed-wave Doppler ultrasound[3], and more recently color Doppler imaging/duplex systems, has allowed us to study the human fetal circulation[4,5]. In normal pregnancy, TAV in most fetal vessels increases with gestation. Vessels examined with Doppler ultrasound include the fetal descending aorta (Figure 2), the common carotid and the middle cerebral artery (Figure 3). The rise in TAV probably reflects a progressive increase in cardiac output to fulfil the demands of the growing fetus, as TAV and vessel diameter are the parameters used to determine volume flow.

The PI, primarily reflecting downstream resistance, remains relatively constant in the aorta, but steadily falls in the common carotid and

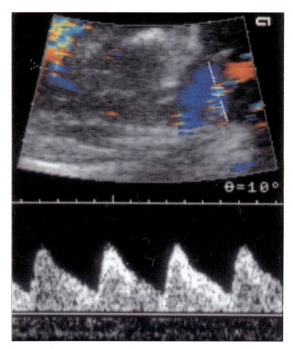

Figure 1 *Normal umbilical artery flow velocity waveform from the second half of pregnancy with abundant diastolic flow*

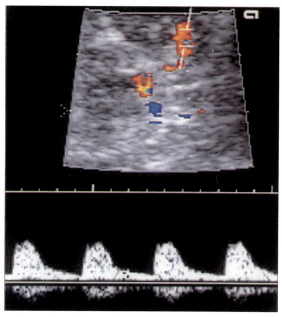

Figure 3 *Normal middle cerebral artery waveform, obtained from an appropriately grown fetus at 32 weeks*

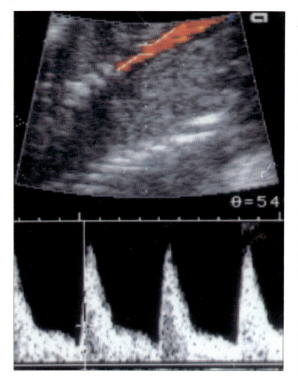

Figure 2 *End-diastolic frequencies present in the aorta during the second half of normal pregnancy*

middle cerebral arteries. These findings suggest that in the latter part of pregnancy a proportionally greater fraction of the cardiac output is directed to the fetal brain, presumably to compensate for the progressive fall in fetal blood pO_2 and increase in pCO_2.

The characteristic pattern or pulsatility of venous FVWs reflects events in the cardiac cycle of the fetal heart. There is a typical triphasic pattern, reflecting ventricular systole, passive filling of the atrium in early diastole, and atrial contraction in late diastole. Venous flow is much more sensitive to changes in the fetal behavioral state, in particular when the fetus is breathing. As with arterial Doppler, this must be taken into consideration when interpreting venous flow waveforms. During the second half of pregnancy, changes in Doppler-derived indices of the fetal venous circulation are similar to those of the arterial system; there is a tendency for velocities to increase, and resistance to fall[6]. The fall in resistance most likely reflects the increasing compliance of the fetal heart. The ductus venosus has the highest velocities in the venous vessels. This allows well-oxygenated blood to be directed towards the foramen ovale and the left ventricle, and consequently to the fetal brain.

PATHOPHYSIOLOGY – THE FETAL RESPONSE TO HYPOXEMIA

Animal studies have demonstrated that during artificially induced hypoxia there is a preferential perfusion of the fetal brain, heart and adrenal glands at the expense of the corpus, gut and kidneys, termed the 'brain-sparing' effect[7]. Doppler ultrasound has allowed us to study the small-for-gestational-age fetus, and to provide evidence of the brain-sparing effect in human pregnancies. It is also possible to document the sequence of changes in the fetal circulation, and correlate these changes with established tests of fetal well-being, such as the amniotic fluid volume and fetal heart trace[8]. Figure 4 illustrates the typical sequence of changes in antenatal investigations in the growth-retarded fetus born small for gestational age.

Umbilical circulation

There is a reduction in the number of arterioles in the tertiary stem villi in pregnancies complicated with fetal growth retardation[9] and it is probable that high-resistance waveforms in the umbilical artery reflect this finding. Persistent high-resistance umbilical artery FVWs have been associated with an increased risk of a fetal chromosomal anomaly[10], and a poor perinatal outcome[11], although the use of the umbilical artery FVWs as a screening test has not been shown to be of value. With cordocentesis, alterations in abnormal umbilical artery FVWs have been correlated with fetal blood oxygen tension in small-for-gestational-age fetuses[12]. An analysis of 207 pregnancies with small-for-gestational-age fetuses has found that the end-diastolic frequencies in FVWs from the umbilical artery were absent in 119 cases, and in 87 (73%) the fetal blood pO_2 was below the 2.5th centile of the normal range[13] (Figure 5).

An abnormal umbilical artery PI will not identify all the compromised fetuses in a population, especially near or at term, but in the small-for-gestational-age fetus, umbilical artery Doppler measurements are now an essential part of determining the etiology of fetal smallness. A randomized study suggests that the management of the small-for-gestational-age fetus with umbilical artery Doppler appears to confer a benefit over management by cardiotocographic criteria[14], although in practice both investigations are utilized.

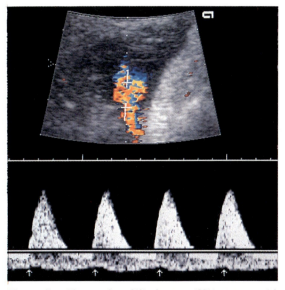

Figure 5 *Abnormal umbilical artery (UA) pattern with loss of end-diastolic frequencies. Abnormal UA waveforms identify an at-risk group, but to ascertain how the fetus is coping with the abnormal UA supply, the fetal circulation should be investigated. Although there is some variability in the UA flow velocity waveforms, they are clearly abnormal*

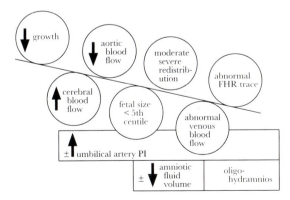

Figure 4 *Diagrammatic representation of the typical sequence of changes in investigations of the fetus compromised by chronic uteroplacental insufficiency. FHR, fetal heart rate*

Umbilical vein pulsations are a normal finding in first-trimester human fetuses[15], whereas later in pregnancy, they are an ominous sign that indicates alterations in cardiac function. They are associated with severe growth retardation, absent end-diastolic velocities in the umbilical artery, abnormal fetal heart rates, and non-immune hydrops[16–18]. Abnormal waveforms were also found in the inferior vena cava, with an increase in the percentage of blood flowing in a reverse direction during atrial contraction.

Fetal arterial circulation

If the blood supply to the head and neck is doubled, there is a relative reduction in aortic blood supply to the rest of the body of about 20%. The relationship between fetal acid–base status (obtained at cordocentesis), and the PI and TAV of the fetal aorta and common carotid artery was therefore examined with pulsed-wave Doppler ultrasound[19].

A total of 41 fetuses that were small, and 10 that were appropriate for gestational age were studied. Although there were significant correlations between the blood-gas result and both the PI and TAV in the individual vessels, better correlations were found with the ratios of the common carotid artery and descending thoracic aorta. The best predictor of asphyxia (as judged by an asphyxia index calculated from the pH, pCO_2 and pO_2) was the aorta TAV/carotid artery PI index. When the aortic–carotid index was abnormal all fetuses had an asphyxia index above the mean, 89% of the fetuses had an asphyxia index one standard deviation above the mean and 60% had an index more than two standard deviations above the mean. A normal index was always associated with normal blood gases. Thus, the aortic–carotid index appears to be a sensitive indicator of the chemoreceptor response to falling blood oxygen tension.

In a separate study investigating fetuses that were small for gestational age (< 5th centile) a significant relationship between fetal acidemia and absence of end-diastolic frequencies in the aorta was found (Figure 6). It is proposed that

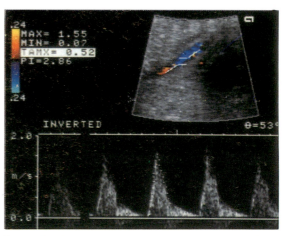

Figure 6 *Loss of end-diastolic frequencies and reduced velocities in the fetal aorta is an ominous sign that indicates severe distribution and probable fetal acidemia. This finding can occur in the presence of a normal umbilical artery flow velocity waveform*

the aortic changes reflect the 'lower-limb' or 'hind-quarter' reflex seen in animal studies[20]. It is thought that this is an end-stage mechanism designed to ensure adequate supply of nutrients to the brain as a result of a diminished supply, and it is considered an ominous sign. Furthermore, the finding of absent end-diastolic frequencies in the fetal descending thoracic aorta is associated with an increased incidence of neonatal necrotizing enterocolitis and hemorrhage[21].

The common carotid artery supplies the tissues of the head and neck in addition to the brain, but the cerebral circulation is likely to give more precise information about changes within the fetal brain itself[22]. With the introduction of colour Doppler the fetal cerebral vascular (middle cerebral artery) response to hypoxia was studied, and correlated with changes in acid–base balance from umbilical cord blood obtained at cordocentesis[23]. The PI and TAV of the middle cerebral artery were measured in 81 small-for-gestational-age fetuses (abdominal circumference < 2.5th centile) prior to cordocentesis. The PI of FVWs from the fetal middle cerebral artery was significantly lower than the reference range (Figure 7), and in the 58 fetuses that had middle cerebral artery TAV measured, the values were significantly higher than the reference range. These data provide evidence of vasodilatation in the cerebral vasculature during mild-to-moderate hypoxia. With severe degrees of hypoxia (2–4 standard deviations below the normal mean for gestation), usually with associated acidosis, the reduction in PI reached a maximum, which probably represents maximum vessel dilatation. In extreme hypoxia (a pO_2 value of > 4 standard deviations below the normal mean for gestation), the reduction in PI was proportionally less. This may reflect the vasodilatation-mediated decrease in PI being blunted by increased intracranial pressure, possibly due to cerebral edema, or perhaps an alteration in cardiac output. This phenomenon has been noted in monkey fetuses deprived of oxygen[24].

Fetal venous circulation

Animal experiments suggest that severe hypoxemia combined with acidosis causes redistribution of umbilical vein blood flow towards the ductus venosus, at the expense of hepatic blood flow, and that fetal systemic vascular resistance has a major influence on venous return and filling patterns of the right heart[25]. The proportion of umbilical vein blood contributing to the fetal cardiac output increased from 27% during normoxemia to 39% during hypoxemia, resulting in a doubling of umbilical vein-derived oxygen delivery to the myocardium. In term primate fetuses, there was an increase of the proportion of umbilical vein blood flow entering the ductus venosus from 53% to 90%, although actual umbilical blood flow decreased by more than 50% during fetal hypoxia and acidosis[26]. We can conclude from these animal experiments that severe hypoxemia combined with acidosis causes redistribution of umbilical vein blood towards the ductus venosus at the expense of hepatic blood flow.

Arterial blood flow redistribution in fetal hypoxia provides sufficient oxygen to the brain and the myocardium. As long as the fetus is able to compensate in this way, preferential myocardial oxygenation prevents the development of right heart failure, despite an increase afterload. In a study in humans, the fetal heart and

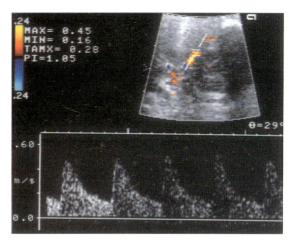

Figure 7 Low-resistance waveform (PI < 5th centile) obtained from the middle cerebral artery of a growth-retarded hypoxic fetus. Redistribution of blood to the fetal brain identifies the fetus that is adapting to reduced substrate supply and thereby at risk, but alone does not identify the optimum time for delivery of an at-risk fetus

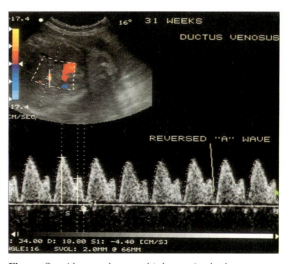

Figure 8 Abnormal reversed 'a' wave in the ductus venosus of a hypoxic fetus. Changes in the waveform of the ductus venosus and inferior vena cava suggest right heart failure. These changes usually occur after there is evidence of arterial redistribution but prior to the onset of an ominous fetal heart rate pattern. This information may be of use in the management of the very premature fetus.

venous circulation were investigated in fetuses with severe arterial redistribution (absent end-diastolic frequencies in the aorta). There was an increase in the ratio of the right to left ventricular end-diastolic diameters, and a decrease in right ventricular fractional shortening[27]. These findings suggest that right ventricular dysfunction can occur as a result of chronic intrauterine hypoxia, and these changes can occur without changes in left ventricular function.

Changes in the venous circulation therefore indicate failure of the compensatory circulatory mechanisms (Figure 8), implying the development of right heart failure secondary to an increase in afterload (the ductus arteriosus allows the right heart to communicate with the systemic circulation). The worsening myocardial hypoxia and ischemia may already be evident as a suboptimal cardiotocogram at this time, and within days the cardiotocogram will develop a terminal pattern. For this reason fetal venous Doppler studies may have a role to play in the timing of delivery for the very premature fetus.

SUMMARY

The value of uterine Doppler ultrasound for the early prediction of the fetus at risk of developing hypoxia has already been reported[28]. If the fetus becomes growth-retarded or compromised, fetal Doppler ultrasound allows us to assess the onset, progression and severity of prenatal hypoxia. The fetal Doppler findings have been corroborated with values obtained at cordocentesis. Umbilical artery Doppler is of help in the management of the small-for-gestational-age fetus, identifying a subpopulation with increased morbidity and mortality, but the umbilical artery FVW can be normal when a fetus is compromised, especially if the problems develop at or near term. Umbilical venous pulsations carry a poor prognosis in the growth-retarded fetus.

The reduction in fetal growth and evidence of mild redistribution of its arterial circulation are typically the initial responses of a fetus with a compromised supply of nutrients/oxygen from the placenta. A slowing in growth reduces metabolic demand whilst maintaining basal metabolism. Redistribution of blood to the head ensures that the total nutrient supply to the brain is sufficient to meet the demand of the growing brain. As the fetus can demonstrate changes in growth and cerebral blood supply in the presence of normal oxygenation, these are suitable criteria for identifying a compromised fetus, but not alone sufficient to determine the timing of delivery.

Maximal cerebral redistribution of flow is reached on average approximately two weeks before the onset of fetal heart-rate decelerations, but systemic changes in blood flow redistribution continue until delivery[29]. Increased resistance in the fetal systemic arterial circulation (absent end-diastolic frequency in the fetal aorta) suggests a deterioration in the fetal condition and the onset of acidemia. This is useful in identifying the small, sick fetus, whereas changes in the fetal venous circulation indirectly signal right heart failure and precede the onset of an abnormal cardiotocogram. Fetal Doppler ultrasound therefore allows a more accurate determination of the deteriorating fetal condition *in utero*.

The degree of compromise suffered *in utero*, especially the presence of prolonged acidemia, may influence the neurodevelopmental potential of a fetus after birth[30]. We already use Doppler ultrasound to help us identify and monitor the small sick fetus as early as possible in the pregnancy. If there is a significant fall-off in growth velocity, or if the fetus is found to be small for gestational age on scan, we will look at the fetal circulation to decide on the frequency of follow-up and/or delivery.

The information derived from fetal Doppler studies complements other tests of fetal well-being, and is already an essential part of our practice. It is not yet clear whether fetal Doppler will allow us ultimately to replace other, less sensitive, tests of well-being (e.g. fetal heart rate testing), or simply remain as a core part of our assessment. Future studies will address this issue.

References

1. Stuart, B., Drumm, J., Fitzgerald, D. and Duignan, N. M. (1980). Fetal blood velocity waveforms in normal pregnancy. *Br. J. Obstet. Gynaecol.*, **88**, 865–9
2. Kaufman, P., Senn, D. K. and Schweikhart, G. (1979). Classification of human placental villi. *Cell Tissue Res.*, **200**, 400–23
3. Bilardo, C. M., Campbell, S. and Nicolaides, K. H. (1988). Mean blood velocities and flow impedance in the fetal descending thoracic aorta and common carotid artery in normal pregnancy. *Early Hum. Dev.*, **18**, 213–18
4. Meerman, R. J., Van Bel, F., Van Zwieten, P. H. T. *et al.* (1990). Fetal and neonatal cerebral blood flow velocity in the normal fetus and neonate: a longitudinal Doppler study. *Early Hum. Dev.*, **24**, 209–17
5. Arudini, D. and Rizzo, G. (1990). Normal values of pulsatility index from fetal vessels: a cross sectional study on 1556 healthy fetuses. *J. Perinat. Med.*, **18**, 165–71
6. Hecher, K., Snijders, R., Campbell, S. and Nicolaides, K. (1994). Reference ranges for fetal venous and intracardiac blood flow parameters. *Ultrasound Obstet. Gynecol.* in press
7. Peters, L. L. H., Sheldon, R. E., Jones, M. D., Makowski, E. L. and Meschisa, G. (1979). Blood flow to fetal organs as a function of arterial oxygen content. *Am. J. Obstet. Gynecol.*, **135**, 637–42
8. Harrington, K., Hecher, K. and Campbell, S. (1993). Doppler ultrasound in obstetrics. In Studd, J. and Jardine-Brown, C. (eds.) *RCOG Yearbook 1993*, pp. 247–59. (London: RCOG Press)
9. Giles, W. B., Trudinger, B. J. and Baird, P. J. (1985). Fetal umbilical artery flow velocity waveforms and placental resistance: pathological correlation. *Br. J. Obstet. Gynaecol.*, **92**, 31–8
10. Wenstrom, K. D., Weiner, C. P. and Williamson, R. A. (1991). Diverse maternal and fetal pathology associated with absent diastolic flow in the umbilical artery of high risk fetuses. *Obstet. Gynecol.*, **77**, 374–8
11. Trudinger, B. J., Cook, C. M. *et al.* (1991). Fetal umbilical artery velocimetry waveforms and subsequent neonatal outcome. *Br. J. Obstet. Gynaecol.*, **98**, 378–84
12. Nicolaides, K. H., Bilardo, C. M., Soothill, P. W. and Campbell, S. (1988). Absence of end diastolic frequencies in the umbilical artery: a sign of fetal hypoxia and acidosis. *Br. Med. J.*, **297**, 1026–9
13. Campbell, S., Vyas, S. and Nicolaides, K. H. (1991). Doppler investigation of the fetal circulation. *J. Perinat. Med.*, **19**, 21–6
14. Almstrom, H., Axelson, O., Cnattinghius, S. *et al.* (1992). Comparison of umbilical-artery velocimetry and cardiotocography for surveillance of small for gestational age fetuses. *Lancet*, **340**, 936–40
15. Rizzo, G., Arudini, D. and Romanini, C. (1992). Umbilical vein pulsations: a physiologic finding in early gestation. *Am. J. Obstet. Gynecol.*, **167**, 675–7
16. Reed, K. L., Appleton, C. P., Anderson, C. F., Shenker, L. and Sahn, D. J. (1990). Doppler studies of vena cava flows in human fetuses. Insights into normal and abnormal cardiac physiology. *Circulation*, **81**, 498–505
17. Indik, J. H., Chen, V. and Reed, K. L. (1991). Association of umbilical venous with inferior vena cava blood flow velocities. *Obstet. Gynecol.*, **77**, 551–7
18. Nakai, Y., Miyazaki, Y. *et al.* (1992). Pulsatile umbilical venous flow and its clinical significance. *Br. J. Obstet. Gynaecol.*, **99**, 997
19. Bilardo, C. M., Nicolaides, K. H. and Campbell, S. (1990). Doppler measurement of fetal and uteroplacental circulations: relationship with umbilical venous blood gases measured at cordocentesis. *Am. J. Obstet. Gynecol.*, **162**, 115–20
20. Akalin-Sel, T., Nicolaides, K. and Campbell, S. (1992). Understanding the pathophysiology of intrauterine growth retardation: the role of the lower limb reflex in redistribution of blood flow. *Eur. J. Obstet. Gynecol. Reprod. Biol.*, **46**, 2–4
21. Hackett, G. A. S., Campbell, S., Gamsu, W. Cohen-Overbeck, T. and Pierce, J. M. F. (1987). Doppler studies in the growth retarded fetus and prediction of neonatal necrotising enterocolitis hemorrhage and neonatal morisidity. *Br. Med. J.*, **294**, 13–16
22. Van den Wijngaard, J. A. G. W., Greenenberg, I. A. L., Wladimiroff, J. W. and Hop, W. C. J. (1989). Cerebral Doppler ultrasound in the human fetus. *Br. J. Obstet. Gynaecol.*, **96**, 845–9
23. Vyas, S., Nicolaides, K. H., Bower, S. and Campbell, S. (1990). Middle cerebral artery flow velocity waveforms in fetal hypoxemia. *Br. J. Obstet. Gynaecol.*, **97**, 797–803
24. Myers, R. E., de Courtney-Myers, G. M. and Wagner, K. R. (1984). Effects of hypoxia on fetal brain. In Beard, R. W. and Nathanielsz, P. W. (eds.) *Fetal Physiology and Medicine*, pp. 419–36. (London: Butterworths)
25. Reuss, M. L. and Rudolph, A. M. (1980). Distribution and recirculation of umbilical and sys-

temic venous blood flow in fetal lambs during hypoxia. *J. Dev. Physiol.*, **2**, 71–84
26. Behrman, R. E., Lees, M. H., Peterson, E. N., de Lannoy, C. W. and Seeds, A. E. (1970). Distribution of the circulation in the normal and asphyxiated fetal primate. *Am. J. Obstet. Gynecol.*, **108**, 956–69
27. Rasanen, J., Kirkinen, P. and Jouppila, P. (1989). Right ventricular dysfunction in human fetal compromise. *Am. J. Obstet. Gynecol.*, **161**, 136–40
28. Harrington, K., Campbell, S., Bewley, S. and Bower, S. (1991). Doppler velocimetry studies of the uterine artery in the early prediction of pre-eclampsia and intrauterine growth retardation. *Eur. J. Obstet. Gynecol.*, **42**, S14–20
29. Arduini, D., Rizzo, G. and Romanini, C. (1992). Changes of pulsatility index from fetal vessels preceding the onset of late decelerations in growth-retarded fetuses. *Obstet. Gynecol.*, **79**, 605–10
30. Soothill, P. W., Ajayi, R. A., Campbell, S. *et al.* (1992). Relationship between fetal acidemia at cordocentesis and subsequent neurodevelopment. *Ultrasound Obstet. Gynecol.*, **2**, 80–3

The effect of maternal vasoactive agents on uterine and fetal hemodynamics

P. Jouppila, J. Räsänen, S. Alahuhta and R. Jouppila

During the last few years Doppler and color Doppler methods have enabled the exact non-invasive examination of human uterine and fetal hemodynamics. These methods have not only opened up quite new possibilities for the elucidation of physiological and pathophysiological problems in hemodynamic regulation but have also provided a new model for the study of fetal wellbeing. One interesting topic for Doppler examinations is the increasing knowledge which can be obtained on the circulatory effects of different maternal vasoactive agents during pregnancy.

The main interest in hemodynamic studies has focused into the arterial blood flow velocities and waveforms in the main uterine and arcuate arteries, umbilical arteries and fetal cerebral and renal arteries. Also, the examination of fetal cardiac function and recently that of venous blood flow in the umbilical vein, inferior vena cava and ductus venosus have been points of interest. Most studies are based on the use of indices (pulsatility, resistance and systolic/diastolic) obtained from the arterial velocity curve which reflects peripheral vascular resistance distal to the point of measurement. Although it is impossible in human studies to measure many other central parameters, such as fetal blood pressure and details of oxygen metabolism which also reflect hemodynamic changes, it is still possible to obtain reliable new knowledge on the effects and safety of different vasoactive agents. Many of these factors could potentially modify fetal circulation either indirectly through changes in the maternal uterine blood flow or by direct effects on the fetal hemodynamics.

ANTIHYPERTENSIVE DRUGS

Pregnancy-induced hypertension is associated with increased peripheral vascular resistance which can lead to a reduction in uteroplacental blood flow by 40–70% compared with normal pregnancies. Opinions regarding the advantages and disadvantages of different antihypertensive drugs on the uteroplacental and fetal hemodynamics before Doppler were controversial. Vasodilator agents have been accepted universally as drugs of choice for the treatment of pregnancy-induced hypertension but there are still problems involved in assessing their actual benefits and potential hemodynamic hazards. One critical point is the placental circulation reaction to a decreased maternal blood pressure and peripheral vascular resistance which raises the question: do the originally compromised uteroplacental hemodynamics react similarly with arterial vasodilatation or with a compensatory vasoconstriction?

The first reports dealing with the effects of antihypertensive drugs on the uteroplacental circulation were based on isotope methods. No changes were observed in short-term conditions using labetalol[1,2] or dihydralazine[3,4] despite a significant decrease of maternal blood pressure. Similarly, infusions of pindolol, metoprolol and prostacyclin did not cause any changes in placental blood flow[5–7].

Recently, the short- and long-term effects of different antihypertensive drugs on umbilical and fetal circulation have been studied using Doppler methods. No significant changes on the blood flow volume in the umbilical vein were observed after labetalol[2] and prostacyclin[6] infusion whereas an increase was observed following dihydralazine administration[4]. Metoprolol, which is a β1-adrenoreceptor antagonist increased the peripheral vascular resistance, and elevated the resistance index in the fetal descending thoracic aorta, while labetalol, a combined α-, β-adrenergic blocker, did not have any effect in corresponding short-term conditions[7]. Montan and colleagues have observed that atenolol, a cardioselective β-blocker, increased the uteroplacental vascular resistance[8] and also increased indices in the fetal descending aorta and umbilical artery in long-term conditions[9]. Pindolol, a non-selective β-blocker with vasodilatory effects, did not change resistance in any fetal arteries[9]. Our recent unpublished results also support the different response of the fetal circulation and cardiac function to atenolol and pindolol in short-term conditions. No effects on the vascular resistance of the umbilical artery, fetal cerebral and renal circulation and on fetal cardiac function were observed after intravenous labetalol in short-term conditions[10]. This also holds true in groups with the most marked decrease in maternal blood pressure and in originally pathological umbilical vascular resistance. Correspondingly, no changes in vascular resistance of umbilical arteries were observed after one week of peroral labetalol treatment[11]. Contrary to these findings, Harper and Murnaghan observed increased pulsatility index values in the umbilical artery after labetalol infusion[12]. A single dose of nifedipine, a calcium blocking agent, did not alter vascular resistance in the umbilical or middle cerebral arteries in hypertensive pregnancies[13].

The Doppler method has markedly increased our ability to study, in detail, the hemodynamic effects of maternal antihypertensive agents on the uterine and fetal circulation under real clinical conditions in hypertensive pregnancies. It seems that a moderate decrease in maternal blood pressure by these drugs has no detrimental effect on these parameters. This may signify broad safety margins in the uteroplacental circulation and a good fetal tolerance to changes in maternal blood pressure and to drug concentrations in the fetal circulation. On the other hand, no clear improvement, i.e. a decrease of vascular resistance in the uterine arteries has been observed as a consequence of the decreased blood pressure produced by these agents. Thus, according to our knowledge, the indications for the use of antihypertensive drugs during pregnancy should be mainly maternal ones: the prevention of cerebrovascular accidents and placental abruption and the prolongation of pregnancy until better fetal maturity. It seems that the fetal concentrations of these agents are great enough to produce some modifying effects on the fetal circulation and therefore the use of β-blockers with vasoconstrictory capacities during pregnancy may be reconsidered. This may be especially true in cases with compromised fetal circulation in chronic asphyxia where the avoidance of any iatrogenic changes to fetal cardiac function and hemodynamic redistribution is important.

OBSTETRIC ANALGESIA AND ANESTHESIA

The different forms of obstetric analgesia and anesthesia provide an interesting topic for Doppler studies due to the threat of maternal hypotension that often accompanies regional blocks and to the potentially vasoactive character of the anesthetic agents. Also, adrenaline added to the local anesthetics and the use of vasopressors in treating maternal hypotension may cause changes in the uterine and fetal circulation.

Epidural analgesia during labor with bupivacaine seems to cause no changes in uteroplacental and umbilical blood flow in healthy parturients if maternal hypotension can be avoided with preventive methods (lateral position, prehydration)[14,15]. Also, epidurally administered opioids did not modify the vascular resistance in uterine or umbilical arteries during labor[16]. A significant increase in intervillous blood flow[17] or a decrease in originally pathological indices in the uterine[18] and umbilical arteries[19] was observed after epidural analgesia during labor in severe pre-eclampsia. Paracervical block with bupivacaine did not change indices in the uterine and umbilical arteries, but in some cases of fetal bradycardia after epidural block the vascular resistance of umbilical arteries showed a marked increase[20]. This may be due to the direct vasoconstrictory effect of bupivacaine on the umbilical vessels in high, accidental concentrations.

The methods of regional anesthesia in Cesarean sections (epidural and spinal) have become the most commonly used anesthetic techniques. Their benefits include avoidance of maternal complications related to general anesthesia and the obvious advantages to the fetus/neonates. Both of these anesthetic methods, however, produce an extensive sympathetic block leading to peripheral vasodilatation and maternal hypotension if sufficient preventive methods are not used. This effect could lead to hazards in the uterine and fetal circulation. It has been demonstrated using Doppler methods that the pulsatility index in the maternal femoral artery decreased by 68% following epidural anesthesia for Cesarean section[21] signifying a great decrease of vascular resistance in the legs.

In some papers, an increase in vascular resistance in the uterine but not in the umbilical arteries after epidural block with bupivacaine has been observed[22]. In the majority of recent reports, however, no deleterious effect on the uterine or umbilical circulation has been found[22–25]. Adrenaline added to the anesthetic agent may in theory reduce the uteroplacental blood flow due to its vasoconstrictory capacities. However, no changes in the vascular resistance of uterine and umbilical arteries have been observed using Doppler after epidural anesthesia with adrenaline added to bupivacaine[24,26,27]. The fetal myocardial function seems also to be unaltered in connection with epidural anesthesia for Cesarean section in healthy mothers[25–27]. In our recent paper[28] the hemodynamic effects of epidural anesthesia were studied in hypertensive pregnancies with signs of chronic fetal asphyxia. In the subgroup who received bupivacaine alone as an anesthetic agent no changes were measured, whereas in the group receiving bupivacaine–adrenaline an increase in the blood velocity indices in the uterine arteries and a decrease of the values in the fetal renal and middle cerebral artery were observed.

Spinal anesthesia at Cesarean section with a more sudden onset of autonomic blockade can, in theory, lead to even more marked disturbances in the uterine and fetal circulation. In fact, Robson and co-workers[29] measured increased index values in the umbilical artery after induction of spinal anesthesia. This finding of increased vascular resistance was attributed to a simultaneous decrease of maternal cardiac output. According to many other studies[30,31], however, no changes have been found in uteroplacental and umbilical hemodynamics after spinal anesthesia if profound maternal hypotension is avoided. In these prophylactic procedures, uterine displacement plays a central role in avoiding aortocaval compression. Our team has recently studied the effect of tilt produced by either wedge or a mechanical uterine displacer under spinal anesthesia. Blood velocity indices for the underlying uterine artery increased significantly when using a mechanical displacer while no changes were observed for the wedge[32].

Different vasopressors are commonly used as prophylactic medication or in the treatment of hypotension at spinal anesthesia. Both ephedrine and ephrine significantly increased vascular resistance in the uterine arteries if they were used for treatment of maternal hypotension[33]. No changes were observed in the umbilical circulation but ephedrine decreased indices in the fetal middle cerebral and renal arteries and increased fetal right ventricular contractility. Ephedrine used as a low dosage prophylactic infusion at spinal anesthesia did not, however, modify uterine or fetal hemodynamic parameters[34] but phenylephrine, a more potent arterial vasoconstrictor, increased index values in the uterine arteries and decreased those in fetal renal arteries. The clinical outcomes for all these fetuses/newborns, however, were uneventful. Wright and associates[35] noted a brief increase in pulsatility indices of uterine arteries after methoxamine administration (a pure α-agonist) used as a vasopressor during epidural anesthesia. They still concluded that the choice of vasopressor is of minor importance compared with the avoidance of maternal hypotension.

It can be stated conclusively that properly managed obstetric regional analgesia and anesthesia do not have any significant effects on uterine and fetal hemodynamics. It is possible to detect changes in uterine and fetal hemodynamics using sensitive Doppler methods caused by some vasoactive drugs, external maternal agents or due to the lack of preventive methods at obstetric anesthesia. These effects seem to occur mainly as an increase in vascular resistance in the uterine arteries, but some regulatory alterations can also be detected in fetal hemodynamics or cardiac function. Clinically they are obviously harmless, reflecting a great fetal tolerance to minor hemodynamic alterations. They are, however, signs of the potential vasoregulatory dangers associated with obstetric anesthesia. Doppler techniques can be evaluated as a method to be used in the safety testing of new anesthetic drugs and the modifications of methods also in the future.

PROSTAGLANDIN SYNTHETASE INHIBITORS

Prostaglandins play a significant physiological role in the augmentation of uterine contractions. On the other hand, prostaglandin synthetase inhibitors such as indomethacin, naproxen and sulindac decrease this activity by competing with arachidonic acid for cyclooxygenase enzyme. These drugs therefore have a potential role in the treatment of premature labor during pregnancy and data from several studies suggest that indomethacin is more effective than betamimetics[36]. The problem is that indomethacin has been associated with transient constriction of the fetal ductus arteriosus[37,38] and also causes other changes in the fetal circulation.

According to experimental studies on fetal lambs, increased systolic (>140 cm/s) and diastolic (>35 cm/s) ductal velocities reflect the constriction of the fetal ductus arteriosus[37]. The incidence of ductal constriction during indomethacin therapy seems to be as frequent as 50–86%[38,39]. It is also obvious that the fetal ductus becomes more reactive to indomethacin with increasing gestational age[39], but can still occur as early as week 24. Regurgitation at the tricuspid valve level as a sign of increased afterload in the right ventricle has been observed simultaneously in 22–50% of cases[37,39]. The signs of ductal constriction and tricuspid regurgitation disappear within 72 h after indomethacin treatment[39], but perinatal problems are especially common in cases where premature delivery occurs during or immediately after indomethacin therapy. In fact, bronchopulmonary dysplasia has been reported in 33% of these babies. Some reports on pulmonary hypertension in newborns after long-term indomethacin therapy have been published[36,40].

The effect of indomethacin on various other fetal, umbilical and uterine arteries has also been studied. When both ductal constriction and tricuspid regurgitation occur simultaneously, the vascular resistance in the fetal middle cerebral artery is decreased[41]. This suggests a compensatory increase in cerebral blood flow. No changes in the uterine and umbilical artery indices have been found[42,43]. Indomethacin also seems to have no effect on the vascular resistance in the fetal renal arteries[44] although it decreases fetal urine output and the amount of amniotic fluid.

What about the role of other prostaglandin synthetase inhibitors with regard to the effects on fetal hemodynamics? Low-dose aspirin therapy has been used during pregnancy to prevent pre-eclampsia and fetal growth retardation and in cases with anticardiolipin antibodies. In two longitudinal studies[45,46], no effect on the blood flow velocities or pulsatility indices of the fetal ductus arteriosus and the umbilical artery were observed during aspirin treatment. Interestingly, sulindac, a prostaglandin synthetase inhibitor closely related to indomethacin, seems to differ from indomethacin regarding its effect on the fetal ductus arteriosus. In a recent randomized study[47] a trend towards higher ductus velocities noted in the indomethacin group was not seen during sulindac treatment. Our own recent unpublished data support these findings. Sulindac seems, however, to be as effective for refractory preterm labor. The difference in the fetal hemodynamic effects may be based on the negligible or non-existent placental transfer of sulindac.

The frequency of occurrence of ductal constriction with other negative circulatory and adaptation consequences in the fetus and newborn justifies a close follow-up of these cases during indomethacin therapy. Despite the obvious transient character of ductal constriction, a critical attitude to the routine use of this drug or at least in long-term therapy for premature contractions has been aroused.

EFFECTS OF MATERNAL OXYGENATION

Intrauterine fetal growth retardation in the presence of impaired utero- and fetoplacental circulation is often associated with fetal hypoxemia and acidemia. In this condition, the fetal circulation can be redistributed favoring the brain at the expense of the viscera and musculoskeletal system, and these changes can be registered by Doppler studies in human fetuses. Maternal oxygen inhalation and hyperoxygenation have been used recently as a treatment or as a test in pregnancies with hypoxic or growth retarded fetuses. Arduini and colleagues[48] studied the fetal hemodynamic response to maternal hyperoxygenation in growth retarded fetuses which had pathological index values in the umbilical artery, the fetal descending aorta and the internal carotid artery. They observed that those fetuses which did not respond to oxygen therapy by normalization of vascular resistance later developed acute fetal distress more often. The authors suggested that such fetuses would require early delivery. Good responders can benefit from continuing maternal oxygen therapy and the prolongation of pregnancy. Bilardo and co-workers[49] also studied the effect of maternal hyperoxygenation in severely growth retarded hypoxemic fetuses at 22–30 weeks' gestation. In the surviving subgroup, the originally low mean velocity in the fetal descending aorta increased, whereas in intrauterine deaths there was a trend towards continuing deterioration of this velocity during oxygenation. The fetal carotid and umbilical artery indices did not change. On the contrary, Mori and associates[50] observed a decrease of flow velocities in the fetal middle cerebral artery in connection with increased fetal aorta velocities during oxygen inhalation.

In the study by de Rochambeau and colleagues[51] the most marked finding was that in cases with absent end-diastolic velocity in the umbilical artery with a brain-sparing effect in the cerebral arteries. The outcome was strongly dependent on the oxygen test response. If the test is negative (no normalization of index values) the authors suggest an urgent delivery in this group of fetuses. A positive response, on the other hand, suggests some placental reserve and may indicate that the pregnancy can still be managed. Increased velocities in the fetal ductus venosus were found during maternal hyperoxygenation, suggesting constriction of this vessel in correlation with increasing blood oxygen levels[52]. In a longitudinal study of four intrauterine growth retarded fetuses with fetal heart rate declarations, Ribber and associates[53] could not demonstrate any index changes in the fetal carotid artery during maternal hyperoxygenation. Although blood gas abnormalities were less frequent in the fetuses/neonates of mothers treated with oxygen, they concluded that a positive clinical effect of oxygen therapy is uncertain. The potential detrimental effects of this monotherapy due to prolongation of intrauterine malnutrition have not yet been excluded.

In some recent studies a significant improvement in perinatal mortality rate of growth retarded fetuses has been observed in an oxygen treated group[54]. It is clear, however, that the ideal intrauterine therapy for these fetuses should not be limited to the supply of oxygen but should also include other nutrients, such as glucose and amino acids. This is not yet possible in practice. Therefore, before the results obtained by randomized studies can be analyzed, maternal oxygen therapy must be characterized for test purposes only when considering either the immediate delivery or prolongation of pregnancy in chronic fetal distress.

OTHER VASOACTIVE AGENTS

Maternal smoking is associated with many adverse fetal effects such as reduced birth weight. It appears to decrease intervillous blood flow[55] and increase fetal heart rate[56]. The effects on the fetal hemodynamics as assessed by Doppler methods, however, have been somewhat controversial. No effects on the blood flow volume in the fetal descending aorta and umbilical vein were observed by Jouppila and associates[57] and Pijpers and colleagues[58], whereas Sindberg Eriksen and Marsál[59] found a significant increase in fetal aortic and umbilical artery blood flow. Lindblad and co-workers[60] measured the maternal plasma concentrations of nicotine and carbon monoxide simultaneously with fetal Doppler methods. They noted that an increased blood flow in the fetal aorta and umbilical vein and decreased pulsatility indices in these vessels correlated with maternal nicotine levels but were unaffected by carbon monoxide. Contrary to these results, Morrow and associates[61] observed increased vascular resistance in the umbilical artery after smoking one cigarette. The indices of maternal uterine arteries were unaffected. The conflicting results may be due to the different nicotine concentrations of a 'standard' cigarette. At any rate, the detrimental fetal effects of smoking seem to be reflected in some way by changes in fetal hemodynamics, according to the majority of Doppler studies.

β-Adrenergic agonists, widely used for the treatment of premature labor, cause clear changes in maternal hemodynamics, i.e. an increase in heart rate and cardiac output and a decrease in systemic vascular resistance and blood pressure. No changes in intervillous or umbilical blood flow volume were observed after 1 h of ritodrine infusion[62]. In a more detailed study, Räsänen[63] found a significant increase in fetal pulse rate and blood velocities in the fetal aorta. The indices were unchanged in the fetal aorta and umbilical artery but decreased in the middle cerebral and renal arteries. The parameters for fetal myocardial function were unchanged after a 2.5 h ritodrine infusion. Subcutaneous terbutaline decreased vascular resistance in the umbilical artery and this effect persisted after correction for the increase of fetal heart rate[64]. No index changes were observed in the same study in patients treated with intravenous magnesium. Indices in the uterine and umbilical arteries have also been demonstrated to decrease in association with increasing dose of ritodrine infusion[65]. Sharif and associates stated that the fetal stroke volume was constant during increased heart rate at the time of maternal terbutaline infusion[66]. Nylidrin for treatment of premature labor did not cause any constriction of the fetal ductus arteriosus or tricuspid regurgitation[67]. In addition, antenatal dexamethasone administration for prevention of respiratory distress syndrome in newborns had no constrictive effects on the ductus arteriosus of the fetus between 24 and 31 weeks of pregnancy[68]. These partly conflicting results may be due to the different dosages used in drug administration as well as the methodological problems associated with using the Doppler technique, such as the effect of changing pulse rate on blood velocity waveforms and thus on the index values.

The angiotensin infusion test has been used to predict the development of pregnancy hypertension. Erkkola and Pirhonen[69] observed a significant increase in vascular resistance in the uterine arteries, whereas Jones and Sanchez-Ramos[70] did not find any changes. In both these studies, the umbilical artery indices were unaltered. No effect on the vascular resistance of the uterine and umbilical arteries was registered using vaginal application of prostaglandin E_2 analogs for the induction of labor during late pregnancy[71,72]. In the first trimester, however, this treatment used in legal abortions markedly increased pulsatility index values in the uterine arteries[73].

Single oral doses of alcohol during the last trimester of pregnancy did not cause any significant changes in pulsatility index values of the umbilical artery[74] suggesting that the untoward fetal effects of alcohol may be mediated by some other mechanism than acute alteration in umbilicoplacental vascular resistance.

CONCLUSIONS

The Doppler method enables the simultaneous assessment of the effect of various maternal vasoactive agents on uterine and fetal circulation as well as on fetal cardiac function in a very comprehensive manner. Experiences with this technique over the last 10 years demonstrate that many potentially disturbing clinical factors such as maternal drugs, anesthesia, maternal position etc., which could theoretically have a negative effect, do not hinder the uteroplacental and fetal circulation. If these factors are strong enough, the changes seem to begin with an increased vascular resistance in the uterine arteries without any immediate compromises in fetal hemodynamics. Some regulatory changes do occur, however, in the fetal cerebral and renal arteries and in fetal myocardial contractility with, for example, maternal adrenergic drugs. This obviously signifies that the fetal concentrations of some vasoactive drugs may modify the fetal hemodynamics in a manner which could lead to problems especially in an already compromised fetal circulation. Perhaps the most significant detailed example of the detection of this type of effect is with indomethacin. It is obvious that without the Doppler method the constrictory effects of indomethacin on the fetal ductus arteriosus could not have been found so early and so indisputably. The circulatory safety aspects of many vasoactive agents can now be tested with the Doppler method more reliably than before. This increasing understanding of uterine and fetal hemodynamic regulation in many different clinical conditions has been of great benefit to perinatal practice.

References

1. Lunell, N. O., Nylund, L. and Lewander, R. (1982). Acute effect of an antihypertensive drug, labetalol, on uteroplacental blood flow. *Br. J. Obstet. Gynaecol.*, **89**, 640–4
2. Jouppila, P., Kirkinen, P., Koivula, A. and Ylikorkala, O. (1986). Labetalol does not alter the placental and fetal blood flow or maternal prostanoids in pre-eclampsia. *Br. J. Obstet. Gynaecol.*, **93**, 543–7
3. Lunell, N. O., Lewander, R. and Nylund, L. (1983). Acute effect of dihydralazine on uteroplacental blood flow in hypertension during pregnancy. *Gynecol. Obstet. Invest.*, **16**, 274–8
4. Jouppila, P., Kirkinen, P., Koivula, A. and Ylikorkala, O. (1985). Effects of dihydralazine infusion on the fetoplacental blood flow and maternal prostanoids. *Obstet. Gynecol.*, **65**, 115–8
5. Lunell, N. O., Nylund, L., Lewander, R., Sarby, B. and Wager, J. (1984). Uteroplacental blood flow in pregnancy hypertension after the administration of a beta-adrenoreceptor blocker, pindolol. *Gynecol. Obstet. Invest.*, **18**, 269–74
6. Jouppila, P., Kirkinen, P., Koivula, A. and Ylikorkala, O. (1985). Failure of exogenous prostacyclin to change placental and fetal blood flow in pre-eclampsia. *Am. J. Obstet. Gynecol.*, **151**, 661–5
7. Jouppila, P. and Kirkinen, P. (1986). The effect of labetalol and metoprolol on the placental and fetal hemodynamics. In Jung, H. and Fendel, H. *Doppler Techniques in Obstetrics*, pp. 82–5. (Stuttgart-New York: Georg Thieme Verlag)
8. Montan, S., Liedholm, H., Lingman, G., Marsál, K., Sjöberg, N. O., and Solum, T. (1987). Fetal and uteroplacental haemodynamics during short term atenolol treatment in pregnancy hypertension. *Br. J. Obstet. Gynaecol.*, **94**, 312–17
9. Montan, S., Ingemarsson, I., Marsál, K. and Sjöberg, N. O. (1992). Randomised controlled trial of atenolol and pindolol in human pregnancy: effects on fetal haemodynamics. *Br. Med. J.*, **304**, 946–9
10. Jouppila, P. and Räsänen, J. (1993): Effect of labetalol infusion on uterine and fetal hemodynamics and fetal cardiac function. *Eur. J. Obstet. Gynecol. Reprod. Biol.*, **51**, 111–17
11. Mahmoud, T. Z. K., Bjornsson, S. and Calder, A. A. (1993). Labetalol therapy in pregnancy induced hypertension: the effects on fetoplacental circulation and fetal outcome. *Eur. J. Obstet. Gynecol. Reprod. Biol.*, **50**, 109–13
12. Harper, A. and Murnaghan, G. A. (1991). Maternal and fetal haemodynamics in hypertensive pregnancies during maternal treatment with intravenous hydralazine or labetalol. *Br. J. Obstet. Gynecol.*, **98**, 453–9
13. Pirhonen, J. P., Erkkola, R. U. and Ekblad, U. U. (1990). Uterine and fetal flow velocity waveforms in hypertensive pregnancy: the effect

of a single dose of nifedipine. *Obstet. Gynecol.*, **76**, 37–41
14. Jouppila, R., Jouppila, P., Hollmen, A. and Kuikka, J. (1978). Effect of segmental extradural analgesia on placental blood flow during normal labour. *Br. J. Anaesth.*, **50**, 563–7
15. Patton, D. E., Lee, W., Miller, J. and Jones, M. (1991). Maternal, uteroplacental and fetoplacental hemodynamics and Doppler velocimetric changes during epidural anesthesia in normal labor. *Obstet. Gynecol.*, **77**, 17–19
16. Alahuhta, S., Räsänen, J., Jouppila, P., Jouppila, R. and Hollmen, A. (1993). Epidural sufentanil and bupivacaine for labor analgesia and Doppler velocimetry of the umbilical and uterine arteries. *Anesthesiology*, **78**, 231–6
17. Jouppila, P., Jouppila, R., Hollmen, A. and Koivula, A. (1982). Lumbar epidural analgesia to improve intervillous blood flow during labor in severe preeclampsia. *Obstet. Gynecol.*, **59**, 158–61
18. Ramos-Santos, E., Devoe, L. D., Wakefield, M. L., Sherline, D. M. and Metheny, W. P. (1991). The effects of epidural anesthesia on the Doppler velocimetry of umbilical and uterine arteries in normal and hypertensive patients during active term labor. *Obstet. Gynecol.*, **77**, 22–6
19. Mires, G. J., Dempster, J., Patel, N. B. and Taylor, D. J. (1990). Epidural analgesia and its effect on umbilical artery flow velocity waveform patterns in uncomplicated labour and labour complicated by pregnancy-induced hypertension. *Eur. J. Obstet. Gynecol. Reprod. Biol.*, **36**, 35–41
20. Räsänen, J. and Jouppila, P. (1993). Does a paracervical block with bupivacaine change vascular resistance in uterine and umbilical arteries. *J. Perinat. Med.*, (in press)
21. Kinsella, S. M., Lee, A. and Spencer, A. D. (1991). Maternal peripheral arterial resistance changes following lumbar epidural anesthesia for Cesarean section: validation of Doppler ultrasound pulsatility index. *J. Matern. Fetal Invest.*, **1**, 25–8
22. Baumann, H., Alon, E., Atanassoff, P., Pasch, Th., Huch, A. and Huch, R. (1990). Effect of epidural anesthesia for Cesarean delivery on maternal femoral arterial and venous, uteroplacental, and umbilical blood flow velocities and waveforms. *Obstet. Gynecol.*, **75**, 194–8
23. Turner, G. A., Newnham, J. P., Johnson, C. and Westmore, M. (1991). Effects of extradural anaesthesia on umbilical and uteroplacental arterial flow velocity waveforms. *Br. J. Anaesth.*, **67**, 306–9
24. McLintic, A. J., Danskin, F. H., Reid, J. A. and Thornburn, J. (1991). Effect of adrenaline on extradural anaesthesia, plasma lignocaine concentrations and the fetoplacental unit during elective Caesarean section. *Br. J. Anaesth.*, **67**, 683–9
25. Alahuhta, S., Räsänen, J., Jouppila, R., Jouppila, P., Kangas-Saarela, T. and Hollmen, A. I. (1991). Uteroplacental and fetal haemodynamics during extradural anaesthesia for Caesarean section. *Br. J. Anaesth.*, **66**, 319–23
26. Morrow, R. J., Rolbin, S. H., Ritchie, J. W. K. and Haley, S. (1989). Epidural anaesthesia and blood flow velocity in mother and fetus. *Can. J. Anaesth.*, **36**, 519–22
27. Alahuhta, S., Räsänen, J., Jouppila, R., Jouppila, P. and Hollmen, A. I. (1991). Effects of extradural bupivacaine with adrenaline for Caesarean section on uteroplacental and fetal circulation. *Br. J. Anaesth.*, **67**, 678–82
28. Alahuhta, S., Räsänen, J., Jouppila, R. and Hollmen, A. I. (1993). Uteroplacental and fetal circulation during extradural bupivacaine-adrenaline and bupivacaine for Caesarean section in hypertensive pregnancies with chronic fetal asphyxia. *Br. J. Anaesth.*, **71**, 348–53
29. Robson, S. C., Boys, R. J., Rodeck, C. and Morgan, B. (1992). Maternal and fetal haemodynamic effects of spinal and extradural anaesthesia for elective Caesarean section. *Br. J. Anaesth.*, **68**, 54–9
30. Jouppila, P., Jouppila, R., Barinoff, T. and Koivula, A. (1984). Placental blood flow during Caesarean section performed under subarachnoid blockade. *Br. J. Anaesth.*, **56**, 1379–82
31. Fairlie, F. M., Kirkwood, I., Lang, G. D. and Sheldon, C. D. (1990). Umbilical artery flow velocity waveforms during spinal anesthesia. *Eur. J. Obstet. Gynecol. Reprod. Biol.*, **38**, 3–7
32. Alahuhta, S., Karinen, J., Lumme, R., Jouppila, R., Hollmen, A. I. and Jouppila, P. (1994). Uteroplacental haemodynamics during spinal anaesthesia for Caesarean section with two types of uterine displacement. *Int. J. Obstet. Anaesth.*, in press
33. Räsänen, J., Alahuhta, S., Kangas-Saarela, T., Jouppila, R. and Jouppila, P. (1991). The effects of ephedrine and etilefrine on uterine and fetal blood flow and fetal myocardial function during spinal anaesthesia for Caesarean section. *Int. J. Obstet. Anaesth.*, **1**, 3–8
34. Alahuhta, S., Räsänen, J., Jouppila, P., Jouppila, R. and Hollmen A. I. (1992). Ephedrine and phenylephrine for avoiding maternal hypotension due to spinal anaesthesia for Caesarean section. *Int. J. Obstet. Anaesth.*, **1**, 129–34
35. Wright, P. M. C., Iftikhar, M., Fitzpatrick, K. T., Moore, J. and Thompson, W. (1992). Vasopressor therapy for hypotension during epidural anesthesia for Cesarean section: effects on maternal and fetal flow velocity ratios. *Anesth. Analg.*, **75**, 56–63

36. Gerson, A., Abbasi, S., Johnson, A., Kalchbrenner, M., Ashmead, G. and Bolognese, R. (1990). Safety and efficacy of long-term tocolysis with indomethacin. *Am. J. Perinatol.*, **7**, 71–4
37. Huhta, J. C., Moise, K. J., Sharif, D. S., Wasserstrum, N. and Martin, C. (1987). Detection and quantitation of constriction of the fetal ductus arteriosus by Doppler echocardiography. *Circulation*, **75**, 406–12
38. Moise, K. J., Huhta, J. C., Sharif, D. S., Ou, C. N., Kirshon, B., Wasserstrum, B. and Cano, L. (1988). Indomethacin in the treatment of premature labor. Effects on the fetal ductus arteriosus. *N. Engl. J. Med.*, **319**, 327–31
39. Eronen, M. (1993). The hemodynamic effects of antenatal indomethacin and a beta-sympathomimetic agent on the fetus and newborn: a randomized study. *Pediatr. Res.*, **33**, 615–19
40. Besinger, R. E., Niebyl, J. R., Keyes, W. G. and Johnson, T. R. B. (1991). Randomized comparative trial of indomethacin and ritodrine for the long-term treatment of preterm labor. *Am. J. Obstet. Gynecol.*, **164**, 891–8
41. Mari, G., Moise, K. J., Deter, R. L., Kirshon, B., Huhta, J. C., Carpenter, R. J. and Cotton, D. B. (1989). Doppler assessment of the pulsatility index of the middle cerebral artery during constriction of the fetal ductus arteriosus after indomethacin therapy. *Am. J. Obstet. Gynecol.*, **161**, 1528–31
42. Mari, G., Kirshon, B., Wasserstrum, N., Moise, K. J. and Deter, R. L. (1990). Uterine blood flow velocity waveforms in pregnant women during indomethacin therapy. *Obstet. Gynecol.*, **76**, 33–6
43. Moise, K. J., Mari, G., Kirshon, B., Huhta, J. C., Walsh, S. W. and Cano, L. (1990). The effect of indomethacin on the pulsatility index of the umbilical artery in human fetuses. *Am. J. Obstet. Gynecol.*, **162**, 199–202
44. Mari, G., Moise, K. J., Deter, R. L., Kirshon, B. and Carpenter, R. J. (1990). Doppler assessment of the renal blood flow velocity waveform during indomethacin therapy for preterm labor and polyhydramnios. *Obstet. Gynecol.*, **75**, 199–201
45. Danti, L., Soregaroli, M., Valcamonico, A., Frusca, T., Zucca, S. and Gastalsi, A. (1992). Ductus arteriosus flow velocities in fetuses exposed to low-dose aspirin. *J. Matern. Fetal Invest.*, **2**, 169–71
46. Forouzan, I., Cohen, A. W., Lindenbaum, C. and Samuels, P. (1993). Umbilical artery and ductal blood flow velocities in patients treated with aspirin and prednisone for presence of anticardiolipin antibody. *J. Ultrasound Med.*, **3**, 135–8
47. Carlan, S. J., O'Brien, W. F., O'Leary, T. D. and Mastrogiannis, D. (1992). Randomized comparative trial of indomethacin and sulindac for the treatment of refractory preterm labor. *Obstet. Gynecol.*, **79**, 223–8
48. Arduini, D., Rizzo, G., Romanini, C. and Mancuso, S. (1989). Fetal haemodynamics to acute maternal hyperoxygenation as predictor of fetal distress in intrauterine growth retardation. *Br. Med. J.*, **298**, 1561–2
49. Bilardo, C. M., Snijders, R. M., Campbell, S. and Nicolaides, K. (1991). Doppler study of the fetal circulation during long-term maternal hyperoxygenation for severe early onset intrauterine growth retardation. *Ultrasound Obstet. Gynecol.*, **1**, 250–7
50. Mori, A., Iwashita, M., Nakabayashi, M. and Takeda, Y. (1992). Effect of maternal oxygen inhalation on fetal hemodynamics in chronic asphyxia with IUGR. *J. Matern. Fetal Invest.*, **2**, 93–9
51. de Rochembeau, B., Poix, D. and Mellier, G. (1992). Maternal hyperoxygenation: a fetal blood flow velocity prognosis test in small-for-gestational-age fetuses. *Ultraound Obstet. Gynecol.*, **2**, 279–82
52. Soregaroli, M., Rizzo, G., Danti, L., Arduini, D. and Romanini, C. (1993). Effects of maternal hyperoxygenation on ductus venosus flow velocity waveforms in normal third-trimester fetuses. *Ultrasound Obstet. Gynecol.*, **3**, 115–9
53. Ribbert, L. S. M., van Lingen, R. A. and Visser, G. H. A. (1991). Continuous maternal hyperoxygenation in the treatment of early fetal growth retardation. *Ultrasound Obstet. Gynecol.*, **1**, 331–5
54. Battaglia, C., Artini, P. G., D'Ambrogio, G., Galli, P. A., Segre, A. and Genazzani, A. R. (1992). Maternal hyperoxygenation in the treatment of intrauterine growth retardation. *Am. J. Obstet. Gynecol.*, **167**, 430–5
55. Lehtovirta, P. and Forss, M. (1978). The acute effect of smoking on intervillous blood flow of the placenta. *Br. J. Obstet. Gynaecol.*, **85**, 729–31
56. Quigley, M. E., Sheehan, K. L., Wilkes, M. M. and Yen, S. S. C. (1979). Effects of maternal smoking on circulating catecholamine levels and fetal heart rates. *Am. J. Obstet. Gynecol.*, **133**, 125–9
57. Jouppila, P., Kirkinen, P. and Eik-Nes, S. (1983). Acute effect of maternal smoking on the human fetal blood flow. *Br. J. Obstet. Gynaecol.*, **90**, 7–10
58. Pijpers, L., Wladimiroff, J. W., McGhie, J. S. and Bom, N. (1984). Acute effect of maternal smoking on the maternal and fetal cardiovascular system. *Early Hum. Dev.*, **10**, 95–105
59. Sindberg Eriksen, P. and Marsál, K. (1984). Acute effects of maternal smoking on fetal blood flow. *Acta Obstet. Gynecol. Scand.*, **63**, 385–90
60. Lindblad, A., Marsál, K. and Andersson, K. E. (1988). Effect of nicotine on human fetal blood flow. *Obstet. Gynecol.*, **72**, 371–82

61. Morrow, R. J., Knox Ritchie, J. W. and Bul, S. B. (1988). Maternal cigarette smoking: the effects on umbilical and uterine blood flow velocity. *Am. J. Obstet. Gynecol.*, **159**, 1069–71
62. Jouppila, P., Kirkinen, P., Koivula, A. and Ylikorkala, O. (1985). Ritodrine infusion during late pregnancy: effects on fetal and placental blood flow, prostacyclin, and thromboxane. *Am. J. Obstet. Gynecol.*, **151**, 1028–32
63. Räsänen, J. (1990). The effects of ritodrine infusion on fetal myocardial function and fetal hemodynamics. *Acta Obstet. Gynecol. Scand.*, **69**, 487–92
64. Wright, J. W., Patterson, R. M., Ridgway, L. E. and Berkus, M. D. (1990). Effect of tocolytic agents on fetal umbilical velocimetry. *Am. J. Obstet. Gynecol.*, **163**, 748–50
65. Brar, H. S., Medearis, A. L., DeVore, G. L. and Platt, L. D. (1988). Maternal and fetal blood flow velocity waveforms in patients with preterm labor: effect of tocolytics. *Obstet. Gynecol.*, **72**, 209–14
66. Sharif, D. S., Huhta, J. C., Moise, K. J., Morrow, R. W. and Yoon, G. Y. (1990). Changes in fetal hemodynamics with terbutaline treatment and premature labor. *J. Clin. Ultrasound*, **18**, 85–9
67. Eronen, M. (1993). The hemodynamic effects of antenatal indomethacin and beta-sympathomimetic agent on the fetus and the newborn: a randomized study. *Pediatr. Res.*, **33**, 615–19
68. Eronen, M., Kari, A., Pesonen, E. and Hallman, M. (1993). The effect of antenatal dexamethasone administration on the fetal and neonatal ductus arteriosus. A randomized double-blind study. *Am. J. Dis. Child.*, **147**, 187–92
69. Erkkola, R. U. and Pirhonen, J. P. (1990). Flow velocity waveforms in uterine and umbilical arteries during the angiotension II sensitivity test. *Am. J. Obstet. Gynecol.*, **162**, 1193–7
70. Jones, D. C. and Sanchez-Ramos, L. (1990). Effect of angiotensin II infusion during normal pregnancy on flow velocity waveforms in the uteroplacental and umbilical circulations. *Obstet. Gynecol.*, **76**, 1093–6
71. Fairlie, F. M., Lang, G. D., Greer, I. A. and McLaren, M. (1990). Umbilical artery Doppler flow velocity waveforms and maternal prostaglandin E2 and F2 alfa metabolite concentrations during cervical ripening with prostaglandin E2. *Eur. J. Obstet. Gynecol. Reprod. Biol.*, **37**, 7–13
72. Rayburn, W. F., Anderson, J. C., Smith, C. V. and Appel, L. L. (1991). Uterine and fetal Doppler flow changes after intravaginal prostaglandin E2 therapy for cervical ripening. *Am. J. Obstet. Gynecol.*, **165**, 125–65
73. Jouppila, P. and Suomalainen-König, S. (1994). Effect of the prostaglandin E1 analogue gemeprost on the blood flow velocity waveforms of uterine arteries during the first trimester of pregnancy. *Br. J. Obstet. Gynaecol.*, in press
74. Erskine, R. L. A. and Ritchie, J. W. K. (1986). The effect of maternal consumption of alcohol on human umbilical artery blood flow. *Am. J. Obstet. Gynecol.*, **154**, 318–21

Assessment of the hypoxic fetus with color Doppler and automated heart-rate analysis

31

N. Montenegro, J. Bernardes and L. Pereira-Leite

INTRODUCTION

Hypoxia is defined as a decreased concentration of oxygen in the tissues, hypoxemia as a low oxygen content of the blood, acidosis as a high tissue pH, acidemia as an elevated blood pH and asphyxia as an insufficiency or absence of respiratory gas exchange leading to different degrees of severity from slight hypoxia to severe acidosis[1].

Perinatal hypoxia, a rather common situation, is a matter of great clinical interest as it is as major cause of morbidity and mortality. However, hypoxemia is only related to poor outcome when associated signs of multi-organ dysfunction are present. This situation has now been clearly defined in the newborn by the American College of Obstetricians and Gynecologists as the simultaneous occurrence of Apgar score < 3, umbilical artery blood pH < 7.00 and signs of multi-organ dysfunction (e.g. CNS, renal). This corresponds to fetal distress, defined as a persistent fetal asphyxia that, if not corrected or circumvented, will result in permanent neurological damage or death[2].

Fetal hypoxia, and conditions leading to it, give rise to a wide range of biochemical, hemodynamic and neurological manifestations[3,4].

The evaluation of biochemical manifestations of fetal hypoxia is at present, limited in clinical practice, because it requires invasive procedures. Moreover, it is generally confined to the evaluation of hypoxia at the blood level (hypoxemia), without the evaluation of associated organ dysfunction[2].

Until now, assessment of the amount of amniotic fluid, considered an indirect evaluation of renal perfusion, was the only way of assessing organ perfusion in clinical practice[5]. It is now possible, with duplex color Doppler, to estimate blood flow non-invasively in human maternal and fetal–placental blood vessels, allowing the clinician to investigate the changes associated with hypoxia that have been described for years in animal studies[6].

Fetal neurological hypoxia-related manifestations have been assessed by the study of fetal movements, changes in tone and heart rate[5]. Changes in fetal heart rate (FHR) have been the most widely researched manifestations and cardiotocography has been the standard method for their detection. It has been demonstrated, however, that visual analysis of cardiotocograms suffers from marked intra- and inter-observer variation which compromises its clinical usefulness and may make its use harmful for the mother and fetus. Therefore, as the abandonment of cardiotocography is unlikely, there is a widespread view that computer analysis of cardiotocograms, which are able to eliminate observer variation in the judgement of tracings, is of important clinical value[7–13].

The aim of this chapter is to provide an overview of the present state of assessment of fetal hypoxia with automated analysis of cardiotocograms and Doppler ultrasound.

HEMODYNAMIC AND FETAL HEART-RATE CHANGES ASSOCIATED WITH HYPOXIA

Hemodynamic changes

Some conditions associated with a high risk of fetal hypoxia lead to maternofetal hemodynamic manifestations, even before the occurrence of fetal hypoxia. For example, it has been widely demonstrated that failure of trophoblastic invasion of spiral arteries in early pregnancy gives rise to an increase in vascular resistance of the uterine artery, that placental vascular pathology results in increased placental vascular resistance, and that both situations are frequently associated with intrauterine growth retardation (IUGR) and oligohydramnios[14]. Whether uterine hypertonus, umbilical cord entanglements, decreased amniotic fluid or fetal anemia, without concomitant fetal hypoxia, can result in changes in fetal blood flow remain in question.

Regarding fetal hypoxia, it has been demonstrated in the lamb that oxygen limitation gives rise to a series of cardiovascular and metabolic adjustments to preserve the most vital organs such as the brain, heart and adrenal glands[15,16]. Initially, selective vasoconstriction takes place in certain organs and vasodilatation occurs in others, with increased blood flow in vital organs and decreased perfusion of the body (brain-sparing effect). Cardiac output remains stable, decreasing with more severe degrees of hypoxia[17]. This reduction can be explained by increased afterload that directly affects stroke volume, namely of the right ventricle[18]. In a second phase overall oxygen consumption de-

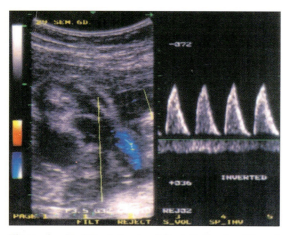

Figure 1 *Umbilical absent end-diastolic flow in a 29-week pregnancy*

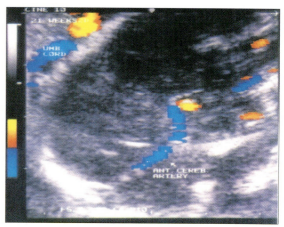

Figure 3 *Color Doppler cerebral blood flow (transvaginal) in a 21-week pregnancy*

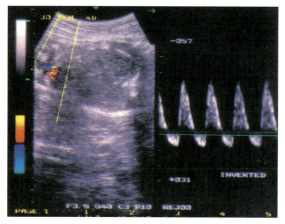

Figure 2 *Reverse end-diastolic flow in a 30-week pregnancy*

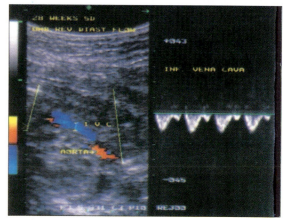

Figure 4 *Inferior vena cava blood flow in a case of reverse end-diastolic flow in umbilical arteries, at 28 weeks' pregnancy*

clines to values as low as 50% of those of controls[19]. These events probably express fetal adaptation to hypoxia. However, if hypoxia persists, intense vasoconstriction of all vascular beds occurs and oxygen delivery to the brain and heart can no longer be maintained. This represents the decompensation phase that precedes bradycardia, hypotension and death[20].

In our experience[6] regarding monitoring of human fetuses with Doppler waveform analysis, we observed a systematic decrease in middle-artery resistance indices before the disappearance of end-diastolic blood flow ($n = 58$) in the descending aorta (Figures 1–3). A later observed sign was pulsatile umbilical venous blood flow and reverse diastolic flow in the inferior vena cava, probably as a reflex of right heart failure (Figure 4)[21]. Finally, the transmitral maximum velocity became greater than in the tricuspid valve, as the output of the left ventricle exceeded that of the right side[22].

Changes in fetal heart rate

FHR depends on intrinsic cardiac activity and on the modulation exerted on it by different effectors, the most important of which is, particularly in the second half of pregnancy, the autonomic nervous system. This is activated by inputs from the central nervous system and from the peripheral chemo- and baroreceptors. Therefore, FHR changes reflect fetal neurocardiac activity[3].

The parasympathetic nervous system exerts a tonic inhibitory action on the sinoatrial and atrioventricular nodes. Its activation leads to a decrease of FHR and an increase in its variability, whereas activation of the sympathetic nervous system results in an increase of FHR.

In the healthy fetus, under stable respiratory and hemodynamic conditions when there are no fetal movements, the FHR exhibits a stable pattern which corresponds to the cardiac intrinsic activity plus the tonic parasympathetic action and is generally designated as basal FHR. Accelerations appear superimposed on this basal pattern, generally associated with fetal movements.

After 34–36 weeks, they arise as a result of fetal behavioral states or as a reflex to different stimuli[3,23–27].

Acute short episodes of hypoxia result in reflex FHR changes such as decelerations and increased variability or periodic accelerations. Prolonged decelerations or bradycardia, with a decrease of FHR variability, are seen with longer acute hypoxic episodes. Long-lasting fetal hypoxia gives rise, at first, to the disappearance of accelerations and a decrease in FHR variability, and, later on, to an increase in FHR without decelerations, to a sinusoidal pattern or to terminal bradycardia and death[5,23,28–33].

METHODS TO ASSESS FETAL BLOOD FLOW AND HEART RATE

Doppler ultrasound

Doppler ultrasound was introduced in obstetrics in the late 1970s. At first, efforts were directed to volumetric blood-flow estimation in fetal vessels, such as the umbilical vein and the descending aorta. However, a wide variation in these calculations was observed, due to methodological problems and to basic principles of the Doppler effect that hamper the rigorous measurement of either the vessel diameter or the insonation angle, leading to the abandonment of volumetric blood-flow assessment. Thus, different Doppler spectral analyses derived ratios of systolic and diastolic frequencies, including the resistance indices of Pourcelot (RI) and of Stuart and Drumm (S/D) and the pulsatility index of Gosling and King (PI). More recently, color Doppler became available, enhancing the possibilities to study blood flow, even in small vessels, with more reproducibility and reducing the time spent on the investigation when compared to conventional duplex imaging[34–38].

Several authors demonstrated that Doppler indices are capable of reflecting downstream vascular impedance to blood flow[39]. Umbilical resistance indices express placental vascular impedance, namely at the level of tertiary stem villi arteries, which falls, in normal pregnancy, as gestational age advances[40]. Resistance indices of

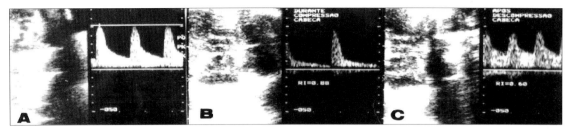

Figure 5 Middle cerebral artery blood flow before (A), during (B), and after (C) compression of fetal head

cerebral arteries also show a continuous drop with advancing normal gestation as a reflex of cerebral angiogenesis, and vasoactive and neuronal maturation, although higher resistance indices are found in the same period than in umbilical arteries[41,42]. In our experience, a slight tendency for an inverse cerebroplacental ratio (CPR) was found after 40 weeks in normal pregnancies. Theoretically, CPRs are expected to express the centralization of blood flow when hypoxia develops[6]. This concept has been validated in human pregnancies in intrauterine growth retardation[43,44].

Umbilical arteries, ascending and descending aorta, and cerebral vessels such as the internal carotid, anterior and middle cerebral arteries, have been widely studied. Reference values for indices in such vessels are widely described in the literature, although different techniques and methodologies have been used by investigators[44,45].

The reproducibility of Doppler waveform analysis has been questioned[46]. Some technical and methodological aspects must be taken into account when performing the examinations to improve the reproducibility of measurements. For example, one should be aware that RIs for cerebral arteries are quite different with and without head compression (Figure 5) and that RIs for umbilical arteries are different in the fetal and placental portions of the umbilical cord[6]. Color Doppler yields additional improvement of reproducibility by permitting correct identification of vessels and the choice of the best insonation angles[37]. In spite of some controversy concerning the quantitative analysis of arterial Doppler waveforms, the resistance index of Pourcelot (RI) seems to be preferable[47–49].

Umbilical resistance indices can accurately predict perinatal compromise, using as 'gold standards' late and severe variable decelerations, and pH of the fetal scalp and umbilical artery[49,50]. However, Copel and colleagues[51] demonstrated, in the lamb, that acute hypoxia cannot be detected by the umbilical S/D ratio. Concerning the fetal cerebrovascular circulation, some studies confirm the potential of the resistance index of the middle cerebral artery to recognize fetal compromise, including hypoxemia at delivery[52,53].

Automated analysis of cardiotocograms

A number of systems for the automated analysis of cardiotocograms (CTGs) have recently become available for clinical practice. They vary considerably, however, and have been differently validated (Tables 1 and 2). The systems are all based on low-cost user-friendly personal computers and can be divided into two main groups: those essentially dedicated to the segmentation of tracings in the FHR baseline, accelerations and decelerations, which leave the clinician the

Table 1 Facilities for ante- and intrapartum use and commercial availability of systems based on personal computers for the automated analysis of cardiotocograms

	Ante-partum	Intra-partum	Commercially available
8000 (68)	+	−	+
2CTG (55)	+	?	+
KOMPOR (56)	+	?	+
Searle (85)	+	−	−
Porto (87)	+	+	−
Toitu (86)	+	+	+
Natali (39)	−	+	+
Hernandez (90)	+	+	−
Turkish (91)	+	−	−

Table 2 Clinical value of visual and automated fetal heart-rate analysis according to the available systems based on personal computers. For detailed explanations, see text

	Internal validity	External validity	Efficacy	Efficiency
Visual analysis[11-13]	−	−	−	−
8000[67-83]	±	±	±	?
2CTG[84]	±	?	?	?
KOMPOR[56]	?	?	?	?
Searle[85]	±	?	?	?
Porto[54]	+	±	?	?
Toitu[86-88]	?	±	?	?
Natali[89]	?	±	?	?
Hernandez[90]	?	±	?	?
Turkish[91]	?	±	?	?

−, Poor or not demonstrated; +, demonstrated; ±, limited evaluation; ?, not evaluated

decision to classify and interpret tracings, and those dedicated to the classification and interpretation of cardiotocograms, which leave the clinician eventually without the information on FHR segmentation. The 2CTG, KOMPOR, Searle, Porto and Turkish systems belong to the former group, the Toitu, Natali and Hernandez systems to the latter; system 8000 provides both segmentation and classification of tracings. Most systems incorporate, at least partially, the FIGO (International Federation of Obstetricians and Gynecologists) criteria for FHR monitoring. However, in some systems new criteria or even concepts were introduced (e.g. 'FHR variation' in system 8000, 'fetal distress score' in the Toitu system, and 'discriminance function' in the Natali system). Some systems can only be used in the ante- or intrapartum period, others in both. Four of them are commercially available[54-56].

Figure 6 shows different FHR patterns as analyzed by the Porto system developed at the Porto University[54,57,58]. In Table 2, the results of the studies on the assessment of the clinical value of the above-mentioned systems for the automated analysis of cardiotocograms are presented, according to an approach described by Grant[59]. Internal validity is defined as the reliability of the system's measurements of the variables they analyze. The standard to evaluate internal validity has been the agreement between the system's and the expert's analysis of tracings. In Table 2, these studies were considered limited if the comparison between experts and systems was not carried out blindly and if the statistical analysis was not performed as described by Bland and Altman for continuous variables and by Grant for categorical variables[60,61]. External validity is defined as the faculty to identify or predict clinical situations. It is expressed as sensitivity, specificity and predictive values. Efficacy is the ability of the test (plus appropriate management) to prevent the clinical situations they are supposed to prevent. Efficiency is the capability of being more efficacious than alternative methods.

ASSESSMENT OF FETAL HYPOXIA WITH COLOR DOPPLER AND AUTOMATED ANALYSIS OF CARDIOTOCOGRAMS

Screening and diagnosis

Analysis of the blood flow of the umbilical artery with continuous Doppler is simple and has high sensitivity and specificity in the detection of IUGR. Several studies suggest its superiority when compared to methods of surveillance in the screening of the fetus at risk of hypoxia, both in the ante- and intrapartum periods. However, its final efficacy and efficiency as a screening or diagnostic tool for conditions leading to fetal hypoxia, or for fetal hypoxia itself, are still to be determined[6].

Automated analysis of CTGs is easy to apply in clinical practice and some studies have suggested a high sensitivity and specificity in the detection of the moderately to severely hypoxic

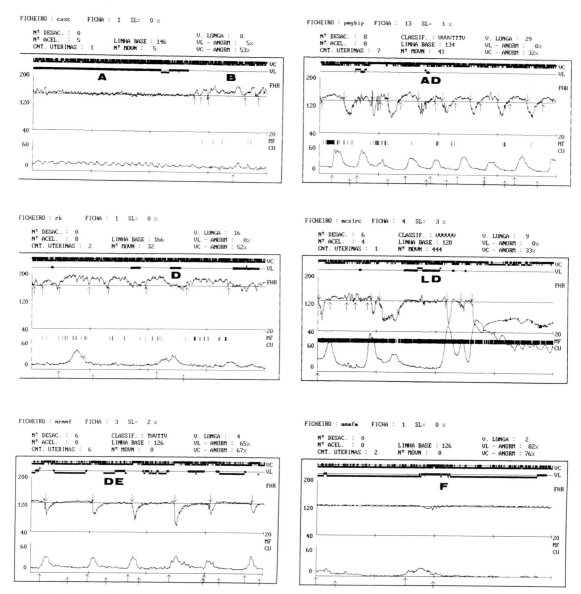

Figure 6 *Patterns of fetal heart rate (FHR) as analyzed by the Porto system: A, behavioral state 1F; B, behavioral state 2F; D, behavioral state 4F; DE, decelerative pattern; AD, accelerative/decelerative pattern; LD, largely decelerative pattern (second stage of labor); F, flat pattern (compare with pattern A in long-term variability). SL, signal loss; N^0 DESAC, decelerations (n); N^0 ACEL, accelerations (n); CNT. UTERINAS, uterine contractions (n); LINHA BASE, basal FHR; N^0 MOVN, fetal movements (n); V. LONGA, modal value of FHR long-term variability; VL-ANORM, abnormal long-term variability (%); VC-ANORM; abnormal short-term variability (%); MF, fetal movements; CU, uterine contractions. Top of CTG registration: VC and VL bars are shifted up or downward when they are increased or reduced, respectively. Basal FHR is indicated as a horizontal straight line at the level of the corresponding value. Beginning of accelerations and decelerations are indicated with vertical ascending and descending arrows, respectively. Fetal movements are indicated by small vertical bars*

or anemic fetus in the ante- and intrapartum periods. Although the results obtained so far are promising there are no studies yet definitely supporting the use of automated analysis of CTGs, either as a screening or as a diagnostic method in the detection of the hypoxic fetus[54].

It is interesting to note that Arduini and associates[62] concluded that the clinical performance of automated analysis of cardiotocograms and Doppler ultrasound as labor admission tests were probably better when they were used together rather than separately.

Monitoring

Antepartum

Visser and co-workers[63–66], engaged in several cross-sectional and longitudinal studies, described sequential changes in Doppler waveforms in fetal heart rate as analyzed by system 8000 and in movement patterns in fetuses with IUGR exhibiting progressive antepartum hypoxia. Although considerable inter-fetal differences in parameters measured were observed, the first changes detected were abnormal umbilical artery waveforms followed by behavioral changes. Heart-rate decelerations and reduced heart-rate variation emerged later and were followed first by reduced body movements and later by reduced breathing movements. Finally, terminal fetal heart-rate patterns and absence of movements could be observed. They concluded that in cases of IUGR, progressive deterioration in fetuses could be monitored by Doppler blood flow assessment and automated analysis of CTGs, and that such a monitoring approach seems to contribute to establishing the ideal time to intervene, despite the fact that the optimal timing of delivery remains to be determined.

Figure 7 summarizes our preliminary experience with antepartum monitoring of the progressive deterioration of very compromised premature fetuses, with Doppler waveform analysis and automated analysis of CTGs based on the Porto system, which closely follows the FIGO guidelines for fetal monitoring. It displays data from seven premature compromised fetuses, which were admitted to our department with absent or reversed end-diastolic umbilical blood flow.

All three fetuses which had suspicious tracings in the 24 h which preceded delivery were born alive without signs of multi-organ dysfunction associated with asphyxia. Moreover, tracings remained suspicious for days to several weeks (5 weeks in one case). This suggests that the finding of a suspicious tracing does not mandate immediate delivery in the extremely premature fetus with absent or reversed end-diastolic umbilical blood flow. Pathological tracings never recovered to a normal pattern (although they were allowed little time to do so). They were always preceded by suspicious tracings and were generally associated with perinatal death or neonatal multi-organ dysfunction associated with asphyxia. In one case, however, a pathological tracing was present for 3 days without the appearance of this outcome. These aspects suggest that it is prudent to intervene before a pathological tracing appears and that it is mandatory to identify pathological tracings as soon as possible, as they represent a perinatal emergency, in such settings as those of fetuses included in this study.

Absent and reversed umbilical artery end-diastolic blood flow on their own were not directly related to perinatal death or neonatal signs of multi-organ dysfunction associated with asphyxia. Furthermore, they were observed in some cases for weeks. These preliminary findings suggest that although absent or reversed umbilical artery end-diastolic blood flow is associated with high perinatal morbidity and mortality it does not mandate for immediate termination of pregnancy with an extremely premature fetus, especially if conditions are not ideal for neonatal survival.

In summary, our results suggest that assessment of blood flow in the umbilical artery associated with automated analysis of cardiotocograms as provided by the Porto system, is able to monitor progressive fetal deterioration. It seems prudent to deliver a fetus as soon as a suspicious tracing appears in the setting of an absent or reversed umbilical artery end-diastolic blood flow. However, when ideal conditions for neonatal survival do not exist, a more expectant attitude can be more appropriate. More extensive studies are needed.

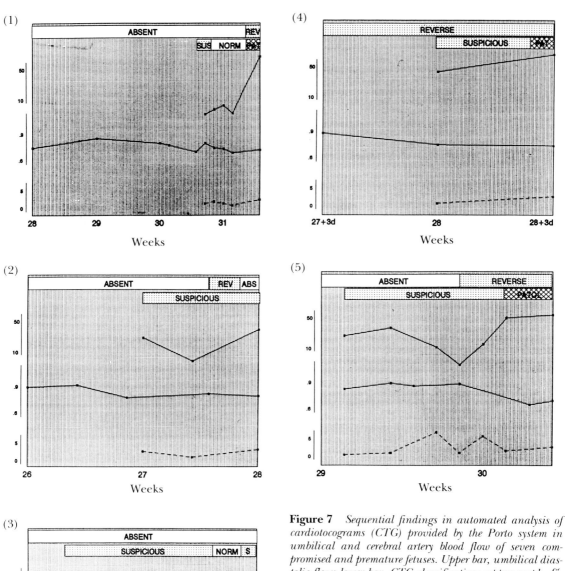

Figure 7 *Sequential findings in automated analysis of cardiotocograms (CTG) provided by the Porto system in umbilical and cerebral artery blood flow of seven compromised and premature fetuses. Upper bar, umbilical diastolic flow; lower bar, CTG classification; upper graph, % tracing with abnormal long-term variability; middle graph, resistance index of middle cerebral artery; lower graph, number of decelerations.*

Outcomes. Case 1: birth weight (BW) 920 g, Cesarean section, Apgar 0/7/9, umbilical artery pH 7.19, intensive care unit (ICU) stay, neurological sequelae. Case 2: BW 800 g, Cesarean section, alive at 28 days. Case 3: BW 1070 g, Cesarean section, Apgar 4/8, ICU stay, alive at 28 days. Case 4: BW 500 g, Cesarean section, Apgar 6/7, umbilical artery pH 7.06, death at 24 h. Case 5: BW 990 g, Cesarean section, Apgar 5/5, ICU stay, alive at 28 days. Case 6: BW 830 g, Cesarean section, Apgar 3/6/7, ICU stay, alive at 28 days. Case 7: BW 700 g, Cesarean section, Apgar 6/9, ICU stay, iatrogenic neonatal death at 72 h

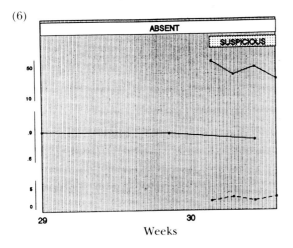

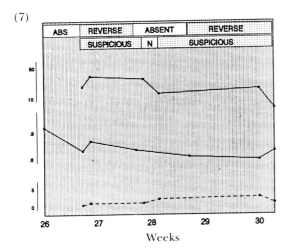

Intrapartum

Preliminary results regarding the application of the Porto system to intrapartum FHR monitoring suggest that it is able to identify normal, moderate and severe fetal compromise. If this is confirmed, this means that the system will indeed be able to monitor the fetus and provide valuable information concerning intervention[54].

CONCLUSIONS

Perinatal hypoxia, when associated with multiorgan dysfunction, remains an important cause of perinatal morbidity and mortality. Doppler materno–fetal blood-flow assessment and automated analysis of cardiotocograms are promising tools to join the clinical evaluation of the potentially hypoxic or hypoxemic fetus. They are expected to improve screening and diagnosis of these conditions. Moreover, they appear useful in monitoring of the hypoxic fetus in order to determine the ideal time to deliver. More studies are, however, needed before their routine use in clinical practice can be advocated. Clinical decisions should not be based solely on maternofetal Doppler blood-flow assessment or automated analysis of cardiotocograms, without the consideration of the clinical context.

ACKNOWLEDGEMENTS

We are indebted to Dr Rosalind Snijders, PhD, for her critical comments. Dr Diogo Ayres de Campos, M.D., is acknowledged for his kind collaboration in figure organization.

References

1. Arias, F. (1992). Birth asphyxia. In Arias, F. (ed.) *Practical Guide to High-Risk Pregnancy and Delivery*, pp. 413–29. (St Louis: Mosby Year Book)
2. American College of Obstetricians and Gynecologists (1993). Technical Bulletin Number 163 – January 1992. Fetal and neonatal neurologic injury. *Int. J. Gynaecol. Obstet.*, **41**, 97–101
3. Arnold-Aldea, S. A. and Parer, J. T. (1990). Fetal cardiovascular physiology. In *Assessment and Care of the Fetus*, p. 29–42. (New York: Prentice-Hall International)
4. Kjellmer, I. (1988). Prenatal and intrapartum asphyxia. In Levene, M., Bennett, M. J. and Punt, J. (eds.) *Fetal and Neonatal Neurology and Neurosurgery*, pp. 357–69 (Edinburgh: Churchill Livingstone)
5. Vintzileos, A. M. (1989). The biophysical profile. Predictor of fetal condition at birth. *Obstet. Gynecol. Rep.*, **1**, 140–51

6. Montenegro, N. (1993). *Anatomo-physiopathology of the Feto-placental Circulation. Clinical Implications of Doppler Flowmetry*, PhD thesis Faculdade de Medicina do Porto
7. Donker, D. K. (1991). *Interobserver Variation in the Assessment of Fetal Heart Rate Recordings*, Thesis. Free University, Amsterdam
8. Borgotta, L., Shrout, P. E. and Divon, M. Y. (1988). Reliability and reproducibility of non-stress test readings. *Am. J. Obstet. Gynecol.*, **159**, 554–8
9. Hage, M. L. (1985). Interpretation of nonstress tests. *Am. J. Obstet. Gynecol.*, **153**, 490–5
10. Lotgering, F. K., Wallenburg, H. C. S. and Schouten, H. J. A. (1982). Interobserver and intraobserver variation in the assessment of antepartum cardiotocograms. *Am. J. Obstet. Gynecol.*, **144**, 701
11. Grant, A. (1989). Monitoring the fetus during labour. In Chalmers, I., Enkin, M. and Keirse, M. J. N. C. (eds.) *Effective Care in Pregnancy and Childbirth*, pp. 846–82. (Oxford: Oxford University Press)
12. Mohide. P. and Keirse, M. J. N. C. (1989). Biophysical assessment of fetal well-being. In Chalmers, I., Enkin, M. and Keirse, M. J. N. C. (eds.) *Effective Care in Pregnancy and Childbirth*, pp. 477–92. (Oxford University Press)
13. Spencer, J. A. D. (1993). Clinical overview of cardiotocography. *Br. J. Obstet. Gynaecol.*, **100** (Suppl. 9), 4–7
14. Greiss, F. C. (1989). Uterine blood flow and fetal growth. In Spencer, J. A. D. (ed.) *Fetal Monitoring*, pp. 9–14. (Southampton: Castle House Publications)
15. Cohn, H. E., Sacks, E. J., Heyman, M. A. and Rudolph, A. M. (1974). Cardiovascular responses to hypoxemia and acidemia in fetal lambs. *Am. J. Obstet. Gynecol.*, **135**, 637–46
16. Peters, L. L. H., Sheldon, R. E., Jones, M. D., Makousk, E. L. and Meschia, G. (1979). Blood flow to fetal organs as a function of arterial oxygen content. *Am. J. Obstet. Gynecol.*, **135**, 637–46
17. Cohn, H. E., Piasecki, G. J. and Jackson, B. T. (1980). The effect of fetal heart rate on cardiovascular function during hypoxemia. *Am. J. Obstet. Gynecol.*, **138**, 1190
18. Thornburg K. L., Morton, M. J., Pinson, C. W., Reller, M. D., Giraud, G. D. and Reid, D. L. (1990). Fetal cardiac output and its distribution. In Dawes, G. S., Borruto, F. and Zacutti, A., (eds.) *Fetal Autonomy and Adaptation*, pp. 15–28 (Chichester: John Wiley & Sons)
19. Parer, J. T. (1980). The effect of acute maternal hypoxia on fetal oxygenation and the umbilical circulation in the sheep. *Eur. J. Obstet. Gynecol. Reprod. Biol.*, **10**, 125–36
20. Parer, J. T. and Livingstone, E. G. (1990). What is fetal distress? *Am. J. Obstet. Gynecol.*, **162**, 1421–7
21. Nakai, Y., Miyazaki, Y. and Matsuoka, Y. (1993). Pulsatile umbilical venous flow and its clinical significance. *Br. J. Obstet. Gynaecol.*, **99**, 977–80
22. Fernandez-Pineda, L., Lopez-Zea, M., Rico, F., Cazzaniga, M., Maitre Azcarate, M. J. and Quero Jimenez, M. (1993). Changes in fetal blood flow distribution in small-for-gestational-age fetuses. *J. Matern. Fetal Invest.*, **3**, 155–8
23. Court, D. J. and Parer, J. T. (1984). Experimental studies of fetal asphyxia and fetal heart rate interpretation. In Nathanielsz, P. W. and Parer, J. T. (eds.) *Research in Perinatal Medicine*, pp. 113–69. (New York: Perinatology Press)
24. Nijhuis, J. G. (1989). Fetal behavioural states. In Spencer, J. A. D. (ed.) *Fetal Monitoring*, pp. 24–7. (Southampton: Castle House Publications)
25. Griffin, R. L., Caron, F. J. M. and Van Geijn, H. P. (1985). Behavioral states in the human fetus during labor. *Am. J. Obstet. Gynecol.*, **152**, 828–33
26. Van Woerden, E. E. (1989). *Fetal Heart Rate and Movements. Their Relationship within Behavioural States 1F and 2F*. Thesis, Free University, Amsterdam (Katwijk, The Netherlands: 'All In' B.V.)
27. Van Woerden, E. E., van Geijn, H. P., Mantel, R. and Swartjies, J. M. (1991). Duration, amplitude and shape of accelerations in relation to fetal body movements in behavioural state 2F. *J. Perinat. Med.*, **19**, 73–80
28. Johnson, P. (1989). Fetal distress or physiological response and adaptation? In Spencer, J. A. D. (ed.) *Fetal Monitoring*, pp. 28–33. (Southampton: Castle House Publications)
29. Melchior, J. and Bernard, N. (1989). Second stage fetal heart rate patterns. In Spencer, J. A. D. (ed.) *Fetal Monitoring*, pp. 155–8. (Southampton: Castle House Publications)
30. Nijhuis, J. G., Kruyt, N. and van Wijck J. A. M. (1988). Fetal brain death. Two case reports. *Br. J. Obstet. Gynaecol.*, **95**, 197–8
31. Ribbert, L. S. M., Snijders, R. J. M., Nicolaides, K. H. and Visser, G. H. A. (1990). Relationship of biophysical profile and blood gas values at cordocentesis in severely growth-retarded fetuses. *Am. J. Obstet. Gynecol.*, **163**, 569–71
32. Van Geijn, H. P., Copray, F. J. A., Donkers, D. K. and Bos, M. H. (1991). Diagnosis and management of intrapartum fetal distress. *Eur. J. Obstet. Gynecol. Reprod. Biol.*, **42**, S63–72
33. Visser, G. H. A., Stigter, R. H. and Bruinse, H. W. (1991). Management of the growth-retarded fetus. *Eur. J. Obstet. Gynecol. Reprod. Biol.*, **42**, S71–4
34. Fitzgerald, D. E. and Drumm, J. E. (1977). Quantitative measurement of fetal blood flow

using ultrasound: a new method. *Br. Med. J.*, **2**, 1450–1
35. Gill, R. W. (1978). Quantitative blood flow measurements in deep-lying vessels using pulsed-Doppler with the Octoson. In White, D. and Lyons, E. A. (eds.) *Ultrasound in Medicine*, p. 341–8. (New York: Plenum Press)
36. Eik-Nes, S. H., Brubakk, A. O. and Ulstein, M. (1980). Measurement of human fetal blood flow. *Br. Med. J.*, **1**, 283–4
37. Evans, D. H., McDicken, W. N., Skidmore, R. and Woodcock, J. P. (1989). Doppler systems: a general overview. In *Doppler Ultrasound. Physics, Instrumentation and Clinical Applications*. (Chichester: John Wiley & Sons)
38. Gill, R. W. (1985). Measurement of blood flow by ultrasound: accuracy and sources of error. *Ultrasound Med. Biol.*, **4**, 625–41
39. Maulik, D. (1993). Hemodynamic interpretation of the arterial Doppler waveform. *Ultrasound Obstet. Gynecol.*, **3**, 219–27
40. Giles, W. B., Trudinger, J. B. and Baird, P. J. (1985). Fetal umbilical artery velocity waveforms and placental resistance: a pathological correlation. *Br. J. Obstet. Gynaecol.* **92**, 31–8
41. Arbeille, Ph., Montenegro, N., Tranquart, F., Berson, M., Ronan, A. and Pourcelot, L. (1990). Assessment of the main cerebrovascular areas by ultrasound color-coded Doppler. *Echocardiography*, **7**, 629–34
42. Cowan, W. M., Fawcet, J. W., O'Leary, D. D. M. and Stanfield, B. B. (1984). Regressive events in neurogenesis. *Science*, **225**, 1258–65
43. Arbeille, Ph., Roncin, A., Berson, M., Patat, F. and Pourcelot, L. (1987). Exploration of the fetal cerebral blood flow by duplex Doppler-linear array system in normal and pathological pregnancies. *Ultrasound Med. Biol.*, **6**, 329–37
44. Gronenberg, I. A. L., Hop, W. C. J., Bogers, J. W., Santema, J. G. and Wladimiroff, J. W. (1993). The predictive value of Doppler flow velocity waveforms in the development of abnormal fetal heart traces in intrauterine growth retardation: a longitudinal study. *Early Hum. Dev.*, **32**, 151–9
45. Wladimiroff, J. W., Huisman, T. W. A. and Stewart, P. A. (1992). Intracerebral, aortic and umbilical artery flow velocity waveforms in the late first trimester fetus. *Am. J. Obstet. Gynecol.*, **166**, 46–51
46. Scherjon, S. A., Kok, J. H., Oosting, H. and Zondervan, H. A. (1993). Intra-observer and inter-observer reliability of the pulsality index calculated from pulsed Doppler flow velocity waveforms in three fetal vessels. *Br. J. Obstet. Gynecol.*, **100**, 134–8
47. Hoskins, P. R., Haddad, N. G., Johnstone, F. D., Chambers, S. E. and McDicken, W. N. (1989). The choice of the index for umbilical artery Doppler waveforms. *Ultrasound Med. Biol.*, **15**, 107–11
48. Thompson, R. S., Trudinger, B. J. and Cook, C. M. (1988). Doppler ultrasound waveform indices: A/B ratio, pulsality index and Pourcelot ratio. *Br. J. Obstet. Gynaecol.*, **95**, 581–8
49. Maulik, D., Yaralagadda, P., Youngblood, J. P. and Ciston, P. (1991). Comparative efficacy of umbilical arterial Doppler indices for predicting adverse perinatal outcome. *Am. J. Obstet. Gynecol.*, **164**, 1434–40
50. Maulik, D., Yarlagadda, P., Youngblood, J. P. and Ciston, P. (1990). The diagnostic efficacy of the umbilical arterial systolic/diastolic ratio as a screening tool: a prospective blinded study. *Am. J. Obstet. Gynecol.*, **162**, 1518–25
51. Copel, J. A., Woudstra, B. R., Schlafer, D., Hobbins, J. C. and Nathanielz, P. W. (1991). Hypoxia cannot be detected by the umbilical S/D ratio in fetal lambs. *J. Matern. Fetal Invest.*, **1**, 219–21
52. Satoh, S., Koyanagi, T., Fukuhara, M., Hara, K. and Nakano, H. (1989). Changes in vascular resistance in the umbilical and middle cerebral arteries in the human intrauterine growth-retarded fetus, measured with pulse Doppler ultrasound. *Early Hum. Dev.*, **20**, 213–20
53. Chandran, R., Serra-Serra, V., Sellers, S. M. and Redman, C. W. G. (1993). Fetal cerebral Doppler in the recognition of fetal compromise. *Br. J. Obstet. Gynecol.*, **100**, 139–44
54. Bernardes, J. (1993). *Automated reading of cardiotocograms. Development and evaluation*, PhD Thesis. Faculdade de Medicina do Porto
55. Arduini, D., Rizzo, G., Gianni, P., Bonalumi, A., Brambilla, P. and Romanini, C. (1993). Computerized analysis of fetal heart rate: I. Description of the system (2CTG) *J. Matern. Fetal Invest.*, **3**, 159–63
56. Jezewski, J. and Wróbel, J. (1993). *Fetal Monitoring with Automated Analysis of Cardiotocogram: the Kompor System* (Zabrze (Poland): Obream Aparatury Medycznej)
57. Bernardes, J., Moura, C., Marques-de-Sá, J. P. and Pereira-Leite, L. (1991). The Porto system for automated cardiotocographic signal analysis. *J. Perinat. Med.*, **19**, 61–5
58. Bernardes, J., Moura, C., Marques-de-Sá, J. P. and Pereira-Leite, L. (1994). The Porto system. In van Geijn, H. P. and Copray, F. J. A. (eds.) *A Critical Appraisal of Fetal Surveillance* (in press)
59. Grant, A. (1984). Principles for clinical evaluation of methods of perinatal monitoring. *J. Perinat. Med.*, **12**, 227
60. Grant, J. M. (1991). The fetal heart rate is normal, isn't it? Observer agreement of categorical assessments. *Lancet*, **337**, 215–18

61. Bland, J. M. and Altman, D. G. (1986). Statistical methods for assessing agreement between two methods of clinical measurement. *Lancet*, **1**, 307–10
62. Arduini, D., Rizzo, G., Caforio, L. and Romanini, C. (1992). Umbilical artery velocimetry versus fetal heart monitoring as labor admissions tests. *J. Matern. Fetal Invest.*, **2**, 37–9
63. Snijders, R. J. M., Ribbert, L. S. M., Visser, G. H. A. and Mulder, E. J. H. (1992). Numeric analysis of heart rate variation in intrauterine growth-retarded fetuses: a longitudinal study. *Am. J. Obstet. Gynecol.*, **166**, 22–7
64. Visser, G. H. A. and Bekedam, D. (1989). Monitoring the growth-retarded fetus. In Spencer, J. A. D. (ed.) *Fetal Monitoring*, pp. 112–17. (Southampton: Castle House Publications)
65. Visser, G. H. A., Bekedam, D. J. and Ribbert, L. S. M. (1990). Changes in antepartum heart rate patterns with progressive deterioration of the fetal condition. *Int. J. Biomed. Comput.*, **25**, 235–7
66. Visser, G. H. A., Stigter, R. H. and Bruinse, H. W. (1991). Management of the growth-retarded fetus. *Eur. J. Obstet. Gynecol. Reprod. Biol.*, **S73–8**
67. Dawes, G. S., Redman, C. W. G. and Smith, J. H. (1985). Improvements in the registration and analysis of fetal heart rate records at the bedside. *Br. J. Obstet. Gynecol.*, **92**, 317–25
68. Dawes, G. S., Moulden, M. and Redman, C. W. G. (1990). Criteria for the design of fetal heart rate analysis systems. *Int. J. Biomed. Comput.*, **25**, 287–94
69. Dawes, G. S., Rosevear, S. K., Pello, L. C., Moulden, M. and Redman, C. W. G. (1991). Computerized analysis of episodic changes in fetal heart rate variations in early labor. *Am. J. Obstet. Gynecol.*, **165**, 618–24
70. Dawes, G. S., Moulden, M. and Redman, C. W. G. (1992). Short-term fetal heart rate variation, decelerations, and umbilical flow velocity waveforms before labor. *Obstet. Gynecol.*, **80**, 673–8
71. Dawes, G. S., Lobb, M., Moulden, M., Redman, C. W. G. and Wheeler, T. (1992). Antenatal cardiotocogram quality and interpretation using computers. *Br. J. Obstet. Gynecol.*, **99**, 791–7
72. Cheng, L. C., Gibb, D. M. F., Ájayi, R. A. and Soothill, P. W. (1992). A comparison between computerised (mean range) and clinical visual cardiotocographic assessment. *Br. J. Obstet. Gynecol.*, **99**, 817–20
73. Economides, D. L., Selinger, M., Ferguson, J., Bowell, P. J., Dawes, G. S. and Mackenzie, I. Z. (1992). Computerized measurement of heart rate variation in fetal anemia caused by rhesus alloimmunization. *Am. J. Obstet. Gynecol.*, **167**, 689–93
74. Henson, G., Dawes, G. S. and Redman, C. W. G. (1984). Characterization of the reduced heart rate variation in growth-retarded fetuses. *Br. J. Obstet. Gynecol.*, **91**, 751–5
75. Hiett, A. K., Devoe, L. D., Youssef, A., Gardner, P. and Black, M. (1993). A comparison of visual and automated methods of analyzing fetal heart rate tests. *Am. J. Obstet. Gynecol.*, **168**, 1517–21
76. Mantel, R., van Geijn, H. P., Caron, F. J. M., Swartjes, J. M., van Woerden, E. E. and Jongsma, H. W. (1990). Computer analysis of antepartum fetal heart rate: 1. Baseline determination. *Int. J. Biomed. Comput.*, **25**, 261
77. Mantel, R., Van Geijn, H. P., Ververs, I. A. P. and Copray, F. J. A. (1991). Automated analysis of near-term antepartum fetal heart rate in relation to fetal behavioral states: the Sonicaid System 8000. *Am. J. Obstet. Gynecol.*, **165**, 57–65
78. Pello, L. C., Dawes, G. S., Smith, J. and Redman, C. W. G. (1988). Screening of fetal heart rate in early labour. *Br. J. Obstet. Gynecol.*, **95**, 1128
79. Schneider, E., Schulman, H., Farmakides, G. and Chan, L. Clinical experience with antepartum computerized fetal heart rate monitoring. *J. Matern. Fetal Invest.*, **2**, 41–4
80. Schneider, E., Schulman, H., Farmakides, G. and Paksima, S. (1991). Comparison of the interpretation of antepartum fetal heart rate tracings between a computer program and experts. *J. Matern. Fetal Invest.*, **1**, 205–8
81. Smith, J. H., Dawes, G. S. and Redman, C. W. G. (1987). Low human fetal heart rate variation in normal pregnancy. *Br. J. Obstet. Gynecol.*, **94**, 656
82. Smith, J. H., Anand, K. J. S., Cotes, P. M., Dawes, G. S., Harkness, R. A., Howlett, T. A., Rees, L. H. and Redman, C. W. G. (1988). Antenatal fetal heart rate variation in relation to the respiratory and metabolic status of the compromised human fetus. *Br. J. Obstet. Gynaecol.*, **95**, 980–9
83. Street, P., Dawes, G. S., Moulden, M. and Redman, C. W. G. (1991). Short-term variation in abnormal antenatal fetal heart rate records. *Am. J. Obstet. Gynecol.*, **165**, 515–23
84. Arduini, D., Rizzo, G., Giannini, F., Garzetti, G. G. and Romanini, C. (1993). Computerized analysis of fetal heart rate: II. Comparison with the interpretation of experts. *J. Matern. Fetal Invest.*, **3**, 165–8
85. Searle, J. R., Devoe, L. D., Phillips, M. C. and Searle, N. S. (1988). Computerized analysis of resting fetal heart rate tracings. *Obstet. Gynecol.*, **71**, 407
86. Maeda, K., Tatsumura, M., Nakajima, K. and Nagata, N. (1989). Computerized assessment of fetal wellbeing. In Belfort, P., Pinotti, J. A. and Eskes, T. K. A. B. (eds.) *Advances in Gynecology*

and *Obstetrics Series. The Proceedings of the XIIth World Congress of Gynecology and Obstetrics.* (Carnforth, UK: Parthenon Publishing Group)

87. Maeda, K. (1990). Computerized analysis of cardiotocograms and fetal movements. *Baillière's Clin. Obstet. Gynecol.*, **4**, 797

88. Parsons, R. J., Chandler, C. J., Palmer, A. and Maeda, K. (1985). The automatic diagnosis of fetal distress by microcomputer. In Van Geijn, H. P. (ed.) *Perinatal Monitoring, 4th Progress Report*, pp. 203–4. EEC Concerted Action Project no. I.1.1

89. Krause, W. (1989). Natali, a computer aided system for supervision of labour. In *The 2nd World Symposium Computers in the Care of the Mother, Fetus and Newborn.* (Blaustein, Germany: Niess Elecktromedikin)

90. Hernandez, C. and Arias, J. E. (1984). Syntactic pattern recognition of fetal stress. *J. Biomed. Eng.*, **6**, 97

91. Beksaç, M. S., Özdemir, K., Karakas, Ü., Yalçin, S. and Karaagaoglu, E. (1990). Development and application of a simple expert system for the interpretation of the antepartum fetal heart rate tracings (version 88/2.29). *Eur. J. Obstet. Gynecol. Reprod. Biol.*, **37**, 133–41

Doppler velocimetry of the great vessels in fetuses with intrauterine growth retardation: correlation with blood biochemistry and perinatal outcome

E. Ferrazzi, M. Bellotti, A. M. Marconi, G. D. Orta and G. Pardi

INTRODUCTION

Cardiovascular adaptations to hypoxemia have been studied in fetal sheep[1]. Hypoxemia in the mature fetus of the sheep is associated with cerebral and coronary vasodilatation, with general somatic vasoconstriction[1,2] and with a decrease in cardiac output[3]. Fetal right ventricular stroke volume is normally larger than its left counterpart but is profoundly reduced during episodes of acute hypoxemia when associated with an increase in arterial pressure[4]. Moreover, different adaptations to hypoxemic conditions were observed in sheep fetuses in the second and third trimesters[5].

In recent years important parameters of fetal adaptation to chronic substrate deprivation have been studied in the human fetus by means of pulsed Doppler velocimetry. Using this technology, several authors[6-9] have reported that cerebral vasodilatation and splanchnic and renal vasoconstriction are often found with severe intrauterine growth retardation (IUGR) in the human fetus. Important parameters of cardiac function have also been studied: atrioventricular filling characteristics[10], peak velocities and acceleration time of the outflow tract of the great vessels[11], flow measurements[12] and other parameters such as ventricular force development[13]. For clinical purposes accurate and reproducible measurements are welcomed. This is especially true when dealing with growth-retarded fetuses whose conditions are often associated with oligohydramnios. The measurement of the peak velocity is probably one of the parameters that can meet these requirements. Moreover, this parameter can be considered to be directly correlated with blood flow without being biased by the error in estimating the cross-sectional area of the great vessels. As a matter of fact, experimental findings in the fetal lamb by Trudinger and co-workers[14] have shown a highly significant correlation ($r = 0.84$) between aortic peak velocity and aortic flow under different conditions of cardiac contractility. Of course, the peak velocity of the outflow tract does not represent all the many variables of the afterload and myocardial contractility. However, the hypothesis is intriguing that in the human fetus, the cardiac performance, as it is represented by this parameter, could correlate with the fetal adaptation to placental insufficiency. This hypothesis has been investigated in our perinatal unit.

METHODS OF DOPPLER INVESTIGATION OF THE PEAK VELOCITY OF THE OUTFLOW TRACT OF THE GREAT VESSELS

A coaxial pulsed Doppler color-flow-imaging system (Hitachi 590), equipped with a 3.5 or 5.0 MHz transducer, was used in our laboratory. Peak velocities in the aorta, pulmonary artery and ductus arteriosus were measured, with a sample volume of < 3 mm. The Doppler sample volume was placed immediately distal to the valve leaflets. The angle between the Doppler beam and direction of blood flow was always less than 30°. Once the angle cursor was set manually, angle corrections were performed automatically. Recordings were performed during phases of fetal rest without breathing movements. Doppler cardiac examinations never exceeded 30 min. The pulsatility index of the umbilical artery and the middle cerebral arteries were measured on the same occasion. Our reference values were collected from a control group of 200 normal singleton pregnancies previously dated in the second trimester by ultrasound. All these fetuses were studied between 20 and 36 weeks of gestation and accurate sonographic biometry and fetal weight estimation were performed. The circumference of the head and the abdomen were used to estimate fetal weight *in utero*.

All fetuses were of normal weight and were uneventfully delivered at term. Doppler measurements of peak velocities were obtained in about 85% of normal fetuses. We analyzed the velocity measurements of the great vessels as a function of estimated fetal weight rather than gestational age. Therefore, we were able to compare the velocities in fetuses with IUGR with velocities in normal fetuses of comparable weight.

The analysis of our findings in normal fetuses showed a progressive increase in peak ejection velocities from both ventricles, which correlated with increasing fetal body mass during gestation.

CORRELATION WITH FETAL GROWTH AND FETAL DISTRESS *IN UTERO*

Seventy-nine consecutive growth-retarded fetuses with sonographic assessment of gestational age before 24 weeks of gestation, no congenital anomalies and a sonographic diagnosis of IUGR (abdominal circumference below the 5th centile and abnormal umbilical Doppler velocimetry) were included in the study.

The last sonographic and Doppler examination of the peak velocity of the great vessels was performed within 3 days of delivery. The clinical staff was unaware of the cardiac Doppler studies. Timing of delivery was decided upon fetal biophysical and biochemical parameters and according to worsening maternal condition. Fetal distress was defined as non-reactive heart rate[15], acidemia at cordocentesis[16] and lack of growth of abdominal circumference on serial ultrasound examinations associated with oligohydramnios[15].

The ratio of head to abdominal circumference was measured and compared with the reference values of our laboratory. Long-standing substrate deprivation causes a progressive cardiovascular adaptation that is generally believed to result in asymmetry of the growth profile. The adaptation to chronic substrate deprivation was assessed in the fetuses of this study by the combination of fetal morphometric criteria and the brain-sparing effect, evaluated on the basis of the waveforms of the cerebral vessels.

The results of 48 fetuses fell above the confidence limits determined for our normal population and they were diagnosed to be asymmetrically growth retarded. A total of 31 fetuses were diagnosed as symmetrically growth retarded, because they fell within the 95% confidence limits. More precisely, all these fetuses fell between the 50th and 95th centile. This suggested a continuum between the two groups of fetuses with IUGR, which were separated by the 95th centile of the head-to-abdomen ratio in order to identify a possible cut-off for a condition of severity in the process of adaptation. The pulsatility index of the middle cerebral arteries was 1.34 ± 0.5 in asymmetrical growth-retarded fetuses and 1.59 ± 0.5 in symmetrical growth-retarded fetuses ($p < 0.02$).

Peak velocities of the outflow tracts of the great vessels in fetuses with symmetrical IUGR within 3 days of delivery were similar to those of normal fetuses of comparable weight (aorta, $p = 0.4$; pulmonary artery, $p = 0.9$; ductus, $p = 0.7$). The mean age of delivery was 34 ± 4 weeks, and the mean weight at birth was 1296 ± 537 g. No intrauterine death occurred in this group. There were 26 elective Cesarean sections in this group, but only six cases were decided for genuine fetal indication, as considered by the clinical staff.

The group of fetuses with IUGR with the head-to-abdomen circumference ratio above the 95th centile (fetuses with asymmetrical IUGR) showed significantly lower peak velocities than normal fetuses of comparable weight for the three vessels which were investigated (aorta, $p = 0.001$; pulmonary artery, $p = 0.03$; ductus, $p = 0.003$) (Figure 1). In this group, there were six intrauterine deaths, 20 Cesarean sections (out of 37) for genuine fetal distress, and six neonatal deaths. The mean age at delivery was 33 ± 4 weeks, and the mean weight at birth was 1266 ± 461 g. The comparison between aortic and pulmonary peak velocity in each fetus showed a trend towards a more severe impairment of the right ventricle. This is shown in Figure 2. This is in agreement with the results reported by Rizzo and Arduini[17] on growth-retarded fetuses in which aortic peak velocities were less affected than pulmonary velocities. These human data support the finding of Pinson and colleagues[18] that the fetal right ventricle is less able to eject in the face of a pressure load than is the left ventricle.

The peak velocities of fetuses with IUGR in our study were observed within 3 days of delivery. The age of gestation, newborn weight, and number of elective Cesarean sections were not significantly different in the two groups. However, interestingly, the number of intrauterine deaths and the number of Cesarean sections for genuine fetal distress were significantly higher in the group of asymmetrically growth-retarded fetuses. Five of the six intrauterine deaths which occurred in this group showed abnormal peak velocities of the outflow tract of the aorta. The lower peak velocities in the right and left outflow tracts in fetuses with asymmetrical IUGR suggest that asymmetrically growth-retarded fetuses are more prone to a deterioration of cardiac performance. The poor outcome of these fetuses suggests that abnormal peak velocities of the great vessels identify fetuses at risk of intrauterine distress. It is likely that longitudinal monitoring of this parameter could be of great value in monitoring the transition from adaptation to distress of growth-retarded fetuses.

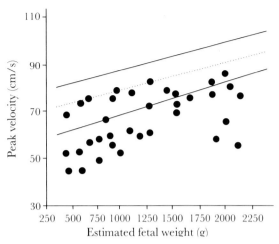

Figure 1 *Peak velocity of the aortic outflow tract in fetuses with asymmetrical growth retardation compared with normal reference values (dotted line, median; solid lines, 25th and 75th centiles). Velocimetric findings are correlated with estimated fetal weight*

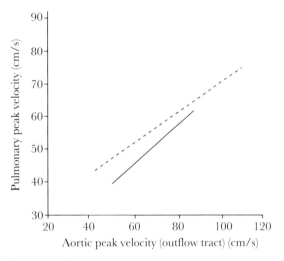

Figure 2 *Regression between the pulmonary and proximal aortic peak velocities ($p < 0.0001$) in fetuses with asymmetrical growth retardation. The slope of the observed linear regression (dashes) is lower than that of the identity line obtained by the expected correlation in normal fetuses between the pulmonary and aortic peak velocities*

CORRELATION WITH ABSENT END-DIASTOLIC FLOW IN THE UMBILICAL ARTERY

The absence of flow in diastole observed by Doppler velocimetry is strongly correlated with severe perinatal prognosis. According to some management protocols, this finding after 34 weeks of gestation demands prompt delivery by Cesarean section. Before this gestational age, the absent end-diastolic flow is a major prognostic factor that greatly helps in the decision of a strict monitoring protocol but cannot be used in order to decide a proper timing of delivery. Cordocentesis for assessment of acid–base balance[16], venous flow pulsations[19] and computerized monitoring of the fetal heart rate[20] can be used for a timely identification of fetal distress.

In 23 fetuses with persistently absent end-diastolic flow from 28 to 34 weeks of gestation, we were able to obtain the peak velocity of the outflow tract of the aorta and of the pulmonary artery. In six fetuses, both the aortic and pulmonary peak velocity were normal. However, in 11 fetuses, both vessels showed abnormal findings. These data were obtained within 3 days of delivery. All the six fetuses with absent end-diastolic flow but still normal velocimetry of the great vessels did well. On the other hand, of the fetuses with abnormal velocimetry in both the outflow tracts, four died *in utero*, three died in the neonatal intensive care units, one suffered permanent brain damage, and only three were dismissed from the neonatal intensive care units in good health. These findings provided further evidence of the close correlation between the worsening cardiac function and the severe perinatal prognosis of the growth-retarded fetus.

CORRELATION WITH THE ACID–BASE STATUS AND OXYGENATION OF THE GROWTH-RETARDED FETUS

Fetal blood sampling for the assessment of the acid–base balance is usually performed when the traditional biophysical parameters show a questionable worsening of fetal condition[16]. In our diagnostic work-up these parameters are fetal growth, umbilical artery Doppler velocimetry, amniotic fluid evaluation, and fetal heart-rate recordings[15]. In our experience[16], the prevalence of fetal acidemia in two groups of fetuses with IUGR with abnormal umbilical velocimetry and reactive or non-reactive heart rate was 16% and 64%, respectively. These data are well in agreement with another reported series that showed the presence of acidemia in 88% of fetuses with an abnormal heart rate pattern assessed by an automatic computerized analysis[20]. These observations suggest that Doppler velocimetry of the great vessels performed at the time of fetal blood sampling could show the cardiac performance in a group of fetuses with IUGR at risk of intrauterine acidemia.

In 31 asymmetrically growth-retarded fetuses the peak velocities of the outflow tract of the aorta and pulmonary artery and of the ductus arteriosus were measured before percutaneous umbilical blood sampling. These fetuses represent a subgroup of the larger series in which this research was performed. Reliable measurements of the aortic, pulmonary and ductal velocities were obtained in 100%, 82%, and 46% of cases, respectively. The mean gestational age at percutaneous umbilical blood sampling was 31 ± 3 weeks. The mean gestational age at delivery was 33 ± 3 weeks; the mean weight at birth was 1174 ± 463 g.

Fetal blood, obtained from the umbilical vein under sonographic guidance according to standard procedures[16], was collected into heparinized syringes and stored in ice. Blood pH, lactate concentrations, pCO_2 and pO_2 were measured, and oxygen saturation and hemoglobin concentration were analyzed, to calculate oxygen content.

In this subgroup, as well as in the larger series of fetuses with IUGR, the peak velocities of the outflow tract of the aorta, the pulmonary artery and the ductus arteriosus were significantly lower ($p < 0.002$, $p < 0.004$, and $p < 0.03$ respectively) than in normal fetuses of comparable weight. Similarly, we found a significant correlation between decreasing values of aortic and pulmonary peak velocities ($p < 0.0001$, $r = 0.84$). The resulting regression line was lower than the identity line, i.e. the normal expected correlation between aortic outflow velocities and pulmonary velocities observed in normal fetuses. A similar highly significant correlation was observed between the peak velocities in the pulmonary artery and in the ductus ($p < 0.002$, $r = 0.74$). Kamitom and co-workers[21] showed, in chronic hypoxemic fetal sheep, that both right and left ventricular outputs were decreased, but with a prevalence of the decrease of the right output. In a large series of fetuses with IUGR and cerebral vasodilatation, Rizzo and Arduini[17] proved that the left heart ejection velocity was privileged compared with the right peak velocity.

Figure 3 shows the values of oxygen content observed in this series of fetuses. Fetuses with abnormal aortic peak velocity had significantly lower values than fetuses with normal aortic peak velocity ($p < 0.004$). Similar highly significant differences were observed for lactate concentration, pH and pCO_2 ($p < 0.007$; $p < 0.01$; $p < 0.01$) in fetuses with abnormal aortic peak velocity (lactate concentration, 1.41 ± 0.6 mmol/l; pH, 7.32 ± 0.03; pCO_2, 46 ± 5 mmHg) and normal aortic peak velocity (lactate concentration, 0.96 ± 0.3 mmol/l; pH, 7.35 ± 0.04; pCO_2, 42 ± 4 mmHg). The hemoglobin concentration in the two groups was 15.7 ± 1.5 and 15.3 ± 2.0 mg/ml, respectively ($p = 0.3$). These biological differences between the two groups were further emphasized by the significant correlation found between the reduction of aortic peak velocities and lactate concentrations ($p < 0.0001$, $r = 0.71$), pH ($p < 0.01$, $r = 0.42$) and oxygen content ($p < 0.01$, $r = 0.42$).

In experimental studies by Richardson and co-workers[22] in fetal sheep, electrocortical activity, electro-ocular activity and breathing movements were only marginally decreased with chronic hypoxemia alone; a significant decrease appeared only with the onset of acidemia.

Our results show that growth-retarded fetuses with abnormal peak velocity of the aortic outflow tract had significantly lower oxygen content and pH and higher lactate concentration and pCO_2 than did growth-retarded fetuses with normal aortic peak velocity. This suggests that the proximal aortic peak velocity helps to identify two different groups of growth-retarded fetuses

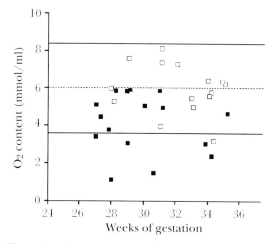

Figure 3 *Oxygen content of blood at cordocentesis in fetuses with intrauterine growth retardation and abnormal (filled squares) and normal (empty squares) peak velocity of the aortic outflow tract. Normal references values are shown for comparison (dotted line, median; solid lines, 25th and 75th centiles)*

as far as their acid–base balance and oxygenation is concerned.

These findings help us to focus on the transitional period from adaptation to distress, in which a reproducible non-invasive technique could help to identify a break-point associated with fetal acidemic hypoxemia.

The venous blood sampled at cordocentesis from the umbilical vein goes directly via the ductus venosus, inferior vena cava and foramen ovalis to the left heart and hence to the coronary circulation, which supplies the myocardial metabolism. The hemodynamic characteristics of the acidemic fetuses of our series are therefore in agreement with the expected metabolic impairment of cardiac contractility.

In conclusion, measurement of acid–base and oxygen content at percutaneous umbilical blood sampling provides direct evidence that, in the human fetus with intrauterine growth retardation, abnormally low peak velocities in the outflow tract of the great vessels is associated with a significant risk of fetoplacental metabolic acidemia and hypoxemia and an impaired exchange of CO_2.

References

1. Thornburg, K. L. (1991). Fetal response to intrauterine stress. *The Childhood Environment and Adult Disease*, Ciba Foundation Symposium 156, pp. 17–37 (Chichester: Wiley)
2. Jensen, A., Roman, C. and Rudolph, A. M. (1991). Effects of reducing uterine blood flow on fetal blood flow redistribution and oxygen delivery. *J. Dev. Physiol.*, **15**, 309
3. Chon, H. E., Sacks, E. J., Heymann, M. A. and Rudolph, A. M. (1974). Cardiovascular response to hypoxemia and acidemia in fetal lamb. *Am. J. Obstet. Gynecol.*, **120**, 817
4. Reller, M. D., Morton, M. J., Giraud, G. D., Reid, D. L. and Thornburg, K. L. (1989). The effect of acute hypoxemia on ventricular function during beta-adrenergic and cholinergic blockade in the fetal sheep. *J. Dev. Physiol.*, **11**, 263
5. Iwamoto, H. S., Kaufman, T., Keil, L. C. and Rudolph, A. M. (1989). Responses to acute hypoxemia in fetal sheep at 0.6–0.7 gestation. *Am. J. Physiol.*, **256**, 613
6. Jouppila, P. and Kirkinen, P. (1984). Increased vascular resistance in the descending aorta of the human fetus in hypoxia. *Br. J. Obstet. Gynecol.*, **91**, 853–6
7. Mari, G. Moise, K. J., Deter, R. L., Kirshon, B., Carpenter, R. J. and Huhta, J. C. (1989). Doppler assessment of the pulsatility index in the cerebral circulation of the human fetus. *Am. J. Obstet. Gynecol.*, **160**, 698–703
8. Rizzo, G. and Arduini, D. (1991). Fetal renal artery velocity waveforms and amniotic fluid volume in growth retarded and post-term fetuses. *Obstet. Gynecol.*, **77**, 370
9. Al Gazali, W., Chita, S. K., Chapman, G. and Allan, L. D. (1989). Evidence of redistribution of cardiac output in asymmetrical growth retardation. *Br. J. Obstet. Gynaecol.*, **96**, 697–704
10. Rizzo, G., Arduini, D., Romanini, C. and Mancuso, S. (1988). Doppler echocardiographic assessment of atrioventricular velocity waveforms in normal and small-for-gestational-age fetuses. *Br. J. Obstet. Gynaecol.*, **95**, 65–9
11. Van Der Mooren, K., Barendregt, L. G. and Wladimiroff, J. W. (1965). Fetal atrioventricular velocity waveforms during normal second half of pregnancy. *Am. J. Obstet. Gynecol.*, **3**, 669–74
12. Reed, K. L., Anderson, C. F. and Shenker, L. (1987). Changes in intracardiac doppler blood flow velocities in fetuses with absent umbilical artery diastolic flow. *Am. J. Obstet. Gynecol.*, **157**, 774–9
13. Sutton, M. S., Gill, T., Plappert, T., Saltzman, D. H. and Doubilet, P. (1991). Assessment of right and left ventricular function in terms of force development with gestational age in the normal human fetus. *Br. Heart J.*, **66**, 285–9
14. Trudinger, B. J., Thompson, R. S., Connelly, A. J., Reed, V. D. and Ng, A. (1992). The influence of cardiac contractility on the aortic flow velocity waveform. *39th Meeting of the Society for Gynecological Investigation*, (Abstr.) p. 387, San Antonio, Texas
15. Ferrazzi, E., Vegni, C., Bellotti, M., Borboni, A., Della Peruta, S. and Barbera, A. (1991). The role of umbilical Doppler velocimetry in the biophysical assessment of the growth retarded fetus: answers from neonatal morbidity. *J. Ultrasound Med.*, **10**, 309
16. Pardi, G., Cetin, I., Marconi, A. M., Lanfranchi, A., Bozzetti, P., Ferrazzi, E., Buscaglia, M. and Battaglia, F. C. (1990). Diagnostic value of blood sampling in fetuses with growth retardation. *N. Engl. J. Med.*, **328**, 692–6
17. Rizzo, G. and Arduini, D. (1991). Fetal cardiac function in intrauterine growth retardation. *Am. J. Obstet. Gynecol.*, **165**, 876–82
18. Pinson, C. W., Morton, M. J. and Thornburg, K. L. (1987). An anatomical basis for fetal right ventricular dominance and arterial pressure sensitivity. *J. Develop. Physiol.*, **9**, 253–69
19. Rizzo, G., Arduini, D., and Romanini, C. (1992). Interior vena cava flow velocity waveforms in appropriate- and small-for-geatational-age fetuses. *Am. J. Obstet. Gynecol.*, **116**, 1271–80
20. Ribbert, L. S. M., Snijders, R. J. M., Nicolaides, K. H. and Visser, G. H. A. (1991). Relation of blood gases and data from computer-assisted analysis of fetal heart rate patterns in small for gestational age fetuses. *Br. J. Obstet. Gynaecol.*, **98**, 820–3
21. Kamitomo, M., Longo, L. D. and Gilbert, R.D. (1992). Right and left ventricular function in fetal sheep exposed to long-term high-altitude hypoxemia. *Am. J. Physiol.*, **262**, 399–405
22. Richardson, B. S., Carmichel, L., Homan, J. and Patrick, J. E. (1992). Electrocortical activity, electroocular activity, and breathing movements in fetal sheep with prolonged and graded hypoxemia. *Am. J. Obstet. Gynecol.*, **167**, 553–8

Doppler velocimetry of the uterine artery and ischemic–hemorrhagic lesions of the placenta

G. P. Bulfamante, E. Ferrazzi, A. Barbera, E. Pollina and G. Pardi

INTRODUCTION

Ischemic–hemorrhagic lesions of the placenta can be found in both normal and abnormal pregnancies[1]. These changes are frequently related to maternal hypertension or to maternal 'vasculolesive' pathologies, such as autoimmune disease, diabetes, or heavy cigarette smoking, which can decrease the maternal blood supply to the placenta. In these conditions the placental damage is usually severe (infarctions with or without centrocotyledonary hemorrhage) and widespread (involving more than 5% of the parenchyma).

Uneventful pregnancies usually show only small placental infarctions or minimal ischemic damage (e.g. hyperplastic cytotrophoblast, thickening of villous basement membranes and excess of syncytial knot formation), probably related to occasional endovascular alterations producing the obstruction of one or some uteroplacental arteries.

In contrast with this general trend, there are some hypertensive pregnancies in which the placenta is normal, some normal pregnancies in which the ischemic–hemorrhagic damage of the placenta is particularly severe, and many pregnancies of apparently healthy women associated with asymmetrical growth-retarded fetuses, where the placental damage is extensive and severe. Recently, several studies have suggested that these not-so-rare 'exceptions to the rule' could result from a different grade of adaptation, achieved during the first half of the pregnancy, by the uterine spiral arteries[2–6].

Morphological analysis of biopsies of the uterine placental bed (decidual and internal myometrial layer) has suggested that in the normal late pregnancy the spiral arteries should all be modified into uteroplacental arteries, thus producing an adequate maternal blood supply to the placenta. Nevertheless, this adaptive process can be absent or partial, thus causing an abnormal blood flow in the placental bed and, probably, placental ischemic–hemorrhagic changes. The failure of the conversion of the distal uterine arteries into uteroplacental arteries seems to be very frequent in hypertensive pregnancies but can also be observed in normotensive pregnancies, particularly if associated with an asymmetrical growth-retarded fetus (so-called 'idiopathic intrauterine fetal growth retardation'). Indeed, biopsy of the uterine placental bed has been a precious tool for building a reliable hypothesis on the developmental mechanisms of the uteroplacental vascular bed.

Unfortunately, one cannot go beyond the hypothesis, because (a) this tool is not suitable for use on a large scale, because of the possible risks to the patient, and (b) it allows the investigation of no more than 1–2 distal uterine arteries. This fact is a serious limitation to the evaluation of the biological role of the pathology (the defective adaptation to the pregnancy of the uterine spiral arteries) that, most often, seems to occur in only some tracts of the single artery, and in only a part of the uterine spiral artery complex within the placental bed.

In order to better evaluate the patterns of maternal blood supply to the placenta in each specific pregnancy, we chose to correlate the pathological uteroplacental findings with those of Doppler velocimetry of the uterine arteries, to evaluate the velocimetric profile of the blood flow in the whole uterus. Our attention was directed to pregnancies of apparently healthy women with asymmetrical fetal growth retardation, a group in which the finding of severe placental ischemic lesions is frequent, and where uterine biopsies have given the most variable results. Moreover, several clinical series have shown that abnormal uterine Doppler velocimetry can be found in both hypertensive and normotensive pregnant women giving birth to growth-retarded fetuses[7].

The main aims of these studies were to evaluate the correlation between abnormal Doppler velocimetry of the uterine arteries and ischemic–hemorrhagic placental lesions and decidual arterial changes, to investigate whether this relationship was different in women with pregnancy-induced hypertension and in normotensive women also having fetal growth retardation, and to analyze the correlations of uterine velocimetric abnormalities and decidual–placental lesions with perinatal outcome.

MATERIALS AND METHODS

For our studies we used the following procedures[8,9].

Patients

Only women without evidence of maternal 'vasculolesive' diseases before pregnancy were accepted for the studies. Pregnancies with idiopathic asymmetrical defective fetal growth were included, but only if in accordance with the following criteria: (a) there was longitudinal sonographic monitoring of fetal growth; (b) there was longitudinal Doppler velocimetric examination (at least three examinations from 20–24 weeks of gestation to the last week before delivery); (c) there was absence of maternal diseases (autoimmune disease, diabetes) and smoking; and (d) there was absence of congenital malformations, and no sonographic evidence of prenatal infection *in utero* and/or clinical evidence of infection after birth.

Uneventful pregnancies with normal fetuses and normal uterine Doppler velocimetric findings, selected according to the same criteria, were used as controls, after informed consent was obtained.

Diagnostic criteria

Asymmetrical intrauterine growth retardation was diagnosed when serial abdominal circumference measurements showed a decrease to below the 10th centile and the head-to-abdomen ratio increased above the 90th centile. Each pregnant woman was retrospectively classified as normotensive or affected by pregnancy-induced hypertension.

Pregnancy-induced hypertension (PIH) was diagnosed when values of systolic–diastolic blood pressure were persistently above 140/90 mmHg[10]. The occurrence and severity of PIH was monitored together with its related disorders (renal function, coagulation homeostasis and liver function).

Doppler velocimetric examinations were made with a sonographic scanner with pulsed Doppler. The ascending branches of the left and right uterine arteries and the umbilical artery were examined with a Doppler sample volume of 5 mm, wall filters were set at 50 Hz, while the Doppler carrier frequency was 3.5 MHz. Both examinations were performed on each patient on the same occasion from 20–24 weeks of gestation to the last week before delivery. The minimum number of Doppler examinations per patient was three. Abnormal uterine velocimetry was defined by a mean left–right systolic/diastolic ratio of > 2.6 and/or a dicrotic notch. Abnormal umbilical pulsatility index varies throughout gestation and was defined according to our reference values[11].

Oligohydramnios was diagnosed when the maximum fluid pocket was less than 2 cm in mean diameter.

A diagnosis of fetal distress was made on the basis of acidemia at cordocentesis (lactate concentration above 1.5 mmol/ml, and pH below 7.30)[12] and/or non-reactive fetal heart-rate tracing and/or oligohydramnios with less than two body/limb movements in 30 min of sonographic examination after 34 weeks of gestation.

Timing of delivery was decided if there was the occurrence of fetal distress or worsening maternal conditions in pregnancies affected by PIH. Doppler velocimetry of the uterine arteries never influenced the timing of delivery.

The same monitoring procedures, except for cordocentesis, were performed on the control cases (uneventful pregnancies with normal fetuses and normal uterine velocimetry without hypertension, resulting in the birth of fetuses that were appropriate for gestational age).

Placental morphology

The volume of the placentas was measured using the water-displacement method[6] after thorough removal of the amniochorionic membranes, umbilical cord and superficial clots. Placentas were fixed for 10 days in 10% formalin. Placentas were cut into serial coronal slices of 1 cm and on gross examination all lesions were identified and measured, using the point-counting method (1000 points in each placenta)[6]. Large infarctions (more than 5% of placental parenchyma) and abruptio placentae were defined as severe lesions, because of their association with poor fetal nutrition and perinatal outcome[1]. All identified gross lesions were sampled and confirmed by histological examinations. A thorough histological examination was then performed on blocks of placental tissue sampled under the insertion of the cord, on one grossly normal central cotyledon and on ten full-thickness placental samples randomly selected. Sections were routinely stained with hematoxylin–eosin and, where necessary, with periodic acid-Schiff, Gomori's stain for reticulum and Hart's method for elastic fibers, to help the identification of decidual vessels in the placental maternal plate. The decidual arterial evaluation was performed only when at least two-thirds of the blocks of a single case contained decidua. The term 'minimal ischemic damage' was used to identify all extensive histological villous ischemic changes, e.g. hyperplastic cytotrophoblast, thickening of villous basement membranes and excessive syncytial knot formation.

The Mann–Whitney test was used to compare independent groups with a non-normal distribution of data; Fisher's exact test was used to analyze different frequencies in the groups of these series.

RESULTS

In our studies, all the patients with fetal growth retardation affected by PIH showed abnormal uterine Doppler velocimetry (mean parity: 1.9 ± 1; group 1). The time of diagnosis of systemic hypertension always followed that of the Doppler velocimetric abnormality (by an average of 5 weeks). The same abnormal velocimetric profiles characterized 80% of the patients with fetal growth retardation but without PIH (mean parity: 2.1 ± 1; group 2). The remaining 20% of the patients with fetal growth retardation but without PIH showed normal values of uterine Doppler velocimetry (mean parity: 2.1 ± 1; group 3).

Notching of the Doppler uterine waveform was observed both in normotensive (65%) and hypertensive patients (64%). The control cases (mean parity: 1.8 ± 1) always showed normal values of uterine Doppler velocimetry.

Group 1 and group 2 were not significantly different in the prevalence of infarctions (approximately 90% vs. 70%; $p < 0.2$) and in large infarctions (55% vs. 45%; $p < 0.9$), extensive minimal ischemic damage (100% vs. 85%; $p < 0.3$), abruptio placentae (18% vs. 10%; $p < 0.9$), and defective response to placentation of decidual arteries (80% vs. 78%; $p < 0.9$). The prevalence of these lesions in the control cases was, respectively, 6%, 0%, 13%, 0%, and 0%. All these percentages were significantly lower ($p < 0.0001$) than in groups 1 and 2. The prevalence of these lesions in the pregnancies of group 3 was, respectively, 0%, 0%, 20%, 0%, and 0%.

In pregnant women with fetal growth retardation, the positive predictive value of abnormal uterine Doppler velocimetry for placental ischemic damage proved to be 100% in hypertensive pregnancies and 85% in normotensive pregnancies. The frequency of large infarcts was not significantly higher in patients with notching of the uterine waveform (50%) than in patients without notching (55%). The evaluation of the distal tract of the uterine arteries showed that defective response to placentation (i.e. incomplete conversion of the spiral arteries of the non-pregnant uterus to the uteroplacental arteries[13]) and acute atherosis were found only in cases with abnormal uterine velocimetry. The distribution of these lesions was not significantly different in normotensive and hypertensive patients with growth-retarded fetuses and abnormal uterine velocimetry.

Additional placental changes (subchorial or intervillous thrombosis and perivillous fibrin deposition) and thrombosis of arteries that were well adapted to pregnancy were also found. These decidual–placental changes were randomly distributed among all the studied cases, not showing any correlation with uterine blood-flow waveforms, maternal blood pressure or type of fetal growth.

The frequency of abnormal umbilical velocimetry in fetuses from normotensive and hypertensive pregnancies with abnormal Doppler uterine waveforms was, respectively, 60% and 72% (no significant difference).

With reference to the perinatal outcomes, no neonatal deaths occurred in the studied series. The mean weight of growth-retarded fetuses with maternal PIH (group 1) was significantly lower than that of growth-retarded fetuses without maternal PIH (group 2), but this difference was explained by the covariance of gestational age. In fact, the percentage of babies weighing below the 50th centile was not significantly different in the two groups with asymmetrical growth retardation. Intrauterine death (concerning about 25% of the cases) was observed only in group 1, and was associated with abnormal umbilical velocimetry. The distribution of the other perinatal outcomes, i.e. oligohydramnios, preterm deliveries and/or Cesarean sections, and fetal distress, was not significantly different in groups 1 and 2.

Conversely, in group 3, the fetal weight was always much higher than in groups 1 and 2; umbilical Doppler velocimetry, amniotic fluid and fetal heart rate were normal and all the fetuses were vaginally delivered at term.

DISCUSSION

The comprehensive correlation among abnormal uterine Doppler velocimetry, placental ischemic–hemorrhagic changes, and defective response to the placentation of the uterine spiral arteries, observed in our studies, suggests the following considerations.

The abnormalities of the waveforms of the uterine arteries, documented by Doppler velocimetry, reflect an important pathogenetic mechanism of the placental ischemic–hemorrhagic changes. As a matter of fact, the prevalence of these placental changes was significantly higher in pregnancies with growth-retarded fetuses and abnormal uterine Doppler velocimetry than in pregnancies with growth-retarded or normal fetuses and normal uterine Doppler velocimetry. Moreover, severe placental damage was never observed in these latter pregnancies.

The abnormalities of the uteroplacental arteries, previously observed with the uterine biopsy method, seem to be very important in the production of the abnormalities of the uteroplacental blood flow. In fact, the histological examination of placental decidual tissue demonstrated a defective response to placentation and acute atherosis of decidual vessels only in pregnancies with abnormal uterine Doppler velocimetry. This vascular damage, in any case, does not seem to be a rule in pregnancies with a growth retarded fetus, and pregnancies with normal uterine arteries and Doppler velocimetry can be observed. The variability in the arterial damage, moreover, can explain the different grade of increased resistance to blood flow in the uterine arteries documented by Doppler velocimetry and, consequently, the different grade of placental ischemic damage.

The defective placentation and the alterations of the uterine blood flow are not specific PIH-related abnormalities; in fact, they also involve the majority of so-called 'fetal growth retardation'. In pregnant women with fetal growth retardation, the positive predictive value of abnormal uterine Doppler velocimetry for placental damage was very high (100% in hypertensive pregnancies and 85% in normotensive pregnancies). These data suggest that the finding of abnormal Doppler velocimetry of the uterine arteries in pregnancies with fetal growth retardation should be considered a risk factor for severe placental damage, even in patients without PIH. These findings confirm that Doppler examination of the uterine arteries is able to detect abnormal uteroplacental conditions that sometimes develop into a maternal systemic disease (PIH), but more frequently are able to induce placental changes and poor perinatal outcome.

In our studies we found a small number of growth-retarded fetuses in normotensive pregnancies with normal uterine Doppler velocimetry. The rates of placental and decidual ischemic lesions were significantly lower than those found in patients with abnormal uterine velocimetry and not significantly different from the control cases. Therefore, causes other than placental–decidual lesions observed in the present study can determine fetal growth retardation and these conditions are not detectable by Doppler examination of the uterine arteries. The causes of fetal growth retardation without maternal hypertension are mostly unknown. In the growth-retarded fetuses without maternal hypertension, the term 'idiopathic' could well be used only for the cases with normal uterine blood-flow velocimetry, whereas those showing Doppler velocimetric abnormalities of the uterine arteries would be better classified as 'growth-retarded fetuses with hemodynamic abnormality confined to the uterus'.

Uterine Doppler velocimetry seems to be a good tool for an early evaluation of the risk of placental ischemic–hemorrhagic damage. Indeed, in our experience, the delay between finding the Doppler velocimetric abnormality and the clinical appearance of PIH was 5 weeks.

Concerning the perinatal outcomes, we observed that the severity of fetal growth retardation was similar in the two studied groups with abnormal uterine Doppler velocimetry regardless of its association with PIH. The mean percentage of weight below the 50th centile in the two groups was in fact 39% and 44%. On average, fetal growth retardation occurred earlier, and the timing of delivery was also significantly earlier, in pregnant patients with PIH than in patients without maternal hypertension. This obviously suggests that when maternal adaptation to pregnancy is upset by uteroplacental–fetal disease, the disease itself tends to be more severe. However, cases of similar severity in weight deprivation and gestational age of birth occurred in both groups. Moreover, the number of fetuses with abnormal umbilical pulsatility index and oligohydramnios, and the number of fetuses with a diagnosis of intrauterine distress, was not significantly different in the two groups. Only a few fetuses were admitted to vaginal delivery. It is important to highlight that normal umbilical waveforms were found in both groups, but that there were no cases of fetal distress or perinatal death in those fetuses with normal umbilical findings. This finding is in agreement with the larger series that we have monitored in the past, in which not only perinatal mortality but also morbidity proved to be significantly worse in fetuses with abnormal umbilical velocimetry[14]. However, the severity of fetal growth retardation suggests that proper fetal and maternal monitoring is required in pregnancies with persistently abnormal uterine waveforms, even if umbilical velocimetry remains within normal limits.

Summarizing our experiences, it is possible to conclude that persistently abnormal uterine velocimetry in pregnancies with asymmetrical fetal growth retardation identifies similar placental damage, which is significantly correlated with poor perinatal outcome, regardless of maternal pregnancy-induced hypertension. These findings suggest that the sonographic finding of fetal growth retardation with abnormal velocimetry of the uterine arteries allows the clinician to diagnose the same fetoplacental disease as in pregnancies with hypertension and with abnormal uteroplacental velocimetry. Growth-retarded fetuses with abnormal uterine velocimetry must be carefully monitored, even if maternal blood pressure and fetal umbilical velocimetry are normal.

References

1. Fox, H. (1978). Pathology of the placenta. In Bennington, J. L. (ed.) *Major Problems in Pathology*, vol. 7, pp.104–23. (London, Philadelphia, Toronto: W. B. Saunders)
2. Sheppard, B. L. and Bonnar, J. (1981). The ultrastructure of the arterial supply of the human placenta in pregnancy complicated by fetal growth retardation. *Br. J. Obstet. Gynaecol.*, **83**, 948–59
3. Brosens, I., Dixon, H. G. and Robertson, W. B. (1977). Fetal growth retardation and the arteries of the placental bed. *Br. J. Obstet. Gynaecol.*, **84**, 656–63
4. Robertson, W. B., Khong, T. Y., Brosens, I., De Wolf, F., Sheppard, B. L., Phil, D. and Bonnar, J. (1986). The placental bed biopsy: review from three European centers. *Am. J. Obstet. Gynecol.*, **155**, 401–12
5. Voigt, H. J. and Becker, V. (1992). Uteroplacental insufficiency. Comparison of uteroplacental blood flow velocimetry and histomorphology of placental bed. *J. Matern. Fetal Invest.*, **2**, 251
6. Aherne, W. A. and Dunnill, M. S. (1966). Quantitative aspects of placental structure. *J. Pathol. Bacteriol.*, **91**, 123–39
7. McCowen, L. M., Ritchie, K., Mo, L. Y., Bascom, P. A. and Sherret, H. Uterine artery flow velocity waveforms in normal and growth retarded pregnancies. *Am. J. Obstet. Gynecol.*, **158**, 499–504
8. Bulfamante, G., Ferrazzi, E., Barbera, A., Moneghini, L. and Pavesi, A. (1993). Uterine blood flow velocimetry and placental changes in hypertensive and normotensive pregnancies with growth retarded fetuses: a pilot study (part 1). *J. Matern. Fetal Invest.*, **3**, 239–43
9. Ferrazzi, E., Bulfamante, G. P., Barbera, A., Pavesi, A., Moneghini, L. and Pardi, G. (1993). Perinatal outcome of growth retarded fetuses with abnormal uterine Doppler velocimetry and placental ischemic hemorrhagic damage and decidual arterial lesions, a pilot study (part 2). *J. Fetal Matern. Invest.*, **3**, 244–9
10. Davey, D. and MacGillivray, I. (1988). The classification and definition of the hypertensive disorders of pregnancy. *Am. J. Obstet. Gynecol.*, **158**, 892–8
11. Ferrazzi, E., Gementi, P., Bellotti, M., Della Peruta, S. and Pardi, G. (1990). Critical analysis of umbilical cerebral and aortic reference values. *Eur. J. Obstet. Gynecol. Reprod. Biol.*, **38**, 189–96
12. Pardi, G., Cetin, I., Marconi, A. M., Buscaglia, M., Ferrazzi, E. and Battaglia, F. (1993). Diagnostic value of blood sampling in fetuses with growth retardation. *N. Engl. J. Med.*, **328**, 692–6
13. Brosens, I., Robertson, W. B. and Dixon, H. G. (1967). The physiological response of the vessels of the placental bed to normal pregnancy. *J. Pathol. Bacteriol.*, **93**, 569–79
14. Ferrazzi, E., Chiara, V., Bellotti, M., Borboni, A., Della Peruta, S. and Barbera, A. (1989). Role of umbilical Doppler velocimetry in the biophysical assessment of the growth retarded fetus. Answers from neonatal morbidity. *J. Ultrasound Med.*, **10**, 309–15

Venous return in the human fetus

J. W. Wladimiroff and T. W. A. Huisman

The introduction of non-invasive methods like ultrasonography and Doppler measurements has enormously accelerated and increased our insights into the normal and abnormal fetal circulation. This chapter describes the physiological aspects of fetal venous vasculature and blood flow with the emphasis on venous return.

PRELOAD PHYSIOLOGY

It is remarkable that most published reports have concentrated on the physiology of the left heart and the arterial vascular system. This is also reflected in the data available on fetal cardiology and on venous return.

One of the pioneers in the field of venous return in adults was Arthur C. Guyton[1], who was the first to determine cardiac output by equating venous return curves with cardiac response curves. It was pointed out that the heart could only perform properly under conditions of normal venous return. Many situations that result in cardiac compromise have their origin in an abnormal preload. The function of veins mainly depends on their specific physical properties; since they have a large cross-sectional area, blood flow experiences low resistance, resulting in a small pressure drop from venous capillaries to the right heart as compared with the reduction in blood pressure from the aorta towards the arterial capillaries[2]. Another important factor is venous compliance. Increases in volume and pressure impose very little stretch on the thin-walled, elastic vessel structure. Because of its cross-section, compliance and length, the veins can contain a large proportion (60% to 80% in adults) of the circulating blood volume. Their capacity and compliance are optimally utilized in the role of a variable blood reservoir that receives or releases blood with only small changes in pressure.

Whereas the functional role of the foramen ovale and ductus arteriosus shunt has been reasonably well-established, the role of the ductus venosus is less clear. It has been suggested that the ductus venosus serves as a bypass of the hepatic microcirculation for well-oxygenated umbilical venous blood[3,4]. The anatomical relationship of the distal end of the inferior vena cava, ductus venosus and foramen ovale implies that well-oxygenated umbilical venous blood in the human fetus seems to follow a preferential pathway through the ductus venosus towards the foramen ovale and left heart[5,6].

FLOW VELOCITY WAVEFORMS IN THE DUCTUS VENOSUS, UMBILICAL VEIN AND INFERIOR VENA CAVA IN NORMAL HUMAN FETUSES AT 12–15 WEEKS OF GESTATION

The introduction of transvaginal Doppler ultrasound has allowed flow velocity waveform studies at fetal cardiac and extra-cardiac arterial level as early as 11–12 weeks of gestation[7,8]. The ductus venosus is a blood vessel functioning exclusively in the fetal circulation as a shunt between the umbilical vein and inferior vena cava, thus bypassing the hepatic micro-circulation[4]. Well-oxygenated blood from the umbilical vein will course almost directly through the ductus venosus towards the foramen ovale and left heart, favoring flow to the fetal cerebrum and trunk.

Data on inferior vena cava flow velocity waveforms, collected by transvaginal Doppler ultrasound between 12 and 16 weeks of gestation, demonstrate a significantly higher percent-

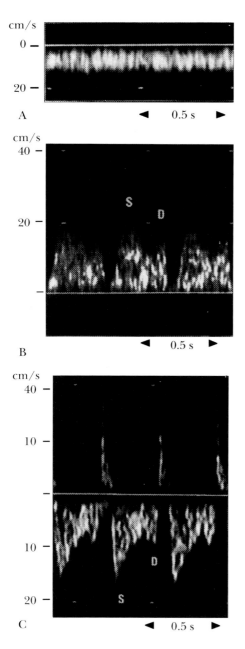

Figure 1 Flow velocity waveform in (A) the umbilical vein, (B) the ductus venosus, and (C) the inferior vena cava in a normal pregnancy at 12 weeks of gestation. S, systole; D, diastole

The question arises as to whether this is also reflected in the flow velocity waveform pattern from the ductus venosus and umbilical vein. Moreover, a marked drop in heart rate as a result of parasympathetic nerve maturation has been demonstrated in late first-trimester fetuses[11].

Between 12 and 15 weeks of gestation, flow velocity waveforms in the umbilical vein are characterized by a continuous forward pattern, in the ductus venosus by a pulsatile systolic and diastolic forward component, and in the inferior vena cava by a pulsatile systolic and early diastolic forward component and a late diastolic retrograde component[12] (Figure 1). The mean (± SD) value for the time-averaged velocity in the ductus venosus was 28.8 (± 6.1) cm/s, in the umbilical vein 9.7 (± 2.9) cm/s and in the inferior vena cava 10.9 (± 2.5) cm/s. In the inferior vena cava the mean percentage (± SD) of retrograde flow was 23.3 (± 5.9)%. The mean (± SD) value for the ductus venosus/umbilical vein ratio was 3.2 (± 0.8) and for the ductus venosus/inferior vena cava ratio 2.7 (± 0.6). The peak systolic/diastolic velocity ratio was 1.1 (± 0.1) for the ductus venosus and 1.6 (± 0.2) for the inferior vena cava. The mean fetal heart rate (± SD) was 160 (± 8) bpm. No statistically significant correlation could be established between the different venous flow velocities and cardiac cycle length ($r = 0.1–0.45$).

Of interest is the abrupt change of a non-pulsatile flow pattern in the umbilical vein into a clearly pulsatile flow pattern in the ductus venosus, which is also seen in late pregnancy[13]. During ventricular systole, the right atrium unfolds after its contraction. This will lead to a passive suction in compliant vessels resulting in a pulsatile profile in both the inferior vena cava and the ductus venosus. The absence of pulsations in the umbilical vein, although it is situated further away from the right atrium, is not properly understood. However, umbilical venous pulsations may be observed both in normal first-trimester pregnancies up to 9–10 weeks[14] and in third-trimester cases of intrauterine growth retardation[15], probably reflecting a high placental vascular resistance.

age of retrograde flow during atrial contraction than is observed in late pregnancy[9,10]. This has been attributed to a relatively low cardiac ventricular compliance in the late first and early second trimesters of pregnancy.

No retrograde flow was established in the ductus venosus. This is in spite of the fact that during the late first and early second trimester of pregnancy, the percentage of retrograde flow in the inferior vena cava is approximately five-fold of that seen near term[9,10]. In addition, the peak systolic/diastolic velocity (S/D) ratio remains constant throughout pregnancy in the ductus venosus (1.1 ± 0.1)[13]. This, together with the absence of retrograde flow, permits its differentiation from the flow pattern in the inferior vena cava (peak S/D ratio throughout pregnancy 1.7 ± 0.3)[9]. The most likely explanation for the presence of only forward flow in the ductus venosus is the single direct connection between the umbilical vein and the fetal venous cardiac inflow, ensuring a sufficient supply of well-oxygenated blood to the fetus under continuous pressure. Late diastolic reversal of ductus venosus flow has been observed only in late pregnancy in a case of fetal supraventricular tachycardia and congestive heart failure[16].

With the use of microspheres, it has been demonstrated in fetal sheep that approximately 50% of umbilical vein blood volume preferentially streams through the ductus venosus towards the foramen ovale without mixing with less-oxygenated blood from the superior and inferior vena cava[5]. Study in the human fetus does not allow volumetric measurements. However, the difference in blood-flow velocities in the ductus venosus, inferior vena cava and umbilical vein, as shown by this study, may also indicate a tendency not to mix. High-velocity blood flow from the ductus venosus as part of venous return will mainly be channelled directly to the foramen ovale, while the lower velocity bloodstream originating from the superior and inferior vena cava will mainly be directed to the tricuspid valve.

THE SUBDIAPHRAGMATIC VENOUS VESTIBULUM ESSENTIAL FOR FETAL VENOUS DOPPLER ASSESSMENT

During Doppler studies of the inferior vena cava immediately proximal to the right atrium, other flow velocity waveforms were often encountered, in particular from the left hepatic vein and ductus venosus. Also, an unexplained large standard deviation was found while analyzing inferior vena cava waveform parameters from this site[9]. Two studies suggest a clinical importance of these parameters in cases of arrhythmias and growth retardation[17,18].

To ascertain the exact anatomical relationship between inferior vena cava, ductus venosus and the hepatic veins in the human fetus in the diaphragmatic and subdiaphragmatic areas, post-mortem specimens of four human fetuses at 18, 26, 28 and 34 weeks of gestation, taken at random, were examined.

The abdominal cavity had been opened in all fetuses during autopsy. The various vessel orifices all entered a funnel-like cavity situated just below the diaphragm. This funnel, or even better this vestibulum, therefore received the abdominal part of the inferior vena cava, the ductus venosus and the orifices of the hepatic veins[19]. In the 18-week specimen as well as in the 34-week specimen, there was a separate orifice for a phrenic vein. The vestibulum continued through the diaphragm where it connected to the right atrium as the thoracic part of the inferior vena cava.

The sagittal ultrasound scan from a 28-week fetus indicated that the ductus venosus, the right hepatic vein and the inferior vena cava showed confluence at the level of the diaphragm before entering the right atrium (Figure 2). The right hepatic vein seemed to have approximately the same diameter as the ductus venosus, while the umbilical sinus and inferior vena cava demonstrated slightly wider vessel sizes. Examination of the 36-week fetus showed a similar situation (Figure 3). The ductus venosus arose from the umbilical sinus, which is an important landmark for measurement of the fetal abdomen circumference[20], to join the inferior vena cava. At that site, a clear widening of the venous structure could be detected before its termination in the right atrium. This image also gives a well-defined sonographic visualization of the fetal portal vasculature. The right portal vein, which is continuous with the left portal vein, split up into an anterior and a posterior branch.

For the clinical evaluation it is important that the presence of the observed vestibulum implies that the data obtained prenatally by Doppler assessment at the inlet of the right atrium provide information on changes in general venous return rather than information on inferior vena cava blood flow alone. Moreover, a considerable variability in flow recording could result from the influence of blood flow from the various vessels propelling into the vestibulum. It was proposed in fetal sheep that blood streams, with negligible mixing, via the venae cavae and ductus venosus into the right atrium[21]. One can imagine that small changes in the scanning plane (such as may be the case during fetal, maternal or examiner movements) may cause variation in blood flow measurements at the site of this vestibulum. This has been observed in a previous study[9].

It is suggested that information on blood flow velocities in the hepatic and subdiaphragmatic area should be obtained more distally in the separate vessels and not at the venous entrance into the right atrium. The possible clinical importance of inferior vena cava flow velocity waveforms should be reconsidered in the light of these new anatomical insights.

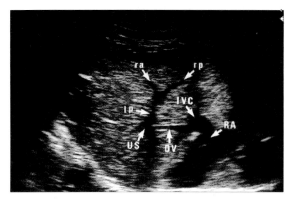

Figure 3 *Ultrasonic image from a normal fetus at 36 weeks of gestation in a transverse-to-oblique scanning phase. Landmarks are the anteriorly situated umbilical sinus (US) and the left portal vein (lp). IVC, inferior vena cava; DV, ductus venosus; RA, right atrium; ra, anterior branch of the right portal vein; rp, posterior branch of the right portal vein*

NORMAL FLOW VELOCITY WAVEFORMS FROM FETAL VENOUS INFLOW DURING THE SECOND HALF OF PREGNANCY

Flow velocity waveforms in the fetal vena cava

Table 1 presents the values for time-averaged velocity, peak S/D, time velocity integral (TVI) S/D and % reverse flow in the fetal inferior vena cava at 19–22, 27–30 and 36–39 weeks of gestation. A statistically significant positive correlation ($r_s = +0.58$; $p < 0.001$) existed between time-averaged velocity and gestational age and a statistically significant negative correlation ($r_s = -0.67$; $p < 0.001$) was established between % reverse flow and gestational age. Peak S/D and TVI S/D did not significantly change with gestational age. Reverse flow was absent in 5 out of 48 women (10%), all at 36–39 weeks of gestation. There was no statistically significant correlation between different inferior vena cava flow velocity waveform parameters and fetal heart rate.

The nearly two-fold increase in time-averaged velocity in the inferior vena cava may be accounted for by increased volume flow in this

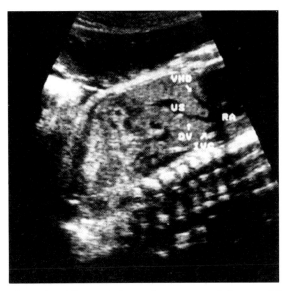

Figure 2 *Ultrasonic image from a normal fetus at 28 weeks of gestation in a sagittal scanning phase. The posteriorly situated fetal spine and the umbilical sinus (US) serve as landmarks. IVC, inferior vena cava; DV, ductus venosus; RA, right atrium; VHD, right hepatic vein*

Table 1 Mean (± 1 SD) values for time-averaged velocity, peak systolic/diastolic ratio (S/D), time velocity integral (TVI) S/D and % reverse flow in the fetal inferior vena cava at 19–22, 27–30 and 36–39 weeks of gestation

Women (n)	Gestational age (weeks)	Time-averaged velocity (cm/s)	Peak S/D	TVI S/D	% reverse flow
13	19–22	14.2 ± 3.1	1.8 ± 0.3	3.5 ± 1.1	16.6 ± 6.2
18	27–30	23.1 ± 4.0	1.7 ± 0.3	3.7 ± 1.0	11.3 ± 3.7
17	36–39	25.6 ± 5.0	1.8 ± 0.2	3.7 ± 1.1	5.2 ± 3.6

Table 2 Normal mean (± SD) values for time-averaged velocity, peak systolic and peak diastolic velocity and peak systolic/diastolic ratio (S/D) in the fetal ductus venosus at 19–22, 27–30 and 36–39 weeks of gestation

Women (n)	Gestational age (weeks)	Time-averaged velocity (cm/s)	Peak systolic velocity (cm/s)	Peak diastolic velocity (cm/s)	Peak S/D
14	19–22	36.4 ± 8.0	47.1 ± 9.3	42.3 ± 8.8	1.12 ± 0.06
18	27–30	43.7 ± 6.9	55.4 ± 8.4	49.2 ± 6.9	1.13 ± 0.05
16	36–39	51.0 ± 7.4	64.2 ± 8.3	57.9 ± 8.4	1.13 ± 0.05

vessel, raised cardiac contractility and reduced cardiac afterload. Age-related reduction in afterload has been established as a result of the physiological decrease in placental vascular resistance during the second half of pregnancy[22,23].

The % reverse flow in the inferior vena cava demonstrated a three-fold reduction with advancing gestational age, which may be explained by the increase in ventricular compliance. Only data on % reverse flow obtained during the latter weeks of gestation were comparable with those obtained by Reed and colleagues[17].

The ratios of systolic to diastolic flow, both for peak velocity and time-velocity integral, did not significantly change during the study period. Both this observation and slightly higher absolute values for the TVI S/D (3.4 ± 1.1–3.7 ± 1.1) are at variance with data reported by Reed and colleagues[17], who found a reduction in the TVI S/D with advancing gestational age and an absolute value for this ratio of 2.8 ± 0.2[9]. This discrepancy may be determined by the limited number of subjects and the different gestational age distribution in their study. However, we found a rather large standard deviation for the TVI S/D and the % reverse flow during all three gestational age periods. As has been discussed before, data on the anatomical relationship between the fetal inferior vena cava and adjacent vessels, e.g. the ductus venosus and hepatic veins at the level of venous entrance in the right atrium, suggest that all three vessels constitute a funnel-like structure, in which the distance between the individual vessels only varies between 2 and 5 mm, depending on gestational age[19].

This implies that at the sonographic scanning level employed by Reed and associates[17] and ourselves, flow velocity waveform recordings may actually originate from the inferior vena cava, the ductus venosus or hepatic veins. This is further supported by our preliminary observation that waveforms obtained from well-defined sonographic images of the hepatic veins closely resemble those obtained at the venous entrance into the right atrium (Figure 4). Of interest is the observation that in contrast to the inferior vena cava and hepatic veins, waveforms originating from the ductus venosus do not display reverse flow.

Ductus venosus blood flow velocity waveforms

The ductus venosus flow velocity waveform depicts a pulsatile pattern, which consists of two forward components. Table 2 presents the values for time-averaged velocity, peak systolic and peak diastolic velocity and peak S/D. A statistically significant positive correlation with

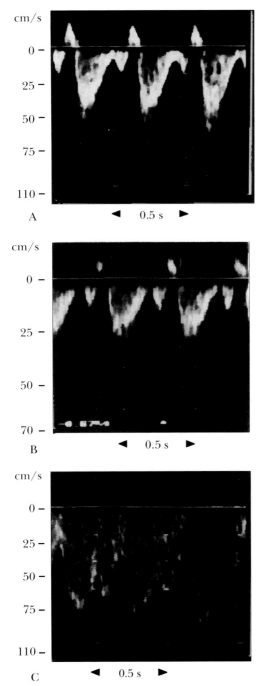

Figure 4 Flow velocity waveform recordings from (A) the fetal 'inferior vena cava', (B) the left hepatic vein, and (C) the ductus venosus, at 38 weeks of gestation

gestational age existed for the time-averaged velocity ($r_s = +0.50$; $p < 0.001$), the peak systolic velocity ($r_s = +0.66$; $p < 0.001$), and the peak diastolic velocity ($r_s = +0.58$; $p < 0.001$). No such correlation could be established for peak S/D. Also, no statistically significant correlation could be demonstrated between the different ductus venosus flow velocity waveform parameters and fetal heart rate.

Of interest is the abrupt change of a non-pulsatile flow pattern in the umbilical vein into a clearly pulsatile flow pattern in the ductus venosus. It is, therefore, very plausible to consider the pump function of the fetal heart in the final formation of the ductus venosus blood flow velocity waveform. During ventricular systole the right atrium relaxes, which may cause a change in the blood flow in the inferior vena cava as well as in the ductus venosus, resulting in a pulsatile profile. The absence of reverse flow in the ductus venosus, present in the inferior vena cava[17], could be the indirect result of the placental pressure gradient over the ductus venosus and umbilical vein. The ductus venosus is the only direct connection between the umbilical vein and fetal circulation, so that a sufficient supply of well-oxygenated blood through the umbilical vein is directed through the ductus venosus under continuous pressure. This supports the view that the faint late-diastolic Doppler shift, observed in some recordings, is not reflecting reverse flow, but is determined by mechanical influence from surrounding tissues.

The results of this study show an increase of peak systolic, peak diastolic and time-averaged flow velocity in the ductus venosus with advancing gestation. This comes as no surprise, since the same development has been demonstrated in other vessels, for example in the descending aorta and the cardiac outflow tract[24,25]. Several factors may play a role in the observed rise in flow velocities in the ductus venosus, such as increased volume flow, increased cardiac compliance and stroke volume or reduced afterload. Age-related reduction in afterload may occur in the human fetus as a result of the physiological decrease in placental vascular resistance[22].

A striking observation is the high amplitude of the blood flow velocity waveform in the ductus venosus. Peak systolic velocities in the range of 40–80 cm/s indicate that ductus venosus velocities appear to be the highest when compared with flow velocities in the umbilical vein, hepatic vein and inferior vena cava[9,26]. Also of interest is the fact that the peak S/D ratio remains rather constant during gestation. The similar rate of increase in peak systolic and peak diastolic velocity can be explained by an increase in volume blood flow through the ductus venosus with advancing gestation. This gestational-age-dependent increase occurs during both cardiac phases without the influence of other cardiac factors such as compliance and stroke volume. Whether these observations will be helpful in discovering pathological cases needs further investigation.

INFLUENCE OF FETAL VARIABLES ON VENOUS DOPPLER WAVEFORMS

For a proper interpretation of recorded Doppler data it is important to take into account the influence of intrinsic fetal factors. Variability in flow measurements can be caused by biological variance within the patient, different fetal behavioral states, fetal (breathing) movements and cardiac arrhythmia. Here, we focus on changes in venous return and venous blood flow velocities relative to different fetal behavioral states.

Fetal behavioral states and ductus venosus flow velocity waveforms

It has been demonstrated that changes dependent on fetal behavioral state occur at both arterial and cardiac level in normal human fetuses at term[27-30]. A significant decrease of the pulsatility index in blood flow velocities during active sleep (fetal behavioral state 2F) as compared with passive sleep (fetal behavioral state 1F) has been observed in the descending aorta and internal carotid artery. This observation suggests increased perfusion of the fetal skeletal musculature and brain to meet raised energy requirements during state 2F[27,28]. During this active sleep period blood flow velocities also appeared to be reduced in the ductus arteriosus[29], but raised at the level of the foramen ovale[31], suggesting increased blood flow to the left heart through this shunt. The question arises as to whether the flow velocity changes dependent on these behavioral states are a result of changed cardiac preload.

Data from the behavioral-state study are presented in Table 3. Peak systolic, peak diastolic and time-averaged velocity demonstrated a statistically significant decrease ($p < 0.001$) in state 1F as compared with state 2F (Figures 1 and 2). Differences did not tend to increase or decrease if the mean level changed. Peak systolic/diastolic ratio and period time were not statistically different between the two behavioral states.

A decrease of approximately 30% was established for both the ductus venosus peak systolic and peak diastolic velocity as well as time-averaged velocity during behavioral state 1F. This decrease may be determined by either a dilatation of the ductal diameter, a reduction in volume flow through the ductus venosus, or a combination of both.

The equal reduction in peak systolic and peak diastolic flow velocity during fetal behavioral state 1F suggests decreased volume flow through the ductus venosus during this behavioral state. If this is true, a redistribution of volume flow at the level of the umbilical sinus

Table 3 Data (mean ± SD) from ductus venosus waveform recording in fetal behavioral state 2F compared with 1F in 15 normal fetuses

	Fetal behavioral state		
	2F	1F	Difference (%)
Time-averaged velocity (cm/s)	56.1 ± 9.2	38.3 ± 7.1	31.7
Peak systolic velocity (cm/s)	70.1 ± 9.5	47.6 ± 7.7	32.1
Peak diastolic velocity (cm/s)	61.6 ± 9.9	42.7 ± 8.1	30.7
Peak systolic/diastolic ratio	1.12 ± 0.08	1.14 ± 0.07	1.8
Period time (ms)	436 ± 36	428 ± 34	1.8

should be considered. More volume flow through the ductus venosus during behavioral state 2F as compared with state 1F would be consistent with earlier reports on a rise in volume flow at the level of the foramen ovale[31] and mitral valve[30], related to behavioral state. Increased volume flow through the left heart would be necessary to ensure raised cerebral blood flow during behavioral state 2F as has been demonstrated in animal studies[32] and has also been suggested from data on reduced vascular resistance at the cerebral level in the human fetus[28].

CONCLUSIONS

Present transvaginal Doppler techniques allow detailed information to be obtained on fetal waveform characteristics and velocities as early as 10 weeks of gestation.

A pulsatile flow pattern was observed in the ductus venosus and inferior vena cava, whereas only the latter demonstrated a retrograde flow component during right atrial contraction. The reduction in inferior vena cava flow reversal with advancing gestational age may be a result of raised ventricular compliance or increased ventricular relaxation rate as well as reduction in afterload. The time-averaged flow velocity in the ductus venosus is 2.7 and 3.2 times higher than that in the inferior vena cava and umbilical vein in early pregnancy. The marked difference in flow velocity between the ductus venosus and inferior vena cava may result in a tendency not to mix, and supports the assumption that two channels of venous return exist. Inferior vena cava blood flow will be mainly directed towards the right ventricle.

This is supported by our study on the anatomical relationships between the venous vessels in the fetal hepatic region in the second half of pregnancy. The abdominal inferior vena cava terminates in a funnel-like venous structure, a subdiaphragmatic vestibulum, which contains the orifices of the hepatic veins as well as the ductus venosus. It is suggested that information on blood flow velocities in the individual vessels in the hepatic and subdiaphragmatic area should be obtained more distally to the right atrium and not at the level of the venous vestibulum.

In fetuses in the second and third trimester, the inferior vena cava flow velocity waveform displays a systolic and early diastolic forward component with reversed flow during late diastole. Waveform recording at the level of the inferior venous entrance into the right atrium provides information on changes in venous return rather than changes in the inferior vena cava *per se*.

The ductus venosus shows a pulsatile flow pattern consisting of a systolic and diastolic forward component without the late diastolic reverse component demonstrated in the inferior vena cava. Ductus venosus peak systolic velocities as high as 40–80 cm/s were observed. A statistically significant increase in time-averaged velocity, peak systolic and peak diastolic velocity in the inferior vena cava and ductus venosus with advancing gestational age was established. This may be caused by increased volume flow, increased cardiac compliance and stroke volume or reduced afterload. Age-related reduction in afterload may occur in the human fetus as a result of the physiological decrease in placental vascular resistance.

A fetal decrease of 30% dependent on behavioral state was observed in the ductus venosus peak systolic, peak diastolic and time-averaged velocity, suggesting a redistribution of umbilical venous blood through the ductus venosus shunt during the passive sleep state as compared with the active sleep state in the term fetus. The fetal behavioral state should be taken into account in future studies on ductus venosus flow velocity waveforms in normal term pregnancies.

References

1. Guyton, A. C. (1991). Cardiac output, venous return and their regulation. In Guyton, A. C. *Textbook of Medical Physiology*, 8th edn., pp. 221–33. (Philadelphia: W. B. Saunders)
2. Scher, A. M. (1989). The veins and venous return. In Patton, H. D., Fuchs, A. F., Hille, B., Scher, A. M. and Steiner, R. (eds.) *Textbook of Physiology*, 21st edn., vol. 2, pp. 879–86. (Philadelphia: W. B. Saunders)
3. Peltonen, T. and Hirvonen, L. (1965). Experimental studies on fetal and neonatal circulation. *Acta Paediatr. Scand.*, **161** (Suppl.), 5–55
4. Rudolph, A. M. (1983). Hepatic and ductus venosus blood flows during fetal life. *Hepatology*, **3**, 254–8
5. Edelstone, D. I. and Rudolph, A. M. (1979). Preferential streaming of ductus venosus blood to the brain and heart in fetal lambs. *Am. J. Physiol.*, **23**, H724–9
6. Kiserud, T., Eik-Nes, S. H., Blaas, H. G. and Hellevik, L. R. (1992). Foramen ovale: an ultrasonographic study of its relation to the inferior vena cava, ductus venosus and hepatic veins. *Ultrasound Obstet. Gynecol.*, **2**, 389–96
7. Wladimiroff, J. W., Huisman, T. W. A. and Stewart, P. A. (1991). Fetal cardiac flow velocities in the late first trimester of pregnancy; a transvaginal Doppler study. *J. Am. Coll. Cardiol.*, **17**, 1357–9
8. Wladimiroff, J. W., Huisman, T. W. A., Stewart, P. A. and Stijnen, Th. (1992). Normal fetal Doppler inferior vena cava, transtricuspid and umbilical artery flow velocity waveforms between 11 and 16 weeks' gestation. *Am. J. Obstet. Gynecol.*, **160**, 921–4
9. Huisman, T. W. A., Stewart, P. A. and Wladimiroff, J. W. (1991). Flow velocity waveforms in the fetal inferior vena cava during the second half of normal pregnancy. *Ultrasound Med. Biol.*, **17**, 679–82
10. Wladimiroff, J. W., Huisman, T. W. A., Stewart, P. A. and Stijnen, T. (1992). Fetal Doppler inferior vena cava, transtricuspid and umbilical artery flow velocity waveforms in normal late first and early second trimester pregnancies. *Am. J. Obstet. Gynecol.*, **166**, 921–4
11. Wladimiroff, J. W. and Seelen, J. C. (1972). Doppler tachometry in early pregnancy. Development of fetal vagal function. *Eur. J. Obstet. Gynaecol. Reprod. Biol.*, **2**, 55–63
12. Huisman, T. W. A., Stewart, P. A., Wladimiroff, J. W. and Stijnen, T. (1993). Flow velocity waveforms in the ductus venosus, umbilical vein and inferior vena cava in normal human fetuses at 12–15 weeks of gestation. *Ultrasound Med. Biol.*, **19**, 441–5
13. Huisman, T. W. A., Stewart, P. A., Wladimiroff, J. W. (1992). Ductus venosus blood flow velocity waveforms in the human fetus; a Doppler study. *Ultrasound Med. Biol.*, **18**, 33–7
14. Rizzo, G., Arduini, D. and Romanini, C. (1992). Umbilical vein pulsations: a physiologic finding in early gestation. *Am. J. Obstet. Gynecol.*, **167**, 675–7
15. Indik, J. H., Chen, V. and Reed, K. (1991). Association of umbilical venous with inferior vena cava flow velocities. *Obstet. Gynecol.*, **77**, 551–7
16. Kiserud, T., Eik-Nes, S. H., Blaas, H. G. and Hellevik, L. R. (1991). Ultrasonographic velocimetry of the fetal ductus venosus. *Lancet*, **338**, 1412–4
17. Reed, K. L., Appleton, C. P., Anderson, C. F., Shenker, L. and Sahn, D. J. (1990). Doppler studies of vena cava flows in human fetuses; insights into normal and abnormal cardiac physiology. *Circulation*, **81**, 498–505
18. Chan, F. Y., Woo, S. K., Ghosh, A., Tang, M. and Lam, C. (1990). Prenatal diagnosis of congenital fetal arrhythmias by simultaneous pulsed Doppler velocimetry of the fetal abdominal aorta and inferior vena cava. *Obstet. Gynecol.*, **76**, 200–4
19. Huisman, T. W. A., Gittenberger-de Groot, A. C. and Wladimiroff, J. W. (1992). Recognition of a fetal subdiaphragmatic venous vestibulum essential for fetal venous Doppler assessment. *Pediatr. Res.*, **32**, 338–41
20. Campbell, S. and Wilkin, D. (1975). Ultrasonic measurement of fetal abdomen circumference in the estimation of fetal weight. *Br. J. Obstet. Gynaecol.*, **82**, 689–97
21. Reuss, M. L., Rudolph, A. M. and Heymann, M. A. (1981). Selective distribution of microspheres injected into the umbilical veins and inferior venae cavae of fetal sheep. *Am. J. Obstet. Gynecol.*, **141**, 427–32
22. Trudinger, B. J., Cook, C. M., Giles, W. B. and Connely, A. (1987). Umbilical artery flow velocity waveforms in high-risk pregnancy: randomized controlled trial. *Lancet*, **2**, 188–90
23. Reuwer, P. J. H. M., Sijmons, E. A., Rietman, G. W., Van Tiel, M. W. M. and Bruinse, H. W. (1987). Intrauterine growth retardation: prediction of perinatal distress by Doppler ultrasound. *Lancet*, **1**, 415–9
24. Marsal, K., Lindblad, A., Lingman, G. and Eik-Nes, S. H. (1984). Blood flow in the fetal descending aorta; intrinsic factors affecting fetal blood flow, i.e. fetal breathing movements and

cardiac arrhythmia. *Ultrasound Med. Biol.*, **10**, 339–48
25. Groenenberg, I. A. L., Wladimiroff, J. W. and Hop, W. C. J. (1989). Fetal cardiac and peripheral arterial flow velocity waveforms in intrauterine growth retardation. *Circulation*, **80**, 1711–7
26. Gill, R. W., Kossoff, G. and Warren, P. S. (1984). Umbilical venous flow in normal and complicated pregnancy. *Ultrasound Med. Biol.*, **10**, 349–63
27. Van Eyck, J., Wladimiroff, J. W., Noordam, M. J., Tonge, H. M. and Prechtl, H. F. R. (1985). The blood flow velocity waveform in the fetal descending aorta; its relationship to fetal behavioural states in normal pregnancy at 37–38 weeks of gestation. *Early Hum. Dev.*, **14**, 99–107
28. Van Eyck, J., Wladimiroff, J. W., Van den Wijngaard, J. A. G. W., Noordam, M. J. and Prechtl, H. F. R. (1987). The blood flow velocity waveform in the fetal internal carotid and umbilical artery; its relationship to fetal behavioural states in normal pregnancy at 37–38 weeks of gestation. *Br. J. Obstet. Gynaecol.*, **94**, 736–41
29. Van der Mooren, K., Van Eyck, J. and Wladimiroff, J. W. (1989). Human fetal ductal flow velocity waveforms relative to behavioural states in normal term pregnancy. *Am. J. Obstet. Gynecol.*, **160**, 371–4
30. Rizzo, G., Arduini, D., Valensise, H. and Romanini, C. (1990). Effects of behavioral states on cardiac output in the healthy human fetus at 36–38 weeks of gestation. *Early Hum. Dev.*, **23**, 109–15
31. Van Eyck, J., Stewart, P. A. and Wladimiroff, J. W. (1990). Human fetal foramen ovale flow waveforms relative to behavioral states in normal term pregnancy. *Am. J. Obstet. Gynecol.*, **163**, 1239–42
32. Richardson, B. S., Patrick, J. E. and Abduljabbar, H. (1985). Cerebral oxidative metabolism in the fetal lamb: relationship to electrocortical state. *Am. J. Obstet. Gynecol.*, **153**, 426–31

Early pregnancy hemodynamics assessed by transvaginal color Doppler

A. Kurjak, F. A. Chervenak, D. Zudenigo and S. Kupešić

INTRODUCTION

Early pregnancy is a period in which many important landmarks with regard to the ultimate outcome of pregnancy are defined. Until the introduction of ultrasound techniques, direct investigation of this period of pregnancy was impossible.

Remarkable progress in diagnostic ultrasound has been made with the introduction of the transvaginal color Doppler technique. This not only provides new physiological data, but also enables us to observe *in vivo* the features classically described by the embryologist. Precise investigation of the blood flow changes in maternal and fetal circulation in early pregnancy is now possible.

In 1987, our group published the first paper on the successful use of color Doppler in clinical obstetrics[1]. Two years later a paper on the use of transvaginal color Doppler appeared[2], followed by several studies on normal and abnormal blood flow in the first trimester of pregnancy[3-10], early cerebral blood flow[11], vascularization of the fetal plexus choroideus[12], gestational trophoblastic disease[13] and fetomaternal circulation in patients with threatened abortion[14].

It is the purpose of this chapter to discuss most of the currently available data from our own studies as well as published studies of other authors.

ANATOMY OF THE HUMAN PLACENTA

The placenta consists of a fetal portion developed from the embryonic chorion and a maternal portion formed by the pregnant endometrium or decidua. The anatomy of the human placenta mainly relates to the fetal circulation, with its connective tissue supports and trophoblastic covering. At the end of the first trimester the placenta can be separated clearly into three basic structures – the chorionic or fetal plate, the placental villous tissue and the basal or maternal plate[15].

Uteroplacental circulation

The maternal portion of the placental circulation consists of the main uterine arteries and their branches that spread throughout uterus until they reach the decidual plate of the placenta. The main uterine arteries originate from the iliac arteries, and give off branches which extend inward for about one-third of the thickness of the myometrium without significant branching. They then subdivide into an arcuate wreath encircling the uterus. From this network, smaller branches arise: these are the radial arteries that are directed towards the uterine lumen, and they become the endometrial spiral arteries as they pass the myometrial–endometrial border[16]. The human uterine circulation is very rich in arterial anastomoses. Branches of the uterine arteries anastomose with branches of the ovarian and vaginal arteries to establish a vascular arcade perfusing the internal genital organs. Vascular connections are also found between the main uterine arteries and their largest branches, or joining the uterine circulation with the systemic circulation[17].

After implantation, the spiral arteries become large tortuous channels as the normal musculoelastic wall is replaced with fibrinoid material and fibrous tissue. Such changes ensure an adequate blood supply to the growing embryo. The vascular changes which convert the spiral arteries into a low-resistance vascular bed are well defined by the 18th week of gestation, and are closely related to the trophoblastic infiltration of the placental bed[18,19]. It is generally accepted that most of these migrating cells are of the cytotrophoblastic type. There is probably only one continuous wave of trophoblastic activity, lasting from the 8th to the 18th week. This vascular transformation is probably also influenced by variations in circulating steroid and protein hormones. Doppler measurements show a significant influence of levels of factors such as intact human chorionic gonadotropin (hCG), free α- and β-hCG subunits and 17β-estradiol on the uterine resistance index[20].

Classically, as soon as the blastocyst has implanted, a number of endometrial vessels are opened by the phagocytic activity of the trophoblast, and maternal blood enters the future intervillous space, bringing nutrients and oxygen to the growing embryo[21]. Recently, Hustin and colleagues, using transvaginal sonography, intervillous hysteroscopy and examination of material obtained by chorionic villous sampling, have been unable to detect continuous blood flow in the intervillous spaces before 13 weeks of gestation[22,23]. The same authors have also perfused pregnant hysterectomy specimens with the embryo *in situ* with barium sulfate and have demonstrated that, during the first 3 months of gestation, the growing embryo is totally separated from the maternal circulation by the trophoblastic shell. At this time the tips of the spiral arteries are obstructed by intravascular trophoblastic plugs and the intervillous space is bathed by a clear fluid, possibly filtered maternal plasma and uterine gland secretions, and not by maternal blood. The spiral arteries widen progressively and, around the 12th gestational week, the trophoblastic plugs are eventually loosened and dislocated, allowing a free circulation of blood in the intervillous space. These findings are surprising and may be decisive in the development of the understanding of the pathophysiology of early pregnancy.

Doppler analysis of uteroplacental circulation

The color Doppler technique easily shows blood flow through the uteroplacental blood vessels (Figure 1). Pulsed Doppler waveform profiles for uterine arteries are characteristic, comprising a high peak-systolic component with a characteristic notch at the descending slope of the systole and very low end-diastolic flow (Figure 2). Doppler sonograms of the arcuate and radial arteries are very similar – moderate peak-systolic and end-diastolic components of blood flow are seen (Figures 3 and 4). A difference is seen in the peripheral vascular impedance, impedance values being lower in the radial arteries than in the arcuate arteries. Pulsed Doppler waveform signals obtained from spiral arteries show low

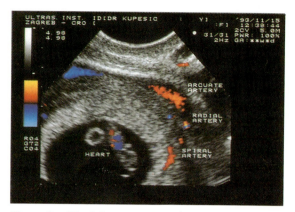

Figure 1 *Blood flow through different segments of uteroplacental circulation (arcuate, radial and spiral artery) and fetal heart*

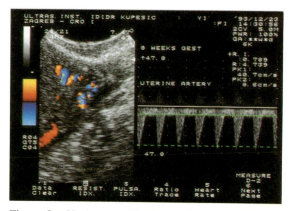

Figure 2 *Uterine artery blood flow at 8th gestational week. Flow velocity waveforms show high peak-systolic and low end-diastolic velocity*

EARLY PREGNANCY HEMODYNAMICS

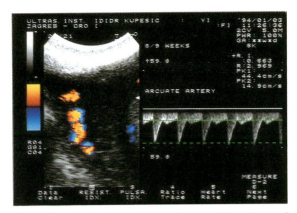

Figure 3 *Arcuate artery blood flow at 9th gestational week. Pulsed Doppler examination shows moderate peak-systolic and end-diastolic velocity*

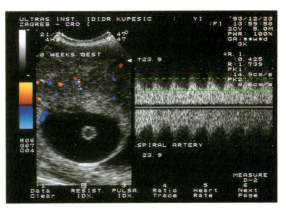

Figure 5 *Spiral artery blood flow at 10th gestational week. Pulsed Doppler waveform signal indicates high end-diastolic velocities and characteristic spiky outline which is a consequence of low impedance to blood flow*

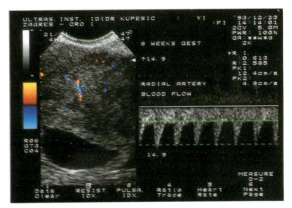

Figure 4 *Color signal in myometrium belongs to the radial artery. Flow velocity waveforms demonstrate lower peak-systolic and higher end-diastolic velocity compared to arcuate artery*

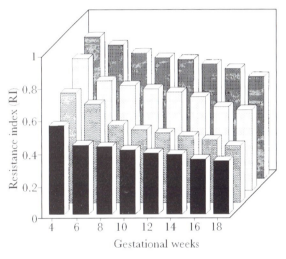

Figure 6 *Mean resistance index in uteroplacental vessels in normal early pregnancy. ■ Spiral arteries, ▨ radial arteries, ▥ arcuate arteries, ▧ uterine artery*

impedance to blood flow and a characteristic spiky outline (Figure 5). Pulsed Doppler studies require a sample volume not less than 1 mm^2, and the diameter of the spiral arteries in the first trimester of pregnancy is only 0.5–0.7 mm. However, this type of waveform is indicative of high turbulence and a tortuous vessel with an irregular wall, which are the features of spiral arteries. Intraplacental sonolucent spaces identified by real-time imaging contain continuous non-pulsatile flow on color imaging with a venous pattern on spectral analysis, which corresponds to maternal intervillous blood flow.

Around 13 weeks, a continuous intervillous flow pattern is observed in all pregnancies, associated with an abrupt increase in blood flow velocity in the main uterine artery, possibly corresponding to the complete dislocation of the trophoblastic plugs, which allows an uninhibited blood circulation in the entire intervillous space[24].

During pregnancy, impedance to blood flow decreases from the main uterine artery to the spiral arteries and with advanced gestational age[4–6,24–31] (Figures 6 and 7). At the same time increasing blood flow seen, as a peak-systolic

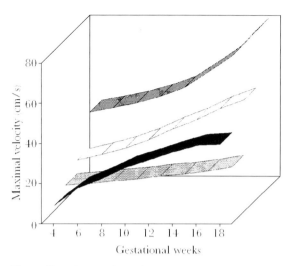

Figure 7 *Mean peak-systolic values in uteroplacental vessels in normal early pregnancy.* ■ *Spiral arteries,* ▨ *radial arteries, arcuate arteries,* ▨ *uterine artery*

Doppler shift, is observed. Decreasing vascular impedance with increasing gestation is probably a consequence of the dilatation of spiral arteries induced by trophoblast infiltration, hormone-mediated vasodilatation and decreased viscosity of maternal blood. However, Dillon and colleagues found no correlation between peripheral vascular impedance, blood flow velocity and gestational age in uterine vessels[32]. Table 1 presents results of Doppler studies of the uteroplacental circulation from different authors.

Although resistance index is independent of the angle of insonation, it indicates only the impedance of a particular signal and thus is unable to characterize the waveform fully, since two vastly different levels of flow can have the same RI if the impedance of the vessels is the same. The actual peak-systolic and end-diastolic frequency shifts or velocities must be reported to describe a waveform more fully.

Dillon and colleagues measured peak-systolic velocity in spiral arteries in an attempt to differentiate abnormal intrauterine pregnancies from pseudogestational sacs associated with ectopic pregnancies[33]. In that study, a peak-systolic velocity > 21 cm/s was 100% specific for the presence of an intrauterine pregnancy, thus excluding the diagnosis of pseudogestational sac and ectopic pregnancy. Flow > 21 cm/s was detected in all intrauterine pregnancies after 36 days. Before that period, the signals detected from intrauterine pregnancies did not exceed this level, and they could not, therefore, be distinguished from pseudosacs. Altieri and coworkers used endovaginal Doppler to evaluate the peritrophoblastic region in pregnancies at less than 6 weeks gestational age[34]. All had a peak-systolic velocity > 10 cm/s when a gestational sac could be visualized. This flow was detectable before a fetal pole could be visualized. Since the sac cannot be visualized until 31 days, there is a 5-day period during which the sac can be visualized and some flow can be seen, but that flow will not be high enough to allow differentiation from myometrial flow surrounding a pseudosac.

Umbilical – placental circulation

The junction between the amnion and the ectoderm is known as the primitive umbilical ring.

Table 1 Summary of recent studies of Doppler measurements in uteroplacental circulation

Author	Number of patients	Comment
Deutinger et al.[26]	88	
Merce et al.[25]	25	
Jurkovic et al.[24]	45	Decrease of vascular impedance with
Kurjak et al.[4]	108	advanced gestational age
Arduini et al.[27]	330	
Montenegro et al.[31]	141	
Dillon et al.[32]	23	No correlation between vascular impedance and gestational age
Jaffe and Warsof[28]	50	

At the fifth week of development this ring is pierced by:

(1) The connecting stalk containing the allantois and the umbilical vessels consisting of two arteries and one vein;
(2) The yolk sac stalk accompanied by the vitelline vessels; and
(3) The canal, connecting the intra- and extra-embryonic coelomic cavities.

During further development the amniotic cavity enlarges rapidly at the expense of the chorionic cavity, and the amnion begins to envelop the connecting and yolk sac stalks, resulting in the formation of the primitive umbilical cord[21].

The umbilical artery branches into the chorionic arteries, and together these form the umbilical–placental circulation. The umbilical artery can be located by transvaginal color Doppler sonography as early in pregnancy as the 6th week. By the end of the 10th gestational week there is no end-diastolic component of blood flow (Figure 8). Between the 10th and the 14th week diastolic velocities begin to emerge, but these are incomplete and inconsistently present. After this time, pandiastolic frequencies are consistently present[35]. Chorionic arteries and intraplacental arterioles can be visualized in a significant proportion of pregnancies. Hsieh and colleagues, using a sensitive color flow mapping system, detected intraplacental arterioles in the upper two-thirds of the placenta, beneath the chorionic plate[36]. Their results show that resistance to flow in the umbilical artery is highest on the fetal side, becoming progressively lower towards the placental side, and being lowest in the arteries within the placenta.

Similar results were obtained by Jauniaux and colleagues (Table 2)[29]. There are no significant changes in umbilical artery blood flow until the 12th gestational week, when a significant decrease in vascular impedance is noticed. Table 3 shows the results of Doppler investigations of blood flow in the umbilical artery in early pregnancy by different authors.

The anatomical changes in the villous vasculature are characterized by the progressive increase of the number and the surface area occupied by the fetal vessels, must have a key role in the gradual fall of blood flow impedance in the umbilical circulation.

FETAL CIRCULATION

Around 21 days after ovulation, corresponding to the end of the 5th week after the last menstrual period, the primitive heart begins to beat. Activity of the embryonic heart has been documented *in utero* as early as 36 days post-menstrual age[37] (Figures 1 and 9). Heart rate increases from 80 to 90 beats/min to 150–170 up to the end of the 9th week. Arrhythmias in the first trimester can precede fetal loss[38], and color Doppler could become the main tool for the detection and screening of such disturbances.

Table 2 *Resistance index (RI) and pulsatility index (PI) for umbilical–placental vessels (mean ± SD)*[29]

	RI	PI
Fetal circulation		
umbilical artery	0.662 ± 0.027	1.145 ± 0.050
chorionic artery	0.564 ± 0.017	0.848 ± 0.035
intraplacental arteriole	0.461 ± 0.014	0.692 ± 0.040

Table 3 *Summary of recent studies of Doppler*

Author	Number of patients	Comment
Kurjak et al.[14]	90	Decrease of vascular impedance with gestational age
Arduini et al.[35]	214	
Den Ouden et al.[30]	85	No correlation between vascular impedance and gestational age in first trimester
Montenegro et al.[31]	96	Increase in pulsatility index until week 11, followed by decrease until 13 weeks

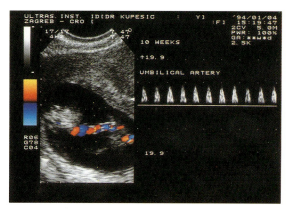

Figure 8 *Color flow imaging and flow velocity waveforms of the umbilical artery at 10 weeks' gestation. End-diastolic velocity is absent*

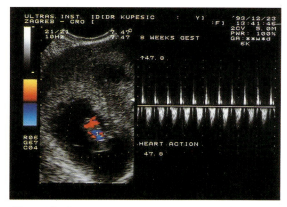

Figure 9 *Transvaginal color imaging and spectral analysis of signals from fetal heart at 8 weeks' gestation*

This technique has also been shown to be helpful in the visualization of normal early fetal cardiac anatomy during the late first and early second trimester of pregnancy. Doppler flow velocities can be measured at the level of the atrioventricular and outflow tracts[39,40]. Up to 11–12 weeks of gestation it is not always possible to differentiate between the two atrioventricular valves. An atrioventricular waveform recording at 10 weeks consists of the early diastolic or E-wave component and late diastolic or A-wave component, demonstrating that differentiation between passive diastolic filling and atrial contraction is already feasible at this very early stage of gestation. Of interest is the relatively low peak E-wave velocity compared with the peak A-wave velocity, resulting in an E/A ratio of approximately 0.5, as opposed to E/A ratios ranging between 0.8 and 0.9 in late pregnancy. The clear A-wave dominance at the atrioventricular level reflects the relative stiffness of the cardiac ventricles in early gestation. At 11–12 weeks mean peak E-wave and A-wave velocities of 20.5 ± 3.2 cm/s and 38.6 ± 4.7 cm/s have been established. There is a marked rise in peak E-wave velocities and E/A ratios of both the mitral and tricuspid level with advancing gestational age. This suggests a shift of blood flow from late towards early diastole, which may be due to increased ventricular compliance and/or raised ventricular relaxation rate.

Aortic and pulmonary artery flow velocities may also be recorded at the outflow tract level as early as 10–11 weeks of gestation. At 11–12 weeks, peak and time-averaged flow velocities are lower than those observed in late pregnancy, with mean values of 32.1 ± 5.4 cm/s and 11.2 ± 2.2 cm/s in the ascending aorta, and 29.6 ± 5.1 cm/s and 10.8 ± 2.1 cm/s in the pulmonary artery. In both vessels a gestational age-related rise in peak velocities can be demonstrated during the early second trimester of pregnancy, the highest velocities being reached in the ascending aorta. A difference in left and right cardiac blood flow in favor of the right side was calculated during the first half of the second trimester of pregnancy. The higher peak-systolic velocities in the ascending aorta compared with the pulmonary artery may be a result of a difference in semilunar valve area between the two vessels, as has been suggested on the basis of similar findings in late pregnancy.

Fetal vessels usually analyzed for assessment of fetal well-being are the aorta, carotid arteries and middle cerebral artery. Pulsations from the fetal aorta can be identified as early as the 6th week of gestation (Figure 10).

In the fetal aorta, as in the umbilical artery, there are no significant changes in blood flow until the end of the 12th gestational week. There is then a significant decrease in peripheral impedance to blood flow. The decrease of peripheral vascular impedance is accompanied by an increase in blood flow velocities in all investigated vessels.

EARLY PREGNANCY HEMODYNAMICS

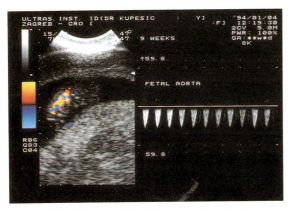

Figure 10 *Color flow imaging and flow velocity waveforms of the fetal aorta at 9th gestational week. End-diastolic flow is absent*

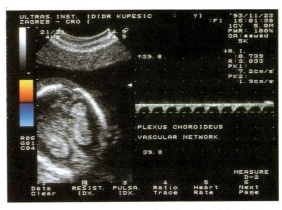

Figure 12 *Transverse scan of the fetal head At the inner edge of the choroid plexus a pulsed Doppler signal is obtained*

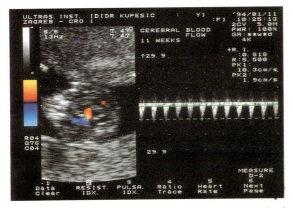

Figure 11 *Transvaginal color Doppler scan of the fetal head at 11 weeks' gestation. Blood flow through middle cerebral artery with constant end-diastolic flow is visible*

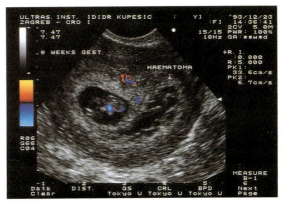

Figure 13 *Anechogenic area below gestational sac represents subchorionic hematoma. Color flow through fetal heart and spiral arteries (subtrophoblastic area) is present*

Fetal cerebral circulation

The intracranial circulation is visible as early as the 8th week of gestation, when discrete pulsations of intracranial parts of the internal carotid arteries are detectable at the base of the skull. During the 9th and the 10th gestational weeks colored patterns representing blood flow can be visualized in the antero-lateral quadrant of the skull base. From the 10th gestational week the morphology of intracranial structures becomes more pronounced. Arterial pulsations can be detected on transverse sections, lateral to the mesencephalon and the cephalic flexure. The distance between the internal carotid artery and middle cerebral artery is a few millimeters or even less: it is, therefore, difficult to distinguish between blood flow in these two arteries. Because of its position this arterial blood flow is presumed to be the middle cerebral artery (Figure 11).

Wladimiroff and colleagues established the appearance of end-diastolic flow velocities in over 50% of intracerebral artery flow velocity waveforms between 10 and 12 weeks of gestation, whereas in the umbilical artery and descending aorta end-diastolic velocities were still absent[41]. These data are in accordance with our observations that decreased vascular impedance in terms of pulsatility index exists earlier in cerebral blood vessels than in the fetal aorta or umbilical artery. These data suggest a relatively low cerebral vascular impedance which could be due to the establishment of circulatory mechanisms which ensure an adequate oxygen and glucose supply to the embryonic brain.

Our recent study showed no significant differences in blood flow in the middle cerebral arteries of fetuses in normal pregnancies and in pregnancies complicated by vaginal bleeding[11]. Results obtained suggest that Doppler studies of the middle cerebral artery in early pregnancy are unlikely to be of value in identifying cerebral hemodynamic disorders in the fetus in early pregnancy. Hemodynamic mechanisms which ensure adequate blood supply to the brain in hypoxic states probably only become active in later pregnancy.

Fetal choroid plexus blood flow

The choroid plexus is a highly vascularized tissue which bathes the exterior of the central nervous system and fills the ventricles, the four large cavities inside the brain. The choroid plexus and arachnoid membrane act together as barriers between the blood and the cerebrospinal fluid. In effect, the choroid plexus acts like a 'kidney' for the brain. It is not simply an excretory organ for creating cerebrospinal fluid: it also provides the cerebrospinal fluid with nutrients extracted from the blood. The network of the choroid plexus is characteristic, each frond consisting of capillaries and other small blood vessels surrounded by a single layer of epithelial cells[42].

The fetal choroid plexus is proportionately larger than that of an adult human and fills more of the space in the ventricles[13]. This suggests that the choroid plexus plays a major role in brain development.

From the 10th gestational week the choroid plexus is clearly visualized in the lateral ventricles of the fetal brain. Pulsed Doppler signals can be obtained at the inner edge of the lateral ventricle choroid plexuses as early as 10 weeks and 3 days[12] (Figure 12). The waveform profile is characteristic: the systolic component of blood flow within a cardiac cycle is not pronounced, and the slope from the systolic peak to the end of the cycle is very gradual. End-diastolic flow can be consistently observed from the 11th–12th gestational week. There is a significant difference between the vascular impedance of the choroid plexus and that of the middle cerebral artery. Small blood vessels surrounded by a single layer of epithelial cells, such as the choroid plexus, create low vascular impedance to blood flow, characterized by moderate systolic and relatively high end-diastolic components of blood flow.

EARLY PREGNANCY FAILURE

Early pregnancy failure is defined as a pregnancy that end spontaneously before the fetus has reached a viable gestational age. The causes of such miscarriages may be genetic, anatomical, infective, endocrine or immunological, but in the majority of cases a detailed investigation fails to identify a cause. The clinical management of these patients requires improvements and better understanding of the mechanisms underlying early pregnancy failure. One of the diagnostic tools which could provide accurate assessment of hemodynamic changes in early pregnancy is transvaginal color and pulsed Doppler.

Threatened abortion and subchorionic hematoma

Threatened abortion is characterized by vaginal bleeding and a closed cervical os with or without lower abdominal pain. Subchorionic hematoma is defined as a sonographically detected intra-uterine echo-free area located between the membranes and the uterine wall (Figure 13). Physiologically, this represents a separation of the chorionic plate from the underlying decidua with a resultant collection of blood between the chorion and the decidua. The pathophysiological basis of this event remains unclear. Table 4 demonstrates the results of 15 studies in which pregnancies with subchorionic hematoma were analyzed[14,44–58].

The incidence of subchorionic hematoma among patients presenting with a threatened abortion is quite variable, ranging from 4 to 40%. The only study in which the incidence of subchorionic hematoma at varying gestational ages was addressed documented an equal distribution of this complication in both the first and second trimester[48]. Patients presenting in the second trimester were more likely to have larger hematomas (> 30 ml). Stabile and colleagues[57] studied only patients in the first trimester and found an incidence of 8%. Interestingly, the volume of the hematomas in their patients was always less than 16 ml. These two studies suggest that subchorionic hematomas in early pregnancy tend to be smaller. It is possible that hematomas of larger volume in the first trimester end in spontaneous abortion, and thereby go unrecognized.

Of the 15 studies reviewed, four assessed the pregnancy outcome solely in patients presenting with bleeding during the first trimester[14,16,47,57]. The rate of spontaneous abortion in these patients ranged from 0 to 23%. No preterm deliveries were documented in this group. The majority of the patients studied had small hematomas (< 30 ml).

Two studies reviewed the outcome during the second trimester[48,51]. In these patients, the incidence of spontaneous abortion ranged from 0 to 11%, and the incidence of preterm delivery ranged from 16 to 25%, a rate exceeding that

Table 4 *Clinical outcome of pregnancies complicated by subchorionic hematoma (SCH)*

Author	Number of patients	Outcome of pregnancy	Comment
Abu-Yousef et al.[45]	21	7 spontaneous abortion, 3 preterm delivery, 5 severe bleeding, therapeutic abortion	large SCH associated with increased risk of poor outcome
Baxi and Pearlstone[46]	5	1 preterm delivery at 24 weeks	selected group of patients with autoantibodies
Bloch et al.[47]	31	3 spontaneous abortion, 2 preterm delivery, 26 full-term delivery,	size of SCH not related to pregnancy outcome
Borlum et al.[48]	86	19 spontaneous abortion	volume of SCH < 30 ml in 85% of the patients
Goldstein et al.[49]	10	2 spontaneous abortion	size of SCH not related to pregnancy outcome
Jouppilla[50]	33	6 spontaneous abortion 3 preterm delivery	size of SCH not related to pregnancy outcome
Mantoni and Pedersen[51]	12	2 spontaneous abortion 1 preterm delivery	large SCH associated with increased risk of poor outcome
Nyberg et al.[52]	46	3 fetal mortality 6 termination of pregnancy 12 preterm delivery	size of SCH not related to pregnancy outcome
Pedersen and Mantoni[53]	23	1 spontaneous abortion 2 preterm delivery	large SCH (> 50 ml) not associated with increased risk of poor outcome
Pedersen and Mantoni[54]	62	7 spontaneous abortion 7 preterm delivery	
Sauerbrei and Pham[55]	30	3 spontaneous abortion 4 stillbirth 7 preterm delivery	large SCH (> 60 ml) associated with increased risk of poor outcome
Spirit et al.[56]	4	2 preterm delivery 2 full-term delivery	
Stabile et al.[57]	20	0 spontaneous abortion	volume of SCH in all study patients < 16 ml
Ylostalo et al.[58]	16	5 placental abruption	median duration of pregnancy shorter in patients with a hematoma
Kurjak et al.[14]	21	3 spontaneous abortion	higher resistance index in spiral arteries on the side of hematoma

documented in control groups. These patients tended to have larger hematomas, although the number studied was small.

If the data are analyzed collectively, the incidence of spontaneous abortion was 14% for patients with a threatened abortion, a subchorionic hematoma, and a live fetus, regardless of trimester. The incidence of preterm deliveries was 12% overall.

In conclusion, small subchorionic hematomas tend to be more common in the first trimester and appear to pose no added risk to the ongoing pregnancy. Conversely, such hematomas in the second trimester are often larger and may be associated with an increased risk of preterm delivery[48,51].

Stabile and colleagues[59] were the first to investigate uteroplacental circulation in patients with threatened abortion, and found no difference between patients with poor outcome (spontaneous abortion) and patients with normal outcome. However, their study was a conventional Doppler study of blood flow in 'subplacental blood vessels just within myometrium': they could not differentiate between radial and spiral arteries. Transvaginal color Doppler, which is more precise in determination of uteroplacental blood flow, could establish some differences in hemodynamic blood flow changes in women with threatened abortion.

In our recent study[14], transvaginal color Doppler was used to investigate fetomaternal circulation in 60 women with threatened abortion and 90 women with normal intrauterine pregnancy. Resistance index (RI) and peak-systolic velocity (PSV) were measured in uteroplacental arteries (uterine, arcuate, radial and spiral artery), while pulsatility index (PI) and PSV were measured in fetal blood vessels (umbilical artery, fetal aorta and cerebral arteries). In the group with threatened abortion, 18 pregnancies were lost before term: eight ended in spontaneous abortion, six in missed abortion and four in blighted ovum. There were no significant differences in RI and PSV between normal pregnancies and threatened abortion (Figures 14 and 15). In nine of 21 women with a visible subchorionic hematoma, the RI in spiral arteries was higher than normal and the PSV was lower than normal (Figure 16). These values were obtained from the spiral arteries on the side of the hematoma and are probably a consequence of compression of the artery walls by the hematoma.

No significant differences in the PI and PSV measured in the fetal circulation were found between normal pregnancies and threatened abortion, regardless of pregnancy outcome.

Missed abortion and blighted ovum

Several studies have used transvaginal color Doppler in the assessment of blighted ovum (Figure 17) and missed abortion (Figure 18). Results of these studies are demonstrated in Table 5. Alfirevic and Kurjak analyzed blood flow in uterine and spiral arteries in cases of missed abortions and blighted ova[9]. These arteries showed a slightly lower RI compared with normal pregnancy values, although the difference failed to reach a level of significance. In pregnancies with blighted ovum and missed abortion flow could not be detected in trophoblastic vessels in two out of six and four out of six cases, respectively. Jaffe and colleagues reported RI values around and above the cutoff point value of 0.63 in cases of missed abortions and below that value in cases of blighted ova[60]. Although the calculated indices did not differ significantly from those found in normal gestation, they detected blood flow more often in spiral arteries in gestations defined as anembryonic than in those defined as missed abortions[61,62]. Although the absence of flow in missed abortions could be a secondary phenomenon, it may indicate that circulatory problems can cause this type of early pregnancy failure. However, the incidence of chromosomal abnormalities was significantly increased in the blighted ova group, indicating that such abnormalities could cause this type of pregnancy failure. Under these circumstances the trophoblast will often develop in the absence of an embryo, and the subplacental circulation is not immediately affected.

Arduini and colleagues[27] found no difference in peripheral vascular impedance between

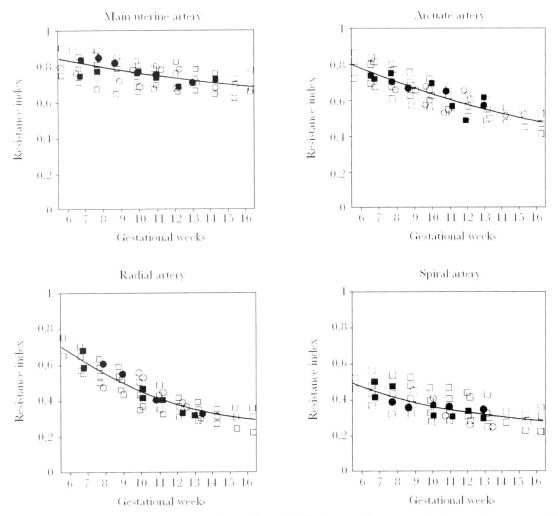

Figure 14 *Reference range of resistance indexes values (± 1 SD) for uteroplacental arteries in normal pregnancy (□), missed abortion (○), spontaneous abortion (■) and blighted ovum (●)*

normal pregnancies and those with blighted ova or missed abortions.

In the study by Kurjak and colleagues[7], RI was higher in a group of patients with blighted ovum and missed abortion than in a control group. Furthermore, in 31% of blighted ova and 26% of missed abortions no blood flow could be detected in the spiral arteries.

Predanic and Kurjak[63] studied blood flow in the spiral arteries in 12 missed abortions and eight blighted ova. There was no mean significant difference in RI between normal and abnormal pregnancies until the end of the 9th gestational week. Significant differences between normal and abnormal pregnancies were found from the 10th gestational week as follows: 10th week, $p < 0.05$; 11th week, $p < 0.05$; 12th week, $p > 0.05$; 13th week, $p > 0.05$; 14th–15th week, $p < 0.05$. Two cases of ultrasonically assessed blighted ova had early molar changes, with an RI below 1 SD of the normal pregnancy curve. In almost all missed abortions, values which were below the confidence limit of the normal pregnancy curve lasted for 3–7 weeks after the embryo's death. This indicates that in most cases of blighted ova and missed abortion

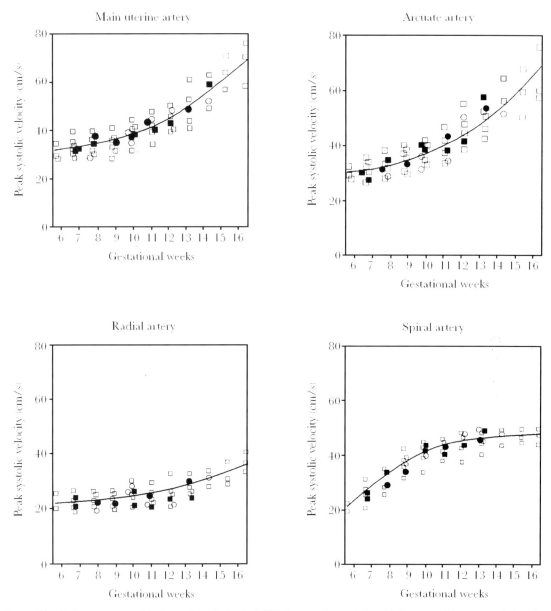

Figure 15 *Reference range of peak-systolic velocity (± 1 SD) for uteroplacental vessels in normal pregnancy (□), missed abortion (○), spontaneous abortion (■) and blighted ovum (●)*

the trophoblast continues its activity. Richly vascularized blighted ova should be followed-up after immediate evacuation.

The histological study of Schaaps and Hustin showed that an intervillous flow could be found before 12 weeks of gestation in all cases of missed abortion[64]. This finding may be a predictor for the development of spontaneous or missed abortion.

Early pregnancy associated with uterine fibroids

Uterine fibroids are known to influence hemodynamic changes in the uterine vascularization by increasing the blood flow. Uterine fibroids may also cause some blood flow changes in the uteroplacental circulation during pregnancy. We assessed hemodynamics in the

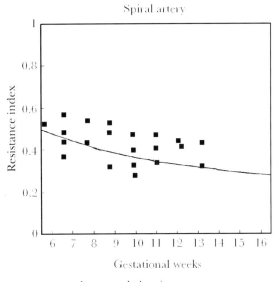

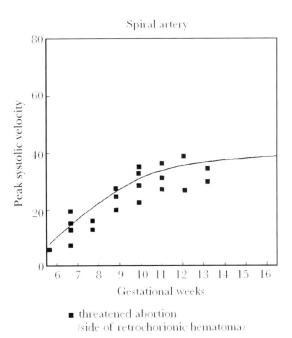

Figure 16 *Resistance index and peak-systolic velocity values (mean ± 1 SD) for spiral arteries in normal pregnancies and on the side of subchorionic hematoma*

uterine arteries and its branches, especially radial arteries (which supply uterine fibroids), in pregnant women with fibroids[6]. No significant difference in vascular impedance was found between women with uterine fibroids and those with normal pregnancy. Uterine fibroids do not influence the hemodynamics of either uteroplacental or fetoplacental circulation. The increased blood flow of the uterine vessel network (especially main arteries), due to hormonal placental and luteal body activity, disguises the subtle degree of increased flow caused by metabolism of the myoma. However, a significant difference in the blood velocity of radial arteries ($p < 0.01$, from the 10th to the 13th gestational week) was noticed. Such increased blood flow in the radial arteries supplying the myoma may be caused by higher levels of estriol, which is metabolized in the placenta[65]. This hormone directly influences the increased metabolism of fibroids cells, causing increased blood velocity in their supplying arteries.

Gestational trophoblastic disease (GTD)

Ultrasound is one of the most valuable non-invasive methods for the diagnosis of GTD. Molar pregnancy can be easily diagnosed by ultrasound with its typical snow-storm pattern, and ultrasound is felt to distinguish reliably between hydatidiform mole and gestational trophoblastic neoplasia. Other diagnostic methods, such as β-hCG level and dynamics, or even an invasive procedure such as pelvic arteriography, are performed to confirm clinical suspicion. Recently, transvaginal color Doppler ultrasound has been reported to be a useful diagnostic tool in evaluating GTD[7,8,13].

Complete or partial mole appears as prominent zones of vascularization inside the uterine cavity as well as in the peritrophoblastic area (Figure 19). These blood vessels belong to the enlarged spiral arteries.

In invasive mole and choriocarcinoma, trophoblastic invasion into myometrial tissue can be recognized as prominent color-coded zones in the myometrium (Figure 20). These zones correspond to enlarged spiral arteries as well as to newly formed vessels feeding the tumor. Since choriocarcinoma is a malignant tumor, it probably produces its own vessels, contributing to the neovascularization. All of these vessels are

Table 5 Review of Doppler findings in uteroplacental vessels in cases of missed abortions and blighted ova

Author (reference)	Number of patients	Outcome of pregnancy	Comment
Alfirevic and Kurjak[9]	6	missed abortion, blighted ovum	slightly lower resistance index than in normal pregnancies. In 2 missed abortion and 4 blighted ova blood flow in spiral arteries could not be detected
Jaffe and Warsof[61]	25 20	missed abortion blighted ovum	no difference for resistance index and S/D values between normal and abnormal pregnancies. A higher rate of blood flow detection in blighted ovum than in missed abortion.
Arduini et al.[27]	8 11	missed abortion blighted ovum	no difference in S/D and pulsatility index between normal and abnormal pregnancy
Kurjak et al.[7]	19	missed abortion blighted ovum	significantly lower resistance index in cases of missed abortion and blighted ovum compared to normal pregnancy
Predanic and Kurjak[63]	13 8	missed abortion blighted ovum	no significant difference in mean resistance index between normal and abnormal pregnancies up to the end of 9th gestational week

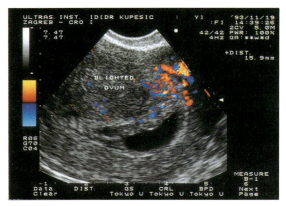

Figure 17 Blighted ovum: extensive blood flow surrounding gestational sac could correspond to early molar changes

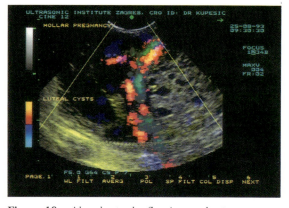

Figure 19 Abundant color flow in a molar pregnancy

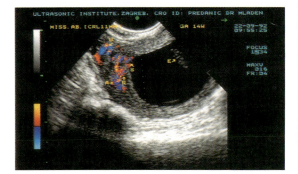

Figure 18 Missed abortion at 14 weeks' amenorrhea. Blood flow through uteroplacental vessels is visible (U, uterine artery; A, arcuate artery; R, radial artery; S, spiral artery)

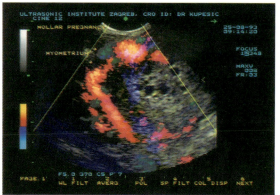

Figure 20 Abundant color flow in myometrium as a consequence of its invasion by trophoblastic tissue

characterized by a high-velocity, low-impedance blood flow pattern. Anatomical identification of the normal spiral and radial vessels is not possible in invasive mole or choriocarcinoma due to the presence of newly formed vessels.

Our own results have shown that uteroplacental blood vessels show lower impedance to blood flow in GTD than in normal pregnancy. The highest impedance is seen in complete mole; that in invasive mole is lower, and the lowest occurs in choriocarcinoma (Tables 6 and 7; Figure 21). Other authors have also found a significantly reduced vascular impedance in uterine arteries in GTD compared with normal pregnancy[62,66,67]. Shimamoto and colleagues stated that invasive mole is the best indication for color flow mapping because there are no false-negative results[68]. Hata and co-workers reported a decrease in the size of color-coded blood flow area detected by color Doppler following chemotherapy[69]. Color Doppler also allows other conditions, such as postabortal uterus and other endometrial pathologies, to be recognized, differentiating these pathological conditions from GTD[70].

Prediction of pregnancy complications

Studies have been performed on the possible predictive value of color Doppler. Arduini and colleagues studied blood flow through uterine, arcuate, spiral and umbilical arteries in 330 pregnancies at 7–16 weeks of gestation[27]. A total of 282 patients has an uneventful pregnancy outcome, 19 developed an early pregnancy failure (eight missed abortion, 11 anembryonic pregnancy) and 29 developed later complica-

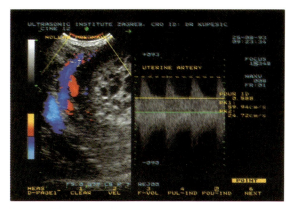

Figure 21 *Color flow imaging and flow velocity waveforms of uterine artery in molar pregnancy. Pulsed Doppler analysis shows very low resistance of blood flow (resistance index = 0.59)*

Table 6 Mean resistance index in uteroplacental blood vessels in molar pregnancy

	Uterine artery	Arcuate artery	Radial artery	Spiral artery	Tumor
Normal pregnancy ($n = 23$)	0.82	0.68	0.52	0.48	—
Hydatidiform mole ($n = 22$)	0.75	0.62	0.47	0.39	—
Gestational trophoblastic neoplasia ($n = 9$)	0.66	—	—	—	0.30

Table 7 Blood flow characteristics of the maternal circulation in normal and abnormal pregnancy[8]. Resistance index (RI) and pulsatility index (PI) ± 2 SD

	Uterine artery		Arcuate artery		Radial artery		Spiral artery	
Patients	RI	PI	RI	PI	RI	PI	RI	PI
Normal pregnancy	0.78 (0.10)	1.91 (0.61)	0.65 (0.14)	1.31 (0.47)	0.52 (0.13)	0.88 (0.34)	0.40 (0.07)	0.60 (0.11)
Molar pregnancy	0.74 (0.09)	1.64 (0.48)	0.61 (0.09)	1.12 (0.34)	0.51 (0.21)	0.77 (0.27)	0.35 (0.05)	0.54 (0.18)
Threatened abortion	0.81 (0.06)	2.13 (0.48)	0.66 (0.07)	1.43 (0.33)	0.54 (0.07)	1.22 (0.56)	0.42 (0.07)	0.52 (0.12)
Anembryonic pregnancy	0.78 (0.03)	2.21 (0.52)	0.66 (0.01)	1.82 (0.44)	0.56 (0.03)	1.28 (0.54)	0.45 (0.02)	0.64 (0.06)
Pregnancy with myoma	0.75 (0.15)	1.97 (0.76)	0.66 (0.17)	2.00 (1.54)	0.57 (0.15)	1.26 (0.63)	0.42 (0.11)	0.67 (0.47)

tions such as hypertension (10), fetal growth retardation (13) or both (6). When the results of Doppler studies of patients with early pregnancy failure or later complications were compared with those of normal pregnancies, no evident differences were found in either of the vascular areas considered.

In another study, the same authors considered 44 patients who had previously developed severe second-trimester pre-eclampsia[71]. They found no significant differences in uterine artery velocity waveforms during the menstrual cycle between women who had developed severe second-trimester pre-eclampsia and a control group. Moreover, 11 of 25 patients (44%) who had a further pregnancy again developed pre-eclampsia. In these pregnancies the S/D ratio from both uterine arteries and the presence of bilateral uterine notch were higher than in the remaining 14 patients with normal outcome. These data indicate that in selected populations with a high prevalence of pre-eclampsia, uterine artery Doppler may be useful to identify pregnancies at an increased risk of developing complications. Such pregnancies may benefit from early treatment.

SAFETY ASPECTS

The use of ultrasound for diagnostic purposes in obstetrics probably carries some risks for the developing fetus. Currently, the major concern is being expressed in the thermal effects of diagnostic ultrasound. Animal studies indicate that cell death, interruption of proliferative activity and vascular damage occur in embryonic tissues when the temperature is raised by 1.5°C. This may result in both developmental defects and abortion. The spatial peak-temporal intensity (ISPTA) is a parameter which correctly expresses thermal effect of diagnostic ultrasound. This parameter should be less than 100 mW/cm^2 if the equipment is to be used for fetal studies.

In transvaginal scanning, the transducer is placed close to the fetus. Concern has been expressed that if the same acoustic output was used with the transvaginal route as is used in the transabdominal technique, the fetus would be insonated with more energy. In general, transvaginal examinations are performed at a higher acoustic frequency and the increased absorption by tissues reduces the anticipated fetal exposure. Therefore, the *in situ* intensity is approximately the same in these two techniques. According to the recently published statement on thermal effects of diagnostic ultrasound by the World Federation for Ultrasound in Medicine and Biology[72], the possibility of any biologically significant effect in transabdominal and transvaginal gray-scale imaging is unlikely.

In pulsed Doppler examination, in contrast to gray-scale imaging where the ultrasonic beam is scanned, the beam is kept stationary to receive the signal emanating from a fixed location. The pulsed repetition rate is also increased to a value as high as is practical to allow measurement of high-velocity flow. As a result, the ISPTA is significantly higher than that used in gray-scale imaging, and in some equipment exceeds the limits quoted in the FDA document.

The recommendation of the World Federation for the use of pulsed Doppler is to use a minimum output and to keep the time for which the beam passes through any one point of tissue as short as possible[73].

The ISPTA in color Doppler is 2–10 times less than that in pulsed Doppler. Consequently, the use of color Doppler carries a significantly lower risk of heating the embryo[73].

CONCLUSION

Since the introduction of diagnostic ultrasound to obstetrics, there has been a dramatic increase in the quantity and quality of the information that can be obtained regarding the normality or abnormality of an early pregnancy. As a direct result, much of the mystique that has long surrounded the early weeks of pregnancy has been dispelled. Ultrasound is undoubtedly the most valuable ancillary aid currently available for the assessment of early pregnancy. It allows the clinician to make many diagnoses that would not be tenable with any other technique and allows him to manage his patient with a degree of assurance that would otherwise be impossible.

Although 35 years have passed since ultrasound was introduced into clinical medicine, new refinements, techniques and modalities are still being developed. The latest, and perhaps most exciting is color Doppler imaging. The greatest advantage of this technique is the recognition of blood vessels, with indications of their anatomical location plus direction and velocity of flow.

With conventional ultrasound it is often difficult to identify the same vessel reproducibly and it may be impossible to differentiate small vessels from other soft-tissue areas or fluid-filled structures. Color Doppler overcomes this because flow is displayed over the whole scanning plane, rather than in a single line of sight, as with pulsed Doppler. This technique has opened new fields in the investigation of the physiology and pathophysiology of pregnancy.

References

1. Kurjak, A., Breyer, B., Jurkovic, D., Alfirevic, Z. and Miljan, M. (1987). Color flow mapping in obstetrics. *J. Perinat. Med.* **15**, 271–81
2. Kurjak, A., Miljan, M., Jurkovic, D., Alfirevic, Z. and Zalud, I. (1989). Color Doppler in the assessment of fetomaternal circulation. *Rech. Gynecol.*, **1**, 269–73
3. Kurjak, A., Crvenkovic, G., Salihagic, A., Zalud, I. and Miljan, M. (1993). The assessment of normal early pregnancy by transvaginal color Doppler ultrasonography. *J. Clin. Ultrasound*, **21**, 3–8
4. Kurjak, A., Zudenigo, D., Funduk-Kurjak, B., Shalan, H., Predanic, M. and Sosic, A. (1993). Transvaginal color Doppler in the assessment of the uteroplacental circulation in normal early pregnancy. *J. Perinat. Med.*, **21**, 25–34
5. Kurjak, A., Kupesic, S., Predanic, M. and Salihagic, A. (1992). Transvaginal color Doppler assessment of uteroplacental circulation in normal and abnormal early pregnancy. *Early. Hum. Dev.*, **29**, 385–9
6. Kurjak, A., Predanic, M., Kupesic, S., Zudenigo, D., Matijevic, R. and Salihagic, A. (1992). Transvaginal color Doppler in the study of early normal pregnancies and pregnancies associated with uterine fibroids. *J. Maternal Fetal Invest.*, **2**, 81–3
7. Kurjak, A., Zalud, I., Salihagic, A., Crvenkovic, G. and Matijevic, R. (1991). Transvaginal color Doppler in the assessment of abnormal early pregnancy. *J. Perinat. Med.*, **19**, 155–65
8. Kurjak, A., Zalud, I., Predanic, M. and Kupesic, A. (1994). Transvaginal color and pulsed Doppler study of uterine blood flow in the first and early second trimester of pregnancy: normal vs. abnormal. *J. Ultrasound Med.*, **13**, 43–7
9. Alfirevic, Z. and Kurjak, A. (1990). Transvaginal color Doppler ultrasound in normal and abnormal early pregnancy. *J. Perinat. Med.*, **18**, 173–80
10. Kurjak, A., Zudenigo, D., Predanic, M. and Kupesic, S. (1993). Recent advances in the Doppler study of early fetomaternal circulation. *J. Perinat. Med.*, **21**, 136–40
11. Kurjak, A., Predanic, M., Kupesic-Urek, S., Salihagic, A. and Demarin, V. (1992). Transvaginal color Doppler study of middle cerebral artery blood flow in early normal and abnormal pregnancy. *Ultrasound Obstet. Gynecol.*, **2**, 424–8
12. Kurjak, A., Predanic, M. and Kupesic, S. (1994). Fetal choroid plexus vascularization assessed by transvaginal color Doppler. *J. Ultrasound Med.*, in press
13. Matijevic, R., Kurjak, A. and Shalan, H. (1992). New approach to diagnose gestational trophoblastic disease by transvaginal color Doppler. *Ultrasound Obstet. Gynecol.*, **2**, 133–7
14. Kurjak, A., Zudenigo, D., Predanic, M. and Kupesic, S. (1994). Transvaginal color Doppler assessment of the fetomaternal circulation in threatened abortion. *Fetal Diagn. Ther.*, in press
15. Fox, H. (1978). *Pathology of Placenta*. (Philadelphia: WB Saunders)
16. Ramsey, E. M. and Donner, N. W. (1980). *Placental Vasculature and Circulation*. (Stuttgart: Georg Thieme)
17. Itskovitz, J., Lindenbaum, E. S. and Brandes, J. M. (1980). Arterial anastomosis in the pregnant human uterus. *Obstet. Gynecol.*, **55**, 67–70
18. Pijnenborg, R., Dixon, G., Robertson, W. B. and Brosens, I. (1980). Trophoblastic invasion of human decidua from 8 to 18 weeks of pregnancy. *Placenta*, **1**, 3–19
19. Pijnenborg, R., Dixon, G., Robertson, W. B. and Brosens, I. (1981). The pattern of interstitial invasion of the myometrium in early human pregnancy. *Placenta*, **2**, 303–16
20. Jauniaux, E., Jurkovic, D., Delogne-Desnoek, J. and Meuris, S. (1992). Influence of human chorionic gonadotropin, oestradiol and pro-

gesterone on uteroplacental and corpus luteum blood flow in normal early pregnancy. *Hum. Reprod.*, **7**, 1467–73

21. Langman, J. (1981). Fetal membranes and placenta. In Langman, J. (ed.) *Medical Embryology*, pp. 93–4. (Baltimore/London: Williams & Wilkins)
22. Hustin, J. and Schaaps, J. P. (1987). Echographic and anatomic studies of the maternotrophoblastic border during the first trimester of pregnancy. *Am. J. Obstet. Gynecol.*, **157**, 162–8
23. Hustin, J., Schaaps, J. P. and Lambotte, R. (1988). Anatomical studies of the utero-placental vascularization in the first trimester of pregnancy. *Trophoblast Res.*, **3**, 49–60
24. Jurkovic, D., Jauniaux, E., Kurjak, A., Hustin, J., Campbell, S. and Nicolaides, K. H. (1991). Transvaginal color Doppler assessment of uteroplacental circulation in early pregnancy. *Obstet. Gynecol.*, **77**, 365–9
25. Merce, L. T., Barco, M. J. and de La Fuente, F. (1989). Doppler velocimetry measured in retrochorionic space and uterine arteries during early human pregnancies. *Acta Obstet. Gynecol. Scand.*, **68**, 603–7
26. Deutinger, J., Rudelstorfer, R. and Bernaschek, G. (1988). Vaginosonographic velocimetry of both main uterine arteries by visual vessel recognition and pulsed Doppler method during pregnancy. *Am. J. Obstet. Gynecol.*, **159**, 1072–6
27. Arduini, D., Rizzo, G. and Romanini, C. (1991). Doppler ultrasonography in early pregnancy does not predict adverse pregnancy outcome. *Ultrasound Obstet. Gynecol.*, **1**, 180–5
28. Jaffe, R. and Warsof, S. L. (1991). Transvaginal color Doppler imaging in the assessment of uteroplacental blood flow in the normal first-trimester pregnancy. *Am. J. Obstet. Gynecol.*, **164**, 781–5
29. Jauniaux, E., Jurkovic, D., Campbell, S., Kurjak, A. and Hustin, J. (1991). Investigation of placental circulations by color Doppler ultrasound. *Am. J. Obstet. Gynecol.*, **164**, 486–8
30. Den Ouden, M., Cohen-Overbeek, T. E. and Wladimiroff, J. W. (1990). Uterine and fetal umbilical artery flow velocity waveforms in normal first trimester pregnancies. *Br. J. Obstet. Gynecol.*, **97**, 716–9
31. Montenegro, N., Beires, J. and Carrera, J. M. (1994). Quantitative and combined color Doppler and hormonal assessment of first trimester hemodynamics. In Kurjak, A. (ed.) *An Atlas of Transvaginal Color Doppler* (Carnforth: Parthenon Publishing)
32. Dillon, E. H. and Taylor, K. J. W. (1993). Endovaginal pulsed and color Doppler in first-trimester pregnancy. *Ultrasound Med. Biol.*, **19**, 517–25
33. Dillon, E. H., Feyock, A. L. and Taylor, K. J. W. (1990). Pseudogestational sacs: Doppler US differentiation from normal or abnormal pregnancies. *Radiology*, **176**, 359–64
34. Altieri, L. A., Cartier, M. S., Emerson, D. S. et al. (1990). Endovaginal color flow Doppler in the early intrauterine pregnancy: Correlation with peritrophoblastic velocities, sac size, and HCG. *Radiology*, **177**, 193A
35. Arduini, D. and Rizzo, G. (1991). Umbilical artery velocity waveforms in early pregnancy: a transvaginal color Doppler study. *J. Clin. Ultrasound*, **19**, 335–9
36. Hsieh, F. J., Kuo, P. L., Ko, T. M., Chang, F. M. and Chen, H. Y. (1991). Doppler velocimetry of intraplacental fetal arteries. *Obstet. Gynecol.*, **77**, 478–82
37. Neiman, H. L. (1990). Transvaginal ultrasound embryography. *Sem. Ultrasound, CT, NMR*, **11**, 22–33
38. Birnholz, J. C. (1990). First trimester fetal arrhythmias. *Fetal Diagn. Ther.*, **8** (Suppl. 2), 6
39. Rizzo, G., Arduini, D. and Romanini, C. (1991). Fetal cardiac and extracardiac circulation in early gestation. *J. Maternal Fetal Invest.*, **1**, 73–8
40. Wladimiroff, J. W., Huisman, T. W. A. and Stewart, P. A. (1991). Cardiac Doppler flow velocities in the late first trimester fetus; a transvaginal Doppler study. *J. Am. Coll. Cardiol.*, **17**, 1357–9
41. Wladimiroff, J. W., Huisman, T. W. A. and Stewart, P. A. (1992). Intracerebral, aortic and umbilical artery flow velocity waveforms in the late first trimester fetus. *Am. J. Obstet. Gynecol.*, **166**, 46–9
42. Spector, R. and Johanson, C. E. (1989). The mammalian choroid plexus. *Sci. Am.*, **42**, 48–53
43. Achiron, R. and Achiron, A. (1991). Transvaginal ultrasonic assessment of the early fetal brain. *Ultrasound Obstet. Gynecol.*, **1**, 336–42
44. Pearlstone, M. and Baxi, L. (1993). Subchorionic hematoma: a review. *Obstet. Gynecol. Surv.*, **48**, 65–8
45. Abu-Yousef, M. M., Bleicher, J. J., Williamson, R. A. and Weiner, C. P. (1987). Subchorionic hemorrhage: sonographic diagnosis and clinical significance. *Am. J. Roentgenol.*, **149**, 737–40
46. Baxi, C. and Pearlstone, M. M. (1991). Subchorionic hematoma and the presence of autoantibodies. *Am. J. Obstet. Gynecol.*, **165**, 1423–6
47. Bloch, C., Altchek, A. and Levy-Ravetch, M. (1989). Sonography in early pregnancy: The significance of subchorionic hemorrhage. *Mt. Sinai J. Med.*, **56**, 290–5
48. Borlum, K. G., Thomsen, A., Clausen, L. and Eriksen, G. (1989). Long-term prognosis of pregnancies in women with intrauterine hematomas. *Obstet. Gynecol.*, **74**, 231–3

49. Goldstein, S. R., Subramanyam, B. R., Raghavendra, B. N., Horii, S. C. and Hilton, S. (1983). Subchorionic bleeding in threatened abortion; sonographic findings and significance. *Am. J. Roentgenol.*, **141**, 975–8
50. Joupilla, P. (1985). Clinical consequences after ultrasonic diagnosis of intrauterine hematoma in threatened abortion. *J. Clin. Ultrasound*, **13**, 107–11
51. Mantoni, M. and Pedersen, J. F. (1981). Intrauterine hematoma and ultrasonic study of threatened abortion. *Br. J. Obstet. Gynaecol.*, **88**, 47–52
52. Nyberg, D. A., Mock, L. A., Beneddeti, T. J., Dale, R. C. and Schuman, W. P. (1987). Placental abruption and placental hemorrhage: Correlation of sonographic findings with pregnancy outcome. *Radiology*, **164**, 357–61
53. Pedersen, J. F. and Mantoni, M. (1990). Large intrauterine hematoma in threatened miscarriage. Frequency and clinical consequences. *Br. J. Obstet. Gynecol.*, **97**, 75–80
54. Pedersen, J. F. and Mantoni, M. (1990). Prevalence and significance of subchorionic hemorrhage in threatened abortion: A sonographic study. *Am. J. Roentgenol.*, **154**, 535–8
55. Sauerbrei, E. E. and Pham, D. H. (1986). Placental abruption and subchorionic hemorrhage in the first half of pregnancy: US appearance and clinical outcome. *Radiology*, **160**, 109–12
56. Spirit, B. A., Kagan, E. H. and Rozanski, R. M. (1979). Abruptio placenta: Sonographic and pathologic correlation. *Am. J. Roentgenol.*, **133**, 877–90
57. Stabile, I., Campbell, S. and Grudzinskas, J. G. (1989). Threatened miscarriage and intrauterine hematomas sonographic and biochemical studies. *J. Ultrasound Med.*, **8**, 289–93
58. Ylostalo, P., Ammala, P. and Seppala, M. (1984). Intrauterine hematoma and placental protein 5 in patients with uterine bleeding during pregnancy. *Br. J. Obstet. Gynaecol.*, **91**, 353–8
59. Stabile, I., Grudzinskas, J. G. and Campbell, S. (1990). Doppler ultrasonography evaluation of abnormal pregnancies in the first trimester. *J. Clin. Ultrasound*, **18**, 497–500
60. Jaffe, R. (1992). Uteroplacental blood flow assessment in early pregnancy failure. In Jaffe, R. and Warsof, S. L. (eds.) *Color Doppler Imaging in Obstetrics and Gynecology* (New York: McGraw-Hill)
61. Jaffe, R. and Warsof, S. L. (1992). Color Doppler imaging in the assessment of uteroplacental blood flow in abnormal first trimester intrauterine pregnancies: an attempt to define etiologic mechanisms. *J. Ultrasound Med.*, **11**, 41–4
62. Jaffe, R. (1993). Investigation of abnormal first-trimester gestations by color Doppler imaging. *J. Clin. Ultrasound*, **21**, 521–6
63. Predanic, M. and Kurjak, A. (1993). Transvaginal color and pulsed Doppler in the assessment of the haemodynamic changes from blighted ova to molar pregnancy. *Fetal Diagn. Ther.*, **8** (Suppl. 2), 39
64. Schaaps, J. P. and Hustin, J. (1988). *In vivo* aspect of the maternal–trophoblastic border during the first trimester of gestation. *Trophoblast Res.*, **3**, 39–48
65. Mc Anulty, J. H., Metcalfe, J. and Veland, K. (1982). Cardiovascular disease. In Burow, G. N. and Ferris, T. F. (eds.) *Medical Complications During Pregnancy*, pp. 145–68. (New York: McGraw-Hill)
66. Long, M. G., Boultbee, J. E., Begent, R. H., Hanson, M. E. and Bagshave, K. D. (1990). Preliminary Doppler studies on the uterine artery and myometrium in trophoblastic tumors requiring chemotherapy. *Br. J. Obstet. Gynaecol.*, **97**, 686–9
67. Taylor, K. J. W., Schwartz, P. E. and Kohorn, E. I. (1987). Gestational trophoblastic neoplasia: diagnosis with Doppler US. *Radiology*, **165**, 445–8
68. Shimamoto, S., Sakuma, S., Ishigaki, T. and Makino, N. (1987). Intratumoral blood flow: evaluating with color Doppler echography. *Radiology*, **165**, 683–7
69. Aoki, S., Hata, H., Hata, K., Senoh, D., Miyako, J., Takamiya, O., Iwanari, O. and Kitao, M. (1989). Doppler color flow mapping of an invasive mole. *Gynecol. Obstet. Invest.*, **27**, 52–4
70. Achiron, R., Goldenberg, M., Lipitz, S. and Mashiach, S. (1993). Transvaginal duplex Doppler ultrasonography in bleeding patients suspected of having residual trophoblastic tissue. *Obstet. Gynecol.*, **81**, 507–11
71. Arduini, D., Rizzo, G., Pietropolli, A., Cacciatore, C., Rinaldo, D. and Romanini, C. (1993). Is it really possible to predict pregnancy complications with early uterine artery Doppler? *Fetal Diagn. Ther.*, **8** (Suppl. 2), 68
72. WFUMB Symposium on Safety and Standardisation in Medical Ultrasound (1992). *Ultrasound Med. Biol.*, **9**, V-IX
73. Kossoff, G. (1994). Ultrasonic exposures in transabdominal and transvaginal sonography. In Kurjak, A. (ed.) *An Atlas of Transvaginal Color Doppler*, (Carnforth: Parthenon Publishing)

Doppler velocimetry in monitoring fetal health during late pregnancy

K. Maršál, S. Gudmundsson and H. Stale

INTRODUCTION

The very first reports on the use of Doppler techniques for recording umbilical blood velocity[1,2] aroused hopes among clinicians of a new and more reliable method of evaluating the condition of the fetus *in utero*. Subsequent developments in the field of Doppler velocimetry in obstetrics have vindicated the early optimism. Disregarding some unrealistic expectations, the Doppler method has proved its potential as an indicator of fetal compromise in high-risk pregnancies. Several research groups have systematically evaluated the Doppler method according to general principles of evaluating clinical diagnostic tests[3]. Recently, several randomized clinical trials have been performed as a final step of evaluation. Indeed, Doppler velocimetry seems to have been evaluated better than any previous method used for fetal assessment, and the introduction of the Doppler method into clinical practice has been performed in a careful and proper way.

This does not exclude a need for further intense research in the field of Doppler velocimetry. Many questions still remain unanswered regarding the pathophysiology of fetal hemodynamic changes, interpretation of the results in clinical situations and the establishment of management protocols based on Doppler velocimetry results. The technical development of the method can be expected to continue, resulting in increased reliability. Nevertheless, it is obvious even now a properly conducted Doppler velocimetry test significantly improves the possibilities of monitoring fetal health *in utero*. We will try to support this statement by a review of the recent literature and by presenting our own experience.

BLOOD VELOCITY WAVEFORM ANALYSIS

Both the maximum velocity (the envelope of the spectrum) and the mean velocity (the weighted average Doppler shift frequency) can be estimated from the Doppler spectrum. A time-averaged mean velocity can be used, after correlation for the cosine of the insonation angle, for calculation of volume blood flow. However, this estimation is subject to several errors[4], which have led to the abandonment of flow estimation in obstetrics. In recent years, the interest of researchers and clinicians has instead turned to velocity waveform analysis. Experience of the diagnostic use of Doppler ultrasound in peripheral vessels indicated that important information on circulation might be gained by analyzing the maximum velocity waveforms[5]. Nevertheless the velocity waveform is not directly related to the blood flow. In the future, when the accuracy of estimating volume blood flow is improved, a renewal of interest in measuring flow in obstetrics is to be expected.

The velocity waveform recorded from arteries can be characterized by various indices (Figure 1), practically all of which express the degree of pulsatility of the waveform. The shape of the velocity waveform recorded from fetal arteries is dependent on several factors: heart contractility, blood viscosity, vessel wall compliance, and both proximal and distal resistance to flow. The vascular resistance peripheral to the site of measurement mainly affects the diastolic part of the velocity waveform: an increase in resistance causes a decrease in diastolic flow and, consequently, an increase in the pulsatility index (PI)[5], resistance index (RI)[6] or systolic-to-

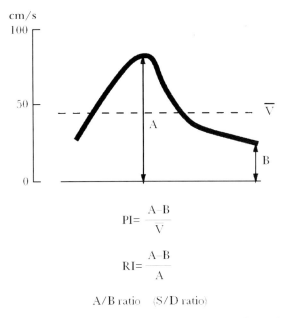

Figure 1 Velocity waveform analysis. A, systolic peak velocity; B, the least diastolic velocity; V, mean velocity over the cardiac cycle; PI, pulsatility index; RI, resistance index; S/D ratio, systolic-to-diastolic ratio

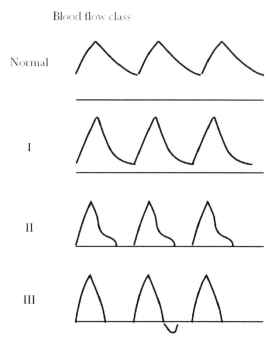

Figure 2 Blood flow classes (BFC) of the blood velocity waveforms recorded from the umbilical artery or fetal descending aorta[14]. BFC normal: positive flow throughout the heart cycle, and a normal pulsatility index (PI); BFC I: positive flow throughout the cycle, and a PI ≥ mean + 2SD of the normals; BFC II: non-detectable end-diastolic velocity; BFC III: absence of positive flow throughout the diastole and/or reverse flow in diastole

diastolic ratio (S/D ratio)[1]. It has been shown both *in vitro*[7] and *in vivo*[8] that the waveform indices reflect changes in the peripheral vascular resistance.

The various waveform indices are often comparable; however, some important differences should be considered. The S/D ratio and RI utilize only two points on the waveform and can thus be easily calculated. The PI considers the whole waveform, but its calculation is more complicated. When resistance is very high, the diastolic velocities disappear: the S/D ratio becomes infinite and thus not operational, and RI = 1.0. In such a situation the PI offers much better resolution as it reflects the area under the curve and continues to increase with the increasing degree of absent end-diastolic flow. Thus, for practical purposes, the PI is superior to the other two indices[9].

Experience from early clinical studies showed that an absent or reverse end-diastolic flow (ARED flow) in the fetal descending aorta[10,11] or umbilical artery[12,13] was associated with unfavorable fetal outcome. Therefore, the end-diastolic part of the waveform is usually qualitatively assessed and the possible absence of diastolic flow looked for. In the early 1980s the Malmö group designed a semiquantitative classification of aortic and umbilical artery waveforms, referred to as blood flow classes[14] (Figure 2). This method has proved to be a versatile and easy way of evaluating the fetal waveforms and has a very good clinical prognostic capacity[15,16]. Several reproducibility studies of waveform indices have been published; a very good reproducibility studies of waveform indices have been published: a very good reproducibility was found for the umbilical artery, in terms of both intra- and interobserver variability[17,18], the coefficients of variation being reported to be below 10%.

The velocity waveforms in fetal vessels are modulated by breathing movements; measurements taken during periods of fetal breathing are therefore unacceptable for the purpose of waveform analysis. Similarly, only periods, without fetal movements should be chosen for Doppler recordings in order to obtain representative and reproducible velocity waveforms.

Waveform indices in both maternal and fetal vessels have been found to be inversely correlated to heart rate. However, for both the fetal descending aorta and the umbilical artery this effect is not too pronounced provided the fetal heart rate is within normal limits (120–160 beats/min)[19,20]. Clinically, the most important possible error in waveform analysis is the false-positive finding of absent end-diastolic velocities. When the diastolic velocity is low, it may fall below the cut-off level of the high-pass filter, and a waveform with erroneously missing end-diastolic flow appears. The risk of this error increases with an increasing insonation angle. Therefore, a finding of missing diastolic flow should always be verified from at least two different insonation angles.

DOPPLER VELOCIMETRY IN UNCOMPLICATED PREGNANCIES

Umbilical artery

In the early first trimester, diastolic blood velocity in the umbilical artery is normally absent[21]. After 15 weeks of pregnancy, umbilical blood flow is maintained throughout diastole, reflecting the low resistance in the fetoplacental circulation (Figure 3). With increasing gestational age, the PI and S/D ratio values fall as a sign of decreasing resistance to blood flow in the placenta[20,22]. The slight variation between published reference values is probably due to differences in processing flow signals in various commercially available Doppler instruments. For the above mentioned reasons, gestational age-related reference curves of waveform indices specific for the Doppler instrument being used should be referred to. Recordings obtained by continuous or pulsed wave Doppler instruments have been compared and no differences in velocity waveforms have been observed[18].

The blood velocity signals recorded in the umbilical artery near the fetal abdomen show higher PI, RI or S/D ratio values than those recorded from the placental end of the umbilical cord[23]. The published reference curves are usually based on signals recorded from the free-floating mid-part of the cord.

Fetal descending aorta

Blood velocity can be recorded in either the thoracic or the abdominal part of the fetal descending aorta. When recording Doppler ultrasound signals from the fetal descending aorta, a duplex system combining pulsed Doppler and real-time imaging is necessary for localization of the vessel and precise sample volume positioning. Aortic velocity waveforms recorded high in the fetal thorax show a high pulsatility with a low proportion of diastolic flow; when recorded in the fetal abdominal aorta, the proportion of the diastolic flow increases. Accordingly, in normal fetuses, the pulsatility index (PI) will always be lower in the abdominal aorta than in the thoracic descending aorta[19].

In uncomplicated late gestation, the PI in the fetal descending aorta is reported to range between 1.83 and 2.49[19,24–26]. The aortic PI is stable throughout the last trimester[19,27] with a slight increase towards term[28]. This finding is contrary to that obtained in the umbilical artery and is probably due to the changes with time in the distribution of aortic blood flow affecting the total vascular impedance. The aortic PI has been reported to vary with fetal behavioral states, at least during the last 4 weeks of gestation[29]. Aortic PI is significantly lower during fetal activity than during the quiet state, and the diastolic velocity is significantly higher. This suggests

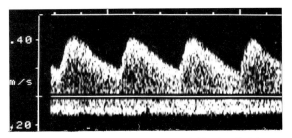

Figure 3 *Doppler shifts spectrum of blood velocities recorded from the umbilical cord of normal fetus. Upper part (above zero): umbilical artery waveforms; lower part (below zero): umbilical vein signals*

decreased peripheral vascular resistance in skeletal muscles, probably due to enhanced perfusion and increased demands on the energy supply. The umbilical artery PI is not related to fetal behavioral states[30].

Fetal renal artery

Fetal lamb kidneys receive 2–3% of the cardiac output, and renal perfusion tends to increase with advancing gestation[31]. Normal fetal renal function is a prerequisite for the maintenance of a normal amniotic fluid volume. In a study of the fetal renal artery velocity waveforms in 121 normal human fetuses Mari and colleagues[32] found the PI, and thereby the renal vascular resistance, to decrease successively towards the end of pregnancy.

Fetal femoral artery

In normal pregnancies, the velocity waveform of the fetal femoral artery changes with advancing gestation from a waveform with forward diastolic flow in the second trimester to a waveform with reverse diastolic flow at term. Consequently, the PI of the fetal femoral artery increases steadily towards term[33,34].

Fetal venous blood velocity

Research on Doppler ultrasound in perinatal medicine was initially focused on fetal or placental arterial blood velocity. More recently, studies of blood velocity in the fetal venous circulation have been reported[35–37] and found to have important clinical implications, since the blood velocity in the systemic venous circulation is a reflection of fetal heart pump function. Fetal venous blood velocity has a characteristic pulsating pattern as a reflection of fetal central venous pressure. The typical blood velocity in the inferior vena cava (IVC) is illustrated in Figure 4. The highest IVC blood velocity towards the heart occurs in ventricular systole; the second peak occurs at the onset of diastole corresponding to the early filling of the ventricles. At the end of diastole, a typical reduction in blood

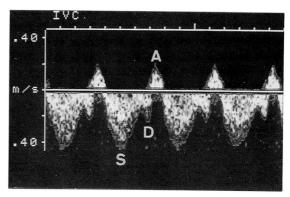

Figure 4 Blood velocity signals recorded from the inferior vena cava of a normal fetus. Velocity signals below zero: blood flow towards the heart. S, peak velocity during systole; D, peak velocity during early diastole corresponding to the opening of atrioventricular valves of the heart; A, moderate reversal of blood flow corresponding to fetal heart atrial contraction

velocities occurs, frequently with reversed blood velocities as a reflection of atrial contraction.

Reference values have been published for the IVC S/D ratio, which does not change with gestational age, the average value being 1.64 (SD, 0.27)[38]. The average proportion of reversed flow during atrial systole decreases with gestational age, being 8.2% (SD 6.2) at 20–25 weeks of gestation and 3.8% (SD 4.0) at term.

Blood velocities in the umbilical vein and portal circulation are normally continuous and without fluctuations. Modulations in blood velocity can be regularly seen during fetal breathing movements. Rhythmic end-diastolic pulsations in umbilical venous blood velocity have been recorded in normal pregnancies up to 13 weeks of gestation[39].

Uteroplacental circulation

The uteroplacental vascular tree branches from the main uterine arteries on each side of the uterus to finally end in the arcuate, radial and spiral arteries. Major morphological changes occur in the uteroplacental blood vessels during early normal pregnancy, facilitating an increase of blood flow to the uterus from about 50 ml/min to 700 ml/min at term[40,41]. Normally, the trophoblast tissue invades the spiral arteries under the placenta. The arterial vessel wall dissolves, leaving the sub-placental arteries as wide channels without contractile potential[42].

During early gestation, the relatively high vascular resistance in the uteroplacental circulation is characterized by a notch in the early diastole of the Doppler velocity waveform recorded from the uterine artery. The notch can be seen in normal pregnancies up to 26 weeks' gestation[43]. Later, the velocity waveforms form the uteroplacental circulation have a characteristic pattern, with high blood velocity during diastole as a sign of low vascular resistance (Figure 5). Arabin and colleagues[44] recorded blood velocities from different parts of the uteroplacental circulation and found that waveforms recorded under the central part of the placenta showed signs of the lowest resistance, followed by blood velocities recorded within the placenta. Blood velocities at the margin of the placenta showed a still lower resistance, followed by recordings from the uterine artery on the same side as the placenta. Signs of the highest vascular resistance were recorded in the uterine artery at the non-placental side of the uterus. This emphasizes that blood velocities should be recorded from a specific location in the uteroplacental circulation using a standard technique. For evaluation of the results, reference charts for each location should be used.

In normal pregnancy, vascular resistance to blood flow in the arcuate arteries seems to fall with gestational age[20]. The uterine artery PI or S/D ratio decreases up to 20–24 weeks of gestation[45,46]. After 24 weeks, the decline in resistance is limited and can be disregarded.

The reproducibility of Doppler signals recorded from the uteroplacental circulation using the 'blind' technique is relatively low. A much better reproducibility can be achieved when color Doppler imaging is used for localization of the main uterine arteries (Figure 6)[47].

COMPLICATED PREGNANCIES

Intrauterine growth retardation

Uteroplacental blood flow is probably the single most effective determinant of fetal growth[48]. Restricted flow through the placental vascular bed can result in intrauterine growth retardation (IUGR)[49]. In the growth-retarded fetus, the umbilical blood flow is reduced[50] and fetal blood flow is redistributed to ensure preferential blood supply to vital organs such as the brain, myocardium and adrenals[51]. The only way of finding a small fetus *in utero* before the era of ultrasound was by manual palpation or by measuring the symphysis fundus height. Ultrasound imaging allowed the abnormally small fetus to be detected, but the examination could not usually determine which small fetuses were unhealthy and needed special surveillance. All pregnancies in which IUGR was suspected were therefore usually monitored by tests that might give information on the oxygen availability to the fetal brain, such as non-stress test of fetal heart rate or a biophysical profile. Doppler velocimetry made it possible to evaluate placental vascular resistance and to detect the signs of redistribution of blood flow within the fetus. Clinical Doppler velocimetry studies in pregnancies with small-for-gestational age (SGA) fetuses have improved our understanding of the pathophysiological processes leading to IUGR and our ability to monitor fetal health.

In SGA fetuses with Doppler signs of increased vascular resistance in the placental circulation – elevated PI, RI or S/D ratio in the umbilical artery and/or uteroplacental vessels – morphological changes indicate a reduction of the fetal vessel bed in the placenta[52] and defective development of spiral arteries in the placental bed[53]. In severely growth-retarded fetuses developing signs of intrauterine distress, the end-diastolic velocity of the aortic and umbilical artery waveform disappears or even becomes reversed (corresponding to blood flow classes II and III)[10–13,54–56].

In a prospective study of 159 fetuses with suspected IUGR, the sensitivity of Doppler velocimetry in predicting IUGR was 41% for aortic PI and 57% for aortic blood flow class; in predicting fetal distress, the corresponding values were 63% and 87%[14]. In another study of 219 high-risk pregnancies, including 141 SGA fetuses, 37 of which suffered intrauterine distress, receiver operating characteristic curves showed the mean velocity of the fetal descending aorta to be the single best parameter in the prediction of adverse fetal outcome[57].

Gudmundsson and Marŝál[54] compared Doppler velocimetry of the umbilical artery and the fetal aorta with regard to their clinical predictive capacity and found that there was only a marginal difference between the two vessels. Umbilical artery velocimetry was slightly more predictive of IUGR and fetal aortic velocimetry was slightly better in identifying fetuses who subsequently developed intrauterine distress. As the Doppler signals of the umbilical artery are easier to record, this vessel seems preferable for clinical examination.

A meta-analysis of 15 published studies comprising more than 4000 pregnancies showed

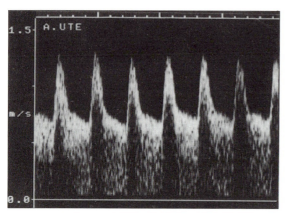

Figure 5 *Normal blood velocity waveforms recorded from the uterine artery in late pregnancy*

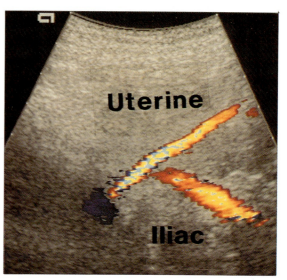

Figure 6 *Color Doppler image of the 'cross-over' of the uterine and external iliac arteries*

Table 1 Predictive capacity of the umbilical, arcuate and uterine artery Doppler velocimetry with regard to small-for-gestational age newborns

Author	Number of patients	Sensitivity (%)	Specificity (%)	Positive predictive value (%)	Negative predictive value (%)
Umbilical artery					
Fleischer et al.[62]	189	78	83	49	95
Trudinger et al.[63]	172	64	77	55	83
Gudmundsson and Marŝál[64]	129	56	84	79	65
Berkowitz et al.[65]	168	45	89	58	86
Al-Ghazali et al.[66]	71	72	87	82	79
Gaziano et al.[67]	256	79	66	79	96
Brar et al.[68]	200	91	91	54	99
Schulman et al.[69]	255	65	91	43	96
Trudinger et al.[59]	2178	91	30	76	58
Arcuate artery					
Trudinger et al.[63]	172	34	81	44	73
Al-Ghazali et al.[66]	71	34	87	69	61
Gudmundsson and Marŝál[64]	129	39	71	59	53
Chambers et al.[70]	145	29	76	66	44
Uterine artery					
Fleischer et al.[43]	71	84	77	57	93
Ducey et al.[71]	136	67	75	42	89
Kofinas et al.[72]	123	78	41	35	82

Table 2 Predictive capacity of the umbilical artery Doppler velocimetry with regard to fetal distress, defined as [a] 5-min Apgar score < 7; [b] operative delivery for fetal distress; [c] late fetal heart rate decelerations; [d] fetal distress in labor; [e] 5-min Apgar score < 7 or low arterial pH

Author	Number of patients	Sensitivity (%)	Specificity (%)	Positive predictive value (%)	Negative predictive value (%)
Trudinger et al.[63a]	172	62	79	63	79
Gudmundsson and Maršál[64b]	129	83	84	68	93
Dempster et al.[73c]	205	70	89	54	94
Brar et al. (123)[74d]	200	95	92	57	99
Maulik et al. (124)[75e]	350	79	93	83	91

Table 3 Umbilical artery blood flow class (BFC) and frequency of small-for-gestational age (SGA) newborns and operative deliveries for fetal distress (ODFD; elective Cesarean sections excluded). Based on the study by Gudmundsson and Maršál (Reference 54)

BFC	n	SGA n	SGA %	ODFD n	ODFD %
Normal	86	30	35	7	10
I	25	17	68	9	45
II–III	28	25	89	23	96

that an abnormal umbilical artery Doppler velocimetry is predictive of IUGR (overall odds ratio 8.1; 95% confidence interval 6.82–9.48)[58]. Trudinger and colleagues[59] reported a highly significant association between increasing abnormality of umbilical artery velocity waveforms in 2178 high-risk pregnancies and fetal size at birth as well as requirements for neonatal intensive care. According to the literature, the average sensitivity of umbilical artery Doppler velocimetry for prediction of SGA newborns is 71% (range 45–91%) (Table 1).

The sensitivity of umbilical artery Doppler velocimetry in predicting the need for operative delivery for fetal distress in pregnancies where IUGR was suspected was 78% (range 62–95%) (Table 2). In our series[54], 10% of fetuses in whom the blood flow velocity in the umbilical artery was normal (blood flow class 0), required operative delivery for fetal distress. This is about the same as for the general population. Nearly all fetuses (96%) in whom the end-diastolic flow was absent (blood flow classes II–III) showed signs of asphyxia at delivery (Table 3). These results are clinically important, as they suggest that Doppler examination of the umbilical artery might detect pregnancies with suspected

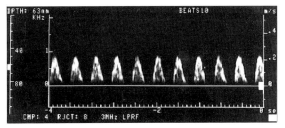

Figure 7 Umbilical artery waveforms with absent end-diastolic velocity (corresponding to blood flow class III)

IUGR in which the fetus is truly at risk for asphyxia and therefore needs special surveillance. Doppler findings seem to be better indicators of fetal health than of fetal size, which is not surprising in view of the multiplicity of determinants of fetal size. It is likely that only fetuses with IUGR of circulatory origin should be expected to be detected by umbilical artery velocimetry.

ARED flow in the umbilical artery (Figure 7) or in the fetal aorta has been shown by many authors to be associated with severe IUGR and a high risk of perinatal death (Table 4). Surviving newborns with ARED flow in utero have a significantly increased frequency of necrotizing enterocolitis[60,61], which might be secondary to severe intestinal vasoconstriction due to fetal

Table 4 Perinatal outcome in pregnancies with absent or reverse end-diastolic blood flow velocity in the umbilical artery according to literature

Author	Number of pregnancies	Perinatal deaths		Perinatal deaths excluding lethal malformations		SGA fetuses	
		n	%	n	%	n	%
Woo et al.[76]	9	8	89	7	78	not available	
Reed et al.[77]	14	6	43	2	14	11	79
Rochelsson et al.[12]	15	8	53	4	27	9	60
Johnstone et al.[78]	24	4	17	4	17	22	92
Brar and Platt[79]	12	7	58	3	25	12	100
McParland et al.[80]	37	15	41	15	41	27	73
Wenstrom et al.[81]	22	12	55	5	23	30	94
Fairlie et al.[82]	43	11	26	11	26	35	81
Mandruzzato et al.[83]	32	7	22	5	16	30	94
Thaler et al.[84]	16	5	31	5	31	13	81
Malcolm et al.[61]	19	7	37	7	37	19	100
Battaglia et al.[85]	26	14	54	13	50	not available	
Schmidt et al.[86]	50	8	16	2	4	44	88
Bell et al.[87]	20	7	35	not available		15	75
Weiss et al.[88]	47	7	15	5	11	36	77
Pattinson et al.[89]	120	63	53	not available		99	83
Arduini et al.[90]	37	14	38	14	38	37	100
Farine et al.[91]	16	9	56	not available		15	94
Valcamonico et al.[92]	31	10	32	not available		31	100
Ertan et al.[93]	93	20	22	not available		62	67
Total	683	242	35	102	25	547	83

redistribution of blood flow during chronic hypoxemia.

The interval between the occurrence of ARED flow in the umbilical artery and cardiotocographic signs of fetal distress varies according to the severity of the blood velocity abnormality and gestational age. The longer the period of absence of end-diastolic blood velocity in the umbilical artery, the sooner a pathological heart rate pattern will develop. In our studies, the median period between the finding of blood flow class III in the umbilical artery and the need for delivery due to signs of fetal asphyxia was 3 days (range 0–21 days)[14,64]. Arduini and co-workers[89] examined serially 37 fetuses with ARED flow and found this interval to be highly variable, between 1 and 26 days, depending on gestational age, presence of maternal hypertension and pulsations in the umbilical vein. These authors suggested that younger fetuses (< 29 weeks of gestation) may have lower oxygen requirements and therefore develop a longer lasting metabolic adaptation.

Analysis of blood gases in the umbilical cord blood taken via cordocentesis or *postpartum* showed that pathological umbilical artery blood velocity waveforms are associated with fetal hypoxemia[94–96]. Fetuses with ARED flow were more often hypoxemic and acidemic than fetuses with positive end-diastolic flow[97]. However, the clinical value of cordocentesis for blood gas analysis in fetuses with ARED flow has been questioned as it did not improve the outcome of the newborns[98].

Abramowicz and colleagues[99] studied 250 high-risk pregnancies and concluded that Doppler umbilical artery velocimetry is as effective as the oxytocin challenge test when applied as a secondary diagnostic test in pregnancies with a non-reactive non-stress test. A comparison of several methods used for surveillance of SGA fetuses showed Doppler velocimetry of the umbilical artery to be a better predictor of perinatal morbidity than the ultrasonically measured fetal abdominal circumference, computerized fetal heart rate variability or biophysical profile score[100]. Similar results were reported by Arduini and associates[101] for low-risk pregnancies.

The results of the studies reviewed above indicate that Doppler velocimetry of the umbilical artery and fetal descending aorta is an excellent method of differentiating between healthy and truly growth-retarded SGA fetuses, and that it may help the clinician in identifying pregnancies that need special surveillance. However, this is true only if the Doppler velocimetry is applied as a secondary diagnostic test in preselected groups of women with high-risk pregnancies[65,67,102]. A recently published review of the few available prospective studies of umbilical artery velocimetry in low-risk populations could not show umbilical Doppler velocimetry to be of any value in the prediction of fetal compromise in unselected pregnancies[103].

The results of the first studies examining velocity waveforms of arcuate and uterine arteries were not as promising as had been expected (Table 1). This was probably due to the relatively poor reproducibility of the 'blind' method of recording Doppler signals[18]. More recently, the use of the color Doppler technique for localization of the uterine artery has improved the predictive capacity of uterine artery velocimetry, which has been found to be as good as that of umbilical artery Doppler velocimetry (Hoffstaetter and colleagues, in preparation).

In a clinical context, as demonstrated above, Doppler velocimetry of the placental and aortic circulation of growth-retarded fetuses gives reliable information on the development of fetal distress, and the finding of ARED flow is accepted by many as an indication for intervention and delivery. This strategy seems to improve the outcome for the fetus when there is no risk of extreme prematurity. However, in pregnancies at a gestational age of < 30–31 weeks, the clinical decision is often difficult, especially when abnormal velocimetry has been reported to last for days or even weeks. An additional parameter is needed to facilitate the clinical management. At present, the potentials of Doppler examination of fetal vessels other than the aorta and umbilical artery are being explored. Doppler examinations of fetal cerebral arteries and the search for

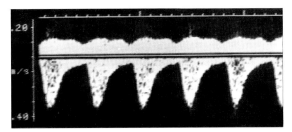

Figure 8 *Abnormal venous pulsations in the umbilical cord. Upper part (above zero): Doppler signals from the umbilical vein; lower part (below zero): pulsatile signals from the umbilical artery with low diastolic velocities*

signs of brain sparing phenomenon is discussed in Chapter 37. So far, insufficient experience has been collected to finally evaluate the potentials of fetal cerebral velocimetry.

Abnormal velocity waveforms have been reported in some studies of the renal artery of SGA fetuses[32,104]. However, the predictive value of this vessel seems to be low (Gunnarsson, personal communication). The same is also true for the fetal femoral artery[33,34], despite the fact that, hypothetically, the femoral artery would reflect vasoconstriction in the fetal body occurring as a part of redistribution of fetal flow in hypoxia.

Abnormal umbilical pulsations have been described in third-trimester fetuses with imminent asphyxia[105] (Figure 8). These venous pulsations may reflect changes in fetal heart function or they might be due to dilatation of the ductus venosus during hypoxia, thus allowing a transmission of pressure waves into the umbilical cord. In the IVC, an increased reversed blood velocity during atrial systole is probably a sign of heart failure or increased afterload. Recording venous blood velocities might be of value in deciding when to deliver the premature IUGR fetus[37].

In a recent study of fetuses with ARED flow in the umbilical artery, an association was found between abnormal end-diastolic umbilical cord venous pulsations and perinatal mortality[104]. Preliminary results from a study in a chronically instrumented fetal lamb model with experimental hypoxia maintained for 90 min have shown that the end-diastolic blood velocity in ductus venosus decreases at the onset of fetal hypoxia and abnormal venous pulsations appear in the intra-abdominal part of the umbilical vein before changes in fetal blood pH occur[105]. However, the venous and arterial blood velocities in the umbilical cord were unaffected during hypoxia. These results suggest that the brain sparing effect and abnormal pulsations in the intra-abdominal part of the umbilical vein might be early signs of fetal hypoxia. Abnormal umbilical cord venous pulsations are probably a late sign of hypoxia, indicating a poor prognosis.

Pre-eclampsia

The normal physiological trophoblast invasion of subplacental spiral arteries with their subsequent dilatation is limited in pre-eclampsia and IUGR[42]. As a consequence, the uteroplacental blood flow is reduced, as has been shown in radioisotope studies[107].

The fetoplacental circulation in pre-eclampsia has been studied by several authors and the predictive value of the blood velocity waveform with regard to perinatal outcome has been found to be similar to that described for IUGR pregnancies[26,108-111]. The uteroplacental circulation has also been examined using Doppler techniques in pre-eclampsia; however, the results were inconsistent. Studies of arcuate artery blood velocity did not find any association between the blood velocity waveform and fetal outcome[108]; this might be due to the fact that one arcuate artery represents only about 10% of the uteroplacental circulation. The blood velocity waveform in the uterine artery seems to be more predictive of outcome in pregnancies complicated by hypertension[72]. The presence of an early diastolic notch is particularly associated with adverse perinatal outcome[43] (Figure 9).

As mentioned above, abnormal uterine blood velocity waveforms are associated with an increased risk of subsequent pre-eclampsia and IUGR[111]. Doppler examination of the uterine artery might therefore play an important role in targeting a subpopulation suitable for prophylactic treatment with low-dose aspirin. Recently, several publications[113,114] have confirmed the beneficial results of the first studies on Doppler screening of the total population[111,114]. In the early publications, the sensitivity of uterine

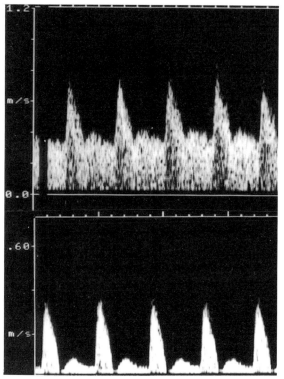

Figure 9 *Two examples of uterine artery waveforms with signs of increased vascular resistance in the uterus and placenta. Upper tracing, slight notch in early diastole; lower tracing, very pronounced diastolic notch*

artery velocimetry was only 25%[112]. By adding the color Doppler technique for vessel localization, the sensitivity for pregnancy-induced hypertension and IUGR has improved substantially, reaching 76%[112]. Abnormal uterine artery blood velocities were recorded in 16% of all pregnancies at 20 weeks of gestation, in 5.4% at 24 weeks and in 4.6% at 26 weeks. Thus, the selected group at risk is of reasonable size, allowing more intense monitoring during the subsequent course of pregnancy. However, the optimal model of Doppler velocimetry screening, subsequent follow-up and prophylactic aspirin treatment, does not seem to have been found yet.

Diabetes mellitus

In one of the very first reports on the use of Doppler techniques to monitor 40 diabetic pregnancies, we were unable to demonstrate any velocity waveform changes in the umbilical artery and fetal descending aorta specific for fetuses of diabetic mothers[116]. Intrauterine fetal distress and IUGR could be predicted from Doppler signals as in non-diabetic pregnancies. Bracero and Schulman[117] reported on a consecutive series of 54 pregnancies complicated by diabetes mellitus. They found a significantly higher prevalence of abnormal uterine artery velocity waveforms than in a non-diabetic population. The diabetic women with abnormal uterine artery Doppler results had a statistically higher incidence of poor glycemic control, chronic hypertension, polyhydramnios, vasculopathy, pre-eclampsia, Cesarean section for fetal distress, and neonatal respiratory distress syndrome. However, there were no differences in the umbilical S/D ratio between the groups with normal and abnormal uterine artery velocity waveforms.

In another cross-sectional study of 65 well-controlled diabetic pregnancies, Doppler measurements of uterine arteries, umbilical artery, fetal descending aorta, and middle cerebral artery were performed[118]. No significant abnormalities of Doppler waveform indices could be demonstrated. It was suggested that the discrepancy between the results of the two studies might be explained by the fact that the former included patients with poor control of their diabetes. In accordance with the study by Salvesen and colleagues[118], no differences in RI in the umbilical artery were found between 128 diabetic and 170 non-diabetic pregnancies[119].

Post-term pregnancy

A decrease in amniotic fluid in association with post-term pregnancy, with or without placental insufficiency, is an important risk factor for fetal morbidity and mortality[120]. The fetal renal system and renal hemodynamics play a major role in the regulation of the amniotic fluid volume. In a study of 50 normal human fetuses at or after 40 gestational weeks, Veille and colleagues[121] reported that the fetal renal artery S/D ratio was significantly higher in pregnancies with oligohydramnios than in those with a normal amniotic fluid volume. Except for contributing to the development of oligohydramnios, the reason for and the importance of this increase in the renal vascular resistance in otherwise healthy and noncompromised fetuses is not clear.

In our prospective study of 102 pregnancies past 294 gestational days with no complication other than prolongation of pregnancy, serial Doppler examinations were performed[122]. Velocity waveforms of the umbilical artery, the fetal descending aorta and common carotid artery, and the maternal uterine artery did not change. Abnormal waveforms had no significant relationship with fetal asphyxia. In another study[123], fetal heart rate monitoring, ultrasonic evaluation of the amniotic fluid volume, and Doppler velocimetry of the umbilical and uterine arteries were used prospectively for surveillance of 140 post-term pregnancies. All methods were characterized by a low sensitivity and positive predictive value regarding fetal compromise: for Doppler velocimetry the values were 17% and 29%, respectively. Used in combination and considering any one abnormal test as a positive result, the sensitivity increased to 67% and the positive predictive value to 33%. The limited value of umbilical and uterine artery Doppler velocimetry for surveillance of prolonged pregnancies was also reported from another study, in which the possible role of the cerebral–placental RI ratio was evaluated[124].

Pregnancy and autoimmune disease

Of the autoimmune diseases, systemic lupus erythematosus (SLE) holds an exceptional position because of the high rate of various fetal complications, including pre-eclampsia, prematurity, IUGR and intrauterine fetal death. In a retrospective study of 27 pregnancies in 26 women with SLE, a pathological uteroplacental and umbilical Doppler velocimetry was reported to facilitate identification of the fetuses at risk of adverse perinatal outcome. Prediction of perinatal outcome from the results of velocimetry was better than that using antiphospholipid antibodies[125]. In a study of 56 pregnant women positive for lupus anticoagulant, the finding of ARED flow predicted accurately fetal distress and delivery by Cesarean section[126]. Pregnant women with SLE treated with aspirin and glucocorticosteroids were reported to have a normal Doppler velocimetry[127].

Placental abruption

Placental abruption is not only a common cause of fetal morbidity and mortality but can also be life-threatening for the mother. Even though heavy smoking and pre-eclampsia are well known risk factors, the etiology and the pathophysiological mechanisms are still incompletely understood.

Except for occasional case reports, few studies of Doppler velocimetry for the surveillance of late pregnancies with clinical suspicion of placental abruption have been published. In a prospective study of 67 third-trimester pregnancies complicated by vaginal bleeding and suspicion of placental abruption, weekly Doppler examinations of the umbilical artery and maternal arcuate artery were performed[128]. The odds ratio for placental abruption occurring was 2 : 1 in pregnancies with an abnormally elevated PI in the arcuate artery, compared with 1 : 7 when the Doppler velocimetry was normal.

RANDOMIZED CONTROLLED TRIALS

As demonstrated above, there is a convincing body of evidence indicating that Doppler umbilical artery velocimetry is a good predictor of antenatal fetal compromise. To estimate the possible benefit of using the Doppler method in clinical management of pregnancies, randomized controlled trails should be performed. During recent years, several have been published and more are in progress.

The first randomized controlled trial evaluating Doppler velocimetry in a group of 300 high-risk pregnancies was published by Trudinger and co-workers in 1987[129]. This study showed that when the traditional methods of fetal surveillance were supplemented with umbilical artery velocimetry, the number of emergency Cesarean sections was significantly lower, the newborns stayed in the intensive care unit for a shorter time and they needed less respiratory support. This was despite the lack of any standardized management protocol based on the results of Doppler velocimetry.

So far, only a few randomized controlled trials have evaluated the use of Doppler velocimetry in a general, low-risk pregnant population. Davies and colleagues[130] recruited 2475 women into their study, and showed no improvement in obstetrical management or perinatal outcome with the use of routine Doppler ultrasound. Unexpectedly, there were more perinatal deaths in the Doppler group, a finding probably due to chance.

Johnstone and associates[131] randomized a large population of 2289 pregnant women referred for fetal monitoring to either routine methods (cardiotocography, fetal biophysical profile, ultrasound fetometry) or to undergo a Doppler examination in addition. There was no difference between the two groups with regard to fetal outcome or frequency of obstetric interventions. The results might suggest that the clinicians managing pregnancies in that study either did not consider Doppler velocimetry to be a reliable method of fetal surveillance or did not have access to the necessary information on how to interpret the Doppler results.

A different, much more positive experience was gained when Doppler examination was used in preselected and well-defined high-risk populations. McParland and Pearce[132] studied 509 pregnant women with hypertension and/or IUGR and concluded that the knowledge of Doppler waveforms had a significant effect on perinatal mortality and also decreased the length of antenatal hospitalization. Omtzigt[133] allocated women early in pregnancy to be managed according to an indicated policy either with or without Doppler velocimetry in case of complications occurring in late pregnancy. In the Doppler group, there were significantly fewer cases of intrauterine deaths; the other indicators of perinatal outcome did not differ between the groups.

Newnham and colleagues[134] examined 505 complicated pregnancies and found that Doppler velocimetry did not result in reduced neonatal morbidity, but did have a small effect on neonatal management. Among 897 pregnant women included in the study by Hofmeyr and co-workers[135] emergency Cesarean sections were less frequent in the group with fetal assessment by Doppler umbilical artery than in the group assessed by computerized fetal heart rate analysis. Surprisingly, Doppler examinations were unsuccessful in 26% of occasions. This is in strong contrast to our experience showing that trained staff succeed in more than 99% of instances in recording umbilical artery signals using 'blind' Doppler techniques similar to that used in the study by Hofmeyr and associates[135].

Almström and colleagues[136] showed, in a randomized comparison of umbilical artery velocimetry and cardiotocography for surveillance of 426 SGA fetuses, that the Doppler group had significantly fewer inductions of labor, emergency Cesarean sections for fetal distress and admissions to neonatal intensive care. The perinatal outcome was equally good in both groups, with the exception of three perinatal deaths in the cardiotocography group and none in the Doppler group. The results of this Swedish study suggest that the use of Doppler velocimetry can make the management of pregnancies with SGA fetuses more cost-effective.

It is difficult to recruit a sufficient number of patients into a randomized controlled trial to prove an effect of any new management technique on perinatal mortality. However, using the statistical technique of meta-analysis, Giles and Bisits[137] reviewed the six trials described above[129,132–136] and found that, in high-risk pregnancies, the use of Doppler ultrasound as a part of obstetrical management leads to a significant reduction in perinatal mortality in comparison with the standard management without Doppler (Figure 10). The typical odds ratio was 0.50 (95% confidence interval 0.34–0.73). The effect was mainly due to the decreased number of stillbirths. Excluding lethal congenital malformations the typical odds ratio was 0.54, 95% (confidence interval 0.32–0.89). A similar conclusion was also arrived at after a meta-analysis of the trials included by Giles and Bisits and additional six trials in press (J.P. Neilson, personal communication).

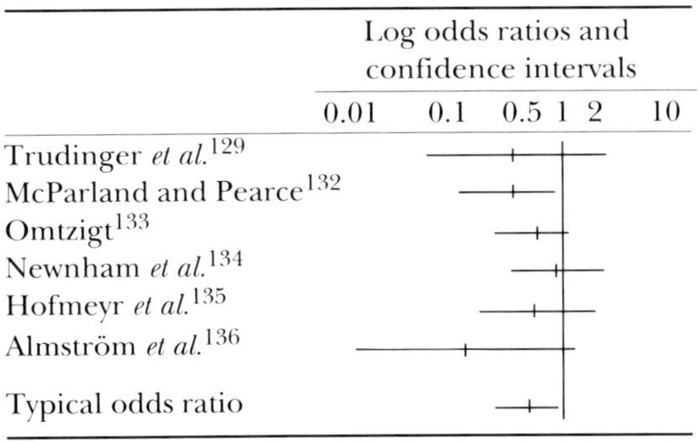

FOLLOW-UP STUDIES

The above review has demonstrated the wealth of studies evaluating the relationship between abnormal intrauterine fetal and umbilical blood flow and the short-term perinatal outcome. Only very few long-term follow-up studies have been performed so far relating the intrauterine hemodynamic situation of fetuses to their postnatal neurological development.

Ertan and colleagues[93] performed repeated neurological examinations up to 3 years of age in 30 infants who showed ARED flow in the umbilical artery *in utero*. Nine of the infants (30%) showed abnormal postnatal neurological development. In the study by Valcamonico and colleagues[92] 31 fetuses with ARED flow were followed. In accordance with other studies, the perinatal mortality was high (Table 4) and survivors had a significantly higher frequency of neurological sequelae than the matched control group at 24 months of age.

In a case-control study, Weiss and co-workers[138] followed 37 fetuses with ARED flow up to 6 months of postnatal age. Eleven of these children showed abnormal neurological symptoms, including cerebral palsy, muscular hypertonia and motor disability. Only three children in the matched control group suffered similar symptoms.

In a group of high-risk infants delivered by Cesarean section before 34 weeks of gestational age the result of cardiotocographic monitoring rather than umbilical Doppler assessment was a

	Log odds ratios and confidence intervals
	0.01 0.1 0.5 1 2 10
Trudinger et al.[129]	
McParland and Pearce[132]	
Omtzigt[133]	
Newnham et al.[134]	
Hofmeyr et al.[135]	
Almström et al.[136]	
Typical odds ratio	

Figure 10 *Effects of umbilical artery Doppler velocimetry vs. standard management on perinatal mortality in high-risk pregnancies. The meta-analysis of six randomized controlled trials was performed by Giles and Bisits*[137]

better discriminator of fetal cognitive development at 2 years of age[139].

In our follow-up study of 147 children, fetal aortic velocity waveforms correlated with the neurological and developmental performance at 7 years of age[140]. Children with an abnormal intrauterine Doppler examination had an increased frequency of minor neurological dysfunction. A logistic regression analysis showed a significant association to exist between abnormal fetal blood flow and minor neurological dysfunction, and between abnormal fetal blood flow and less favorable results of psychological tests (Ley and colleagues, in preparation).

These results suggest that the abnormal adverse fetal blood flow predicts not only perinatal outcome but also future neurological and developmental impairment. Possibly, an earlier obstetric intervention might improve the long-term outcome of fetuses and even prevent minor neurological disorders. However, before adopting this idea in practice, the hypothesis should be tested in prospective and preferably randomized studies.

SUMMARY

Doppler ultrasound velocimetry of uteroplacental, umbilical and fetal vessels provides the clinician with important information on the hemodynamics of the vascular area under study. Gestational age-related reference values have been established for various vessels, including the maternal uterine and arcuate artery, umbilical artery, fetal descending aorta, and fetal renal and femoral artery. Recently, velocimetry of the fetal venous system has gained increasing attention.

In growth-retarded fetuses and fetuses developing intrauterine distress, the umbilical artery blood velocity waveform shows characteristic changes as a result of vascular changes in the placenta. The diastolic velocity of the waveform decreases and eventually disappears. Absent or reverse end-diastolic flow (ARED flow) is associated with high risk of intrauterine demise and adverse perinatal outcome, as has been documented in a number of prospective studies. Applied as a screening test in an unselected pregnant population, umbilical artery velocimetry has not been found useful. In a preselected population of high-risk pregnancies, especially those with SGA fetuses, the method has a high predictive value with regard to diagnosing fetal compromise and can be used for monitoring fetal health. A meta-analysis of randomized clinical trials showed that including Doppler velocimetry in the management of high-risk pregnancies improves perinatal mortality. Follow-up studies, few of which have been published so far, show an association between abnormal intrauterine umbilical and/or fetal blood flow and impairment of postnatal neurological development.

References

1. FitzGerald, D. E. and Drumm, J. (1977). Non-invasive measurement of human fetal circulation using ultrasound: a new method. *Br. Med. J.*, **ii**: 1450–1
2. McCallum, W. D., Williams, C. B., Napel, S. and Diagle, R. E. (1978). Fetal blood velocity waveforms. *Am. J. Obstet. Gynecol.*, **132**, 425–9
3. Grant, A. (1985). Principles for clinical evaluation of methods of perinatal monitoring. In van Geijn, H. P. (ed.) *Perinatal Monitoring, PM 3rd Progress Report*, pp. 267–72 (Amsterdam: Commission of the European Communities)
4. Eik-Nes, S. H., Maršál, K. and Kristoffersen, K. (1984). Methodology and basic problems related to blood flow studies in the human fetus. *Ultrasound Med. Biol.*, **10**, 329–37
5. Gosling, R. G., Dunbar, G., King, D. H., Newman, D. L., Side, C. D., Woodcock, J. P., FitzGerald, D. E., Keates, J. S. and MacMillan, D. (1971). The quantitative analysis of occlusive peripheral arterial disease by a non-intrusive ultrasonic technique. *Angiology*, **22**, 52–5

6. Pourcelot, L. (1974). *Applications Cliniques de L'éxamen Doppler Transcutane*, **34**, pp. 213–40. (Paris: INSERM)
7. Legarth, J. and Thorup, E. (1989). Characteristics of Doppler blood-velocity waveforms in a cardiovascular *in vitro* model. II. The influence of peripheral resistance, perfusion pressure and blood flow. *Scand. J. Clin. Lab. Invest.*, **49**, 459–67
8. Gudmundsson, S., Eik-Nes, S., Lingman, G., Vernersson, E., Grip, A., Kristoffersen, K. and Maršál, K. (1990). Evaluation of blood flow velocity waveform in an animal model. *Echocardiography*, **7**, 647–56
9. European Association of Perinatal Medicine. (1989). *Regulation for the Use of Doppler Technology in Perinatal Medicine. Consensus of Barcelona.* (Barcelona: Instituto Dexeus)
10. Lingman, G., Laurin, J. and Maršál, K. (1986). Circulatory changes in fetuses with imminent asphyxia. *Biol. Neonate*, **49**, 66–73
11. Jouppila, P. and Kirkinen, P. (1984). Increased vascular resistance in the descending aorta of the human fetus in hypoxia. *Br. J. Obstet. Gynaecol.*, **91**, 853–6
12. Rochelson, B., Schulman, H., Farmakides, G., Bracero, L., Ducey, J., Fleischer, A., Penny, B. and Winter, D. (1987). The significance of absent end-diastolic velocity in umbilical velocity waveforms. *Am. J. Obstet. Gynecol.*, **156**, 1213–8
13. Nicolaides, K. H., Bilardo, C. M., Soothill, P. W. and Campbell, S. (1988). Absence of end diastolic frequencies in the umbilical artery: a sign of fetal hypoxia and acidosis. *Br. Med. J.*, **297**, 1026–7
14. Laurin, J., Lingman, G., Maršál, K. and Persson, P. H. (1987). Fetal blood flow in pregnancy complicated by intrauterine growth retardation. *Obstet. Gynecol.*, **69**, 895–902
15. Laurin, J., Maršál, K., Persson, P. H. and Lingman, G. (1987). Ultrasound measurement of fetal blood flow in predicting fetal outcome. *Br. J. Obstet. Gynaecol.*, **94**, 940–8
16. Gudmundsson, S. and Maršál, K. (1991). Receiver operating characteristic curves of fetal, umbilical and uteroplacental blood velocity waveforms as predictors of fetal outcome. *Zentralbl. Gynakol.*, **113**, 601–7
17. Pearce, J. M., Campbell, S., Cohen-Overbeek, T., Hackett, G., Hernandez, J. and Royston, J. P. (1988). Reference ranges and sources of variation for indices of pulsed Doppler flow velocity waveforms from the uteroplacental and fetal circulation. *Br. J. Obstet. Gynaecol.*, **95**, 248–56
18. Gudmundsson, S., Fairlie, F., Lingman, G. and Maršál, K. (1990). Recording of blood flow velocity waveforms in the uteroplacental and umbilical circulation: reproducibility study and comparison of pulsed and continuous wave Doppler ultrasonography. *J. Clin. Ultrasound*, **18**, 97–101
19. Lingman, G. and Maršál, K. (1986). Fetal central blood circulation in the third trimester of normal pregnancy. Longitudinal study. II. Aortic blood velocity waveform. *Early Hum. Dev.*, **13**, 151–9
20. Gudmundsson, S. and Maršál, K. (1988). Umbilical artery and uteroplacental blood flow velocity waveforms in normal pregnancy – a cross-sectional study. *Acta Obstet. Gynecol. Scand.*, **67**, 347–54
21. Wladimiroff, J. W., Huisman, T. W. A. and Stewart, P. A. (1991). Fetal and umbilical flow velocity waveforms between 10–16 weeks' gestation: a preliminary study. *Obstet. Gynecol.*, **78**, 812–4
22. Schulman, H., Fleischer, A., Stern, W., Farmakides, G., Jagani, N. and Blattner, P. (1984). Umbilical velocity wave ratios in human pregnancy. *Am. J. Obstet. Gynecol.*, **148**, 985–90
23. Sonesson, S-E., Fouron, J-C., Drblik, S. P., Tawile, C., Lessard, M. and Scott, A. (1993). Reference values for Doppler velocimetric indices from the fetal and placental ends of the umbilical artery during normal pregnancy. *J. Clin. Ultrasound*, **21**, 317–24
24. Griffin, D., Bilardo, K., Masini, L., Diaz-Recasens, J., Pearce, J. M., Willson, K. and Campbell, S. (1984). Doppler blood flow waveforms in the descending thoracic aorta of the human fetus. *Br. J. Obstet. Gynaecol.*, **91**, 997–1006
25. Tonge, H. M., Struijk, P. C. and Wladimiroff, J. W. (1984). Blood flow measurements in the fetal descending aorta; technique and clinics. *Clin. Cardiol.*, **7**, 323–9
26. Jouppila, P. and Kirkinen, P. (1986). Blood velocity waveforms of the fetal aorta in normal and hypertensive pregnancies. *Obstet. Gynecol.*, **67**, 856–60
27. van Vugt, J. M. G., Ruissen, C. J., Hoogland, H. J. and de Haan, J. (1988). The blood flow velocity waveform index in the fetal thoracic aorta and its ability to detect fetal compromise in the small for gestational age fetus. *Eur. J. Obstet. Gynecol. Reprod. Biol.*, **27**, 105–14
28. Ferrazi, E., Gementi, P., Belloti, M., Rodolfi, M., Peruta, S. D., Barbera, A. and Pardi, G. (1990). Doppler velocimetry: critical analysis of umbili-

cal, cerebral and aortic reference values. *Eur. J. Obstet. Gynecol. Reprod. Biol.*, **38**, 189–96

29. van Eyck, J., Wladimiroff, J. W., Noordam, M. J., Cheung, K. L., van den Wijngaard, J. A. G. W. and Prechtl, H. F. R. (1988). The blood flow velocity waveform in the fetal descending aorta; its relationship to fetal heart rate pattern, eye and body movements in normal pregnancy at 27–28 weeks of gestation. *Early Hum. Dev.*, **17**, 187–94

30. van Eyck, J., Wladimiroff, J. W., van den Wijngaard, J. A. G., Noordam, M. J. and Prechtl, H. F. R. (1987). The blood flow velocity waveform in the fetal internal carotid and umbilical artery; its relation to fetal behavioural states in normal pregnancy at 37–38 weeks. *Br. J. Obstet. Gynaecol.*, **94**, 736–41

31. Rudolph, A. M. and Heyman, M. A. (1970). Circulatory changes during growth in the fetal lamb. *Circ. Res.*, **24**, 289–99

32. Mari, G., Kirshon, B. and Abuhamad, A. (1993). Fetal renal artery flow velocity waveforms in normal pregnancies and pregnancies complicated by polyhydramnios and oligohydramnios. *Obstet. Gynecol.*, **81**, 560–4

33. Mari, G. (1991). Arterial blood flow velocity waveforms of the pelvis and lower extremities in normal and growth-retarded fetuses. *Am. J. Obstet. Gynecol.*, **165**, 143–51

34. Hadijev, C., Ishikawa, M., Sasaki, K., Sengoku, K. and Shimizu, T. (1992). Pulsatility indexes of the fetal middle cerebral, umbilical, internal iliac, and femoral arteries as predictors of intrauterine growth retardation. *J. Maternal Fetal Invest.*, **1**, 271–5

35. Gudmundsson, S., Huhta, J. C., Wood, D. C., Tulzer, G., Cohen, A. W. and Weiner, S. (1991). Venous Doppler in the fetus with non-immune hydrops. *Am. J. Obstet. Gynecol.*, **164**, 33–7

36. Reed, K. L., Appleton, C. A., Anderson, C. F., Shenker, L. and Sahn, D. J. (1990). Doppler studies of vena cava flows in human fetuses – insights into normal and abnormal cardiac physiology. *Circulation*, **81**, 498–505

37. Rizzo, G., Arduini, D. and Romanini, C. (1992). Inferior vena cava velocities in appropriate- and small for gestational age fetuses. *Am. J. Obstet. Gynecol.*, **166**, 1271–80

38. Huisman, T. W. A., Stewart, P. A. and Wladimiroff, J. W. (1991). Flow velocity waveforms in the fetal inferior vena cava during the second half of normal pregnancy. *Ultrasound Med. Biol.*, **17**, 679–82

39. Rizzo, G., Arduini, D. and Romanini, C. (1992). Umbilical vein pulsation: a physiologic finding in early gestation. *Am. J. Obstet. Gynecol.*, **167**, 675–7

40. Assali, N. S., Rauramo, L. and Peltonen, T. (1960). Measurement of uterine blood flow and uterine metabolism. *Am. J. Obstet. Gynecol.*, **79**, 86–98

41. Metcalfe, J., Romney, S. L., Ramsey, L. H., Reid, D. E. and Burvell, C. S. (1955). Estimation of uterine blood flow in normal human pregnancy at term. *J. Clin. Invest.* **34**, 1632–8

42. Sheppard, B. L. and Bonner, J. (1976). The ultrastructure of the arterial supply of the human placenta in pregnancy complicated by fetal growth retardation. *Br. J. Obstet. Gynaecol.*, **83**, 948–59

43. Fleischer, A., Schulman, H., Farmakides, G., Bracero, L., Grunfeld, L., Rochelson, B. and Koenigsberg, M. (1986). Uterine artery Doppler velocimetry in pregnant women with hypertension. *Am. J. Obstet. Gynecol.*, **154**, 806–13

44. Arabin, B., Bergmann, P. L. and Saling, E. (1987). Qualitative Analyse von Blutflusspektren uteroplazentarer Gefässe, der Nabelarterie, der fetalen Aorta und der fetalen Arteria carotis communis in normaler Schwangerschaft. *Ultraschall Klin. Prax.*, **2**, 114–9

45. Schulmann, H., Fleisher, A., Farmakides, G., Bracero, L., Rochelson, B. and Grunfeld, L. (1986). Development of uterine artery compliance in pregnancy as detected by Doppler ultrasound. *Am. J. Obstet. Gynecol.*, **155**, 1031–6

46. Oosterhof, H. and Aarnoudse, J. G. (1992). Ultrasound pulsed Doppler studies of the uteroplacental circulation: the influence of sampling site and placenta implantation. *Gynecol. Obstet. Invest.*, **33**, 75–9

47. Arduini, D., Rizzo, G., Boccolini, M. R., Romanini, C. and Mancuso, S. (1990). Functional assessment of uteroplacental and fetal circulations by means of color Doppler ultrasonography. *J. Ultrasound Med.*, **9**, 249–53

48. Wootton, R., McFayden, I. R. and Cooper, J. E. (1977). Measurement of placental blood flow in the pig and its relation to placental and fetal weight. *Biol. Neonate*, **31**, 333–9

49. Brosens, I., Dixon, H. G. and Robertson, W. B. (1977). Fetal growth retardation and the arteries of the placental bed. *Br. J. Obstet. Gynaecol.*, **84**, 656–63

50. Clapp, J. F., II, Szeto, H. H., Larrow, R., Hewitt, J., and Mann, L. I. (1980). Umbilical blood flow

response to embolization of the uterine circulation. *Am. J. Obstet. Gynecol.*, **138**, 60–7

51. Creasy, R. K., DeSwiet, M., Kahanpää, K. V., Young, W. P. and Rudolph, A. M. (1973). Pathophysiological changes in the foetal lamb with growth retardation. In Comline, K. W., Cross, G. S., Dawes, G. S. and Nathanielsz, P. W. (eds.) *Fetal and Neonatal Physiology.* Sir Joseph Bacroft Centenary Symposium, pp. 398–402. (Cambridge: University Press)
52. Giles, W. B., Trudinger, B. J. and Baird, P. J. (1985). Fetal umbilical artery flow velocity waveforms and placental resistance: pathological correlation. *Br. J. Obstet. Gynaecol.*, **92**, 31–8
53. Olofsson, P., Laurini, R. N. and Marsál, K. (1993). A high uterine artery pulsatility index reflects a defective development of placental bed spiral arteries in pregnancies complicated by hypertension and fetal growth retardation. *Eur. J. Obstet. Gynecol. Reprod. Biol.*, **49**, 161–8
54. Gudmundsson, S. and Marsál, K. (1991). Fetal aortic and umbilical artery blood velocity waveforms in prediction of fetal outcome – a comparison. *Am. J. Perinatol.*, **8**, 1–6
55. Arabin, B., Siebert, M., Jimenez, E. and Saling, E. (1988). Obstetrical characteristics of a loss of end-diastolic velocities in the fetal aorta and/or umbilical artery using Doppler ultrasound. *Gynecol. Obstet. Invest.*, **25**, 173–180
56. Illyés, M. and Gati, M. (1988). Reverse flow in the human fetal descending aorta as a sign of severe fetal asphyxia proceeding intrauterine death. *J. Clin. Ultrasound*, **16**, 403–7
57. Arabin, B., Mohnhaupt, A., Becker, R. and Weitzel, H. K. (1992). Comparison of the prognostic value of pulsed Doppler blood flow parameters to predict SGA and fetal distress. *Ultrasound Obstet. Gynecol.*, **2**, 272–8
58. Divon, M. (1992). Ultrasound and Doppler Diagnosis. Paper presented at the 2nd Congress of Ultrasound in Obstetrics and Gynecology, Bonn, June 28–July 3, 1992
59. Trudinger, B., Cook, C. M., Giles, W. B., Ng, S., Fong, E., Connelly, A. and Wilcox, W. (1991). Fetal umbilical artery velocity waveforms and subsequent neonatal outcome. *Br. J. Obstet. Gynaecol.*, **98**, 378–84
60. Hacket, G., Campbell, S., Gamsu, H., Cohen-Overbeck, T. and Pearce, J. M. F. (1987). Doppler studies in growth retarded fetuses predict neonatal death, necrotizing enterocolitis and haemorrhage. *Br. Med. J.*, **294**, 13–6
61. Malcolm, G., Ellwood, D., Devonald, K., Beilby, R. and Henderson-Smart, D. (1991). Absent or reversed end diastolic flow velocity in the umbilical artery and necrotising enterocolitis. *Arch. Dis. Childhood*, **66**, 805–7
62. Fleischer, A., Schulman, H., Farmakides, G., Bracero, L., Blattner, P. and Randolph, G. (1985). Umbilical artery velocity waveforms and intrauterine growth retardation. *Am. J. Obstet. Gynecol.*, **151**, 502–5
63. Trudinger, B. J., Giles, W. B. and Cook, C. M. (1985). Flow velocity waveforms in the maternal uteroplacental and umbilical placental circulations. *Am. J. Obstet. Gynecol.*, **152**, 155–63
64. Gudmundsson, S. and Marsál, K. (1988). Umbilical and uteroplacental blood flow velocity waveforms in pregnancies with fetal growth retardation. *Eur. J. Obstet. Gynecol. Reprod. Biol.*, **27**, 187–96
65. Berkowitz, G. S., Mehalek, K. E., Chitkara, U., Rosenberg, J., Cogswell, C. and Berkowitz, R. L. (1988). Doppler umbilical velocimetry in the prediction of adverse outcome in pregnancies at risk for intrauterine growth retardation. *Obstet. Gynecol.*, **71**, 742–6
66. Al-Ghazali, W., Chapman, M. G. and Allan, L. D. (1988). Doppler assessment of the cardiac and uteroplacental circulations in normal and complicated pregnancies. *Br. J. Obstet. Gynaecol.*, **95**, 575–80
67. Gaziano, E., Knox, G. E., Wager, G. P., Bendel, R. P., Boyce, D. J. and Olson, J. (1988). The predictability of the small-for-gestational-age infant by real-time ultrasound-derived measurements combined with pulsed Doppler umbilical artery velocimetry. *Am. J. Obstet. Gynecol.*, **158**, 1431–9
68. Brar, H. S., Medearis, A. L., DeVore, G. R. and Platt, L. D. (1988). Fetal umbilical velocimetry using continuous-wave and pulsed-wave doppler ultrasound in high-risk pregnancies: A comparison of systolic to diastolic ratios. *Obstet. Gynecol.*, **72**, 607–10
69. Schulman, H., Winter, D. and Farmakides, G. (1989). Pregnancy surveillance with Doppler velocimetry of uterine and umbilical arteries. *Am. J. Obstet. Gynecol.*, **160**, 192–6
70. Chambers, S. E., Hoskins, P. R., Haddad, N. G., Johnstone, F. D., McDicken, W. N. and Muir, B. B. (1989). A comparison of fetal abdominal circumference measurements and Doppler ultrasound in the prediction of small-for-dates babies and fetal compromise. *Br. J. Obstet. Gynaecol.*, **96**, 803–8
71. Ducey, J., Schulman, H., Farmakides, G., Rochelson, B., Bracero, L., Fleischer, A., Guzman,

E., Winter, D. and Penny, B. (1987). A classification of hypertension in pregnancy based on Doppler velocimetry. *Am. J. Obstet. Gynecol.*, **157**, 680–5

72. Kofinas, A. D., Penry, M., Simon, N. V. and Swain, M. (1992). Interrelationship and clinical significance of increased resistance in the uterine arteries in patients with hypertension or preeclampsia or both. *Am. J. Obstet. Gynecol.*, **166**, 601–6

73. Dempster, J., Mires, G. J., Taylor, D. J. and Patel, N. B. (1988). Fetal umbilical artery flow velocity waveforms: prediction of small for gestational age infants and late decelerations in labour. *Eur. J. Obstet. Gynecol. Reprod. Biol.*, **29**, 21–5

74. Brar, H. S. and Platt, L. D. (1989). Relationship of systolic/diastolic ratios from umbilical velocimetry to fetal heart rate. *Am. J. Obstet. Gynecol.*, **160**, 188–91

75. Maulik, D., Yarlagadda, P., Youngblood, J. P. and Ciston, P. (1990). The diagnostic efficacy of the umbilical arterial systolic/diastolic ratio as a screening tool: a prospective blind study. *Am. J. Obstet. Gynecol.*, **162**, 1518–25

76. Woo, J. S. K., Liang, S. T. and Lo, R. L. S. (1987). Significance of an absent or reversed end diastolic flow in Doppler umbilical artery waveforms. *J. Ultrasound Med.*, **6**, 291–7

77. Reed, K. L., Anderson, C. F. and Schenker, L. (1987). Changes in intracardiac Doppler blood flow velocities in fetuses with absent umbilical artery diastolic flow. *Am. J. Obstet. Gynecol.*, **157**, 774–9

78. Johnstone, F. D., Haddad, N. G., Hoskins, P., McDicken, W., Chambers, S. and Muir, B. (1988). Umbilical artery Doppler flow velocity waveform: the outcome of pregnancies with absent end diastolic flow. *Eur. J. Obstet. Gynecol. Reprod. Biol.*, **28**, 171–8

79. Brar, H. S. and Platt, L. D. (1988). Reverse end-diastolic flow velocity on umbilical artery velocimetry in high-risk pregnancies; an ominous finding with adverse pregnancy outcome. *Am. J. Obstet. Gynecol.*, **159**, 559–61

80. McParland, P., Steel, S. and Pearce, J. M. (1990). The clinical implications of absent or reversed end-diastolic frequencies in umbilical artery flow velocity waveforms. *Eur. J. Obstet. Gynecol. Reprod. Biol.*, **37**, 15–23

81. Wenstrom, K. D., Weiner, C. P. and Williamson, R. A. (1991). Diverse maternal and fetal pathology associated with absent diastolic flow in the umbilical artery of high-risk fetuses. *Obstet. Gynecol.*, **77**, 374–8

82. Fairlie, F. M., Moretti, M., Walker, J. J. and Sibai, B. M. (1991). Determinants of perinatal outcome in pregnancy-induced hypertension with absence of umbilical artery end-diastolic frequencies. *Am. J. Obstet. Gynecol.*, **164**, 1084–9

83. Mandruzzato, P., Bogatti, L., Fischer, L. and Gigli, C. (1991). The clinical significance of absent or reverse end-diastolic flow in the fetal aorta and umbilical artery. *Ultrasound Obstet. Gynecol.*, **1**, 192–6

84. Thaler, I., Wiener, Z., Itskovitz, J. and Brandes, J. M. (1991). Uterine blood flow patterns in patients with absent or reverse end-diastolic flow velocity in umbilical artery waveforms. *J. Maternal Fetal Invest.*, **1**, 83–6

85. Battaglia, C., Artini, P. G., Galli, P. A., D'Ambrogio, G., Droghini, F. and Genazzani, A. R. (1993). Absent or reversed end-diastolic flow in umbilical artery and severe intrauterine growth retardation. *Acta Obstet. Gynecol. Scand.*, **172**, 167–71

86. Schmidt, W., Rühle, W., Ertan, A. K., Boos, R. and Gnirs, J. (1991). Doppler-Sonographie-Perinatologische Daten bei Fällen mit enddiastolischem Block bzw. Reverse Flow. *Geburtsh. Frauenheilkd.*, **51**, 288–92

87. Bell, J. G., Ludomirsky, A., Bottalico, J. and Weiner, S. (1992). The effect of improvement of umbilical artery absent end-diastolic velocity on perinatal outcome. *Am. J. Obstet. Gynecol.*, **167**, 1015–20

88. Weiss, E., Ulrich, S. and Berle, P. (1992). Condition at birth of infants with previously absent or reverse umbilical artery end-diastolic flow velocities. *Arch. Gynecol. Obstet.*, **252**, 37–43

89. Pattinson, R. C., Odendaal, H. J. and Kirsten, G. (1993). The relationship between absent end-diastolic velocities of the umbilical artery and perinatal mortality and morbidity. *Early Hum. Dev.*, **33**, 61–9

90. Arduini, D., Rizzo, G. and Romanini, C. (1993). The development of abnormal heart rate patterns after absent end-diastolic velocity in umbilical artery: analysis of risk factors. *Am. J. Obstet. Gynecol.*, **168**, 43–50

91. Farine, D., Ryan, G., Kelly, E. N., Morrow, R. J., Laskin, C. and Ritchie, K. J. W. (1993). Absent end-diastolic flow velocity waveforms in the umbilical artery – the subsequent pregnancy. *Am. J. Obstet. Gynecol.*, **168**, 637–40

92. Valcamonico, A., Dante, L., Soregaroli, M., Frusca, T., Abrami, F., Tibertis, A. and Zucca,

S. (1992). Absent end diastolic velocity in umbilical artery and risk of neonatal brain damage. *J. Maternal Fetal Invest.*, **2**, 135
93. Ertan, A. K., Ballestrem, C. L. V., Rühle, W., Lauer, S. and Schmidt, W. (1992). Perinatal events and postpartal neurological development of children with end-diastolic zero flow in the umbilical artery and/or fetal aorta in the last trimester of pregnancy. *J. Maternal Fetal Invest.*, **2**, 132
94. Bilardo, C. M., Nicolaides, K. H. and Campbell, S. (1990). Doppler measurements of fetal and uteroplacental circulations: relationship with umbilical venosus blood gases measured at cordocentesis. *Am. J. Obstet. Gynecol.*, **162**, 115–20
95. Gudmundsson, S., Lindblad, A. and Maršál, K. (1990). Cord blood gases and absence of end-diastolic blood velocities in the umbilical artery. *Early Hum. Dev.*, **24**, 231–7
96. Weiner, C. (1990). The relationship between the umbilical artery systolic/diastolic ratio and umbilical blood gas measurements in specimens obtained by cordocentesis. *Am. J. Obstet. Gynecol.*, **162**, 1198–1202
97. Pardi, G., Cetin, I., Marxoni, A. M., Lanfranchi, A., Bozzetti, P., Ferrazzi, E., Buscaglia, M. and Battaglia, F. (1993). Diagnostic value of blood sampling in fetuses with growth retardation. *New Engl. J. Med.*, **328**, 692–6
98. Nicolini, U., Nicolaidis, P., Fisk, N. M., Vaughan, J. I., Fusi, L., Gleeson, R. and Rodeck, C. H. (1990). Limited role of fetal blood sampling in prediction of outcome in intrauterine growth retardation. *Lancet*, **2**, 768–72
99. Abramowicz, J., Warsof, S. L., Sherer, D. M., Santolaya, J., Nobles, G. and Levy, D. L. (1992). Umbilical artery Doppler velocimetry and oxytocin challenge test in nonreactive nonstress tests. *J. Maternal Fetal Invest.*, **3**, 41–5
100. Soothill, P. W., Ajayi, R. A., Campbell, S. and Nicolaides, K. H. (1993). Prediction of morbidity in small and normally grown fetuses by fetal heart rate variability, biophysical profile score and umbilical artery doppler studies. *Br. J. Obstet. Gynaecol.*, **100**, 742–5
101. Arduini, D., Rizzo, G., Soliani, A. and Romanini, C. (1991). Doppler velocimetry versus nonstress test in the antepartum monitoring of low-risk pregnancies. *J. Ultrasound Med.*, **10**, 331–5
102. Maršál, K. and Persson, P. H. (1988). Ultrasonic measurement of fetal blood velocity waveform as a second diagnostic test in screening for intrauterine growth retardation. *J. Clin. Ultrasound*, **16**, 239–44
103. Beattie, R. B., Hannah, M. E. and Dornan, J. C. (1992). Compound analysis of umbilical artery velocimetry in low-risk pregnancy. *J. Maternal Fetal Invest.*, **2**, 269–76
104. Veille, J. C. and Kanaan, C. (1989). Duplex Doppler ultrasonographic evaluation of the fetal renal artery in normal and abnormal fetuses. *Am. J. Obstet. Gynecol.*, **161**, 1502–7
105. Gudmundsson, S., Tulzer, G., Huhta, J. C. and Maršál, K. (1993). Venous Doppler velocimetry in fetuses with absent end-diastolic blood velocity in the umbilical artery. *J. Maternal Fetal Invest.*, **3**, 196
106. Gudmundsson, S., Gunnarsson, G. Ö., Hökegård, K. H., Kjellmer, I. and Maršál, K. (1993). Fetal lamb ductus venosus and umbilical venous blood velocity during hypoxia. *J. Maternal Fetal Invest.*, **3**, 197
107. Nylund, L., Lunell, N.-O., Lewander, R. and Sarby, B. (1983). Uteroplacental blood flow index in intra-uterine growth retardation of fetal or maternal origin. *Br. J. Obstet. Gynaecol.*, **90**, 16–20
108. Gudmundsson, S. and Maršál, K. (1988). Ultrasound Doppler evaluation of uteroplacental and fetoplacental circulation in pre-eclampsia. *Arch. Gynecol. Obstet.*, **243**, 199–206
109. Cameron, A. D., Nicholson, S. F., Nimrod, C. A., Harder, J. R. and Davis, D. M. (1988). Doppler waveforms in the fetal aorta and umbilical artery in patient with hypertension in pregnancy. *Am. J. Obstet. Gynecol.*, **158**, 339–45
110. Trudinger, B. J. and Cook, C. M. (1990). Doppler umbilical and uterine flow waveforms in severe pregnancy hypertension. *Br. J. Obstet. Gynaecol.*, **97**, 142–8
111. Fairlie, F. M., Moretti, M., Walker, J. J. and Sibai, B. M. (1991). Determinants of perinatal outcome in pregnancy-induced hypertension with absence of umbilical artery end-diastolic frequencies. *Am. J. Obstet. Gynecol.*, **164**, 1084–9
112. Campbell, S., Pearce, J. M. F., Hackett, G., Cohen-Overbeek, T. and Hernandez, C. (1986). Qualitative assessment of uteroplacental blood flow: early screening test for high-risk pregnancies. *Obstet. Gynecol.*, **68**, 649–53
113. Harrington, K. F., Campbell, S., Bewley, S. and Bower, S. (1991). Doppler velocimetry studies of the uterine artery in the early prediction of pre-eclampsia and intra-uterine growth retardation. *Eur. J. Obstet. Gynecol. Reprod. Biol.*, **42**, 14–20

114. Valensise, H., Bezzeccheri, V., Rizzo, G., Tranquilli, A-L., Garzetti, G. G. and Romani, C. (1993). Doppler velocimetry of the uterine artery as a screening test for gestational hypertension. *Ultrasound Obstet. Gynecol.*, **3**, 18–22
115. Steel, S. A., Pearce, J. M., McParland, P. and Chamberlain, G. V. P. (1990). Early Doppler ultrasound screening in prediction of hypertensive disorders of pregnancy. *Lancet*, **335**, 1548–51
116. Olofsson, P., Lingman, G., Sjöberg, N.-O. and Maršál, K. (1987). Ultrasonic measurement of fetal blood flow in diabetic pregnancy. *J. Perinat. Med.*, **15**, 545–53
117. Bracero, L. A. and Schulman, H. (1991). Doppler studies of the uteroplacental circulation in pregnancies complicated by diabetes. *Ultrasound Obstet. Gynecol.*, **1**, 391–4
118. Salvesen, D. R., Higueras, M. T., Mansur, C. A., Freeman, J., Brudenell, J. M. and Nicolaides, K. H. (1993). Placental and fetal Doppler velocimetry in pregnancies complicated by maternal diabetes mellitus. *Am. J. Obstet. Gynecol.*, **168**, 645–52
119. Johnstone, F. D., Steel, J. M., Haddad, N. G., Hoskins, P. R., Greer, I. A. and Chambers, S. (1992). Doppler umbilical artery flow velocity waveforms in diabetic pregnancy. *Br. J. Obstet. Gynaecol.*, **99**, 135–40
120. Leveno, K. J., Quirk, J. G. and Cunningham, F. G. (1984). Postterm pregnancy. I. Observations concerning the cause of distress. *Am. J. Obstet. Gynecol.*, **150**, 465–73
121. Veille, J-C., Penry, M. and Mueller-Heubach, E. (1993). Fetal renal pulsed Doppler waveform in prolonged pregnancies. *Am. J. Obstet. Gynecol.*, **169**, 882–4
122. Malcus, P., Maršál, K. and Persson, P. H. (1991). Fetal and uteroplacental blood flow in prolonged pregnancies. *Ultrasound Obstet. Gynecol.*, **1**, 40–5
123. Weiner, Z., Reichler, A., Zlozover, M., Mendelson, A. and Thaler, I. (1993). The value of Doppler ultrasonography in prolonged pregnancies. *Eur. J. Obstet. Gynecol. Reprod. Biol.*, **48**, 93–7
124. Brar, H. S., Horenstein, J., Medearis, A. L., Platt, L. D., Phelan, J. P. and Paul, R. H. (1989). Cerebral, umbilical, and uterine resistance using Doppler velocimetry in postterm pregnancy. *J. Ultrasound Med.*, **8**, 187–91
125. Guzman, E., Schulman, H., Bracero, L., Rochelson, B., Farmakides, G. and Coury, A. (1992). Uterine-umbilical artery Doppler velocimetry in pregnant women with systemic lupus erythematosus. *J. Ultrasound Med.*, **11**, 275–81
126. Kerslake, S., Morton, K. E., Versi, E., Buchanan, N. M. M., Khamashta, M., Baguley, E., Braude, P. and Hughes, G. R. V. (1992). Early Doppler studies in lupus pregnancy. *Am. J. Reprod. Immunol.*, **28**, 172–5
127. Weiner, Z., Lorber, M. and Blumenfeld, Z. (1992). Umbilical and uterine artery flow velocity waveforms in pregnant women with systemic lupus erythematosus treated with aspirin and glucocorticosteroids. *Am. J. Reprod. Immunol.*, **28**, 168–71
128. Malcus, P., Laurini, R. and Maršál, K. (1992). Doppler blood flow changes and placenta morphology in pregnancies with third trimester hemorrage. *Acta Obstet. Gynecol. Scand.*, **71**, 39–45
129. Trudinger, B. J., Cook, C. W., Giles, W. B., Connelly, A. and Thompson, R. S. (1987). Umbilical artery flow velocity waveforms in high-risk pregnancy. Randomised controlled trial. *Lancet*, **1**, 188–90
130. Davies, J. A., Gallivan, S. and Spencer, J. A. D. (1992). Randomised controlled trial of Doppler ultrasound screening of placental perfusion during pregnancy. *Lancet*, **340**, 1299–303
131. Johnstone, F. D., Prescott, R., Hoskins, P. R., Greer, I. A., McGlew, T. and Compton, M. (1993). The effect of introduction of umbilical Doppler recordings to obstetric practice. *Br. J. Obstet. Gynaecol.*, **100**, 733–41
132. McParland, P. and Pearce, J. M. (1988). Doppler blood flow in pregnancy. *Placenta*, **9**, 427–50
133. Omtzigt, A. W. J. (1990). Clinical value of umbilical Doppler velocimetry – a randomized controlled trial. Academic Thesis. (Utrecht: Utrecht University)
134. Newnham, J. P., O'Dea, M., Reid, K. P. and Diepeveen, D. A. (1991). Doppler flow velocity waveform analysis in high-risk pregnancies: a randomized controlled trial. *Br. J. Obstet. Gynaecol.*, **98**, 956–63
135. Hofmeyr, J. G., Pattinson, R., Buckley, D., Jennings, J. and Redman, C. W. G. (1991). Umbilical artery resistance index as a screening test for fetal well-being. II: randomized feasibility study. *Obstet. Gynecol.*, **78**, 359–62
136. Almström, H., Axelsson, O., Cnattingius, S., Ekman, G., Maesel, A., Ulmsten, U., Arström, K. and Maršál, K. (1992). Comparison of umbilical-artery velocimetry and cardiotoco-

graphy for surveillance of small-for-gestational-age fetuses. *Lancet*, **340**, 936–40

137. Giles, W. B. and Bisti, A. (1993). Clinical use of Doppler ultrasound in pregnancy: information from six randomized trials. *Fetal Diagn. Ther.*, **8**, 247–55

138. Weiss, E., Ulrich, S. and Berle, P. (1992). Blood flow velocity waveforms of the middle cerebral artery and abnormal neurological evaluations in live-born fetuses with absent or reverse end-diastolic flow velocities of the umbilical arteries. *Eur. J. Obstet. Gynecol. Reprod. Biol.*, **62**, 93–100

139. Todd, A. L., Trudinger, B. J., Cole, M. J. and Cooney, G. H. (1992). Antenatal tests of fetal welfare and development at age 2 years. *Am. J. Obstet. Gynecol.*, **167**, 66–71

140. Maršál, K. and Ley, D. (1992). Intrauterine blood flow and postnatal neurological development in growth-retarded fetuses. *Biol. Neonate*, **62**, 258–64

Cerebral circulation in the perinatal period

K. Maršál, G. Gunnarsson, D. Ley, A. Maesel and R. N. Laurini

INTRODUCTION

Results from experimental studies in fetal sheep indicate that hypoxic fetuses redistribute their blood flow and give preferential supply to the brain, myocardium and adrenals[1–3]. This redistribution of blood flow has been called the brain sparing phenomenon. The majority of perinatal brain damage in humans arises antenatally, and damage due to abnormal labor and delivery is much less common than previously believed[4]. Naturally, it is of great interest to both clinical perinatologists and fetal physiologists to study blood flow changes in the brain of human fetuses and to elucidate the pathophysiological mechanisms behind perinatal brain damage in relation to the immediate and long-term outcome of pregnancies.

For some time it has been possible to examine the cerebral hemodynamics of newborns using Doppler ultrasound. More recently, the technical development of Doppler ultrasound with colour flow imaging has enabled studies of even very small fetal vessels, such as cerebral arteries. Thus, it is now possible to evaluate the cerebral circulation *in utero*, both antenatally and during labor. As with other vessel areas in the fetus, the present Doppler technique does not allow quantitative measurement of cerebral blood flow: blood velocity waveform analysis offers only an indirect measure of the hemodynamic situation in the fetal brain. However, the information obtained is of considerable interest.

In this chapter an account will be given of the published Doppler ultrasound studies examining the cerebral circulation antenatally, during labor and immediately post-partum in healthy fetuses. Experience gained from the examination of growth-retarded fetuses and fetuses suffering from intrauterine hypoxia will also be reported. The principles of Doppler velocimetry and blood velocity waveform analysis are presented in Chapter 36.

ANTENATAL DOPPLER VELOCIMETRY OF FETAL CEREBRAL VESSELS

Normal pregnancies

Each cerebral hemisphere is supplied by anterior, middle, and posterior cerebral arteries, the first two of which arise by the division of the internal carotid artery, the posterior being the terminal branch of the basilar artery. The Circle of Willis (*circulus arteriosus*) is a seven-sided anastomosis of the main cerebral vessels completed by the short anterior communicating artery, located between the anterior cerebral arteries and, on each side, by the posterior communicating arteries connecting the internal carotid artery with the posterior cerebral arteries[5] (Figure 1).

Middle cerebral artery

Since the use of color-coded Doppler for localizing intracranial vessels became common, most investigators have chosen to study the middle cerebral artery, since this vessel is usually the most accessible major cerebral vessel *in utero* (Figure 2). A prerequisite for the successful recording of Doppler signals is that the fetal head is not too far engaged in the maternal pelvis[6]. Several authors have studied the blood flow velocity waveform in the middle cerebral artery (Figure 3). In a longitudinal study[7], no

Table 1 Regression equations of the middle cerebral artery pulsatility index (PI) in normal fetuses as a function of gestational age (GA)

Authors	Regression equation	Coefficient of determination (r^2)
Årström et al.[11]	$PI = 5.13 - 0.09 \times GA$	0.52
van den Wijngaard et al.[9]	$PI = -3.44 + 0.36 \times GA - 0.006 \times GA^2$	—
Arduini and Rizzo[8]	$PI = -0.006 + 0.144 \times GA - 0.003 \times GA^2$	0.52
Mari and Deter[10]	$PI = -1.97 + 0.327 \times GA - 0.006 \times GA^2$	0.45

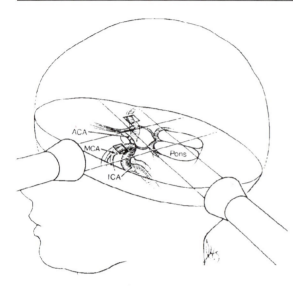

Figure 1 Drawing demonstrating anatomy and insonation by ultrasound of the middle cerebral artery (MCA). ACA, anterior cerebral artery; ICA, internal carotid artery. (Reproduced with permission from Reference 17)

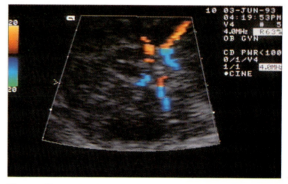

Figure 2 Color Doppler ultrasound image of fetal circle of Willis and the left and right middle cerebral and posterior cerebral arteries

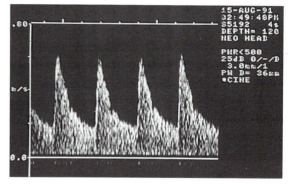

Figure 3 Doppler shift spectrum recorded from the middle cerebral artery of a healthy fetus at term

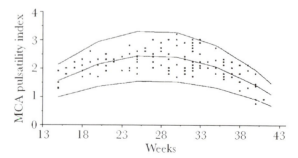

Figure 4 Reference curve of middle cerebral artery (MCA) pulsatility index based on Doppler measurements in 128 healthy fetuses. (Reproduced with permission from Reference 10)

statistically significant decrease in pulsatility index (PI) was found, although the results suggested a increase in cerebral blood flow with advancing gestational age. Arduini and Rizzo[8], van den Wijngaard and co-workers[9] and Mari and Deter[10] studied the middle cerebral artery in the second trimester and found an increasing PI until the late second trimester of pregnancy followed by a decline in the third trimester (Table 1). Only Mari and Deter[10] have proposed a theory for the rise in pulsatility in the second trimester and decline in the third trimester (Figure 4) – they attributed the low PI values at the beginning and end of pregnancy to increased metabolic requirements and therefore lower cerebral vascular impedance to blood flow. In a longitudinal study, Årström and colleagues[11] studied the fetal middle cerebral artery and found no detectable blood flow velocities in end-diastole before 28 weeks of gestation. This finding conflicts with the reports in some more recent studies and might be due to the ultrasound equipment used.

Common carotid artery

In the fetal lamb, *in vitro* examination of the contractile properties of the common carotid artery have shown that this vessel has less dilating capacity in response to hypoxia than do the middle cerebral, posterior communicating, and basilar arteries[12]. Nevertheless, in the exteriorized lamb fetus, using Doppler examination of the flow velocity waveform it has been shown that hypoxia has shown that hypoxia increases the diastolic velocity and, thereby, lowers the PI[13]. In the human fetus suffering from intrauterine growth retardation (IUGR), the ratio of the mean flow velocity in the common carotid artery and that of the fetal aorta predicted a pathological cardiotocogram with a sensitivity of 94% and a specificity of 60%[14]. In a combined cordocentesis and Doppler velocimetry study, the best predictor of asphyxia was an index comprising aortic mean velocity and the common carotid artery PI[15]. Both the common carotid artery PI and the ratio between the PI in the common carotid and in the aorta or umbilical artery have been shown to differ significantly between normal fetuses, growth- retarded fetuses and fetuses with imminent asphyxia[16].

Anterior cerebral artery and posterior cerebral artery

Both the anterior and posterior cerebral artery show a fall in PI in the third trimester of pregnancy. In a study of a relatively small number of subjects, fetuses with IUGR showed a decrease in PI in both these arteries when compared to normal fetuses[9]. The PI of the proximal anterior cerebral artery has been shown to be significantly different from that in the internal carotid artery[17]. This underlines the necessity of knowing exactly which vessel is being insonated.

Intrauterine growth retardation and fetal hypoxia

In accord with previous results obtained in animal fetuses demonstrating a preferential blood supply to the brain in hypoxia[1–3], a change was observed in the waveform of velocities recorded using Doppler ultrasound from the middle cerebral artery of chronically instrumented lamb fetuses during experimental hypoxia (Figure 5a and 5b).

The flow velocity waveforms in the middle cerebral artery of fetuses with IUGR have been studied by several authors[9,10,18–24]. Vyas and colleagues[25] performed Doppler velocimetry and cordocentesis in 81 small-for-gestational age (SGA) fetuses and found a significant relationship between fetal hypoxemia and the degree of reduction in the middle cerebral artery PI. The maximum reduction in PI was reached when the

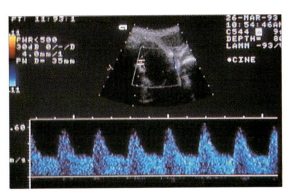 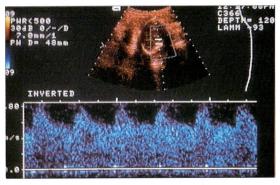

Figure 5 *(a) Doppler shift spectrum recorded from the middle cerebral artery of a normoxemic lamb fetus. (b) Doppler shift spectrum recorded from the middle cerebral artery of a lamb fetus during experimental hypoxia. Observe the pronounced increase in the diastolic flow velocities as an expression of the redistribution of flow (brain sparing phenomenon)*

fetal pO_2 was 2–4 SD below the gestational age-related mean of the normal population. When the oxygen deficit was greater, there was a tendency for the PI to rise. In the study by Arduini and associates[19], a nadir of vasodilatation in fetal cerebral arteries was reached 2 weeks before the onset of antepartum late fetal heart rate (FHR) decelerations, whereas significant changes in the peripheral and umbilical vessel PI occurred close to the onset of abnormal FHR patterns. Mari and Deter[10] found that the SGA fetus with a normal middle cerebral artery PI was at lower risk than the fetus with abnormal PI values. In another comparative study[23], hypoxemia at delivery appeared to be indicated better by fetal middle cerebral artery flow velocity waveform than by FHR analysis. However, the specificity of the method was low. Favre and colleagues[24] found that fetal cerebral velocimetry showed a poor sensitivity and a low positive predictive value for prediction of IUGR and fetal acidosis. In an attempt to improve the diagnostic accuracy, some authors have studied the ratio between Doppler waveform indices in the fetal middle cerebral artery and umbilical artery. Gramellini and co-workers[21] reported the diagnostic accuracy [(true positives + true negatives)/total number of cases] in predicting adverse perinatal outcome for the cerebral–umbilical ratio to be 90%, compared with 79% for the middle cerebral artery and 83% for the umbilical artery. These results, although encouraging, await confirmation.

The internal carotid artery has also been studied in fetuses with IUGR[9,19,26–32]. Arduini and associates[27] used fetal cerebral Doppler ultrasonography as a screening tool at 26–28 weeks' gestation in high-risk pregnancies and found the ratio between PI of the umbilical artery and the internal carotid artery to be an accurate predictor of growth retardation (specificity 92%; sensitivity 78%; positive predictive value 82%; negative predictive value 90%; accuracy 88%). In the study by McCowan and Duggan[29] on 28 SGA fetuses, there was a highly significant association between an abnormal internal carotid waveform and a poor outcome; this was particularly pronounced at a gestational age of less than 34 weeks, when the sensitivity, specificity and predictive values were all 100%. The authors pointed out that whether or not this information should be used clinically is not clear, as the abnormal umbilical and internal carotid waveforms were sometimes present for weeks before delivery was required for fetal indications. In a study of 44 cases of IUGR with eight perinatal deaths, Wladimiroff and colleagues[32] found no correlation between the indicators of fetal well-being (Apgar score at 1 min, FHR patterns, umbilical arterial pH) and the internal carotid artery PI.

Fetal hydrocephaly

Blood flow velocity waveforms in the internal carotid artery have been studied in fetuses with hydrocephaly. Degani and co-workers[33] described four fetuses with hydrocephalus diagnosed at 24–33 weeks of gestation. The velocimetry results showed an inverse relationship with the degree of ventriculomegaly in all four fetuses. A sharp decrease and later a total cessation of blood flow during diastole was observed. Three of the four pregnancies were electively terminated; no neurological follow-up on the surviving infant was presented. Van den Wijngaard and associates[34] presented data on nine fetuses with bilateral symmetrical hydrocephalus and four with unilateral hydrocephalus. An elevated internal carotid artery PI was demonstrated in five cases. The fetal outcome was poor: only one infant seemed to be developing normally at 1 year of age. There was no relationship between PI and fetal outcome. Finally, Kirkinen and colleagues[35] studied flow velocity waveforms from the internal carotid artery in nine hydrocephalic fetuses during the second or third trimester of pregnancy. Normal, increased, and decreased waveform indices were found in these cases; one of the fetuses presented retrograde diastolic flow. Cerebral blood flow patterns in hydrocephalic fetuses therefore seem to vary from case to case, presenting no typical changes in late pregnancy. There was no obvious correlation between the degree of ventricular dilatation and the velocity waveform. The published cases do not justify any definitive conclusions about the prognostic significance of cerebral blood flow measurements in fetuses with hydrocephaly. For assessment of prognosis, the most important factor is the presence of other malformations which may be associated with the cerebral abnormalities[35].

Other complications of pregnancy

Mari and co-workers[36] described flow velocity waveforms in the middle cerebral artery of fetuses before and after amniotic fluid decompression in pregnancies complicated by symptomatic polyhydramnios. After amniocentesis, the PI of the middle cerebral artery was reduced in all fetuses. The authors concluded that the impact of acute amniotic fluid decompression on the fetal circulation, as reflected in the marked PI changes, suggests a possible role of cerebral velocimetry in avoiding large acute changes in pressure during therapeutic amniocentesis.

Ben-Chetrit and colleagues[37] diagnosed antenatally a posterior fossa subdural hematoma in a fetus at 30 weeks of gestation. Doppler velocimetry studies of the middle cerebral artery at that time showed an abnormally high resistance pattern with reverse end-diastolic flow. Ultrasonic assessment of the fetus indicated associated quadriplegia. No cause for the lesion was demonstrated antenatally or at pathological examination postpartum. In the authors' opinion, this case demonstrates the advantage of the determination of cerebral blood flow in fetuses with suspected high intracranial pressure.

Two reports on the terminal patterns of the fetal cerebral blood velocity have been published. Chandran and associates[38] followed a woman with proteinuric pre-eclampsia superimposed on essential hypertension and IUGR diagnosed at 22 weeks of gestation. Starting 14 days before fetal death, the middle cerebral artery was examined on four occasions. A progressive fall in PI was followed by an increase registered 12 h before fetal death. Mari and Wasserstrum[39] reported a similar increase in the middle cerebral PI preceeding fetal death in a pregnant woman with lupus anticoagulant. Preterminal brain edema has been suggested as the underlying cause of this phenomenon[25].

FETAL CEREBRAL VELOCIMETRY DURING LABOR

Fetal cerebral blood flow has been less studied during labor than during the antenatal and neonatal periods. This is partly due to the practical and ethical problems involved in performing Doppler measurements in labor. For the same reason, most human studies during labor describe normal physiological changes.

Uterine contractions, molding of the skull and metabolic changes during labor are factors that might influence fetal cerebral blood flow. Uterine contractions reduce the blood flow velocities in uterine vessels[40-42]. However, the umbilical circulation seems to remain unaffected by the contractions[40,41,43,44]. An experimental animal study has shown that external mechanical compression of the fetal skull leads to a reduction in cerebral blood flow followed by a redistribution of flow with preferential supply to the brain stem[45]. In humans, pressure applied to the maternal abdomen increases vascular resistance in fetal cerebral vessels[46]. Clinical Doppler studies of fetal cerebral circulation in labor have given very varying results. One possible explanation for this is the difficulty in controlling the intensity of uterine contractions. These might have a more pronounced effect on the fetal cerebral circulation in the active phase of labor than in the earlier stage of labor.

For anatomical reasons, i.e., the fetal skull being located behind the symphysis of the mother, transabdominal measurement of fetal cerebral blood flow velocity is difficult to perform during the second stage of labor. The transvaginal approach might be a solution to this problem.

Several published studies have compared fetal cerebral PI values during and between contractions. An increase in vascular resistance was described during uterine contractions in the fetal internal carotid artery[47] and in the anterior cerebral artery[48]. However, other authors found no difference in the anterior cerebral artery[49] and in the middle cerebral artery[50]. An interesting finding in the study by Yagel and co-workers[51] was a reduction of 40% in the vascular resistance in the fetal middle cerebral artery during labor. The authors speculated that this was a protective process aimed at preventing fetal cerebral hypoxia. This finding was further supported by a study demonstrating an increase in fetal aortic blood flow with progress of labor[52].

During normal vaginal delivery, at the moment of birth, decompression of the fetal skull occurs. At this moment, very high cerebral blood flow velocity and low resistance values are found in the middle cerebral artery, suggesting a high cerebral blood flow[53]. In a study of infants delivered by Cesarean section, Ipsiroglu and colleagues[54], reported the highest blood velocities among infants for whom the obstetrician had difficulties in delivering the head.

The mode of delivery is known to influence various neonatal parameters, most of which reflect stress occurring during vaginal delivery. Levels of catecholamines are lower in babies delivered by elective Cesarean section than in those delivered vaginally[55]. The body temperature of newborn infants is also lower after Cesarean section[56]. The mode of delivery does not seem to influence the cerebral blood flow velocity in healthy term newborns as shown by Shuto and co-workers[57] and in our own study comparing blood flow velocity in the middle cerebral artery after vaginal and after elective Cesarean section (Maesel *et al.*, in preparation).

NEONATAL CEREBRAL CIRCULATION

Considerable interest has been paid to neonatal cerebral hemodynamics, as changes in cerebral blood flow have been hypothesized to cause several major types of perinatal brain damage[58].

Physiological regulation

The physiological regulation of cerebral blood flow has been studied using a variety of methods. Two major determinants of cerebral blood flow are perfusion pressure and cerebral metabolic rate. An increase in cerebral metabolism induces an increase in blood flow. Using ^{133}Xe clearance after intravenous injection in preterm infants, Greisen and colleagues[59] found increased cerebral blood flow in the awake state compared with the state of quiet or active sleep.

The ability of the brain to maintain a constant perfusion over a range of varying perfusion pressures is known as cerebral autoregulation. Several studies have demonstrated such autoregulation in newborn experimental animals[60], and the autoregulative capacity has been shown to be disturbed in hypoxic human neonates[61]. Using intra-arterial ^{133}Xe clearance, the cerebral blood flow was found to vary in proportion to systolic blood pressure in stressed newborn infants.

Carbon dioxide is a potent cerebral vasodilator in both preterm[62] and term newborn infants[63]. Small changes in arterial carbon dioxide tension result in changes in cerebral blood flow. Severe hypercarbia will decrease cerebrovascular resistance, increase transmural pressure in the capillary bed and possibly increase the risk of germinal matrix hemorrhage. Severe hyperventilation causing hypocarbia has been suggested to induce cerebral ischemia, resulting in periventricular leukomalacia in preterm infants.

Postnatal cerebral hemodynamic adaptation

The Doppler technique has enabled studies of immediate postnatal cerebral hemodynamic adaptation in human newborns. Head compression and the following decompression of the skull at the moment of birth might influence cerebral blood flow. During the first minutes of life high cerebral blood flow velocities have been recorded[53]. Moreover, a pronounced beat-to-beat variability in this parameter, related to breathing movements, has been observed. In healthy term infants, the variability caused by respiration seems to decrease with increasing postnatal age.

Within the first hours after birth, a significant fall in cerebral blood flow velocity can be observed[64]: this can be mainly explained by blood gas changes, i.e., a fall in pCO_2 and a rise in pO_2. After the initial fall in central blood flow volume, a subsequent increase has been observed during the first weeks of life. The available data suggest that cerebral blood flow increases with gestational age and postnatal age. Doppler studies have suggested a linear increase in cerebral blood flow velocity with increasing postnatal age[65,66]. The physiological closure of the ductus arteriosus and the successive rise in blood pressure are, at least partly, involved in this observed increase.

Perinatal asphyxia

Perinatal asphyxia often results in a combination of changes in blood gases and perfusion. In the initial stage of asphyxia cerebral blood flow is increased[67]; longer lasting asphyxia will produce a decrease. The local distribution of cerebral perfusion appears to be crucial, as the watershed areas between the major cerebral arteries suffer most from a global decrease in cerebral blood flow. Several Doppler studies have shown a low resistance index (RI) in perinatal asphyxia[68,69]. A normal RI was found to be a very sensitive and specific marker of good outcome in infants with postasphyxial encephalopathy[70].

IUGR and neonatal cerebral blood flow

Studies of fetal blood circulation in pregnancies complicated by IUGR have shown signs of a decreased cerebrovascular resistance, probably as a compensatory mechanism for fetal hypoxia (see above). Several studies of SGA neonates have found a decrease in cerebral vascular resistance indices during the first days of postnatal life, suggesting that the fetal brain sparing effect persists into the neonatal period[71,72].

Neonatal cerebral blood flow in various clinical situations

Respiratory distress may affect cerebral blood flow through blood gas changes, systemic hypotension or increased intrathoracic pressure. Artificial ventilation has been associated with a significant decrease in cerebral blood flow in preterm infants[73]. An exaggerated fluctuation in cerebral blood flow velocity was reported by Perlman and colleagues[74] in ventilated babies with respiratory distress and was suggested as a marker of an increased risk of germinal matrix and intraventricular hemorrhage.

The Doppler method, being non-invasive and easily applicable, has been used in studies of cerebral circulation in neonates with apnea and bradycardia[75], seizures[76], endotracheal tube suction[77], and pneumothorax[78]. The observed changes in cerebral Doppler indices were found to reflect changes in blood pressure. Abnormally high RI have been found in infants with hydrocephalus, returning to normal values after drainage[79,80].

A patent ductus arteriosus influences the Doppler waveform in major cerebral arteries, causing an increase in RI[81,82]. Closure of the ductus arteriosus by indomethacin is associated with an increase in RI and a decrease in mean cerebral blood flow velocity[83,84], probably reflecting a reduction in cerebral blood flow induced by the vasoactive effects of the drug. Surgical ligation of the ductus arteriosus causes major changes of the Doppler waveform in the opposite direction to that of indomethacin.

Evaluation of CBF in neonates is an important research tool. However, it has yet not proved to benefit the clinical management.

FUNCTIONAL CEREBRAL VASCULAR MORPHOLOGY

The new non-invasive techniques of modern fetal surveillance allow various fetal functions to be registered. Real-time ultrasound imaging enables studies of fetal behavioral patterns and Doppler ultrasound allows recording of fetal and placental hemodynamics. Hence the morphological findings of the fetus and placenta can be related to both intrauterine structure and function. This dynamic rendering is defined as functional morphology[85].

This concept is of particular importance in studies of cerebral hemodynamics, the distinctive anatomy of the cerebral macro- and microcirculation and their possible role in autoregulation. Autoregulation of cerebral circulation can be defined as the presence of a relatively constant blood flow despite moderate variations in perfusion pressure. It represents the mechanism that protects the brain from hypoxia (low pressure) and edema (high pressure)[86]. The latter definition of autoregulation is of cardinal importance in the context of so-called brain sparing effect.

Preliminary results from systematic post-mortem examinations of fetal and neonatal cerebral vessels support the concept of the unique behavior of this part of the fetal circulation (Laurini, unpublished data). In cases with fetal or perinatal asphyxia, gross examination frequently shows vasodilatation of both anterior and middle cerebral arteries (Figure 6) and veins. These findings are usually accompanied by a considerable dilatation of the vein of Galen. Histological examination of these vessels confirms this dual vasodilatation, which is highly unusual in the extracranial circulation. Moreover, there is a relationship between the diameter of the lumen and the thickness of the wall of the arteries that clearly favors the former (Figure 7): this is the usual pattern for veins but not for muscular arteries. Histological examination demonstrates that these extracerebral arteries have only an internal elastic lamina and have a significantly thinner wall than extracranial muscular arteries of the same calibre.

Furthermore, the inner elastic lamina disappears at the level of the intracerebral arterioles. The unique morphology of the wall of perinatal cerebral arteries might explain the predisposition of intracranial arteries to the development of aneurysms in adulthood[86].

Our preliminary results suggest that extracerebral arteries function in a manner similar to veins. In the presence of hypoxia and hypercapnia and/or with changes in perfusion, vasodilatation reduces the vasomotor capacity of arteries to further adaptation ('vessel paralysis'). The initial arterial vasodilatation is probably a part of the phenomenon of redistribution of blood flow, the known fetal response to stress (Laurini, unpublished observation). Further distress increases the vasodilatation to the point where these particular arteries lose their ability to dilate and constrict, and, consequently, autoregulation is impaired or lost.

The recent review of autoregulation mechanisms by Edvinsson and co-workers[86] underlines the role of myogenic mechanisms and endothelium derived factors. The arteries and arterioles constrict and dilate in response to the changes in transmural pressures. The marked vasodilatation may also affect the intravascular circulation, with changes in both flow velocity and disposition of nucleated cells in circulation, i.e., marginalization of polymorphonuclear leukocytes along the endothelial surface. All of

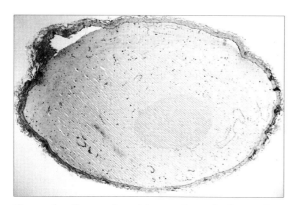

Figure 6 *Cross section of the anterior cerebral artery from a fetus who died in utero at 36 weeks of gestation and had lesions of acute asphyxia and a small placenta. The brain showed meningeal congestion and hemorrhages of the falx and tentorium. Note the marked dilatation of the vessel. Elastin van Gieson, 48×*

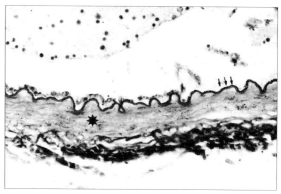

Figure 7 *Vessel wall of middle cerebral artery from a fetus who died at 33 weeks of gestation. The brain showed meningeal congestion and multifocal subarachnoidal hemorrhages. Note the presence of only the inner elastic lamina (arrows) and a muscular media (✱), thin in relation to the calibre of the vessel. Elastin van Gieson, 300×*

these changes can result in damage to the endothelial cells and thus further compromise the vasomotor ability of arteries and veins.

The specific anatomical characteristics of the human perinatal arterial brain circulation play a major role in the autoregulation of cerebral circulation and can, at least partly, explain the events related to its impairment and the possible development of brain damage as a consequence of flow redistribution during asphyxia.

SUMMARY

The Doppler ultrasound technique, combining the spectral and color Doppler mode, has made it possible to evaluate non-invasively the cerebral blood circulation in the perinatal period. The analysis of blood velocity waveforms gives information on the resistance in the cerebral vascular bed, and changes in time-averaged blood velocity reflect the changes in blood flow. Reference values have been established for the main fetal cerebral vessels: the middle cerebral artery, anterior and posterior cerebral arteries, common and internal carotid arteries. In general, during the last trimester of pregnancy, the values of waveform indices (PI, RI) in all fetal cerebral vessels decrease. In Doppler studies of healthy fetuses performed during labor, no significant influence of uterine contractions on fetal cerebral circulation has been observed. Immediately after birth, a decrease in the vascular resistance and an increase in the mean velocity occurs in the middle cerebral artery. There is no difference in cerebral blood flow velocity between infants born vaginally and those delivered by Cesarean section. During the first hours of life, the blood velocity decreases, to increase again during the following weeks.

In growth-retarded fetuses, especially those developing signs of hypoxia, the waveform indices of cerebral vessels are low, indicating the redistribution of flow – the brain sparing effect. This phenomenon is also seen in SGA newborns. The morphological examination of vessels from perinatal brains indicates specific anatomical characteristics which might be of importance in the autoregulation of cerebral circulation.

Some recent clinical reports suggest that the Doppler velocimetry of fetal cerebral vessels might be useful as a clinical test with regard to the prediction of fetal outcome. The same might be also true regarding the neonatal Doppler studies and prediction of the prognosis in cases of various neonatal complications. However, the possible value of cerebral velocimetry in clinical perinatology has not yet been proven.

References

1. Rudolph, A. M. and Heymann, M. A. (1967). The circulation of the fetus in utero. *Circ. Res.*, **21**, 163–84
2. Cohn, H. E., Sacks, E. J., Heymann, M. A. and Rudolph, A. M. (1974). Cardiovascular responses to hypoxemia and acidemia in fetal lambs. *Am. J. Obstet. Gynecol.*, **120**, 817–24
3. Peeters, L. L. H., Sheldon, R. E., Jones, M. D., Makowski, E. L. and Meschia, G. (1979). Blood flow to fetal organs as a function of arterial oxygen content. *Am. J. Obstet. Gynecol.*, **135**, 637–46
4. Nelson, K. B. and Leviton, A. (1991). How much of neonatal encephalopathy is due to birth asphyxia? *Am. J. Dis. Child.*, **145**, 1325–31
5. Lockhart, R. D., Hamilton, G. F. and Fyfe, F. W. (1965). *Anatomy of the Human Body.* pp. 607–9. (London: Faber and Faber)
6. Arbeille, P. H., Tranquart, F., Berson, M., Roncin, A., Saliba, E. and Pourcelot, L. (1989). Visualization of the fetal circle of Willis and intracerebral arteries by color-coded Doppler. *Eur. J. Obstet. Gynecol. Reprod. Biol.*, **32**, 195–8
7. Meerman, R. J., van Bel, F., van Zwieten, P. H. T., Oepkes, D. and den Ouden, L. (1990). Fetal and neonatal cerebral blood velocity in the normal fetus and neonate – a longitudinal Doppler ultrasound study. *Early Hum. Dev.*, **24**, 209–17
8. Arduini, D. and Rizzo, G. (1990). Normal values of pulsatility index from fetal vessels: a cross-

sectional study on 1556 healthy fetuses. *J. Perinat. Med.*, **18**, 165–72
9. van den Wijngaard, J. A. G. W., Groenenberg, I. A. L., Wladimiroff, J. W. and Hop, W. C. J. (1989). Cerebral Doppler ultrasound of the human fetus. *Br. J. Obstet. Gynaecol.*, **96**, 845–9
10. Mari, G. and Deter, R. L. (1992). Middle cerebral artery flow velocity waveforms in normal and small-for-gestational-age fetuses. *Am. J. Obstet. Gynecol.*, **166**, 1262–70
11. Årström, K., Eliasson, A., Hareide, J. H. and Maršál, K. (1989). Fetal blood velocity waveforms in normal pregnancies. A longitudinal study. *Acta Obstet. Gynecol. Scand.*, **68**, 171–8
12. Gilbert, R. D., Pearce, W. J., Ashwal, S. and Longo, L. D. (1990). Effects of hypoxia on contractility of isolated fetal lamb cerebral arteries. *J. Dev. Physiol.*, **13**, 199–203
13. Lingman, G., Maršál, K., Rosen, K. G. and Kjellmer, I. (1984). Blood flow measurements in exteriorized lamb fetuses during asphyxia. In Jung, H. and Fendel, H. (eds.) *Doppler Techniques in Obstetrics*. pp. 36–40. (Aachen, Stuttgart, New York: Georg Thieme Verlag)
14. Arabin, B., Siebert, M. and Saling, E. (1989). The prospective value of Doppler blood flow measurement in uteroplacental and fetal blood vessels – a comparative study of multiple parameters. *Geburtsh. Frauenheilkd.*, **49**, 457–62
15. Bilardo, C. M., Nicolaides, K. H. and Campbell, S. (1990). Doppler measurements of fetal and uteroplacental circulations: relationship with umbilical venous blood gases measured at cordocentesis. *Am. J. Obstet. Gynecol.*, **162**, 115–20
16. Lingman, G. and Maršál, K. (1989). Noninvasive assessment of cranial blood circulation in the fetus. *Biol. Neonate*, **56**, 129–35
17. Mari, G., Moise, K. J., Deter, R. L., Kirshon, B., Carpenter, R. J. and Huhta, J. C. (1989). Doppler assessment of the pulsatility index in the cerebral circulation of the human fetus. *Am. J. Obstet. Gynecol.*, **160**, 698–703
18. Echizenya, N., Kagiya, A., Tachizaki, T. and Saito, Y. (1989). Significance of velocimetry as a monitor of fetal assessment and management. *Fetal Ther.*, **4**, 188–94
19. Ardunini, D., Rizzo, G. and Romanini, C. (1992). Changes of pulsatility index from fetal vessels preceding the onset of late decelerations in growth-retarded fetuses. *Obstet. Gynecol.*, **79**, 605–10
20. Satoh, S., Koyanagi, T., Fukuhara, M., Hara, K. and Nakano, H. (1989). Changes in vascular resistance in the umbilical and middle cerebral arteries in the human intrauterine growth-retarded fetus, measured with pulsed Doppler ultrasound. *Early Hum. Dev.*, **20**, 213–20
21. Gramellini, D., Folli, M. C., Raboni, S., Vadora, E. and Merialdi, A. (1992). Cerebral–umbilical Doppler ratio as a predictor of adverse perinatal outcome. *Obstet. Gynecol.*, **79**, 416–20
22. Veille, J. C. and Cohen, I. (1990). Middle cerebral artery blood flow in normal and growth-retarded fetuses. *Am. J. Obstet. Gynecol.*, **162**, 391–6
23. Chandran, R., Serra-Serra, V., Sellers, S. M. and Redman, C. W. (1993). Fetal cerebral Doppler in the recognition of fetal compromise. *Br. J. Obstet. Gynaecol.*, **100**, 139–44
24. Favre, R., Schonenberger, R., Nisand, I. and Lorenz, U. (1991). Standard curves of cerebral Doppler flow velocity waveforms and predictive values for intrauterine growth retardation and fetal acidosis. *Fetal Diagn. Ther.*, **6**, 113–9
25. Vyas, S., Nicolaides, K. H., Bower, S. and Campbell, S. (1990). Middle cerebral artery flow velocity waveforms in fetal hypoxaemia. *Br. J. Obstet. Gynaecol.*, **97**, 797–803
26. Wladimiroff, J. W., Tonge, H. M. and Stewart, P. A. (1986). Doppler ultrasound assessment of cerebral blood flow in the human fetus. *Br. J. Obstet. Gynaecol.*, **63**, 471–5
27. Arduini, D., Rizzo, G., Romanini, C. and Mancuso, S. (1987). Fetal blood flow velocity waveforms as predictors of growth retardation. *Obstet. Gynecol.*, **70**, 7–10
28. Arduini, D. and Rizzo, G. (1992). Prediction of fetal outcome in small for gestational age fetuses: comparison of Doppler measurements obtained from different fetal vessels. *J. Perinat. Med.*, **20**, 29–38
29. McCowan, L. M. E. and Duggan, P. M. (1992). Abnormal internal carotid and umbilical artery Doppler in the small for gestational age fetus predicts an adverse outcome. *Early Hum. Dev.*, **30**, 249–59
30. Rizzo, G., Arduini, D., Luciano, R., Rizzo, C., Tortorolo, G., Romanini, C. and Mancuso, S. (1989). Prenatal cerebral Doppler ultrasonography and neonatal neurologic outcome. *J. Ultrasound Med.*, **8**, 237–40
31. Wladimiroff, J. W., van den Wijngaard, J. A. G. W., Degani, S., Noordam, M. J., van Eyck, J. and Tonge, H. M. (1987). Cerebral and umbilical arterial blood flow velocity waveforms in normal and growth retarded pregnancies. *Obstet. Gynecol.*, **69**, 705–9
32. Wladimiroff, J. W., Noordam, M. J., van den Wijngaard, J. A. G. W. and Hop, W. C. J. (1988). Fetal internal carotid and umbilical artery blood flow velocity waveforms as a measure of fetal well-being in intrauterine growth retardation. *Pediatr. Res.*, **24**, 609–12
33. Degani, S., Lewinski, R., Shapiro, I. and Sharf, M. (1988). Decrease in pulsatile flow in the in-

ternal carotid artery in fetal hydrocephalus. *Br. J. Obstet. Gynaecol.*, **95**, 138–41
34. van den Wijngaard, J. A. G. W., Reuss, A. and Wladimiroff, J. W. (1988). The blood flow velocity waveform in the fetal internal carotid artery in the presence of hydrocephaly. *Early Hum. Dev.*, **18**, 95–9
35. Kirkinen, P., Muller, R., Baumann, H., Briner, J., Lang, W., Huch, R. and Huch, A. (1988). Cerebral blood flow velocity waveforms in hydrocephalic fetuses. *J. Clin. Ultrasound*, **16**, 493–8
36. Mari, G., Wasserstrum, N. and Kirshon, B. (1992). Reduction in the middle cerebral artery pulsatility index after decompression of polyhydramnios in twin gestation. *Am. J. Perinatol.*, **9**, 381–4
37. Ben-Chetrit, A., Anteby, E., Lavy, Y., Zacut, D. and Yagel, S. (1991). Increased middle cerebral artery blood flow impedance in fetal subdural hematoma. *Ultrasound Obstet. Gynecol.*, **1**, 357–8
38. Chandran, R., Serra, S. V., Sellers, S. M. and Redman, C. W. G. (1991). Fetal middle cerebral artery flow velocity waveforms – a terminal pattern. Case report. *Br. J. Obstet. Gynaecol.*, **98**, 937–8
39. Mari, G. and Wasserstrum, N. (1991). Flow velocity waveforms of the fetal circulation preceding fetal death in a case of lupus anticoagulant. *Am. J. Obstet. Gynecol.*, **164**, 776–8
40. Fleischer, A., Anyaegbunam, A. A., Schulman, H., Farmakides, G. and Randolph, G. (1987). Uterine and umbilical artery velocimetry during normal labor. *Am. J. Obstet. Gynecol.*, **157**, 40–3
41. Brar, H. S., Platt, L. D., De Vore, G. R., Horenstein, J. and Medearis, A. L. (1988). Qualitative assessment of maternal uterine and fetal umbilical artery blood flow and resistance in laboring patients by Doppler velocimetry. *Am. J. Obstet. Gynecol.*, **158**, 952–6
42. Janbu, T., Koss, K. S., Nesheim, B. I. and Wesche, J. (1985). Blood velocities in the uterine artery in humans during labour. *Acta Physiol. Scand.*, **124**, 153–61
43. Fairlie, F. M., Lang, G. D. and Sheldon, C. D. (1989). Umbilical artery flow velocity waveforms in labour. *Br. J. Obstet. Gynaecol.*, **96**, 151–7
44. Stuart, B., Drumm, J., Fitzgerald, N. and Duigan, N. M. (1981). Fetal blood flow velocity waveforms in uncomplicated labor. *Br. J. Obstet. Gynaecol.*, **88**, 865–70
45. O'Brien, W. F., Davis, S. E., Grissom, M., Eng, R. R. and Golden, S. M. (1984). Effect of cephalic pressure on fetal cerebral blood flow. *Am. J. Perinatol.*, **3**, 223–6
46. Vyas, S., Campbell, S., Bower, S. and Nicolaides, K. H. (1990). Maternal abdominal pressure alters fetal cerebral blood flow. *Br. J. Obstet. Gynaecol.*, **97**, 740–2
47. Fendel, H., Funk, A., Jörn, H. and Gans, A. (1990). Zerebraler Blutfluss unter der Geburt. *Z. Geburtsh. Perinat.*, **194**, 272–4
48. Dougall, A., Lang, G. D. and Evans, D. H. (1989). Fetal anterior cerebral flow velocity waveforms during labour. In Gennser, G., Maršál, K., Svenningsen, N. and Lindström, K. (eds.) *Fetal and Neonatal Physiological Measurements*, pp. 301–4. (Malmö: Dept. Obstet. Gynecol., General Hospital)
49. Mirro, R. and Gonzalez, A. (1987). Perinatal anterior cerebral artery Doppler flow indexes: methods and preliminary results. *Am. J. Obstet. Gynecol.*, **156**, 1227–31
50. Maesel, A., Lingman, G. and Maršál, K. (1990). Cerebral blood flow during labor in the human fetus. *Acta Obstet. Gynecol. Scand.*, **69**, 493–5
51. Yagel, S., Anteby, E., Lavy, Y., Ben Chetrit, A., Palti, Z., Hochner-Celnikier, D. and Ron, M. (1992). Fetal middle cerebral artery blood flow during normal active labour and in labour with variable decelerations. *Br. J. Obstet. Gynaecol.*, **99**, 483–5
52. Lindblad, A., Bernow, J. and Maršál, K. (1987). Obstetric analgesia and fetal aortic blood flow during labour. *Br. J. Obstet. Gynaecol.*, **94**, 306–11
53. Maesel, A., Sladkevicius, P., Valentin, L. and Maršál, K. (1994). Fetal cerebral blood flow velocity during labor in the early neonatal period. *Ultrasound Obstet. Gynecol.*, in press
54. Ipsiroglu, O. S., Stöckler, S., Häusler, M. C. H., Kainer, F., Rosegger, H., Weiss, P. A. M. and Winter, R. (1993). Cerebral blood flow velocities in the first minutes of life. *Eur. J. Pediatr.*, **152**, 269–71
55. Lagercrantz, H. and Bistoletti, P. (1973). Catecholamine release in the newborn infant at birth. *Pediatr. Res.*, **11**, 889–93
56. Christensson, K., Siles, C., Cabrera, T., Belaustegui, A., De La Fuente, P., Lagercrantz, H., Puyol, P. and Winberg, J. (1993). Lower body temperature in infants delivered by Caesarean section than in vaginally delivered infants. *Acta Paediatr.*, **82**, 128–31
57. Shuto, H., Yasuhara, A., Sugimoto, T., Iwase, S., Kobayashi, Y. and Nakamura, M. (1987). Longitudinal determination of cerebral blood flow velocity in neonates with the Doppler technique. *Neuropediatrics*, **18**, 218–21
58. Pape, K. E. and Wigglesworth, J. S. (1979). Haemorrhage, ischemia and the perinatal brain. *Clin. Dev. Med. No. 69/70*, pp.11–38. (London: Heinemann)
59. Greisen, G., Hellström-Westas, L., Lou, H., Rosen I. and Svenningsen, N. (1985). Sleep-waking shifts and cerebral blood flow in stable preterm infants. *Pediatr. Res.*, **19**, 1156–9

60. Hernandez, M. J., Brennan, R. V., Boman, G. S. and Vanucci, R. C. (1979). Autoregulation of the cerebral blood flow in newborn dog. *Ann. Neurol.*, **6**, 177–85
61. Lou, H. C., Lassen, N. A. and Friis-Hansen, B. (1979). Impaired autoregulation of cerebral blood flow in the distressed newborn infant. *J. Pediatr.*, **94**, 118–21
62. Leahy, F. A. N., Cates, D., MacCallum, M. and Rigatto, H. (1980). Effect of CO_2 and 100% O_2 on cerebral blood flow in preterm infants. *J. Appl. Physiol.*, **48**, 468–72
63. Costeloe, K., Smyth, D. P. L., Myrdoch, N., Rolfe, P. and Tizard, J. P. M. (1984). A comparison between electrical impedance and strain gauge plethysmography for the study of cerebral blood flow in the newborn. *Pediatr. Res.*, **18**, 290–5
64. Sonesson, S-E., Winberg, P. and Lundell, B. P. W. (1987). Early postnatal changes in intracranial arterial blood flow velocities. *Pediatr. Res.*, **22**, 461–4
65. Gray, P. H., Griffin, E. A., Drumm, J. E., Fitzgerald, D. E. and Duignan, N. M. (1983). Continuous wave Doppler ultrasound in evaluation of cerebral blood flow in neonates. *Arch. Dis. Child.*, **58**, 677–81
66. Archer, L. N. J., Evans, D. H. and Levene, M. I. (1985). Doppler ultrasound examination of the anterior cerebral arteries of normal newborn infants: the effect of postnatal age. *Early Hum. Dev.*, **10**, 255–60
67. Hussman, K. A. and Kleihues, P. (1973). Reversibility of ischaemic brain damage. *Arch. Neurol.*, **29**, 375–85
68. Bada, H. S., Hajjar, W., Chua, C. and Sumner, D. S. (1979). Non-invasive diagnosis of neonatal asphyxia and intraventricular hemorrhage by Doppler ultrasound. *J. Pediatr.*, **95**, 775–9
69. van Bel, F. and Grimberg, M. Th. (1982). Intracraniale bloedingen en asfyxic bil de pasgeborene nadep onderzocht met de Doppler ultrasonoor methode. *Tijdschr. Kindergeneeskd.*, **50**, 1–10
70. Archer, L. N. J., Evans, D. H. and Levene, M. I. (1986). Cerebral artery Doppler ultrasonography predicts outcome in perinatal asphyxia. *Arch. Dis. Child.*, **61**, 632
71. Ley, D. and Maršál, K. (1992). Doppler velocimetry in cerebral vessels of small for gestational age neonates. *Early Hum. Dev.*, **31**, 171–80
72. van Bel, F., van de Bor, M., Stijnen, T. and Ruys, J. H. (1986). Decreased cerebrovascular resistance in small for gestational age infants. *Eur. J. Obstet. Gynecol. Reprod. Biol.*, **23**, 137–44
73. Greisen, G. (1986). Cerebral blood flow in preterm infants during the first week of life. *Acta Pediatr. Scand.*, **75**, 43–51
74. Perlman, J. M., McMenamin, J. B. and Volpe, J. J. (1983). Fluctuating cerebral blood flow velocity in respiratory distress syndrome. *N. Engl. J. Med.*, **309**, 204–9
75. Perlman, J. M. and Volpe, J. J. (1985). Episodes of apnoea and bradycardia in the preterm newborn: impact on cerebral circulation. *Pediatrics*, **76**, 333–8
76. Perlman, J. M. and Volpe, J. J. (1983). Seizures in the preterm infant: effects on cerebral blood flow velocity, intracranial pressure and arterial blood pressure. *Pediatrics*, **102**, 288–93
77. Perlman, J. M. and Volpe, J. J. (1983). Suctioning in the preterm infant: effects on cerebral blood flow velocity, intracranial pressure and arterial blood pressure. *Pediatrics*, **72**, 329–34
78. Hill, A., Perlman, J. M. and Volpe, J. J. (1982). Relationship of pneumothorax to intraventricular hemorrhage in the premature newborn. *Pediatrics*, **69**, 144–9
79. Ando, Y., Takashima, S. and Takeshita, K. (1985). Cerebral blood flow velocity in preterm neonates. *Brain Dev.*, **7**, 385–91
80. Hill, A. and Volpe, J. J. (1982). Decrease in pulsatile flow in anterior cerebral arteries in infantile hydrocephalus. *Pediatrics*, **69**, 4–7
81. Lipman, B., Serwer, G. and Brazy, J. E. (1982). Abnormal cerebral hemodynamics in preterm infants with patent ductus arteriosus. *Pediatrics*, **69**, 778–81
82. Martin, C. G., Snider, A. R., Katz, S. M., Peabody, J. L. and Brady, J. P. (1982). Abnormal cerebral blood flow patterns in patients with a large patent ductus arteriosus. *J. Pediatr.*, **101**, 587–93
83. Archer, L. N. J., Evans, D. H. and Levene, M. I. (1987). The effect of indomethacin on cerebral blood flow velocity in premature infants. In Sheldon, C. D., Evans, D. H. and Salvage, J. R. (eds.) *Obstetric and Neonatal Blood Flow*, pp. 46–7. (London: Biological Engineering Society)
84. Cowan, F. (1986). Acute effects of indomethacin on neonatal cerebral blood flow velocities. *Early Hum. Dev.*, **13**, 343
85. Laurini, R. N. (1990). Abortion from a morphological viewpoint. In Huisjes, H. J. and Lind, T. (eds.) *Spontaneous Abortion*, pp. 79–113. (Edinburgh: Churchill Livingstone)
86. Edvinsson, L., MacKenzie, E. T. and McCulloch, J. (1993). *Cerebral Blood Flow and Metabolism*, pp. 40–56 (New York: Raven Press)

Section 5

Fetal therapy

Aspirin in pregnancy

S. Uzan and B. Haddad

Salicylates were introduced into practice at the end of the 19th century. Since then, they have been used extensively for their analgesic, antipyretic and anti-inflammatory action. Aspirin, or acetylsalicylic acid, is the salicylate most widely used without any prescription (for headache, for instance) and in clinical practice. The pharmacology of salicylates has been elucidated recently, leading to their use in certain diseases where the alteration of prostaglandin production seems to be involved in the pathophysiology. Aspirin may produce a reversal of the pathological process, by interacting with prostaglandin synthesis.

This chapter reviews the pathophysiological changes that occur in pregnancy-induced hypertensive diseases and the current clinical use of low-dose aspirin in pregnancy to improve maternal and perinatal outcome.

RATIONALE FOR OBSTETRIC INDICATIONS

The elucidation of the role of prostaglandins in the control of maternal and fetal adaptation during pregnancy has led to the use of aspirin for some specific obstetric indications. Several studies of the last decade have shown that the adaptation (or maladaptation) of the uteroplacental circulation depends largely on the synthesis of prostaglandins and their regulation during pregnancy, and especially on prostacylin and thromboxane A_2[1], which are metabolites of the arachidonic acid cyclo-oxygenase pathway[2].

Prostacyclin, which is the principal arachidonic acid cyclo-oxygenase product in vascular endothelium, synthesized also in trophoblast cells, causes relaxation of smooth muscle, leading to vasodilatation and the inhibition of uterine contractility. It is also an important inhibitor of platelet aggregation, and it thus prevents thrombosis and placental infarction[3]. Prostacyclin seems also to reduce the sensitivity of the maternal vascular system to angiotensin II[1].

Thromboxane A_2, mainly produced by platelets, is a strong vasoconstrictor agent; it stimulates platelet aggregation and uterine contractility[5]. Thromboxane A_2 is rapidly inactivated by hydrolyze, to produce thromboxane B_2. Its short half-life (30 s) limits its action to the site where it is released[5].

Prostacyclin synthesis seems to be increased in normal pregnancy[1], leading to a dominance of its effect over thromboxane A_2[6], leading then to vasodilatation and to a reduction of systemic vascular resistance, which is characteristic of normal pregnancy.

The mechanism of activation of prostaglandin synthesis in pregnancy remains unknown. Some women fail to develop the physiological adaptation for maintaining a normal pregnancy. In pre-eclamptic women, a decrease in prostacyclin synthesis and an increase in thromboxane A_2 production in both fetoplacental circulation[7] and the circulation of pregnant women has been observed[1,8]. Prostacyclin synthesis is therefore not sufficient, or does not occur, leading to a dominance of the effects of thromboxane A_2. This state is characterized by an increase in vascular sensitivity to angiotensin II, vascular resistance and the development of thrombosis and placental infarction[1,3]. This circulatory maladaptation leads to hypertensive diseases of pregnancy and to an impaired uteroplacental circulation, with intrauterine growth retardation as a consequence[9].

Although this concept contributes to the clarification of the pathophysiology of pregnancy-induced hypertensive diseases, the imbalance of prostacyclin and thromboxane A_2 is unlikely to be the only mechanism involved in this disease. Rees and associates[10] suggested that the endothelium-derived relaxing factor (EDRF) had a major role in physiological vasodilatation in pregnancy. Moreover, the production of EDRF (nitric oxide) was impaired in the umbilical vessels of pre-eclamptic women, compared to that in normotensive pregnant women[11].

Even if the decrease of the production of prostacyclin or EDRF seems to be explained by endothelial cell injury, platelet dysfunction probably plays an important role in pregnancy-induced hypertensive diseases. The impaired production of prostacyclin by the trophoblast–placental vasculature and/or uterine vessels allows surface-mediated platelet activation, resulting in an increase in the secretion by platelets of thromboxane A_2 and serotonin, leading finally to platelet aggregation, occluding the uterine blood circulation in the myometrial–placental bed[12].

Concerning angiotensin-sensitivity, Gant and co-workers[13] showed that patients who developed pre-eclampsia had lost their refractoriness to infusion with angiotensin II several weeks before the onset of the clinical signs of pre-eclampsia. Wallenburg and colleagues[4], in a double-blind placebo controlled study using 60 mg aspirin or a placebo daily for 6 weeks in normotensive primigravid patients who were sensitive to angiotensin-II infusions at 28 weeks, showed that thrombin-induced platelet malondialdehyde production was significantly lower in the aspirin than the placebo group. Moreover, the effective pressor dose of angiotensin II was higher at 34 weeks than at 28 weeks in the aspirin group; in contrast, the placebo had no effect. In addition, seven of the 15 members of the placebo group and none of the 17 members of the aspirin group had a decrease in the effective pressor dose between 28 and 34 weeks. In summary, the increase of the vascular response to angiotensin-II infusion can be mediated by the imbalance of the thromboxane/prostacyclin ratio.

The recognition of the imbalance in the production of prostacyclin and thromboxane A_2 in pregnancy-induced hypertensive diseases, with a dominance in the effect of thromboxane A_2 over prostacyclin, led to the use of aspirin, which is a cyclo-oxygenase inhibitor[14]. It decreases the synthesis of thromboxane A_2 relatively more than that of prostacyclin. This relative decrease of thromboxane A_2 synthesis suppresses the dominance of thromboxane A_2 over prostacyclin in these pregnancy-induced hypertensive diseases, and may then restore the physiological balance of prostacyclin and thromboxane A_2. This concept constitutes the rationale of clinical attempts in the use of the cyclo-oxygenase inhibitor, acetylsalicylic acid (aspirin) in the prevention of hypertensive diseases in women at high risk.

PHARMACOLOGY AND KINETICS

The optimal action of aspirin is as an antithrombotic and an inhibitor of platelet activity. The optimal dose remains unknown. Various doses of aspirin, from as low as 20 mg to as high as 3.5 g daily, are effective in the prevention of thrombosis[12]. Acetylsalicylic acid (which is a nonsteroidal anti-inflammatory drug) acts by an irreversible acetylation and inactivation of the cyclo-oxygenase enzyme (Figure 1), inhibiting prostaglandin synthesis (thromboxane A_2, prostacyclin, prostaglandin E and prostaglandin $F_{2\alpha}$). The duration of this effect depends on the ability of the cells to synthesize cyclo-oxygenase[2]. After the exposure to aspirin and the inactivation of cyclo-oxygenase, platelets, as they are non-nucleated cells, cannot synthesize new

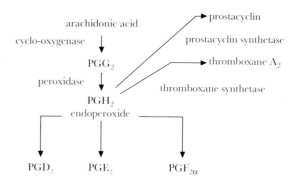

Figure 1 *Arachidonic acid cyclo-oxygenase pathways*

cyclo-oxygenase enzyme. So, the recovery of thromboxane A_2 synthesis requires the production of new platelets by megakaryocytes. Moreover, it seems that platelet cyclo-oxygenase is particularly sensitive to aspirin, and the repeated administration of low-dose aspirin leads to a cumulative inhibition of thromboxane A_2[2]. In contrast the recovery of prostacyclin synthesis is observed relatively rapidly after low-dose aspirin exposure in cultured endothelial cells[15]. The administration of aspirin in doses ranging from 0.3 mg/kg/day to 1.5 mg/kg/day seems to inhibit the cyclo-oxygenase activity in platelets, but much less in endothelial cells[16]. Sibaï and colleagues[17] showed that 60 mg/day or 80 mg/day of aspirin reduced the production of thromboxane A_2 by more than 90% within a few days of therapy. Moreover, in a study by Roberts and co-workers[18], aspirin at 50 mg/day reduced thromboxane A_2 production by more than 95% without any change in prostacyclin production. These authors noted a total inhibition of thromboxane A_2 production, but also a prostacyclin inhibition, when using 100 to 300 mg of aspirin daily.

The combination of these actions therefore gives an explanation of the use of low-dose aspirin in the prevention of pregnancy-induced hypertensive diseases, or of thrombotic events[19] in women with lupus anti-coagulant.

The pharmacokinetics of aspirin should be taken into consideration for understanding its effects. Aspirin is rapidly absorbed from the stomach and upper intestinal tract. The rate of absorption depends on several factors – on the disintegration and dissolution of tablets and capsules, and on the pH of the stomach and upper intestine. Aqueous solutions have a better rate of absorption than plain uncoated tablets or extended-release tablets. After oral administration, plasma salicylate peak levels occur after nearly 30 min[3,20]. Aspirin, a weak acid (pK_a 3.5), is then hydrolyzed to salicylic acid by intestinal, plasma and liver esterases[21]. Aspirin exists in an ionized form in blood and tissues, sodium salicylate[20]. The pharmacokinetics of aspirin or salicylates describe a two-phase curve: the half-lives of aspirin and salicylates are 2.7 and 3.8 min, respectively, in the α-phase and 15 and 238 min in the β-phase[22]. The slow elimination in the β-phase of salicylates is in relation to a high level of plasma-binding protein. Pedersen and Fitzgerald[21] also found that the fractional systemic bioavailability was constant after the use of single oral doses of 20, 40, 325 and 1300 mg of aspirin in non-pregnant patients. These authors noted that platelets were exposed to higher concentrations of aspirin in intestinal capillaries than in the systemic circulation. It has been suggested that, after low-dose aspirin therapy, platelets passing through the pre-systemic portal circulation were exposed to relatively high concentrations of aspirin, leading to the inhibition of their cyclo-oxygenase enzyme, whereas platelets or other cells in the systemic circulation were exposed to a concentration too low to affect their cyclo-oxygenase enzymes. Once inactivated in the portal circulation, platelets remain so for several days after the last ingestion of aspirin.

Salicylates cross the placenta rapidly. After a maternal intravenous administration of aspirin, fetal plasma concentrations reach 80 to 90% of maternal levels 60 to 90 minutes later[23]. However after low-dose oral aspirin ingestion, and after the portal first-pass, the systemic aspirin concentration is too low to expect a significant concentration to reach the placental circulation. To assess the placental transfer of salicylates, several authors studied the fetal production of thromboxane and prostacyclin. Sibaï and colleagues[17] found no modification in the fetal synthesis of platelet thromboxane and prostacyclin after a maternal intake of 20 to 80 mg of aspirin daily for the last 2 weeks before delivery. But for Benigni and associates[24], the long-term administration of 60 mg of aspirin seemed to reduce fetal thromboxane synthesis by 63%.

In conclusion, aspirin inactivates cyclo-oxygenase by acetylation. As aspirin is markedly deacetylated in the hepatic first-pass, its half-life is much lower than that of salicylic acid[9]. Placental transfer depends closely on maternal plasma aspirin concentrations. Thus with low-dose aspirin, the amount of aspirin reaching the placental circulation is low. However, it seems that long-term daily intake of low-dose aspirin

(60–80 mg) reduces thromboxane production by platelets without affecting prostacyclin synthesis.

OBSTETRIC APPLICATIONS
Prevention of pre-eclampsia

Crandon and Isherwood[25], in a retrospective study, suggested that pre-eclampsia occurred less frequently in nulliparous women who took aspirin. Several prospective studies recently published suggest that aspirin therapy might be effective to reduce the incidence of pre-eclampsia in women at high risk. The first (Beaufils and co-workers[26]) was an open prospective randomized study including 102 patients with a poor previous pregnancy or with known hypertension ($\geq 160/95$ mmHg). Patients enrolled were allocated to take aspirin (150 mg) and dipyridamol (300 mg) daily from 3 months ($n = 52$) or no treatment ($n = 50$). Pre-eclampsia was significantly decreased in the aspirin group when compared to the group with no treatment (0 vs. 6, $p < 0.01$).

Wallenburg and colleagues[27] reported the first prospective placebo-controlled double-blind study concerning the possible prevention of pre-eclampsia by low-dose aspirin (60 mg daily) in women at high risk. All patients ($n = 46$) were primigravidae and were selected by testing of angiotensin-II sensitivity at 28 weeks' gestation. The incidence of pre-eclampsia was significantly lower in the aspirin group when compared to the placebo group (0 vs. 7, $p < 0.05$).

Schiff and associates[28] carried out a randomized double-blind placebo-controlled study to investigate the effect of aspirin therapy in preventing pregnancy-induced hypertension in women selected by an abnormal pressor response during a roll-over test performed at 28 to 29 weeks' gestation. A total of 65 patients were enrolled, with 34 women taking 100 mg aspirin daily and 31 a placebo in the third trimester. In this study, the authors found a significant decrease of pre-eclampsia in the aspirin group when compared to the placebo group (1 (2.9%) vs. 7 (22.6%), $p < 0.02$).

McParland and co-workers[29], in a randomized placebo-controlled trial, included 100 patients with a high risk of development of pre-eclampsia, selected by an abnormal uterine Doppler velocity waveform in an examination at 24 weeks' gestation. A total of 48 patients took 75 mg of aspirin daily and 52 took a placebo. Treatment was started after the assessment of the uterine Doppler examination. The frequency of pre-eclampsia decreased significantly in the aspirin group when compared to the placebo group (1/48 (2%) vs. 10/52 (19%), $p < 0.02$).

In summary, low-dose aspirin therapy seems to be effective in the prevention of pre-eclampsia, particularly in women at high risk.

Prevention of intrauterine growth retardation

Recent studies supported the opinion that low-dose aspirin administration may prevent fetal growth retardation in patients at risk. In an open prospective randomized study, Beaufils and colleagues[26] observed a significant reduction of severe intrauterine growth retardation in patients receiving aspirin (150 mg) and dipyridamol (300 mg) daily when compared to the group with no treatment (0 vs. 4, $p < 0.05$).

Wallenburg and Rotmans[30] studied 48 patients with at least two previous poor outcomes, all complicated by intrauterine growth retardation. Of these, 24 had been treated with 1–1.6 mg/kg aspirin and 225 mg dipyridamol daily from 16 to 34 weeks, and 24 others were considered as control. Intrauterine growth retardation occurred in 61% of the control group and only 13% of the treated group.

Trudinger and associates[31] carried out a randomized, placebo-controlled double-blind trial to study the effect of low-dose aspirin (150 mg daily) on neonatal outcome in pregnancies with an impaired umbilical artery Doppler flow velocity waveform. Aspirin treatment was started at about 32 weeks' gestation, after the evaluation of the umbilical Doppler waveform. Aspirin was associated with a significant increase of birth weight (mean difference 526 g) and mean placental weight when compared to the placebo group. However, aspirin therapy did not produce any difference in neonatal outcome when the umbilical Doppler waveform showed an absent diastolic flow. The efficiency of aspirin therapy, given late in pregnancy, and in this indication (impaired umbilical circulation) must be confirmed by other studies.

McParland and associates[29] in a randomized placebo-controlled study, selected their women at high risk of fetal growth retardation by a pathological uterine Doppler examination at 24 weeks' gestation. In 100 patients enrolled, 48 patients had 75 mg of aspirin daily and 52 had a placebo, from 24 weeks' gestation. Fewer aspirin-treated women than placebo-treated women had babies of low birth weight (15% vs. 25%), but this difference was not significant.

Uzan and associates[32], in a randomized placebo-controlled double-blind trial, included 229 patients with histories of at least two poor previous pregnancies. Women were included at 15 to 18 weeks' gestation. They were allocated to receive either a placebo ($n = 73$), aspirin 150 mg daily ($n = 81$), or aspirin 150 mg plus dipyridamol 225 mg daily ($n = 75$). Aspirin therapy ($n = 156$) resulted in a significant decrease in the recurrence of fetal growth retardation (20/156 (13%) vs. 19/73 (26%), $p < 0.02$) and a significantly higher birth weight (2751 g (SD 670) vs. 2526 g (SD 848); difference 225 g (95% CI 129–321 g), $p = 0.029$) when compared to the placebo group.

In conclusion, low-dose aspirin is effective in reducing the incidence of intrauterine growth retardation in patients at high risk for this complication.

A meta-analysis of low-dose aspirin administration for the prevention of pregnancy-induced hypertensive disease

When study designs are similar and criteria and end-points well defined, systemic pooling of the results across trials by means of meta-analysis provides more precise estimates of the effects of treatment[33].

Bréart and colleagues (unpublished data) selected six studies[24,26–29,32] (Table 1) concerning low-dose aspirin therapy in pregnant women at high risk to undergo a meta-analysis. Differences in the end-points of pregnancy-induced hypertension, pre-eclampsia and intrauterine growth retardation between treated and non-treated groups with low-dose aspirin were accumulated and expressed as odds ratios with 95% confidence intervals. The results concerning 324 treated and 240 untreated women with low-dose aspirin are presented in Figure 2. None of the 95% confidence intervals reached 1, which means that pregnancy-induced hypertension, pre-eclampsia and intrauterine growth retardation occurred significantly less frequently in aspirin-treated groups than in controls. Similar findings have been reported by Imperiale and Petrulis[34].

Effects of low-dose aspirin in healthy nulliparous pregnant women

The meta-analysis (see above) showed that aspirin therapy reduced the incidence of pre-eclampsia, intrauterine growth retardation or gestational hypertension, particularly in women at high risk, selected by a poor previous obstetric history, or an abnormal roll-over test or angiotensin-II test, or a pathological early uterine Doppler analysis.

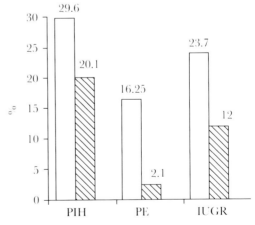

Figure 2 Trials of low-dose aspirin in pregnancies at risk. White bars, placebo; hatched bars, acetylsalicylic acid; PIH, pregnancy-induced hypertension (odds ratio, 0.54; 95% CI, 0.3–0.81); PE, pre-eclampsia (odds ratio, 0.16; 95% CI, 0.09–0.30); IUGR, intrauterine growth retardation (odds ratio, 0.43, 95% CI, 0.27–0.67)

Table 1 *Randomized controlled trials of low-dose aspirin therapy for the prevention of hypertensive disorders in pregnancy in women at high risk*

	Inclusion criteria	Treatment protocol	Number treated	Number control	Placebo	Clinical end-points
Beaufils et al.[26]	poor previous obstetric history	ASA 150 mg/day plus dipyridamol 300 mg/day from 3 months until delivery	48	45	no	PIH, PE, IUGR, BW
Wallenburg et al.[27]	normotensive primigravidae; positive A-II test	ASA 60 mg/day from 28 weeks until delivery	23	23	yes	PIH, PE, IUGR, BW
Benigni et al.[21]	poor previous obstetric history	ASA 60 mg/day from 12 weeks until delivery	17	16	yes	PIH, IUGR, BW
Schiff et al.[28]	positive roll-over test	ASA 100 mg/day in the third trimester	34	31	yes	PIH, PE, IUGR, BW
McParland et al.[29]	nulliparous with abnormal uterine Doppler at 24 weeks	ASA 75 mg/day from 24 weeks until delivery	48	52	yes	PIH, PE, IUGR, BW
Uzan et al.[32]	poor previous obstetric history	ASA 150 mg/day or ASA 150 mg/day plus dipyridamole 225 mg/day from 15–18 weeks until delivery	156	73	yes	PIH, PE, IUGR, BW

A-II, angiotensin-II; ASA, acetylsalicylic acid; PIH, pregnancy-induced hypertension; PE, pre-eclampsia; IUGR, intrauterine growth retardation; BW, birth weight

However, it is important to ask about the effect of aspirin therapy in the prevention of pre-eclampsia in women at low risk. Two recent large randomized placebo-controlled studies seem to give an answer to this question. Hauth and colleagues[35], in a double-blind placebo-controlled study concerning 604 healthy nulliparous women, compared the effect of low-dose aspirin therapy (60 mg daily from 24 weeks until delivery, $n = 302$) to that of a placebo ($n = 302$). Authors found a significant decrease in the incidence of pre-eclampsia in the aspirin group when compared to the placebo group (5 (1.7%) vs. 17 (5.6%); odds ratio 0.29, 95% CI, 0.11–0.79; $p = 0.009$). The incidence of pregnancy-induced hypertension (6.3% vs. 5.6%, respectively) or intrauterine growth retardation (5.6% vs. 6.3%, respectively) were not significantly different in the aspirin and placebo groups. However, these data were suggestive of a positive effect of aspirin on fetal growth, in that the mean birth weight of infants of aspirin-treated women was 3249 g compared with 3169 g in those receiving the placebo ($p = 0.08$).

Sibaï and colleagues[36] reported a study where healthy nulliparous normotensive women with no proteinuria were enrolled at between 13 and 25 weeks' gestation to take aspirin 60 mg ($n = 1485$) or a placebo ($n = 1500$). The incidence of pre-eclampsia was just significantly lower in the aspirin group (69 (4.6%) vs. 94 (6.3%), $p = 0.05$) than in the placebo group. There was no significant difference between the aspirin and placebo groups in the incidence of pregnancy-induced hypertension (6.7% vs. 5.9%, respectively) or intrauterine growth retardation (4.6% vs. 5.8%, respectively).

In these two studies concerning healthy nulliparous women, even though low-dose aspirin did not reduce the incidence of pregnancy-induced hypertension or intrauterine growth retardation, it appeared to be effective in the prevention of pre-eclampsia.

Aspirin to treat pre-eclampsia

Although low-dose aspirin was effective in the prevention of pre-eclampsia, the effects of aspirin therapy in women with established pre-eclampsia or pregnancy-induced hypertension seemed to be less favorable. Schiff and colleagues[37], in a randomized double-blind trial concerning 47 pregnant patients with established pregnancy-induced hypertension between 30 and 36 weeks' gestation, studied the effect of low-dose aspirin 100 mg daily ($n = 23$) compared to placebo ($n = 24$). There were no significant differences found in the occurrence of pre-eclampsia and in birth weight between the two groups, and the authors concluded that low-dose aspirin was not curative.

Prevention of fetal loss in relation to some immunological aspects

An increase of fetal loss has been associated with the presence of antiphospholipid antibodies, including anticardiolipin antibodies and lupus anticoagulant[38]. These antibodies were found in patients with or without systemic lupus erythematosus. They seem to interfere with prostacyclin synthesis in endothelial cells, leading to a relative increase of platelet thromboxane action[39,40]. These pregnancies are associated with an increase of intrauterine growth retardation or fetal death. To prevent these complications, some authors proposed a corticoid and/or low-dose aspirin therapy.

Lockshin and associates[41] reported a study concerning 21 pregnant women with a previous history of fetal death associated with an elevated titer of antiphospholipid antibodies (IgG > 40 phospholipid units). In this study, aspirin therapy of 80 mg ($n = 14$) did not decrease the rate of fetal loss and the authors suggested that aspirin therapy did not improve fetal outcome in asymptomatic pregnant patients with previous fetal loss and a high titer of antiphospholipid antibodies. However, the most important shortcoming of this study was the absence of randomization. Branch and associates[19] identified eight women with a lupus anticoagulant. These patients previously had had collectively 30 spontaneous abortions and fetal deaths out of 31 pregnancies (96.8%). During the current pregnancy, they were treated with 81 mg aspirin and 40–50 mg prednisone daily. Pregnancy loss was reduced to 37.5%; however, all the five patients who gave birth to live infants developed pre-eclampsia and three of the five new-borns were hypotrophic. The authors concluded that the corticosteroid and low-dose aspirin regimen appeared to improve perinatal outcome in cases in which the mother had a lupus anticoagulant. To date, the inhibitory effects of low-dose aspirin therapy in pregnant women have not been established in a randomized placebo-controlled fashion.

In a recent report, Krause and colleagues[12] studied the effects of the induction of the antiphospholipid syndrome in pregnant mice by passive transfer of mouse monoclonal anticardiolipin antibody. The mice with antiphospholipid antibodies had a higher rate of fetal loss ($45.7 \pm 12.2\%$ vs. $2.5 \pm 0.4\%$, $p < 0.001$) when compared to the controls. In the group of mice with antiphospholipid antibodies, those that were treated with low-dose aspirin had a lower resorption rate ($11.1 \pm 9.3\%$ vs. $45.7 \pm 12.2\%$, $p < 0.001$). In this model, the authors concluded that low-dose aspirin had a protective effect against obstetric complications associated with experimental antiphospholipid syndrome.

Prevention of preterm labor

The first-pass deacetylation in the liver is so extensive that high doses of aspirin are needed to obtain a high level of acetylsalicylic acid to inhibit the cyclo-oxygenase enzyme in uterine tissue. Aspirin at high doses (2–3.6 g daily) seems to have a beneficial effect; however, the number of patients studied, without a control group, are too small in these reports to draw a conclusion[13]. Moreover, although low-dose aspirin reduces the incidence of preterm delivery due to intrauterine growth retardation or pre-eclampsia, it does not reduce spontaneous preterm birth. Sibaï and co-workers[36], in a very large randomized placebo-controlled study in healthy nulliparous pregnant women, found no difference in preterm delivery between the aspirin group (60 mg/day) and the placebo group (157 (10.6%) vs. 147 (9.8%), respectively). If the use of cyclo-oxygenase enzyme inhibitor is needed, indomethacin must be preferred to high doses of acetylsalicylic acid.

SAFETY ASPECTS OF ASPIRIN TREATMENT

The association between prenatal aspirin ingestion and adverse effects in the mother, fetus and new-born has been described in several reports. Aspirin and salicylates in pregnant women can cause several general side effects that occur in non-pregnant women. Symptoms of aspirin intolerance, such as nausea, gastric irritation, diarrhea or constipation, bronchospasm, skin rashes and angioedema can occur with high doses of aspirin intake or are signs of aspirin hypersensitivity. Although the potential side effects of aspirin use are not specific for pregnancy, they will be discussed in more detail, as their consequences can be important.

Effects on pregnancy length

In a retrospective study concerning 103 patients taking 3250 mg aspirin daily for at least the last 6 months of pregnancy for a musculoskeletal disease, Lewis and Schulman[44] reported an increase of postmaturity frequency, and mean length of gestation and labor. However, when using lowdose aspirin, Sibaï and colleagues[36] did not observe any difference in postmaturity between patients taking aspirin or placebo.

Teratogenic effects

Saxen[45], when retrospectively analyzing 599 children born with oral clefts, noted that the ingestion of aspirin in the first trimester was three times more frequent in mothers of children with oral clefts than in a control group.

However, Slone and associates[46], in a prospective study of the Collaborative Perinatal Project, concerning 50 282 mother–child pairs, found no difference in the occurrence of congenital malformations when comparing mothers exposed to aspirin in the first four months (14 864) to controls (35 418). No specific malformation occurred more frequently in the group exposed to aspirin. The large number of subjects involved make this prospective study and its conclusion very powerful. More recently, the association between cardiac malformations and aspirin use during the first trimester of pregnancy was assessed by Werler and co-workers[47]. In a large case–control study involving 1381 new-borns with congenital cardiac defects and 6966 infants with other abnormalities, aspirin use did not differ in these two groups, and the authors concluded that aspirin-taking in the first trimester did not increase the risk of congenital heart defects in relation to that of other structural malformations.

Effects on fetal and neonatal hemostasis

Long-term low-dose aspirin use seemed partially to reduce the levels of neonatal serum thromboxane B_2 in a study by Benigni and co-workers[24]. However, Sibaï and associates[17], when studying 30 neonates after low-dose aspirin-taking by mothers (≤ 80 mg/day) in the third trimester for 2 weeks or more, found that the levels of neonatal serum thromboxane B_2 were not affected by any dose of aspirin.

Concerning the clinical side-effects, Rumack and co-workers[48] compared the occurrence of cerebral hemorrhage, detected by computerized tomographic scan, in new-borns with ($n = 17$) and without ($n = 71$) a history of aspirin-taking by mothers within 7 days before delivery. All these new-borns were delivered before 34 weeks of pregnancy. Twelve of the 17 and 31 of the 71 new-borns had evidence of cerebral bleeding; the difference was significant only in a 1-tailed Fisher exact test ($p = 0.041$) and the authors concluded that aspirin taken late in pregnancy caused a significant increase in the risk of intracranial hemorrhage. In contrast, in a prospective study concerning 27 mothers taking aspirin in a high dose of 1 g daily until delivery, Nunez and associates[19] found no evidence of fetal bleeding. Finally, no hemorrhagic complications have been observed in all recent reports[17,24,26,29,32].

In summary, the recent and prospective studies indicate that low-dose aspirin does not induce fetal or neonatal bleeding.

Effects on the ductus arteriosus and pulmonary circulation

Patency of the ductus arteriosus *in utero* is partially dependent on prostaglandins. Prostaglandin E_2 and prostacyclin, produced in the duct wall, have a relaxing effect on the ductus arteriosus. Eicosanoids are also involved in lung vascular relaxation that takes place after birth to ensure an increase of blood flow to the lungs[50]. Therefore, the use of a cyclo-oxygenase inhibitor, such as indomethacin, can close the ductus arteriosus in newborns[51], but can also lead to premature constriction and pulmonary hypertension[52]. Such effects have been noted in the use of a high dose of aspirin, with severe neonatal hypoxemia as a consequence[53]. These complications have not been revealed in a larger clinical study of women taking high doses of aspirin[19]. Moreover, Shapiro and co-workers[54], in the Collaborative Perinatal Project, found no excess of perinatal mortality in infants of mothers taking aspirin during pregnancy. Doppler echocardiography also did not show any evidence of constriction of the ductus arteriosus in 30 women treated with low-dose aspirin in the last 2 or 3 weeks of pregnancy[17].

In conclusion, low-dose aspirin treatment does not seem to be associated with premature closure of the ductus arteriosus.

Effects on the intelligence quotient

The intelligence quotient (IQ) of children exposed *in utero* to aspirin was investigated in two studies. Streissguth and colleagues[55] found a 10-point decrement of the IQ at 4 years of age in children exposed *in utero* to aspirin. However, in a larger study with data collected from the Collaborative Perinatal Project, Klebanoff and Berendes[56] compared the IQ at 4 years of children exposed to aspirin in the first 20 weeks of pregnancy to a control group. These authors found a higher IQ (2.1 points) in children exposed to aspirin. Thus, an adverse effect of aspirin use during pregnancy on children's IQ is unlikely.

Effects of maternal hemostasis

Some reports suggested an increase of bleeding in patients using aspirin. Lewis and Schulman[11], in a retrospective study of 103 patients treated for rheumatoid disease with over 3250 mg of aspirin daily for the last 6 months of pregnancy, reported a greater blood loss at delivery when compared to controls. In a recent report, Taggart and associates[57] found an increase of blood transfusion after coronary bypass grafting in patients receiving prophylactic treatment with aspirin (75–300 mg) when compared to a control group. Baker and colleagues[58] reported two cases of gastrointestinal bleeding, probably related to low-dose aspirin treatment, given once to a pregnant patient for pregnancy-induced hypertension and to another non-pregnant patient in a study on platelet reactivity. In a case–control study, Stuart and colleagues[59] found a decrease of hemoglobin levels after delivery in ten patients who had taken 5 to 10 g of aspirin with 5 days of delivery. However, several prospective and randomized reports studying effects of low-dose aspirin did not find any difference in maternal bleeding at delivery between groups taking aspirin and control groups[17,24,32]. Recently, Sibaï and associates[36] examined the effect of low-dose aspirin (60 mg daily) in healthy women, in a double-blind, placebo-controlled study. There were no differences between the two groups in the incidence of an excessive bleeding at delivery, postpartum hemorrhage, change in the hematocrit or need for blood transfusion. However, the incidence of abruptio placentae was significantly higher among patients who received aspirin (11/1485 vs. 2/1500, $p = 0.01$). Nevertheless, this complication has not been found to be increased in several other reports[29,32]. Uzan and associates[32], in a randomized placebo-controlled double-blind trial, found no difference in the frequency of abruptio placentae between the two groups (7/156 in the aspirin groups vs. 6/73 in the control group). However, this point must be clarified. Even though low-dose aspirin affects platelet functions, it does not seem to induce an increase of spontaneous bleeding in pregnant women, during or after vaginal delivery.

To avoid the potential risk of epidural hematoma following epidural analgesia in women taking aspirin, O'Sullivan[60] recommended stopping aspirin administration 7 to 10 days before delivery and measuring a normal bleeding-time test before performing regional anesthesia.

PRACTICAL APPLICATIONS

It becomes apparent, in view of several double-blind placebo-controlled studies that low-dose aspirin is effective in the prevention of pregnancy-induced hypertensive diseases, especially pre-eclampsia and intrauterine growth retardation, in women at high risk. The high-risk pregnant women can be defined as patients having either a poor past obstetric history (intrauterine growth retardation, pre-eclampsia, eclampsia, and, for some authors, abruptio placentae), or an impaired uterine circulation shown by an early pathological uterine Doppler waveform, or an abnormal angiotensin-II test, or an abnormal roll-over test. In fact, to be effective, aspirin must be started early in pregnancy. Also, the history of poor previous pregnancies or an impaired early uterine Doppler examination constitute the most common practical indications for the use of low-dose aspirin.

The optimal dose of aspirin has not been established. However, a daily single dose of 60 to 100 mg (1 mg/kg) can be an opportune dosage. Low-dose aspirin can be started between 15 to 18 weeks, when the indication is a poor previous history[32], or at 24 weeks after an impaired uterine Doppler waveform[29]. Before starting the therapy, the platelet count must be normal, as must the primary hemostasis Ivy test[61] (under 10 min). Ten to fifteen days after the beginning of treatment, the Ivy test must be controlled for adjusting the drug dose. Most authors will stop this therapy around 35–36 weeks, and the Ivy test will be controlled 10 days later, to ensure normal primary hemostasis when entering labor.

CONCLUSION

Pre-eclampsia and intrauterine growth retardation remain the major cause of maternal and perinatal morbidity and mortality. Pre-eclampsia seems to be related to generalized endothelial cell injury, which can lead to an increase of the thromboxane A_2/prostacyclin ratio, and a decrease of vascular refractoriness to angiotensin II. In such patients, low-dose aspirin seems to reverse the physiological changes, inhibiting relatively selectively the thromboxane A_2 production, and restoring the vascular refractoriness to angiotensin II in angiotensin-sensitive pregnant women.

However, low-dose aspirin is not curative of established pre-eclampsia or intrauterine growth retardation. Its action in women at high risk is to prevent the occurrence of pre-eclampsia and intrauterine growth retardation, but it does not seem to reduce the incidence of pregnancy-induced hypertension. To be effective, low-dose aspirin must be started as early as possible in women at high risk, certainly before the appearance of clinical signs.

Two recent studies have investigated the effect of low-dose aspirin in the prevention of pregnancy-induced hypertensive diseases in low-risk, nulliparous, healthy pregnant women[35,36]. Both studies showed a slight decrease in the incidence of pre-eclampsia, but no beneficial effect on the incidence of pregnancy-induced hypertension or intrauterine growth retardation.

The results of the CLASP trial[62], a multicentric study (involving 9364 women randomly assigned 60 mg aspirin daily or matching placebo) show that overall the use of aspirin was associated with a reduction of only 12% of proteinuric pre-eclampsia (PPE). Aspirin did, however, significantly reduce the likelihood of preterm delivery, with a significant trend towards progressively greater reductions in PPE the more preterm the delivery.

Concerning safety aspects: there was no increase in placental hemorrhage or in bleeding during preparation for epidural anesthesia. A slight increase of blood transfusion after delivery was observed in the aspirin group. Aspirin was generally safe for the fetus and the new born with no evidence of an increased likelihood of bleeding.

This trial supports our opinion that routine prophylactic use of aspirin is not recommended and that aspirin (given early in the second trimester) can be useful in high-risk pregnancies identified either on their past obstetric history or on early markers.

References

1. Friedman, S. A. (1988). Preeclampsia: a review of the role of prostaglandins. *Obstet. Gynecol.*, **71**, 122–37
2. Oates, J. A., FitzGerald, G. A., Brand, R. A., Jackson, E. K., Knapp, H. R. and Roberts, L. J. (1988). Clinical implications of prostaglandin and thromboxane A2 formation. *N. Engl. J. Med.*, **319**, 689–98
3. Walsh, S. W. (1990). Physiology of low-dose aspirin therapy for the prevention of preeclampsia. *Semin. Perinatol.*, **14**, 152–70
4. Wallenburg, H. C. S., Dekker, G. A., Makowitz, J. W. and Rotmans, N. (1991). Effect of low-dose aspirin on vascular refractoriness in angiotensin-sensitive primigravid women. *Am. J. Obstet. Gynecol.*, **164**, 1169–73
5. Moncada, S. and Vayne, J. R. (1979). Pharmacology and endogenous roles of prostaglandin endoperoxides, thromboxane A2 and prostacylin. *Pharmacol. Rev.*, **30**, 293–331
6. Ylikorkala, O. and Mäkilä, U. M. (1985). Prostacyclin and thromboxane in gynecology and pregnancy. *Am. J. Obstet. Gynecol.*, **152**, 318–29
7. Walsh, S. W. (1985). Preeclampsia: an imbalance in placental prostacyclin and thromboxane production. *Am. J. Obstet. Gynecol.*, **152**, 335–40
8. Fitzgerald, D. J., Rocki, W., Murray, R., Mayo, G. and Fitzgerald, G. A. (1990). Thromboxane A2 synthesis in pregnancy-induced hypertension. *Lancet*, **335**, 751–4
9. Bremer, H. A. and Wallenburg, H. C. S. (1992). Aspirin in pregnancy. *Fetal Matern. Med. Rev.*, **4**, 37–57
10. Rees, D. D., Palmer, R. M. J. and Moncada, S. (1989). Role of endothelium-derived nitric oxide in the regulation of blood pressure. *Proc. Natl. Acad. Sci. USA*, **86**, 3375–8
11. Pinto, A., Sorrentino, R., Sorrentino, P., Guerritore, T., Miranda, L., Biondi, A. and Martinelli, P. (1991). Endothelial-derived relaxing factor released by endothelial cells of human umbilical vessels and its impairment in pregnancy-induced hypertension. *Am. J. Obstet. Gynecol.*, **164**, 507–13
12. Dekker, G. A. and Sibaï, B. M. (1993). Low-dose aspirin in the prevention of preeclampsia and fetal growth retardation: Rationale, mechanisms, and clinical trials. *Am. J. Obstet. Gynecol.*, **168**, 214–27
13. Gant, N. F., Daley, G. L., Chand, S., Whalley, P. J. and MacDonald, P. C. (1973). A study of angiotensin II pressor response throughout primigravid pregnancy. *J. Clin. Invest.*, **522**, 2682–9
14. Vayne, J. R. (1971). Inhibition of prostaglandin synthesis as a mechanism of action of aspirin-like drugs. *Nature (London)*, **231**, 232–5
15. Jaffe, E. A. and Wesler, B. B. (1979). Recovery of endothelial cell prostacyclin production after inhibition by low doses of aspirin. *J. Clin. Invest.*, **63**, 532–5
16. Masotti, G., Galanti, G., Poggesi, L., Abbate, R. and Neri-Serneri, G. G. (1979). Differential inhibition of prostacyclin production and platelet aggregation by aspirin. *Lancet*, **2**, 1213–7
17. Sibaï, B. M., Mirro, R., Chesney, C. M. and Leffler, C. (1989). Low-dose aspirin in pregnancy. *Obstet. Gynecol.*, **74**, 551–7
18. Roberts, M. S., Joyce, R. M., Mcleod, L. J., Vial, J. H. and Serville, P. R. (1986). Slow-release aspirin and prostaglandin inhibition. *Lancet*, **2**, 1153–4
19. Branch, D. W., Scott, J. R., Kochenour, N. K. and Hershgold, E. (1985). Obstetrics complications associated with the lupus anticoagulant. *N. Engl. J. Med.*, **313**, 1322–6
20. Kelton, J. G. (1983). Antiplatelet agents: rationale and results. *Clin. Hematol.*, **12**, 311–54
21. Pedersen, A. K. and Fitzgerald, G. A. (1984). Dose-related kinetics of aspirin. *N. Engl. J. Med.*, **311**, 1206–11
22. Rowland, M., Riegelman, S., Harris, P. A. and Sholkoff, S. (1972). Absorption kinetics of aspirin in man following oral administration of an aqueous solution. *J. Pharm. Sci.*, **61**, 379–85
23. Jacobson, R. L., Brewer, A., Eis, A., Siddiqui, T. A. and Myatt, L. (1991). Transfer of aspirin across the perfused human placental cotyledon. *Am. J. Obstet. Gynecol.*, **165**, 939–44

24. Benigni, A., Gregorini, G., Frusca, T., Chiabrando, C., Ballerini, S., Valcamonico, A., Orisio, S., Piccinelli, A., Pinciroli, V., Fanelli, R., Gastaldi, A. and Remuzzi, G. (1989). Effect of low-dose aspirin on fetal and maternal generation of thromboxane by platelets in women at risk for pregnancy-induced hypertension. *N. Engl. J. Med.*, **321**, 357–62

25. Crandon, A. J. and Isherwood, D. M. (1979). Effect of aspirin on incidence of preeclampsia. *Lancet*, **1**, 1356

26. Beaufils, M., Uzan, S., Donsimoni, R. and Colau, J. C. (1985). Prevention of pre-eclampsia by antiplatelet therapy. *Lancet*, **1**, 840–2

27. Wallenburg, H. C. S., Dekker, G. A., Makowitz, J. W. and Rotmans, P. (1986). Low-dose aspirin prevents pregnancy-induced hypertension and preeclampsia in angiotensin-sensitive primigravidae. *Lancet*, **1**, 1–3

28. Schiff, E., Peleg, E., Goldenberg, M., Rosenthal, T., Ruppin, E., Tamarkin, M., Barkaï, G., Ben-Baruk, G., Yahal, I., Blankstein, J., Goldman, B. and Mashiach, S. (1989). The use of aspirin to prevent pregnancy-induced hypertension and lower the ratio of thromboxane A2 to prostacyclin in relatively high risk pregnancies. *N. Engl. J. Med.*, **321**, 351–6

29. McParland, P., Pearce, J. M. and Chamberlain, J. V. P. (1990). Doppler ultrasound and aspirin in recognition and prevention of pregnancy-induced hypertension. *Lancet*, **335**, 1552–5

30. Wallenburg, H. C. S. and Rotmans, N. (1987). Prevention of recurrent idiopathic fetal growth retardation by low-dose aspirin and dipyridamole. *Am. J. Obstet. Gynecol.*, **157**, 1230–5

31. Trudinger, B. J., Cook, C. M., Thompson, R., Gilles, W. B. and Connelly, A. (1988). Low-dose aspirin therapy improves fetal weight in umbilical placental insufficiency. *Am. J. Obstet. Gynecol.*, **159**, 681–5

32. Uzan, S., Beaufils, M., Bréart, G., Bazin, B., Capitant, C. and Paris, J. (1991). Prevention of fetal growth retardation with low-dose aspirin: findings of the EPREDA trial. *Lancet*, **337**, 1427–31

33. Chalmers, I., Hethrington, J., Elbourne, D., Keirse, M. J. N. C. and Enkin, M. (1989). Materials and methods used in synthesizing evidence to evaluate the effect of care during pregnancy and childbirth. In Chalmers, I., Enkin, M. and Keirse, M. J. N. C. (eds.) *Effective Care In Pregnancy and Childbirth*, pp. 39–65. (Oxford: Oxford University Press)

34. Imperiale, T. F. and Petrulis, A. S. (1991). A meta-analysis of low-dose aspirin for the prevention of pregnancy-induced hypertensive disease. *J. Am. Med. Assoc.*, **266**, 261–5

35. Hauth, J. C., Goldenberg, R. L., Parker, R. C., Philips III, J. B., Copper, R. L., DuBard, M. B. and Cutter, G. R. (1993). Low-dose aspirin therapy to prevent preeclampsia. *Am. J. Obstet. Gynecol.*, **168**, 1083–93

36. Sibaï, B. M., Caritis, S. N., Thom, E., Klebanoff, M., McNellis, D., Rocco, L., Paul, R. H., Romero, R., Witter, F., Rosen, M., Depp, R. and the National Institute of Child Health and Human Development Network of Maternal–Fetal Medicine Units. (1993). Prevention of preeclampsia with low-dose aspirin in healthy, nulliparous pregnant women. *N. Engl. J. Med.*, **329**, 1213–8

37. Schiff, E., Barkai, G., Ben-Baruk, G. and Mashich, S. (1990). Low-dose aspirin does not influence the clinical course of women with mild pregnancy-induced hypertension. *Obstet. Gynecol.*, **76**, 742–4

38. Reece, E. A., Gabrielli, S., Cullen, M. T., Zheng, X. Z., Hobbins, J. C. and Harris, E. N. (1990). Recurrent adverse pregnancy outcome and antiphospholipid antibodies. *Am. J. Obstet. Gynecol.*, **163**, 162-9

39. Carreras, L. O., Vermylen, J., Spitz, B. and Van Assche, A. (1981). 'Lupus' anticoagulant and inhibition of prostacyclin formation in patients with repeated abortion, intrauterine growth retardation and intrauterine death. *Br. J. Obstet. Gynaecol.*, **88**, 890–4

40. De Wolf, F., Carreras, L. O., Moarman, P., Vermylen, J., Van Assche, A. and Renaer, M. (1982). Decidual vasculopathy and extensive placental infarction in a patient with repeated thromboembolic accidents, recurrent fetal loss, with a lupus anticoagulant. *Am. J. Obstet. Gynecol.*, **142**, 829–34

41. Lockshin, M. D., Druzin, M. L. and Qamar, T. (1989). Prednisone does not prevent recurrent fetal death in women with antiphospholipid antibody. *Am. J. Obstet. Gynecol.*, **160**, 439–43

42. Krause, I., Blank, N., Brut, B. G. and Shoenfeld, Y. (1993). The effect of aspirin on recurrent fetal loss in experimental antiphospholipid syndrome. *A.J.R.I.*, **29**, 155–61

43. Sibaï, B. M. (1992). An aspirin a day to prevent prematurity. *Clin. Perinatol.* **19**, 305–17

44. Lewis, R. B. and Schulman, J. D. (1973). Influence of acetylsalicylic acid, an inhibitor of prostaglandin synthesis, on the duration of human gestation and labour. *Lancet*, **2**, 1159–61

45. Saxen, I. (1975). Associations between oral clefts and drugs taken during pregnancy. *Int. J. Epidemol.*, **4**, 37–44

46. Slone, D., Siskind, V., Heinonen, O. P., Monson, R. R., Kaufman, D. W. and Shapiro, S. (1976). Aspirin and congenital malformations. *Lancet*, **1**, 1373–5

47. Werler, M. M., Mitchell, A. A. and Shapiro, S. (1989). The relation of aspirin use during the

first trimester of pregnancy to congenital cardiac defects. *N. Engl. J. Med.*, **321**, 1639–42
48. Rumack, C. M., Guggenheim, M. A., Rummack, B. H., Peterson, R. G., Johnson, M. L. and Braithwaite, W. R. (1981). Neonatal intracranial haemorrhage and maternal use of aspirin. *Obstet. Gynecol.*, **58**, 52S–56S
49. Nunez, L., Larrea, J. L., Gil Aguado, M., Reque, J. A., Matorras, R. and Minguez, J. A. (1983). Pregnancy in 20 patients with bioprosthetic valve replacement. *Chest*, **84**, 26–8
50. Cassin, S. (1987). Role of prostaglandins, thromboxane and leukotrienes in the control of the pulmonary circulation in the fetus and newborn. *Sem. Perinatol.*, **11**, 53–63
51. Gersony, W. M., Pecham, G. J., Ellison, R. C., Miettinen, O. S. and Nadas, A. S. (1983). Effects of indomethacin in premature infants with a patent ductus arteriosus: results of a national collaborative study. *J. Pediatr.*, **102**, 895–906
52. Levin, D. L. (1980). Effect of inhibition of prostaglandin synthesis on fetal development, oxygenation, and the fetal circulation. *Sem. Perinatol.*, **4**, 35–44
53. Perkin, R. M., Levin, D. L. and Clark, R. (1980). Serum salicylate levels and right to left ductus shunts in newborn infants with persistent pulmonary hypertension. *J. Pediatr.*, **96**, 721–6
54. Shapiro, S., Siskind, V., Monson, R. R., Heinonen, O. P., Kaufman, D. W. and Slone, D. (1976). Perinatal mortality and birth-weight in relation of aspirin taken during pregnancy. *Lancet*, **1**, 1375–6
55. Streissguth, A. P., Treder, R. P., Barr, H. M., Shepard, T. H., Bleyer, W. A. and Sampson, P. D. (1987). Aspirin and acetaminophen use by pregnant women and subsequent child IQ and attention decrements. *Teratology*, **35**, 211–19
56. Klebanoff, M. A. and Berendes, H. W. (1988). Aspirin exposure during the first 20 weeks of gestation and IQ at four years of age. *Teratology*, **37**, 249–55
57. Taggart, D. P., Siddiqui, A. and Wheatley, D. J., (1990). Low-dose preoperative aspirin therapy, postoperative blood loss, and transfusion requirements. *Ann. Thorac. Surg.*, **50**, 425–8
58. Baker, P. N., Williamson, J. G. and Louden, K. A. (1992). Possible low-dose aspirin-induced gastropathy. *Lancet*, **339**, 550
59. Stuart, M. J., Gross, S. J., Elrad, H. and Graeber, J. E. (1982). Effects of acetylsalicylic-acid ingestion on maternal and neonatal hemostasis. *N. Engl. J. Med.*, **307**, 909–12
60. O'Sullivan, G. (1990). Regional anesthesia and aspirin. *Anaesthesiology*, **73**, 359
61. Ivy, A. D., Nelson, D. and Buches, G. (1941). The standardization of certain factors in the cutaneous venostasis. Bleeding time technique. *J. Lab. Clin. Med.*, **26**, 1812
62. CLASP: a randomised trial of low dose aspirin for the prevention and treatment of pre-eclampsia among 9364 pregnant women (1994). *Lancet*, **343**, 619–29

Diagnosis and management of immune thrombocytopenias

K. A. Eddleman, J. B. Bussel and F. A. Chervenak

INTRODUCTION

The diagnosis of maternal thrombocytopenia (< 150 000 platelets/mm³) is being made with increasing frequency, due to the advent of automated platelet-counting equipment. In a recent surveillance study of over 15 000 pregnancies, maternal thrombocytopenia occurred in 6.6% of all pregnancies and was < 100 /mm³ in 1.2%[1]. In about three-quarters of the cases that have a maternal count of less than 150 000 platelets/mm³, the thrombocytopenia is serendipitously detected and poses little or no risk to the mother or fetus/neonate. Of the remaining one-quarter, the majority of cases are related to hypertensive disorders of pregnancy (pre-eclampsia–toxemia). The neonatal thrombocytopenia associated with maternal hypertension appears to be due to complications of prematurity rather than the underlying maternal thrombocytopenia, as many of these patients require iatrogenic preterm delivery[2]. Approximately 3% of the cases of maternal thrombocytopenia encountered during pregnancy are due to immunological disorders, most commonly immune thrombocytopenic purpura or systemic lupus erythematosus (SLE). The immune-related platelet disorders are the focus of this chapter and will be discussed in depth. Rarer causes of maternal thrombocytopenia include disseminated intravascular coagulation (DIC), familial (hereditary) thrombocytopenia, thrombotic thrombocytopenic purpura (TTP), hemolytic uremic syndrome and type II von Willebrand's disease. The differential diagnosis of maternal thrombocytopenia and laboratory findings are listed in Table 1.

Table 1 *Differential diagnosis of maternal thrombocytopenia*

Cause of thrombocytopenia	Diagnosis
Pre-eclampsia/HELLP syndrome	clinical criteria for pre-eclampsia elevated transaminases, elevated LDH
Systemic lupus erythematosus	American rheumatological association diagnostic criteria, hypocomplementemia
Disseminated intravascular coagulation	elevated fibrin split products, hypofibrinogenemia
Thrombotic thrombocytopenic purpura	microangiopathic hemolytic anemia, elevated haptoglobins, renal dysfunction, neurological symptoms
von Willebrand's disease (type II)	increased sensitivity to ristocetin-induced platelet aggregation
Immune thrombocytopenic purpura	antiplatelet antibodies, clinical history
Gestational thrombocytopenia (incidental thrombocytopenia)	by exclusion
Drug-induced thrombocytopenia	by history
Human immunodeficiency virus (HIV) infection	risk factors, opportunistic infections, positive serological testing for HIV
Familial (hereditary) thrombocytopenia	by history, family platelet counts

HELLP, hemolysis, elevated liver enzymes, low platelets; LDH, lactate dehydrogenase

Thrombocytopenia also occurs commonly in infection with the human immunodeficiency virus (HIV)[3]. It has been estimated that HIV infection may be responsible for at least 10% of all cases of thrombocytopenia in non-pregnant patients[4]. It may mimic classical immune thrombocytopenic purpura in symptoms, signs and pathophysiology. With the increasing heterosexual transmission of HIV in the West, it is likely that HIV-related thrombocytopenia will become of significant concern in pregnant patients.

Thrombocytopenia in the mother, even immune thrombocytopenia, rarely causes significant long-term sequelae. Platelet counts are easy to monitor and usually improve after delivery. The real concern is that some causes of maternal thrombocytopenia can, in turn, cause fetal/neonatal thrombocytopenia and lead to catastrophic intracranial hemorrhage. Life-threatening neonatal thrombocytopenia (< 50 000 platelets/mm^3) is infrequent and occurred in 0.12% of deliveries in one series[1]. About one-half of the cases of neonatal thrombocytopenia are associated with maternal thrombocytopenia.

The most severe cases of neonatal thrombocytopenia are associated with immune thrombocytopenia. The focus of this chapter is therefore the immune-related thrombocytopenias: 'gestational' thrombocytopenia (GTP), autoimmune thrombocytopenia (ITP) and alloimmune thrombocytopenia (AIT). Clinical significance, diagnosis and management will be discussed for each entity.

GESTATIONAL THROMBOCYTOPENIA

Background and incidence

GTP (also called incidentally-detected or asymptomatic thrombocytopenia) is a clinically benign condition for both the mother and fetus[5-7]. The diagnosis of GTP is usually limited to those patients with counts of less than 150 000 platelets/mm^3 but more than 100 000 platelets/mm^3 at delivery. Mothers with counts between 75 000 and 100 000 platelets/mm^3 may have GTP; however, this range of platelet counts overlaps with true ITP. GTP, to a certain extent, is a diagnosis of exclusion and is made only after other immune and non-immune causes of thrombocytopenia have been excluded (see Table 1). However, the three cardinal criteria are:

(1) A mild degree of thrombocytopenia;

(2) No prior history of thrombocytopenia; and

(3) No bleeding symptoms.

As previously indicated, the diagnosis is being made with increasing frequency, due to the advent of automated platelet counting. GTP is the most frequent type of thrombocytopenia encountered in pregnancy[7]. The incidence is approximately 4–8% of 'normal' pregnancies[1,6]. GTP is estimated to account for approximately 75% of all cases of pregnancy-related thrombocytopenia. The major confusion with GTP is the frequent difficulty in distinguishing GTP from true ITP (see below, discussion of anti-platelet antibodies).

Pathogenesis

Patients with GTP may have both direct and indirect anti-platelet antibodies. Samuels and colleagues[8] reported that 62% of patients with GTP had increased levels of indirect (circulating) anti-platelet antibodies. Lescale and associates[9] compared the results of platelet-associated (direct) immunoglobulin (Ig) G, IgM and C3 (third component of complement) and platelet-bindable (indirect) IgG, IgM, and C3 in 250 patients (90 with true ITP and 160 with GTP). Only platelet-bindable IgG was significantly higher in the ITP patients, but overlap between the two groups precluded using this test to distinguish ITP from GTP. Available platelet antibody testing does *not* distinguish GTP from ITP. Based on these studies, we postulate that GTP is a result of non-specific platelet activation, as opposed to true ITP, which is an autoimmune disorder. The cause of that non-specific activation is unknown. Currently, it appears that a history of ITP antedating the pregnancy is the best discriminator between these two causes of thrombocytopenia[8]. More specific platelet anti-

IMMUNE THROMBOCYTOPENIAS

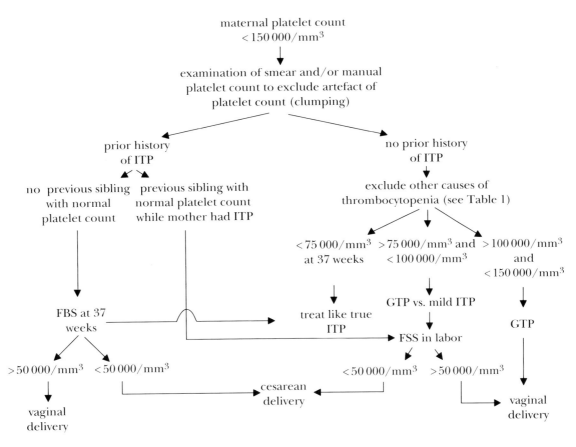

Figure 1 *Management of thrombocytopenia. FBS, fetal blood sampling; FSS, fetal scalp sampling; GTP, gestational thrombocytopenia; ITP, immune thrombocytopenic purpura*

body tests such as those measuring antibodies directed against platelet glycoproteins (GP IIB/IIA, GP IB/IX) may provide better serological distinction[9].

Diagnosis and management

The management of patients with GTP involves excluding other causes of thrombocytopenia and is outlined in Figure 1. When the automated platelet count is less than 150 000 platelets/mm^3, a careful history should be taken to exclude other causes of pregnancy-related thrombocytopenia (pregnancy-associated hypertension, medications, antecedent history suspicious for true ITP, DIC or TTP). The pursuit of earlier platelet counts (for example from employment physical examinations or previous pregnancies) is important. A peripheral smear should be examined to exclude platelet clumping and/or a manual platelet count should be done. If the manual platelet count is less than 75 000 platelets/mm^3 then the patient should be considered as having true ITP (management discussed below). If the manual count is less than 150 000 but more than 100 000 platelets/mm^3 and other causes of thrombocytopenia have been excluded, the diagnosis of GTP is made. Platelet counts should be followed serially throughout pregnancy to ensure that they remain within the range consistent with GTP. No intervention is necessary in these patients. Platelet counts are likely to fluctuate over time. If, at the time of labor, the maternal platelet count is more than 100 000 platelets/mm³, the fetus may be delivered vaginally with or without scalp platelet sampling. In the patient with a platelet count between 75 000 and 100 000, the distinction between mild ITP and GTP cannot be made with current methodology. Mothers in this 'gray zone' are best managed by fetal scalp sampling in labor to identify the rare thrombocytopenic fetus of the mildly-affected mother who actually has true ITP. The advantages and disadvantages of fetal scalp sampling for platelet counts are discussed in depth in the discussion of ITP. Using this management protocol minimizes Cesarean deliveries and fetal blood samplings for fetuses likely to have normal platelet counts, but also optimizes identification of those fetuses at greatest risk for thrombocytopenia.

IMMUNE THROMBOCYTOPENIC PURPURA

Background

ITP is a non-malignant hematological disorder with a predilection for women in the reproductive age-group. The true prevalence of ITP is unknown: it is estimated to be 3–5 cases per 10 000 pregnancies, but it may be higher, depending upon definition, i.e. the distinction from GTP[7]. Because of its predilection for the reproductive age-group and the tendency for ITP to worsen during pregnancy in some women, the initial clinical presentation of ITP may be during pregnancy. Diagnosis during pregnancy does not always indicate onset during pregnancy, as patients with counts as low as 30 000 platelets/mm³ may be asymptomatic in the non-pregnant state. The most common clinical presentation with classical ITP is that of petechiae and ecchymoses.

Pathophysiology

In ITP, platelet-binding autoantibodies are produced, which primarily are directed at glycoproteins (GP) expressed on the platelet surface, especially GP IIB/IIIA. There is no apparent difference in antibody specificity between pregnant and non-pregnant patients; however, this has not been well studied. Based on the disappearance of antibody in certain patients following splenectomy, and on *in vitro* studies demonstrating the presence of mononuclear cells secreting anti-platelet antibody in removed spleens, it is believed that a part of the antibody is made in the spleen. However, the predominant role of the spleen is that of a 'filter' of the blood. Antibody-coated platelets are thought to be removed via interaction with Fc receptors of splenic macrophages, in the same way that antibody-coated bacteria are cleared from the circulation. Generally, in thrombocytopenic patients, increased platelet destruction overwhelms compensatory increases in platelet production, resulting in thrombocytopenia. It has been recently recognized that some of the more chronic refractory cases of ITP in adults have decreased platelet production as well. The role of antibody cross-reactivity with megakaryocytes in the bone marrow, and how this affects platelet production, remains to be clarified.

Several sex-steroid effects are known which may exacerbate disease during pregnancy. Increased expression and avidity of Fc receptors can be induced on mononuclear phagocytes by estrogen. Cyclic thrombocytopenia in non-pregnant patients has been shown to be dependent upon hormonal surges. Additionally, danazol (a modified androgen) has been shown to increase the platelet count in many (non-pregnant) patients with ITP, emphasizing the clinical significance of sex steroids.

Maternal management

The clinical course of characterized by exacerbations of varying severity and frequency. Contemporary treatment of exacerbations has reduced maternal mortality and morbidity to virtually nil. The most common antepartum treatments for maternal thrombocytopenia are corticosteroids and intravenous gamma-globulin[10]. These therapies pose no apparent risk to the fetus. These therapies are usually begun once the maternal platelet count falls below 20 000 to 30 000 platelet/mm³, or at higher counts if there is clinical bleeding or need for an invasive procedure such as amniocentesis. Plasmapheresis has been attempted, with mixed results. Ante- or peripartum splenectomy has been used in the past, but is no longer performed, except in the most exceptional patients refractory to traditional therapy.

In the mother with ITP, platelet counts can be performed easily and as frequently as required. Should the need arise, prompt and rapidly acting treatment can be instituted. The fetus, however, is more of a 'black box', making management more complicated. Some, but not all, mothers with ITP will have their anti-platelet antibodies cross the placenta and 'attack' the fetus' platelets, resulting in fetal thrombocytopenia. It is important to remember that maternal IgG normally crosses the placenta in increasing quantities as gestation progresses, for passive immunization of the neonate against infection in the weeks and months after birth. Also, other fetal neonatal disorders are mediated by transplacental passage of autoantibodies, such as congenital heart block in mothers with collagen vascular diseases, and neonatal hyperthyroidism in mothers with Grave's disease. Therefore, the first goal of management is the identification of the fetus that will be or is affected.

Prediction of fetal platelet count

The major risk due to thrombocytopenia in the fetus is that of intracranial hemorrhage. In a summary of three articles published in 1990 of 182 mothers with ITP, there was an incidence of severe neonatal thrombocytopenia (< 50 000 platelets/mm^3) of 14.7%[11]. The incidence of intracranial hemorrhage in that series was 1.5% and perinatal mortality was 0.5%. It is exceedingly rare to have an antenatal intracranial hemorrhage with ITP. Also, intracranial hemorrhage as a result of thrombocytopenia is exceedingly rare in neonates with a platelet count of more than 50 000, and very uncommon if the platelet count is more than 20 000 platelets/mm^3.

An important consideration in estimating the platelet count is that the platelet count typically falls after birth; it is felt that the count at delivery is the most important platelet count with regards to risk of intracranial hemorrhage, rather than the nadir count, which may occur one to three (or even more) days after birth.

The fundamental problem with management of the pregnant patient with ITP is how to determine antenatally which neonates are at risk of having platelet counts of less than 50 000 platelets/mm^3, and what to do if you succeed in identifying them. The issue is further confounded by uncertainty as to whether Cesarean delivery actually offers protection against intracranial hemorrhage.

It is well accepted that there is no correlation between fetal and maternal platelet counts[13–17]. For example, fetal thrombocytopenia can exist even in cases of apparent maternal remission after splenectomy[18]. Maternal antibodies may exist in these cases but not lead to destruction of maternal platelets, because of absence of the spleen. IgG and IgM platelet-associated (direct) and circulating (indirect) antibodies have been measured in an attempt to estimate the severity of fetal thrombocytopenia. Some studies have shown weak correlations between maternal anti-platelet antibody levels and fetal platelet counts, but at best these tests are of limited help in predicting those fetuses at risk for severe thrombocytopenia[8,15,17,18]. Additionally, as stated above, anti-platelet antibodies are not helpful in distinguishing the more benign gestational thrombocytopenia from ITP.

Direct estimates of fetal platelet counts can be obtained antenatally by either fetal scalp blood sampling or fetal umbilical cord blood sampling. Ayromlooi and colleagues in 1978 introduced fetal scalp sampling as a means to assess fetal platelet count prior to delivery[19]. Scott and associates[12] showed that scalp sampling could be performed accurately in predicting which fetuses have platelet counts below 50 000 platelets/mm^3. Scalp sampling, however, has several drawbacks and has been abandoned in many centers for the following reasons. It is technically difficult, membranes must be ruptured and the cervix must be dilated at least 2–3 cm to obtain a sample. Platelet clumping can lead to falsely low platelet counts and unnecessary obstetric intervention[18–20]. Adams and co-workers[21] recently have reported that scanning the smear for the presence of clumps of ten or more platelets is a more reliable way to predict the platelet count. This, however, requires experience in smear review and has been validated in only one thrombocytopenic neonate. When relying on scalp platelet counts, there is also a theoretical risk of intracranial hemorrhage during early labor before the cervix is dilated enough to obtain the sample. We use fetal scalp sampling in those patients at low to moderate risk of having a fetus with severe thrombocytopenia.

Some centers have advocated utilizing fetal blood sampling in the management of pregnancies complicated by ITP[13,22-24]. The obvious advantage of fetal blood sampling is that it provides an accurate measurement of the fetal platelet count before labor begins and while membranes are intact. Kaplan and colleagues[13] and Daffos and co-workers[22] in the past have advocated fetal blood sampling at 20–22 weeks' gestation to assess fetal platelet counts in order to modify maternal treatment, and again at term to determine mode of delivery. Limitations to this approach include the absence of a reliable antenatal treatment that corrects fetal thrombocytopenia and the risk of loss from the procedure, including catastrophic hemorrhage from the cord puncture site if the fetus is indeed thrombocytopenic[5]. The disadvantage of fetal blood sampling in the third trimester is that it is technically more difficult. We utilize fetal blood sampling at term in those patients who have a prior history of a neonate with a platelet count below 50 000 platelets/mm^3 in order to offer potential treatment. Alternately, one could perform an elective Cesarean delivery without fetal blood sampling, as our current data suggest that these mothers are very likely to have thrombocytopenic fetuses again[25].

Management

Figure 1 provides an algorithm to guide management of delivery. This is not meant to be the only way to manage ITP in pregnancy but, given the pitfalls discussed above, we feel that this algorithm provides a reasonable margin of safety for both mother and fetus. If the history of thrombocytopenia antedates the pregnancy, the patient is considered to have true ITP and the maternal platelet count, while required for maternal management, is superfluous in fetal management.

In these patients we recommend a fetal blood sampling at or about 37 weeks' gestational age. If the fetal platelet count is less than 50 000 platelets/mm^3, a Cesarean delivery is recommended once fetal lung maturity has been documented. This can usually be done by removing an aliquot of amniotic fluid at the time of fetal blood sampling and examining phospholipid ratios. If the fetal platelet count is more than 100 000 platelets/mm^3, then spontaneous labor and vaginal delivery is allowed. If the fetal platelet count is between 50 000 and 100 000 platelets/mm^3 and fetal lung maturity is documented, then induction of labor would seem reasonable, since the platelet count could drop below 50 000 platelets/mm^3 if one waited for spontaneous labor.

In conclusion, true ITP in pregnancy is not an infrequent disorder, but associated significant neonatal thrombocytopenia is uncommon. Fortunately, the incidence of neonatal intracranial hemorrhage as a result of thrombocytopenia is rare and there are no convincing cases of *in utero* intracranial hemorrhage that have definitely been attributed to classical maternal ITP. Considerable controversy exists over the management of the pregnant patient with ITP. The primary goal is to minimize unnecessary Cesarean deliveries and fetal blood sampling procedures in fetuses with normal platelet counts, while preventing intracranial hemorrhages in those rare fetuses who do have low platelet counts. As stated above, Cesarean delivery may not even prevent intracranial hemorrhage[26]. The controversy is compounded by a lack of adequate clinical trials. The outcome variable of interest (neonatal intracranial hemorrhage) is so infrequent, it is unlikely that even a collaborative trial will be able to evaluate management protocols prospectively with adequate statistical power. Until a serological means of prediction of fetal/neonatal thrombocytopenia is available, we feel that the algorithm outlined above strikes a logical balance of safety for both the mother and the fetus.

ALLOIMMUNE THROMBOCYTOPENIA

Background and incidence

AIT occurs as a result of maternal sensitization to paternally-derived fetal platelet antigens. Women who lack these antigens produce antibodies of the IgG subclass, which cross the placenta and attach to the antigen on the fetal platelet. These antibody-coated platelets are then recognized by the fetal reticuloendothelial system and destroyed. A better known pathophysiological analog to AIT is that of rhesus isoimmunization and resultant erythroblastosis fetalis. Maternal–fetal incompatibility for the PLA1 antigen is the most common cause of AIT and is responsible for the majority of cases in Caucasians[27]. This antigen has also been referred to as the Zwa antigen, or more recently as the HPA-1A antigen, and is expressed earlier than 16 weeks of gestation[28]. Transplacental passage of anti-PLA1 antibodies can occur as early as 14 weeks' gestation and fetal thrombocytopenia has been documented as early as 16 weeks' gestation[29,30]. Table 2 lists platelet antigens that have been associated with AIT in order of decreasing frequency[31]. PLA1 has been emphasized in the past, because it is the antigen most frequently tested, and in many cases, the only antigen tested. Additionally, frequency is a function of ethnicity. PLA2 does not occur in Asians or Blacks and Yuk/Pen occurs in Asians but not Caucasians. Finally, Br is the second most commonly reported antigen in Caucasians in Europe, but this may depend upon larger family sizes there and/or HLA (human leukocyte antigen) types, since it is not recognized as frequently in the United States[4]. Although a majority of cases of AIT are caused by PLA1 incompatibility, only 2% of the population lacks the antigen and are at risk of producing antibodies[32]. Only 65 to 80% of those women who are PLA1-negative and deliver thrombocytopenic infants will have detectable antibodies[27,33]. Neither the presence of anti-PLA1 antibodies nor the absolute antibody titer are useful in predicting the severity of fetal or neonatal thrombocytopenia[29]. The production of alloantibodies seems to be related to the concomitant presence of the DW52a haplotype in the maternal major histocompatibility complex[34,35].

Prospective studies of AIT have suggested that the incidence is as high as one in 2000 pregnancies[26]. If one accepts the 0.12% (one in 1200 deliveries) overall incidence of *severe* neonatal thrombocytopenia stated earlier, then AIT would be responsible for half or more of those cases. Inferences such as this are problematic, however, due to the differences in design of the studies involved, but nonetheless, AIT represents a far higher fraction of severe thrombocytopenia than does ITP. Unlike rhesus disease, approximately half of all first cases of AIT in a family occur in the first pregnancy. The most devastating complication of AIT is that of intracranial hemorrhage and occurs in 20–30% of cases[37,38]. Of intracranial hemorrhages, 25–50% occur *in utero*[37–39], and this complication has been reported as early as 20 weeks' gestation[40]. Based on the number of births in

Table 2 *Platelet-specific alloantigen systems. Other antigens, including Mo and Ca/Tu have recently been described. Nomenclature is currently under discussion. Adapted from reference 31, with permission*

System	HPA nomenclature	Alleles	Phenotype frequency	Glycoprotein association
PI^A	HPA-1	1 (a)	98	IIIa
		2 (b)	28	
Bak (Lek)	HPA-3	a	85	IIb
		b	63	heavy chain
Pen (Yuk)	HPA-4	a (b)	> 99	IIIa
		b (a)	1.7	
Ko (Sib)	HPA-2	a	15	?
		b	99	
Br	HPA-5	a	20	Ia
		b	99	

the United States and the incidences indicated above, it has been estimated that 800 to 2000 cases of AIT occur annually in the United States with 160 to 400 resultant intracranial hemorrhages[4]. The classical clinical presentation is that of a healthy mother with a normal platelet count who delivers an infant that develops petechiae and ecchymoses obvious at or within hours of birth. Alternatively, the diagnosis may be made during the evaluation of abnormal bleeding after blood collection or circumcision. Couples whose siblings have had children affected with AIT are also at risk and should be evaluated. The recurrence of AIT in subsequent pregnancies is higher than 99% in antigen-positive fetuses and therefore the recurrence risk depends on the frequencies of the antigens involved and on paternal zygosity. For PLA1, it is approximately 87.5% (3 of 4 fathers are homozygotes)[31]. In those pregnancies, the degree of thrombocytopenia is similar to or worse than that seen in the previously affected sibling and usually progressively worsens with advancing gestational age[37]. In general, the degree of thrombocytopenia in AIT is worse than that seen with ITP. Spontaneous improvement is extremely unlikely[38].

Diagnosis

All neonates with platelet counts less than 30 000 platelets/mm^3, even if they have another possible explanation for the thrombocytopenia, such as ITP, sepsis, DIC or viral infections, should have serological testing. This is especially important if the platelet count is a birth platelet count and not a nadir count from 24 to 48 h post-delivery. When AIT is suspected, parental platelets should be typed for common platelet antigens to determine compatibility. Additionally, maternal serum should be evaluated for the presence of antibodies specific for platelet antigens that react with the neonate's platelets. If antibody testing is negative but PLA1 incompatibility is detected, testing for the antibody can be repeated after the puerperium. HLA-Dwa52a typing may also be useful in those patients, as Dw52a-negative women are much less likely to produce antibodies.

Management – neonate

AIT is a self-limiting disorder in the neonate, typically lasting one to two weeks, and is usually completely resolved by 3 months of age, once the maternal antibodies have disappeared from the neonatal circulation. Neonatal head sonography is important to determine the presence of hemorrhage. Management of the neonate with AIT is aimed at prevention of intracranial hemorrhage if this has not already occurred. The therapy of choice in the neonate with a severely depressed platelet count (< 20 000–50 000 platelets/mm^3) is transfusion with platelets that lack the antigen involved. This is most easily accomplished by transfusion with maternal platelets that have been concentrated to minimize the amount of residual anti-platelet antibody in the plasma. Since the majority of the population is PLA1-positive, and this is the most frequent antigen involved in AIT, random donor platelets should be reserved for management of ongoing intracranial or other serious hemorrhage[38]. Other modalities used to treat AIT include intravenous gammaglobulin (IVGG) with or without concomitant corticosteroids. This should be administered if antigen-negative platelets are not available, or while waiting for them to become available.

Management – fetus

Since a significant number of intracranial hemorrhages occur antenatally, optimal management should begin *in utero*. Management of the fetus at risk for AIT is controversial. Opinions are dichotomous and rest between medical management with IVGG, corticosteroid or both, or management by repeated fetal blood sampling and *in utero* platelet transfusions for thrombocytopenic fetuses. Bussel and colleagues[37] treated seven patients at risk for AIT with weekly maternal IVGG infusions. All seven of the neonates had counts higher than 30 000 platelets/mm^3 at birth. Six of the fetuses underwent fetal blood sampling both before and after institution of therapy and all six demonstrated significant increases in platelet counts. Lynch and associates[38] subsequently reported on an expanded series of patients (including the seven patients mentioned above) treated with either IVGG alone or with corticosteroid. The 18 patients in that series had 21 previously affected infants, of whom ten (48%) had intracranial hemorrhages. Six of those hemorrhages (60%) occurred antenatally. In the subsequent monitored pregnancies, the patients underwent fetal blood sampling at 20–22 weeks, to determine platelet count and type. If the fetal platelet count was below 100 000 platelets/mm^3, treatment was begun with IVGG. Nine patients additionally received steroids. A repeat fetal blood sampling was performed 4–6 weeks after institution of therapy, and thereafter at 6–8-week intervals, to monitor response to treatment. Median fetal platelet counts before treatment and at delivery were 32 000 and 60 000 platelets/mm^3, respectively. Antenatal treatment resulted in a neonatal platelet count higher than 30 000 platelets/mm^3 in 15 of 18 patients (83%), much higher than that of the previous untreated siblings. There were no significant differences between the group that received concomitant corticosteroid and the group that received IVGG alone. There were no intracranial hemorrhages in the 18 neonates, even in the three treatment failures. The authors speculated that even if the platelet count fails to increase, IVGG therapy may protect against intracranial hemorrhage by some unknown mechanism[41].

A further trial involved more than 50 randomized patients and confirmed the previously reported results. The preliminary results are that the mean platelet increase from the first fetal blood sampling to birth was greater than 40 000 platelets/mm^3. Approximately three-quarters of the babies were born with platelet counts higher than 30 000 platelets/mm^3 whereas half had counts at initial fetal blood sampling of 20 000 platelets/mm^3. No infant in the study had an intracranial hemorrhage.

Kaplan and co-workers[29] employed an approach in nine patients that included fetal blood sampling early in gestation to determine if the fetus was affected, and again at 38 weeks to transfuse platelets prior to delivery, in those fetuses with counts below 50 000 platelets/mm^3. Six fetuses received antenatal platelet transfusions and eight of the nine fetuses had platelet counts higher than 100 000 platelets/mm^3 at birth. There were no intracranial hemorrhages. The theoretical risks to this approach are those of antenatal hemorrhage before transfusion and hemorrhage from the puncture site in the cord after the fetal sample is obtained.

An alternative approach, also utilizing fetal blood sampling, is that of weekly *in utero* platelet transfusions. Nicolini and associates[42] reported a case managed in such a manner, where seven prophylactic platelet transfusions were performed at weekly intervals from 26 to 32 weeks' gestation. The fetal platelet count was below 50 000 platelets/mm^3 before and above 150 000 platelets/mm^3 after transfusion in each case. The fetus was delivered electively at 32 weeks' gestation by Cesarean delivery and had a platelet count of 44 000 platelets/mm^3. The neonate required no subsequent platelet transfusions and had no sonographic evidence of intracranial hemorrhage. The major disadvantage to this approach is the need for frequent transfusions, since the half-life of transfused platelets is 4–10 days, and the inherent procedure-related risk to serial fetal blood samplings[38]. Since these fetuses are often profoundly thrombocytopenic, there is a real risk of exsanguination from the cord puncture site after fetal blood sampling (Dr R. L. Berkowitz, personal communication). For that reason, concentrated maternal platelets should be available for transfusion prior to removing the needle from the umbilical cord if the fetus is found to be thrombocytopenic. Alternatively, the maternal platelets can be given empirically after the fetal blood is obtained, if no fetal platelet count is available immediately.

The approach we recommend is outlined in Figure 2. Paternal zygosity testing is recommended prior to invasive testing to assess the possibility of a PLA1-negative fetus[30]. Patients at risk for AIT undergo fetal blood sampling for platelet count and typing at 20 weeks' gestation. Concentrated maternal platelets are prepared prior to the procedure, and either transfused empirically at completion of the procedure or after fetal platelet counts are available, before

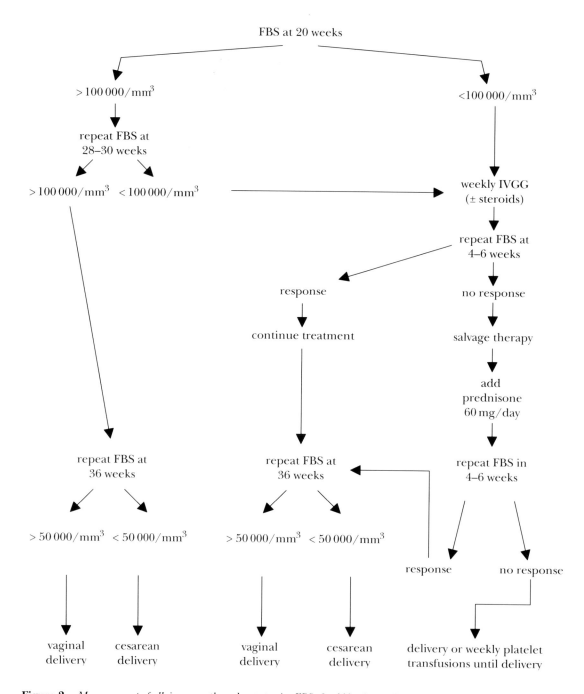

Figure 2 *Management of alloimmune thrombocytopenia. FBS, fetal blood sampling; IVGG, intravenousgammaglobulin*

removal of the needle from the umbilical cord for reasons outlined above. If the fetal platelet count is less than 100 000 platelets/mm³, the patient is begun on weekly infusions of IVGG at a dose of 1 g/kg body weight/week. A subsequent fetal blood sampling is performed 4–6 weeks after institution of therapy, to assess response. If the subsequent fetal platelet count is higher than the previous count or 20 000 platelets/mm^3, then IVGG therapy is continued. A final fetal blood sample is recommended at 36 weeks, to determine mode of delivery. If the fetal platelet count is less than 50 000 platelets/mm^3, then Cesarean delivery is recommended; otherwise, vaginal delivery is allowed (unless there are obstetric indications for Cesarean delivery). If at the time of the second fetal blood sampling the fetal platelet count indicates no response to therapy, then corticosteroids are added (prednisone 60 mg/day). Serial fetal blood sampling at 6–8-week intervals is helpful to guide therapy. Weekly fetal platelet transfusions are used only for those patients who fail 'salvage' therapy with prednisone.

In conclusion, AIT is an important cause of fetal/neonatal thrombocytopenia, which can result in catastrophic intracranial hemorrhage if present. The magnitude and timing of that risk is difficult to assess, but it can occur at any time from 18 weeks' gestation to delivery. In most series using untreated affected siblings as 'historical' controls, it appears that diagnosis using fetal blood sampling combined with treatment using IVGG moderates the severity of the disease, and thus prevents intracranial hemorrhage.

References

1. Burrows, R. F. and Kelton, J. G. (1993). Fetal thrombocytopenia and its relation to maternal thrombocytopenia. *N. Engl. J. Med.*, **329**, 1463–6
2. Burrows, R. F. and Andrew, M. (1990). Neonatal thrombocytopenia in the hypertensive disorders of pregnancy. *Obstet. Gynecol.*, **76**, 234–8
3. Morris, L., Distenfeld, A., Amorosi, E. and Karpaktkin, S. (1982). Autoimmune thrombocytopenic purpura in homosexual men. *Ann. Intern. Med.*, **96**, 714–17
4. Bussel, J. B. and Schreiber, A. D. (1991). Immune thrombocytopenic purpura, neonatal alloimmune thrombocytopenia, and post-transfusion purpura. In Hoffman, R., Benz, E. J., Shattil, S. J., Furie, B. and Cohen, H. J. (eds.) *Hematology: Basic Principles and Practice*, pp. 1485–94. (New York: Churchill Livingstone)
5. Aster, R. H. (1990). 'Gestational' thrombocytopenia: a plea for conservative management. *N. Engl. J. Med.*, **323**, 264–6
6. Burrows, R. F. and Kelton, J. G. (1988). Incidentally detected thrombocytopenia in healthy mothers and their infants. *N. Engl. J. Med.*, **319**, 142–5
7. Burrows, R. F. and Kelton, J. G. (1990). Thrombocytopenia at delivery: a prospective survey of 6715 deliveries. *Am. J. Obstet. Gynecol.*, **162**, 731–4
8. Samuels, P., Bussel, J. B., Braitman, L. E., Tomaski, A., Druzin, M. L., Menutti, M. T. and Cines, D. B. (1990). Estimation of the risk of thrombocytopenia in the offspring of pregnant women with presumed immune thrombocytopenic purpura. *N. Engl. J. Med.*, **323**, 229–35
9. Lescale, K. B., Bussel, J., Eddleman, K. A., Cines, D. and Samuels, P. (1993). Distinguishing chronic ITP from gestational GTP in thrombocytopenic pregnant women. *Am. J. Obstet. Gynecol.*, **168** (Suppl.), **412**, in press
10. Newland, A. C., Boots, M. A. and Patterson, K. G. (1984). Intravenous IgG for ITP in pregnancy (letter). *N. Engl. J. Med.*, **310**, 261–2
11. Bussel, J. B., Druzin, M. L., Cines, D. B. and Samuels, P. (1991). Thrombocytopenia in pregnancy (letter). *Lancet*, **337**, 251
12. Scott, J. R., Cruikshank, D. P., Kochenour, N. K., Pitkin, R. M. and Warenski, J. C. (1980). Fetal platelet counts in the obstetric management of immunological thrombocytopenic purpura. *Am. J. Obstet. Gynecol.*, **136**, 495–9
13. Kaplan, C., Daffos, F., Forestier, F., Tertian, G., Catherine, N., Pons, J. C. and Tchernia, G. (1990). Fetal platelet counts in thrombocytopenic pregnancy. *Lancet*, **336**, 979–82
14. Kelton, J. G. (1983). Management of the pregnant patient with idiopathic thrombocytopenic purpura. *Ann. Intern. Med.*, **99**, 796–800
15. Kelton, J. G., Inwood, M. J., Barr, R. M., Effer, S. B., Hunter, D., Wilson, W. E., Ginsburg, D. A. and Powers, P. J. (1982). The prenatal prediction of thrombocytopenia in infants of mothers with clinically diagnosed immune thrombocytopenia. *Am. J. Obstet. Gynecol.*, **144**, 449–54
16. George, J. N. (1990). Platelet immunoglobulin G: its significance for the evaluation of thrombocytopenia and for understanding the origin of alpha-granule proteins. *Blood*, **76**, 859–70
17. Scott, J. R., Rote, N. S. and Cruikshank, D. P. (1983). Antiplatelet antibodies and platelet counts in pregnancies complicated by autoim-

mune thrombocytopenic purpura. *Am. J. Obstet. Gynecol.*, **145**, 932–9
18. Burrows, R. F. and Kelton, J. G. (1990). Low fetal risks in pregnancies associated with idiopathic thrombocytopenic purpura. *Am. J. Obstet. Gynecol.*, **163**, 1147–50
19. Ayromlooi, J. (1978). A new approach to the management of immunologic thrombocytopenic purpura in pregnancy. *Am. J. Obstet. Gynecol.*, **130**, 235–6
20. Christiaens, G. and Helmerhorst, F. M. (1987). Validity of intrapartum diagnosis of fetal thrombocytopenia. *Am. J. Obstet. Gynecol.*, **157**, 864–5
21. Adams, D. M., Bussel, J. B. and Druzin, M. L. (1994). Accurate intrapartum estimation of fetal platelet count by fetal scalp sample smear. *Am. J. Perinatol.*, **11**, 42–5
22. Daffos, F., Forestier, F., Kaplan, C. and Cox, W. (1988). Prenatal diagnosis and management of bleeding disorders with fetal blood sampling. *Am. J. Obstet. Gynecol.*, **158**, 939–46
23. Moise, K. J., Carpenter, R. J., Cotton, D. B., Wasserstrum, N., Kirshon, B. and Cano, L. (1988). Percutaneous umbilical cord blood sampling in the evaluation of fetal platelet counts in pregnant patients with autoimmune thrombocytopenic purpura. *Obstet. Gynecol.*, **72**, 346–50
24. Scioscia, A. L., Grannum, P. A. T., Copel, J. A. and Hobbins, J. C. (1988). The use of percutaneous umbilical blood sampling in immune thrombocytopenic purpura. *Am. J. Obstet. Gynecol.*, **159**, 1066–8
25. Bussel, J. and Christiens, G. (1993). Birth platelet counts in sequential newborns of mothers with ITP: do the platelet counts change with subsequent babies? *Blood*, **82** (Suppl.), 202a
26. Cook, R. L., Miller, R. C., Katz, V. L. and Cefalo, R. C. (1991). Immune thrombocytopenic purpura in pregnancy: a reappraisal of management. *Obstet. Gynecol.*, **78**, 578–83
27. Mueller-Eckhardt, C., Keifel, V., Grubert, A., Kroll, H., Weishit, M., Schmidt, S., Mueller-Eckhardt, G. and Santoso, S. (1989). 348 cases of suspected neonatal alloimmune thrombocytopenia. *Lancet*, **1**, 363–6
28. Johnson, J. M., McFarland, J. G., Blanchette, V. S., Freedman, J. and Siegel-Bartelt, J. (1993). Prenatal diagnosis of neonatal alloimmune thrombocytopenia using an allele-specific oligonucleotide probe. *Prenat. Diagn.*, **13**, 1037–42
29. Kaplan, C., Forestier, F., Cox, W. L., Lyon-Caen, D., Depuy-Montbrun, M. C. and Salmon, C. (1988). Management of alloimmune thrombocytopenia: antenatal diagnosis and *in utero* transfusion of maternal platelets. *Blood*, **72**, 340–3
30. Lipitz, S., Ryan, G., Murphy, M. F., Robson, S. C., Hueusler, M. C. H., Metcalfe, P., Kelsey, H. and Rodeck, C. H. (1992). Neonatal alloimmune thrombocytopenia due to anti-PLA1 (anti-HPA-1a): importance of paternal and fetal platelet typing for assessment of risk. *Prenat. Diagn.*, **12**, 955–8
31. Kunicki, T. J. (1991). Human platelet antigens. In Hoffman, R., Benz, E. J., Shattil, S. J., Furie, B. and Cohen, H. J. (eds.) *Hematology: Basic Principles and Practice*, pp. 1556–65. (New York: Churchill Livingstone)
32. Skacel, P. O. and Contreras, M. (1989). Neonatal alloimmune thrombocytopenia. *Blood Rev.*, **3**, 174
33. McFarland, J. G., Frenzke, M. and Aster, R. H. (1989). Testing of maternal sera in pregnancies at risk for neonatal alloimmune thrombocytopenia. *Transfusion*, **29**, 128–33
34. Reznikoff-Etievant, M. F., Dangu, C. and Lobert, R. (1981). HLA-B8 antigen and anti-PLA1 alloimmunization. *Tissue Antigens*, **18**, 66
35. Reznikoff-Etievant, M. F., Muller, J. Y., Julien, F. and Patereau, C. (1988). An immune response gene linked to MHC in man. *Tissue Antigens*, **22**, 312
36. Blanchette, V. S., Chen, L., Salomon De Friedberg, Z., Hogan, V. A., Trudel, E. and Decary, F. (1990). Alloimmunization to the Pl^{A1} platelet antigen: results of a prospective study. *Br. J. Haematol.*, **74**, 209–15
37. Bussel, J. B., Berkowitz, R. L., McFarland, J. G., Lynch, L. and Chitkara, U. (1988). Antenatal treatment of neonatal alloimmune thrombocytopenia. *N. Engl. J. Med.*, **319**, 1374–8
38. Lynch, L., Bussel, J. B., McFarland, J., Chitkara, U. and Berkowitz, R. L. (1992). Antenatal treatment of alloimmune thrombocytopenia. *Obstet. Gynecol.*, **80**, 67–71
39. Herman, J. H., Jumbelic, M. I., Ancona, R. J. and Kickler, T. S. (1986). In utero cerebral hemorrhage in alloimmune thrombocytopenia. *Am. J. Pediatr. Hematol. Oncol.*, **8**, 312–7
40. Giovangrandi, Y., Daffos, F. and Kaplan, C. (1990). Very early intracranial hemorrhage in alloimmune thrombocytopenia (letter). *Lancet*, **2**, 310
41. Lynch, L., Bussel, J., McFarland, J. G., Chitkara, U. and Berkowitz, R. L. (1992). Antenatal treatment of alloimmune thrombocytopenia (letter). *Obstet. Gynecol.*, **80**, 1057
42. Nicolini, U., Rodeck, C. H., Kochenour, N. K., Greco, P., Fisk, N. M. and Letsky, E. (1988). *In utero* platelet transfusion for alloimmune thrombocytopenia (letter). *Lancet*, **2**, 506

Fetal therapy

L. K. McLean and M. S. Golbus

INTRODUCTION

Fetal therapy became a reality with Liley's report[1] of intraperitoneal transfusion for the treatment of severe erythroblastosis fetalis in 1963. Since that time, many treatment modalities have been attempted including, but not limited to, vitamin and dietary supplementation, medical pharmacological treatment, ultrasound-guided percutaneous procedures, open fetal surgery, stem-cell transplantation and gene therapy. Many of these modes of treatment are reviewed in this chapter.

MEDICAL INTERVENTION

Maternal conditions

Changes in diet and medications made prior to or during pregnancy may have profound effects on fetal outcome. The goal of this therapy is to prevent fetal anomalies associated with a maternal disease, certain medications or vitamin deficiencies. Many of these therapies need to be instituted prior to conception to achieve maximal benefit. An excellent example is the markedly decreased incidence of fetal anomalies in women with insulin-dependent diabetes mellitus in good control prior to conception[2,3].

Maternal phenylketonuria is another example of a maternal metabolic condition that may have an adverse fetal effect. Phenylalanine is hydroxylated to tyrosine by phenylalanine hydroxylase; classic phenylketonuria occurs when there is less than 10% of this enzyme activity. Children with phenylketonuria develop mental retardation, eczema, hypopigmentation and neurological symptoms, if not maintained on a strict diet low in phenylalanine. Patients have been continued on this diet until 6–8 years of age, and studies have shown intelligence comparable to unaffected sibs[4,5]. Recent studies have proposed that patients continue on the low-phenylalanine diet indefinitely[6]. Over 90% of neonates born to women with phenylketonuria on unrestricted diets have mental retardation, microcephaly, congenital heart and/or vascular problems as well as growth retardation[7,8]. Neonates delivered to women who begin a low-phenylalanine diet during pregnancy have a better prognosis, but are still at risk for low birthweight, small head circumference and congenital malformations[9]. There is some evidence that the neonatal risk is even lower for women who start on a phenylalanine-restricted diet prior to conception.

Any medication that the mother is taking should be evaluated for its necessity. Certain medications must be stopped several months prior to conception to avoid possible malformations (e.g. accutane). The patient should be switched to the least teratogenic agent that treats her condition (e.g. coumadin to heparin, methimazole to propylthiouracil, oral hypoglycemic agents to insulin). Patients on anticonvulsants should be switched to the least teratogenic agent that controls their seizures prior to conception. Phenytoin has long been known to cause fetal anomalies and intrauterine growth retardation. Approximately 10% of phenytoin-exposed fetuses will have the fetal hydantoin syndrome; over 30% of the remaining neonates will have some effects of the disorder evident. A recent study has proposed the measurement of epoxide hydrolase activity as a way to detect the fetuses that are at greatest risk for the fetal hydantoin syndrome[10].

Vitamin and mineral supplementation

An association between neural tube defects (NTD) and dietary deficiencies was supported by an increased incidence of NTD following the famine in Holland in 1944–45, as well as food shortages in Germany after World War II. Animal studies using diets deficient in folic acid combined with aminopterin (a folate antagonist) produced a higher incidence of NTD. These studies led to the proposal that folate supplementation in high-risk patients would decrease the incidence of NTD. The British Medical Research Council published a randomized, double-blind prospective study evaluating the possible benefits of multivitamin and folic-acid supplementation. Almost 1200 women who had a previous fetus with a neural tube defect were enrolled in the study and were randomized to four groups; group A received 4 mg of folic acid, group B received a multivitamin supplement that contained 4 mg of folic acid, group C received placebo and group D received multivitamins without folic acid. The study was stopped in 1991, because a definite benefit from folic acid supplementation had been demonstrated. There was a 70% reduction in the incidence of NTD in high-risk women given high-dose folic acid[11]. Studies are now evaluating the place of folic-acid supplementation in low-risk populations (where 95% of the NTD will occur). The current recommendations in the United States are that every woman who may become pregnant should consume 0.4 mg of folic acid daily. In high-risk patients, the dose should be 1 to 4 mg daily.

Mineral supplementation to decrease the incidence or severity of certain genetic conditions has been evaluated in animal models. These include manganese supplementation in mouse strains with pigmentation and inner-ear abnormalities[12] as well as prenatal copper supplementation to a mouse strain with the 'crinkled' gene mutation[13]. These investigators have noted that the 'crinkled' gene phenotype has many similarities to the phenotype of patients with X-linked Menkes kinky-hair syndrome. Postnatal copper supplementation has not been beneficial in mice with the 'crinkled' gene mutation nor in patients with Menkes syndrome. There have not been any published studies evaluating the prenatal use of mineral supplementation for human mendelian conditions.

Fetal metabolic conditions

There are several fetal conditions that may be treated or ameliorated medically, with the goal of this therapy being to prevent disease progression and/or fetal damage prior to delivery. The transplacental passage, and placental and fetal metabolism of substances must be taken into account when managing these patients. One of the best-studied examples of medical fetal therapy is the administration of maternal corticosteroids for the prevention of respiratory distress syndrome and intraventricular hemorrhage in the premature infant.

Some corticosteroids cross the placenta and suppress the fetal adrenal gland. Evans and colleagues[14] were the first to report the use of maternal dexamethasone therapy in an attempt to avoid masculinization of a female fetus thought to have congenital adrenal hyperplasia. Congenital adrenal hyperplasia may be secondary to 21-hydroxylase deficiency, which results in a block in the metabolic pathway converting cholesterol to cortisol. This block creates a deficiency of cortisol, results in high levels of adrenocorticotropic hormone (ACTH), and a build-up of 17-hydroxyprogesterone. The excessive 17-hydroxyprogesterone is converted to and creates an excess of androstenedione and other adrenal androgens. The high levels of adrenal androgens masculinize female fetuses in ways varying from clitoral hypertrophy to complete formation of a phallus with an apparent scrotum. Several studies have reported giving the mother glucocorticoids beginning in the first trimester (usually before 9 weeks) to suppress the fetal adrenal gland[15–17]. In an excellent review of the cases reported, Pang and associates[17] found that five of the 15 affected female neonates treated *in utero* had normal female genitalia, while the others had varying degrees of virilization. In some of these cases, the glucocorticoid dose was inadequate or started later in gestation. However, in a few cases no explanation for the virilization could be found, which led them to conclude that there are other factors that may determine the effectiveness of the glucocorticoid therapy. Investigators recommend that dexamethasone, 1.5 mg a day divided into two or three doses, be given to the mother starting as early as 5 menstrual weeks. Congenital adrenal hyperplasia may now be diagnosed by chorionic villus sampling so that only mothers carrying affected female fetuses will have prolonged treatment[18].

Methylmalonic acidemia results from an inborn error of metabolism in which there is a defect in the conversion of methylmalonyl coenzyme A to succinyl coenzyme A. This conversion uses methylmalonyl-CoA mutase with vitamin B_{12} (cobalamin) as a coenzyme. There have been five genetically determined causes of a block in this enzymatic step, four of which involve adenosylcobalamin biosynthesis. Some of the patients with a defect in the adenosylcobalamin biosynthesis pathway may improve dramatically with large doses of vitamin B12. It is proposed that giving large doses of vitamin B_{12} may enhance the amount of active enzyme available, thereby increasing the amount of methylmalonic coenzyme A that is converted. There may be an increased frequency of congenital anomalies in fetuses with methylmalonic acidemia and it is proposed that reducing the fetal methylmalonic acid would allow more normal fetal development and improve the neonatal course[19]. Fetal methylmalonic acidemia results in markedly elevated levels of methylmalonic acid in the amniotic fluid as well as in maternal urine. Ampola and associates[20] used the methylmalonic acid levels in maternal urine to diagnose and guide their management of a pregnancy complicated by fetal methylmalonic acidemia. High-dose oral vitamin B_{12} was slowly effective in significantly reducing the maternal urinary excretion of methylmalonic acid. There was a significant decline in excretion to slightly above normal levels prior to delivery, as well as a six-fold increase in maternal vitamin-B_{12} levels when 5 mg daily cyanocobalamin was given intravenously. Postnatally the diagnosis was confirmed and the child has done well on a protein-restricted diet.

Biotin-responsive multiple carboxylase deficiency is a second inborn error of metabolism that has been diagnosed and treated prenatally. In this condition, there are several biotin-dependent mitochondrial enzymes that have diminished activity. Affected patients present with severe metabolic acidosis, neurological abnormalities, a characteristic organic aciduria and dermatitis. Biotin supplementation may correct the metabolic abnormality. Cultured amniocytes have been used to make the diagnosis[21,22]. In these two reports, the mother received oral biotin (10 mg daily) and the neonates did well. Cultured neonatal fibroblasts confirmed the diagnosis in both cases.

There have been several case reports of fetal thyroid abnormalities being treated *in utero*[23,24]. This fetal endocrinopathy may be secondary to maternal disease (maternal antibodies crossing the placenta), or its treatment (propylthiouracil or methimazole crossing the placenta and suppressing the fetal thyroid) or it may be congenital. The development of a large goiter may cause fetal head extension, decreased swallowing resulting in polyhydramnios, and possibly preterm labor. Untreated neonatal hypothyroidism results in mental retardation, myxedema and growth retardation. Animal studies have demonstrated that fetal hypothyroidism and hyperthyroidism result in decreased cerebral development and smaller brains than in controls[25].

Davidson and colleagues[23] reported *in utero* treatment of a fetal goiter associated with maternal Graves disease requiring large doses of propylthiouracil. The fetal goiter was detected by ultrasound at 28 menstrual weeks, and was increased in size on serial examinations. Fetal blood sampling at 35 weeks' gestation revealed an elevated thyroid stimulating hormone level and a decreased serum thyroxine level consistent with fetal hypothyroidism. Serial intraamniotic injections of thyroxine (250 µg) at 35, 36 and 37 weeks resulted in a rapid decrease in the size of the goiter. Spontaneous vaginal delivery occurred at 38 weeks and neonatal thyroid studies were normal.

Fetal arrhythmias

The most common fetal cardiac arrhythmias are isolated premature atrial contractions and supraventricular tachycardia. Isolated premature atrial contractions (PAC) do not require treatment and rarely progress to supraventricular tachycardia[26]. Maternal ingestion of caffeine, nicotine, chocolate and other stimulants should be avoided, because they may exacerbate fetal PAC.

Sustained fetal supraventricular tachycardia (SVT), on the other hand, requires treatment because it may result in cardiac failure, fetal hydrops and possibly demise. A detailed fetal sonogram and echocardiogram are indicated to rule out anomalies. The best therapy if the fetus is near term is delivery with evaluation and treatment in the nursery. If the fetus is premature, then intrauterine therapy is indicated. Digoxin administered orally to the mother is considered the first-line therapy. Because enteral absorption may be decreased, doses of 0.5–0.75 mg daily are often needed to achieve a therapeutic plasma level of 1–2 ng/ml. The mother should be followed closely for any signs of digitalis toxicity. Cases in which fetal SVT does not convert with therapeutic levels of digoxin have been reported, and several other antiarrhythmic agents have been used, including verapamil, flecainide acetate, amiodarone and propranolol[26]. The clearance of digoxin may be decreased by these agents and levels should be followed closely. Procainamide has been used, but fetal toxicity may develop secondary to accumulation of the drug in the fetus[27]. Fetal thrombocytopenia, retinal damage and intrauterine fetal demise have been reported with quinidine[28].

Transplacental passage of antiarrhythmic agents may be erratic and decreased in hydropic fetuses[29]. There have been several case reports of tachyarrhythmias refractory to maternal therapy that have responded to direct administration of antiarrhythmic agents. Weiner and Thompson[30] administered digoxin percutaneously into the fetal thigh and buttocks. Antiarrhythmics have also been administered into the peritoneal cavity[31] and the umbilical vein[32].

Kleinman and Copel[33] reported a series of 43 fetal supraventricular tachydysrhythmias. There were 34 cases of SVT; 32 responded to *in utero* therapy, one fetus had congenital heart disease and there was one fetal demise. Nine cases of fetal atrial flutter-fibrillation were reported; three fetuses had congenital heart defects and there were four fetal demises. Fetal atrial flutter/fibrillation is rare, frequently associated with congenital heart defects and has a high mortality rate. These investigators propose considering the use of procainamide and quinidine in cases of fetal flutter/fibrillation that are unresponsive to digoxin therapy.

Complete atrioventricular block occurs in approximately 1 in 20 000 live births. In a multicenter study, 55 fetuses with complete heart block were identified[34]. Almost half had structural cardiac defects detected on fetal echocardiography. Evidence of a connective-tissue disease or anti-nuclear antibodies were detected in 19 of the 26 fetuses with normal cardiac anatomy. Normal anatomy was found to be a good prognostic sign, with 22 of 26 fetuses surviving. The development of fetal hydrops was a poor prognostic sign, and none of the 22 fetuses with hydrops survived in this study. Treatment with terbutaline, ritodrine and isoproterenol has not been shown to be beneficial. Glucocorticoids may be beneficial in the patient with antinuclear antibodies.

SURGICAL INTERVENTIONS

Fetal transfusion therapy

Fetal transfusion therapy began in 1963 when Liley described the first successful intraperitoneal transfusion for hemolytic disease in the fetus[1]. Since that time, it has been used to correct fetal anemia due to red cell alloimmunization, fetomaternal hemorrhage, and parvovirus infection, as well as thrombocytopenia secondary to platelet alloimmunization. This topic is covered elsewhere in this book and will not be covered further here.

Stem cell transplantation

Bone-marrow transplantation can successfully treat a wide variety of diseases, including Wiskott-Aldrich syndrome, the leukemias, severe combined immunodeficiency, hemoglobinopathies, and several metabolic conditions such as the Hurler syndrome. Postnatal transplantation requires a human leukocyte antigen (HLA)-compatible donor as well as immunosuppression of the recipient. It may be complicated by side-effects of the chemotherapy and/or radiation, graft-versus-host disease (GVHD), graft rejection and any disease sequelae that occurred prior to transplantation.

Hematopoietic stem cells originate in the yolk sac and migrate to the fetal liver and spleen during the 6–7th gestational week (Figure 1). The bone marrow is seeded by stem cells from the fetal liver between 18 and 20 weeks' gestation. These multipotent cells continuously renew themselves as well as differentiating into the various hematopoietic cell lineages. In postnatal bone marrow the concentration of stem cells is approximately 1 in 100 000 cells.

Initially the fetal immune system is 'tolerant'; it is unable to distinguish 'self' from 'foreign' and the only protection the fetus has from foreign cells is the placenta. The first evidence that cells crossing the placenta are tolerated by the fetus was a naturally occurring chimera in bovine twins with intrauterine vascular connections[35]. Stem-cell transplantation in humans was first documented by Turner and associates[36] in a follow-up study of 65 children who had received transfusions *in utero*, of whom five had circulating donor leukocytes 1 year after birth.

The fetus is considered the ideal donor as well as the ideal recipient of stem cells. Fetal stem cells are the ideal donor cells because early in gestation the T cells are immature and incapable of causing GVHD. Immature T cells migrate to the thymus at approximately 8 weeks' gestation and T cells within the thymus are capable of responding to antigen-stimulation at 11–12 weeks' gestation. Mature T lymphocytes capable of causing GVHD have been detected within the fetal liver after 18 weeks' gestation. The fetus is the ideal recipient of stem cells because the bone marrow is prepared for seeding by stem cells and the fetus will accept the cells as 'self', and therefore does not require HLA-compatible donors or immunosuppression.

Fetal stem-cell transplantation, postnatal and *in utero*, has been successful in several animal models, including mice, sheep and primates[37–39]. Animal studies have shown that fetal liver cells are a better source of donor stem cells than is bone marrow[40].

Postnatal fetal liver stem cell transplantation has been used extensively in Europe to correct several conditions, including severe combined immunodeficiency (SCID). The only case of GVHD was seen when the transplantation used cells from a 16-week fetus[41]. Investigators advise using fetal liver cells from gestations less than 14 menstrual weeks to avoid the risk of GVHD.

Approximately one dozen cases of *in utero* transplantation for several different conditions have been reported in the literature[42,43]. The seven cases that used parental bone marrow as the source of stem cells were all unsuccessful. Touraine and co-workers[43] have reported four fetuses who received fetal-liver stem-cell transplants. Their first case was of 30 weeks' gestation, diagnosed with bare lymphocyte syndrome, and in which fetal liver and thymic cells were transplanted into the umbilical vein. The donors were two fetuses of approximately 9 menstrual weeks. Almost 10% engraftment was documented following delivery and the child is doing well, albeit after several postnatal trans-

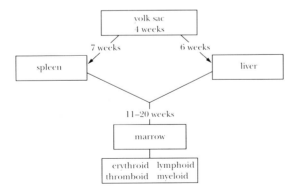

Figure 1 *Diagram of embryology of hematopoietic stem-cell development and migration*

plants. They have reported three other cases, two fetuses with thalassemia major and one fetus with SCID. Fetal stem cells were transplanted intravascularly in two fetuses (19 and 28 weeks' gestation) and intraperitoneally (at 14 weeks' gestation). The results from two of these cases demonstrated some engraftment and amelioration of the disease. Unfortunately, one of the intravascular transplantations was complicated by fetal bradycardia, and was followed by fetal demise. It is hoped that in the future *in utero* stem-cell transplantation will be able to cure many hematological, immunological and metabolic conditions while avoiding the possible complications of postnatal transplantation.

Fetal surgery

The advent of high-resolution sonography has made it possible to detect a wide array of fetal anomalies. These anomalies may be divided into five broad categories:

(1) Severe disorders, defects or malformations that are lethal or not compatible with prolonged quality of life, best managed by termination or at least non-intervention (e.g. anencephaly, lethal skeletal dysplasias, trisomy 13 and 18);

(2) Defects that are best corrected after delivery, includes almost all correctable malformations;

(3) Defects that may influence the mode of delivery (e.g. conjoined twins, neural tube defects, giant omphaloceles);

(4) Defects that may influence the timing of delivery (e.g. immune hydrops, intrauterine growth retardation, obstructive uropathy); and

(5) Defects that may benefit from intervention *in utero*. There are only a very few anomalies in which correction *in utero* would allow more normal development and a better chance for neonatal survival.

Prior to considering fetal therapy, it is essential to know the natural history of the anomaly. Is it progressive, will it cause organ damage or interfere with normal development? Finally, and most importantly, will fetal therapy improve neonatal outcome? Understanding the pathophysiology of the disease process is vital in designing fetal therapy, and many of these questions must be answered in animal models before fetal therapy in humans is attempted.

Shunt placement

Placement of a shunt *in utero* to decompress a fluid collection may prevent organ damage and allow more normal development. Shunting *in utero* has been performed for ventriculomegaly, obstructive uropathy and hydrothorax. Each of these will be considered separately.

Ventriculomegaly

The diagnosis of ventriculomegaly is based on the demonstration of enlarged lateral ventricles. Nomograms have been developed and published for the various areas of the lateral ventricle, including the atrium and body as well as the frontal, occipital and temporal horns. Various methods have been proposed to diagnose fetal ventriculomegaly. The two most commonly used are measurements of the atrium and the ratio of the lateral ventricle to the hemisphere. A useful observation is the orientation of the choroid plexus within the lateral ventricle. The choroid plexus typically fills the atrium of the lateral ventricle; however, when there is ventriculomegaly, the choroid plexus 'dangles' within the enlarged ventricle. Each of these and many other diagnostic criteria have their supporters and critics.

Enlargement of the ventricles may be secondary to an increase in the amount of cerebrospinal fluid (obstruction of flow, overproduction or decreased resorption) or a decrease in the amount of cortical tissue (underdevelopment or destruction). Obstruction of cerebrospinal fluid flow may be secondary to a neural tube defect and associated Arnold–Chiari malformation, infection causing scarring around the aqueduct of Sylvius or an intracranial mass. Decreased cortical mass may be seen in cases of *in utero* intraventricular hemorrhage. Hydrocephalus may be inherited as a part of a malformation syndrome or as an isolated autosomal or X-linked disorder.

Neonatal shunting of hydrocephalus has enjoyed good success, and in the 1980s, *in utero* shunting of ventriculomegaly to avoid irreversible brain damage was proposed. Birnholz and Frigoletto[44] were the first to report *in utero* cephalocentesis as treatment for hydrocephalus. A ventriculoamniotic shunt was developed and first used by Clewell and co-workers[45]. The Fetal Surgery Registry reported that there had been 44 drainage procedures by 1985[46]. A review of the outcomes of these pregnancies revealed a 10% procedure-related fetal mortality and 83% neonatal survival. However, 18 of the 34 survivors were severely handicapped. Because of these disappointing results, there has been a *de facto* moratorium on *in utero* treatment of ventriculomegaly since the 1980s.

Since that time, several studies evaluating the natural history of prenatally detected ventriculomegaly have been published[47–49]. These studies involved over 300 fetuses with ventriculomegaly, and found that 10% had chromosomal aneuploidy, 70–80% had other anomalies, 40% of which were not detected prenatally, and the prognosis was determined primarily by the associated anomalies and their severity. Fetuses with 'isolated' ventriculomegaly had a better prognosis; 60% survived and were developmentally normal. The fetuses with stable ventriculomegaly had a better prognosis than those with progressive ventriculomegaly. It is in this small group of fetuses with progressive, 'isolated' ventriculomegaly (less than 5% in these studies) that *in utero* management may have a role in the future.

A proposed protocol for the management of a fetus diagnosed with ventriculomegaly should include a detailed fetal survey and amniocentesis (fluid should be sent for karyotyping, assessment of levels of α-fetoprotein and acetylcholinesterase, and viral cultures). If there are other severe anomalies, the prognosis is grim, and aggressive management for fetal interests should not be done. Cephalocentesis (if indicated) and vaginal delivery is in the best interest of the mother in these very difficult cases. In the absence of other detected anomalies, serial ultrasound examinations should be performed to follow the degree of ventriculomegaly. In the absence of progressive, severe hydrocephalus the pregnancy should be allowed to go to term. Vaginal delivery is appropriate in cases without macrocephaly (< 2 SD above the mean) and vertex presentation. When progressive ventriculomegaly is detected, fetal lung maturity should be documented prior to preterm delivery. Corticosteroids may be given to decrease the risk of respiratory distress syndrome in the preterm fetus.

Obstructive uropathy

Dilatation of the renal collecting system may be readily seen on ultrasound examination. There are several different etiologies. Diagnostic clues include the areas of the system affected as well as the severity of the dilatation. Megacystisis with proximal urethral dilatation (a 'keyhole' appearance) is essentially pathognomonic for posterior urethral valves. These are found almost exclusively in male fetuses and are associated with varying degrees of hydroureter, hydronephrosis, oligohydramnios and pulmonary hypoplasia. Renal disease may develop and is thought to be secondary to the obstruction causing increasing back pressure. Pulmonary hypoplasia, when it occurs, is thought to be due to oligohydramnios and thoracic compression, although an associated primary pulmonary malformation has been proposed[50].

Hydronephrosis accounts for 87% of the renal anomalies detected *in utero*. Minimal bilateral hydronephrosis typically resolves in the neonate and is attributed to the high progesterone levels of pregnancy acting as a smooth muscle relaxant. Ureteropelvic-junction obstruction is suspected when there is isolated hydronephrosis; the ureters, bladder and amniotic-fluid volume are normal. Its occurrence is sporadic and most cases are thought to be secondary to a functional obstruction. Over two-thirds of these fetuses had moderate-to-good neonatal renal function and did not require surgical correction[51]. Ureteroceles typically result in hydronephrosis and hydroureter. Most cases are associated with duplication of the collecting system in which the upper pole moiety obstructs and the lower pole refluxes. The diagnosis is confirmed by visualization of the ectopic ureterocele within the bladder.

The diagnosis of a fetal renal-tract anomaly dictates that the contralateral renal collecting system, bladder and amniotic fluid volume be examined closely. Chromosomal aneuploidy and associated anomalies have been reported in 15–40% of pregnancies complicated by obstructive uropathy[52]. Because neonatal prognosis depends on associated anomalies, a detailed fetal survey is indicated. A review of 682 fetuses with renal anomalies revealed that the maternal-age-related risk for chromosomal aneuploidy increased three-fold in fetuses with isolated renal defects and over 30-fold when other anomalies were detected by ultrasound[53].

The prognosis for a fetus with unilateral obstructive uropathy, normal amniotic fluid and karyotype without associated anomalies is good[54]. Fetuses with bilateral urinary obstruction have a variable outcome; some have already experienced irreversible renal and possible pulmonary damage at the time of diagnosis and have a very grim prognosis. Others continue to have good renal and pulmonary development throughout pregnancy and have a reasonably good neonatal prognosis. Finally, some fetuses are destined to develop severe renal and pulmonary damage. It is in this last group that *in utero* decompression may be beneficial. The difficulty is knowing into which group a fetus with bilateral urinary obstruction falls.

Several modalities to evaluate fetal renal function have been proposed, including ultrasound as well as urine electrolytes, β_2 microglobulin levels and protein electrophoresis. Each of these will be reviewed and the protocol presented that is currently used at the University of California, San Francisco (UCSF).

The ability of ultrasound to predict renal function has been evaluated in a series of 31 fetuses with obstructive uropathy[55]. Renal cortical cysts were most predictive of renal dysplasia, with a specificity of 100%. However, the sensitivity was only 44%. Increased renal echogenicity had a specificity of 89% with a sensitivity of 57%. The least predictive ultrasound findings were the degree of hydronephrosis and amniotic fluid volume.

Fetal urine is an ultrafiltrate of fetal serum with selective tubular resorption of electrolytes and proteins. Urine production begins at approximately 13 menstrual weeks; sodium, chloride and osmolality levels in the urine decrease during gestation. It is thought that levels of urine calcium and β_2 microglobulin remain constant throughout gestation[56] and that albumin is the only protein normally found in the urine after approximately 18 weeks[57]. Based on these principles, several studies have evaluated the predictive value of various urinary measurements for renal function.

In a retrospective review of fetal urine samples obtained by bladder aspiration from fetuses with obstructive uropathy (Figure 2), Crombleholme and associates[58] found that urine electrolytes and osmolarity correlated with renal dysplasia. Hypotonic urine and low sodium and chloride levels were associated with a good prognosis. Figure 3 demonstrates the relationship between renal dysplasia, fetal urine electrolytes and osmolarity. The groups with no dysplasia and severe dysplasia were fairly well separated, with only a small amount of overlap. As demonstrated by Wilkins and co-workers[59] in a small study of nine fetuses, fetal urine electrolytes are not predictive of neonatal renal function; these values are only useful in determining renal function at the time of sampling.

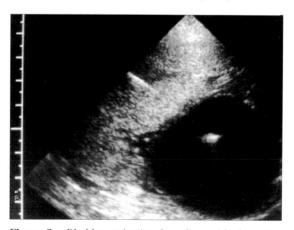

Figure 2 *Bladder aspiration from fetus with obstructive uropathy*

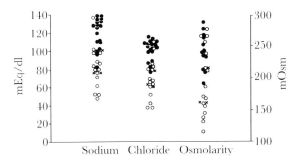

Figure 3 *Fetal urine sodium, chloride, and osmolarity as a predictor of renal status in the fetus with bilateral obstructive uropathy.* ●, *poor function;* ○, *good function;* ×, *pending*

The assessment of β_2 microglobulin has been reported to be a valuable addition to the fetal urinary analysis[56,60]. In a study of 100 consecutive fetuses with bilateral obstructive uropathy, Muller and associates[60] found that an elevated fetal urine β_2 microglobulin level was most predictive of elevated serum creatinine levels during the second year of life. The elevated β_2 microglobulin level was both specific (83%) and sensitive (80%), while urine sodium, chloride and urea levels were sensitive (70% or better) but lacked specificity (less than 65%).

Holzgreve and colleagues[57] were the first to report the use of protein electrophoresis to detect fetal proteinuria and predict fetal renal function. They reported a fetus at 19 menstrual weeks with severe oligohydramnios, megalocystis and unfavorable urine electrolytes that had a normal protein electrophoresis (the only protein detected was albumin). Therapy *in utero* was performed with a good neonatal outcome. This group has subsequently reported 22 cases of fetal obstructive uropathy in which urine electrolytes and protein electrophoresis were performed[61]. In four cases, the electrolytes were unfavorable while the protein electrophoresis was reassuring; in all four cases, decompression *in utero* was performed and all had a good neonatal outcome.

The protocol at UCSF for the management of a fetus with bilateral urinary obstruction is presented in Figure 4. In pregnancies over 32 menstrual weeks with severe fetal hydronephrosis or decreasing amniotic fluid volume, betamethasone (if indicated) is given and labor is induced. Patients whose fetuses have unfavorable urinary studies and oligohydramnios are offered pregnancy termination or non-intervention, because the prognosis is so grim. There have not been any survivors from this group in our series.

Fetal therapy is offered to patients with fetuses of less than 32 weeks' gestation that have decreased amniotic fluid volume and favorable urinary studies. The goal of fetal therapy is to allow urine to enter the amniotic cavity, thereby decreasing the pressure within the renal collecting system, and allowing more normal pulmonary development. Typically, a Rocket catheter is placed under ultrasound guidance with one end of the catheter in the bladder and the other end in the amniotic fluid space. Antibiotic prophylaxis is given to decrease the incidence of chorioamnionitis. Unfortunately, these catheters may become displaced or blocked, requiring recatheterization. The International Fetal Surgery Registry 1985 Update[46] reported that 72 fetuses had undergone *in utero* treatment of urinary obstruction by chronic vesicoamniotic shunt placement. The overall survival rate was 42% with a procedure-related perinatal mortality of 4%. There was a high incidence of shunt migration and blockage. Several fetuses have undergone open fetal surgery for urinary tract obstruction at UCSF and these results will be presented in that section.

Hydrothorax

As is the case for most fetal anomalies, the detection of a fetal pleural effusion demands a search for other anomalies. Evaluation should include a detailed sonogram, echocardiogram, karyotype and cytomegalovirus culture. Up to one-third of fetuses with hydrothoraces have chromosomal aneuploidy[52]. The prognosis in fetuses with isolated pleural effusions is quite variable. In some cases, the effusion spontaneously resolves or is well tolerated and the neonatal outcome is good. In other instances, the hydrothorax results in pulmonary hypoplasia, mediastinal shift, fetal hydrops and fetal demise. The natural history of 24 cases of primary fetal hydrothorax has been reported by

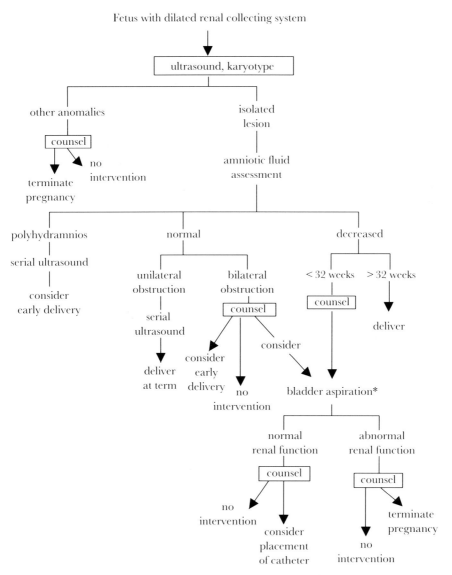

Figure 4 *Protocol of University of California, San Francisco for management of a fetus with bilateral urinary tract obstruction. *Evaluate urine sodium, chloride, osmolality, β_2-microglobulin*

Longaker and associates[62] with an overall perinatal mortality of 53%. This group found that unilateral effusions without mediastinal shift, spontaneous resolution of the effusion and the absence of fetal hydrops were all good prognostic signs, associated with a 100% survival rate. In cases that developed signs of hydrops fetalis the survival rate was less than 40%. Detection of pleural effusions early in pregnancy (< 33 weeks) and preterm delivery were associated with a poor outcome.

Preterm fetuses with large pleural effusions resulting in mediastinal shift and/or hydrops have a poor prognosis and may benefit from therapy *in utero*. Because rapid reaccumulation of these effusions frequently occurs following needle aspiration, long-term drainage by a catheter is indicated. Nicolaides and Azar[63] reported the results of thoraco-amniotic shunting in 51 singleton pregnancies. Forty-seven pregnancies were complicated by fetal pleural effusions, three fetuses had pulmonary cysts and one had a pericardial effusion. In all cases there was a large pleural effusion (or pulmonary cyst) and hydrops fetalis, polyhydramnios or mediastinal shift. All patients had a detailed sonogram and fetal karyotype. Five fetuses had chromosomal abnormalities (four, trisomy 21, one, monosomy X), and four of these pregnancies were terminated. Following placement of the thoraco-amniotic catheter, polyhydramnios resolved in 20 of the 30 affected pregnancies, fetal hydrops resolved in 13 of the 28 hydropic fetuses. All of the non-hydropic fetuses survived (18 patients), half of the hydropic fetuses survived (14 of 28). Poor prognostic factors included associated malformations, bilateral effusions, or persistence of hydrops or polyhydramnios following placement of the catheter. Five fetuses with chromosomal abnormalities, two with congenital diaphragmatic hernias and two with congenital cardiac defects within this series underlines the importance of a rapid karyotype and thorough search for associated anomalies in these cases. Some heart defects may be undetectable until the mediastinal shift resolves.

Based on these results and other studies with similar results, we recommend serial sonograms in pregnancies complicated by fetal hydrothorax without mediastinal shift or hydrops. Thoracentesis *in utero* just prior to delivery of a fetus with a large pleural effusion may be considered to assist neonatal resuscitation. Preterm fetuses with large pleural effusions resulting in mediastinal shift and/or hydrops are screened with detailed examinations by ultrasound, echocardiogram, karyotype, cultures and analysis of maternal antibody screen. Patients may be offered thoracoamniotic shunting *in utero* in an effect to improve neonatal prognosis.

Twins

Twinning occurs in approximately 1 in 90 births in the United States and is associated with an increased rate of complications. The incidence of dizygotic twinning varies with maternal age, race and parity, while monozygotic twinning has a fairly constant incidence of 1 in 250 births. The perinatal mortality rate for diamnionic–dichorionic twins is approximately 10%. This increased rate compared to singletons is secondary to an increased incidence of preterm deliveries, intrauterine growth retardation, congenital anomalies and an increased incidence of maternal complications. Monochorionic twins have a 25% perinatal mortality; their risk is increased because monochorionic twins may share vascular anastomoses within the placenta. These anastomoses may result in the twin-to-twin transfusion syndrome, fetal damage or demise of a twin secondary to demise of its co-twin or acardiac twinning. The 50% perinatal mortality rate seen in monoamnionic–monochorionic twins is primarily due to these risks plus the risk of entanglement of the umbilical cord.

Twin-to-twin transfusion syndrome

The twin-to-twin transfusion syndrome complicates approximately 5–30% of monochorionic twin gestations and occurs when blood shunts from one twin to the other via an arteriovenous anastomosis. This may result in an anemic, growth-retarded fetus with oligohydramnios and a plethoric, fluid-overloaded fetus with hydrops and polyhydramnios. The natural history of the twin-to-twin transfusion syndrome has been reported by Bebbington and Wittman[64]. They reported 25 cases diagnosed between 14 and 35 menstrual weeks. The mean age at delivery was 28 menstrual weeks, with an overall survival of only 41%. None of the fetuses with hydrops survived. When twin-to-twin transfusion syndrome is diagnosed prior to 28 weeks, the survival has been reported to be only 21%[65].

Because of the very dismal prognosis for pregnancies complicated by severe twin-to-twin transfusion syndrome, many different treatment modalities have been attempted. Maternal digoxin therapy to treat signs of fetal congestive heart failure has been reported[66]. Fetocide by intracardiac injection of normal saline has been reported[67] but concerns have been raised about possible damage or demise of the co-twin. DeLia and co-workers[68] have performed fetoscopy with laser coagulation of the communicating vessels. Encouraging results have been reported with serial amniocentesis; over 170 cases with severe twin-to-twin transfusion syndrome diagnosed before 28 weeks' gestation have been reported, with an overall survival of approximately 50%[69].

Two pregnancies complicated by severe twin-to-twin transfusion syndrome that failed to respond to aggressive serial amniocentesis underwent hysterotomy, with removal of the twin within the oligohydramniotic sac at the University of California, San Francisco Fetal Treatment Center. In one case the remaining twin died *in utero* and in the other case the co-twin required delivery at 27 weeks' gestation and had a pro- longed neonatal hospitalization, but survived.

Acardiac twinning

One of the most bizarre complications of multifetal gestations is acardiac twinning. It is a very rare occurrence, complicating approximately 1 in 25 000 pregnancies and is primarily seen in monochorionic twins. The acardiac twin may not have any vascular connections with the placenta, and is totally dependent on its co-twin for perfusion. Umbilical arterial-to-arterial and venous-to-venous anastomoses allow blood to circulate from the normal twin to the acardiac twin. The very abnormal development of the acardiac twin is thought to be secondary to hypoxia and the reversed blood flow (lower extremities are better perfused than the head and upper extremities). The acardiac twin is non-viable. Moore and colleagues[70] reported the perinatal outcome of 49 pregnancies complicated by acardiac twinning. The overall perinatal mortality was 55%, the major perinatal problems included pump-twin congestive heart failure, polyhydramnios and preterm delivery. Poor prognostic factors included a high acardiac to pump twin weight ratio, development of congestive heart failure and hydramnios in the pump twin as well as preterm labor.

Selective removal of the acardiac twin is an experimental procedure to try to improve the chances of survival in the normal co-twin. There have been six hysterotomy procedures to remove the acardiac twin reported[71,72]. One fetus died postoperatively secondary to placental abruption; three fetuses were delivered preterm (27, 28 and 33 weeks' gestation) and two were delivered at 35 weeks; all five had good neonatal outcomes.

Open fetal surgery

There has been extensive experimental work performing open fetal surgery in animals to correct certain congenital anomalies. Much has been learned from these experiments and the human cases done thus far; however, this work must still be considered experimental. General guidelines for fetal surgery have been developed at UCSF[73]:

(1) The natural history of the disease has been defined;

(2) The pathophysiology of the disorder has been evaluated in animal models;

(3) The safety and feasibility of the treatment has been evaluated in animal models;

(4) The patient and family have been fully informed;

(5) A multidisciplinary team, involved in the care of the patient, includes a perinatologist skilled in intrauterine procedures, a geneticist, a sonologist experienced in evaluating fetal anomalies, a pediatric surgeon and a neonatologist;

(6) Approval of the institutional review board has been obtained;

(7) A level-III high-risk obstetric and neonatal unit is available; and

(8) Bioethical and psychosocial consultation is available.

A team approach involving all of the subspecialities must be utilized in a fetal treatment program. The patient and her family need to receive all available information to make the decision that is best for them. They must weigh the risks of surgery to the fetus and mother against the possible neonatal complications and debilitating disease associated with an uncorrected lesion.

At UCSF we are currently investigating open fetal correction of congenital cystic adenomatoid malformations and congenital diaphragmatic hernias. Detailed ultrasound, echocardiogram and karyotype examinations are performed. Extensive counseling is provided, which includes meetings with anesthetists, pediatric surgeons, neonatologists, perinatologists, geneticists, social workers and nurses involved in the fetal-treatment group. Patient deciding to proceed with open fetal surgery are scheduled depending on the anomaly, presence of hydrops and gestational age. Typically, fetal surgery is performed between 24 and 25 menstrual weeks. The patient is admitted the night before surgery and started on indomethacin preoperatively. Epidural catheters for postoperative pain control are used frequently. Preterm labor has been a major problem and its management has been a source of maternal morbidity. Animal studies have shown[74] that nitric oxide donors are effective tocolytic agents and, based on this work, intravenous nitroglycerine is used as a tocolytic agent in these patients. Central and arterial lines are placed. Aggressive hydration to maintain a satisfactory mean arterial pressure is frequently required when patients are on intravenous nitroglycerine.

A Mallard incision allows adequate exposure. Intraoperative, sterile ultrasound examination locates the placenta and determines fetal position. Placement of the uterine incision avoids the placenta while allowing access to the desired fetal parts. A trocar is placed under ultrasound guidance and some of the amniotic fluid is withdrawn. The uterine incision is made by the Lactomer stapler while the trocar is elevating the uterine wall and fetal membranes. The stapled incision is hemostatic and attaches the membranes to the uterine wall. Continuous fetal monitoring is accomplished by placing a pulse oximeter on the fetal hand and attaching a radio telemeter to the fetal back with EKG leads placed subcutaneously. A small pressure catheter extends from the radio telemeter into the amniotic fluid and measures amniotic fluid pressure post-operatively to help guide tocolytic therapy.

The necessary fetal parts are then elevated out of the uterine incision and the fetal surgery is performed. Throughout the surgery the fetus and uterus are bathed by a warm saline infusion. The fetal parts are then returned to the uterus and the uterine incision closed in layers with careful incorporation of the fetal membranes. Fibrin glue may be applied to the incision to decrease the risk of amniotic fluid leakage. Warm Ringer's lactate solution with 500 mg of vancomycin is used to replenish the amniotic fluid.

Postoperatively the maternal and fetal conditions are monitored closely in the intensive care unit. The most troublesome problem continues to be preterm labor. In 1 to 3 days the patients are weaned off nitroglycerine, started on another tocolytic agent (terbutaline, nifedipine or magnesium sulfate) and moved out of the intensive care unit. Activity and diet are slowly advanced. Frequent ultrasound examinations to evaluate any changes in the fetal status are performed. Indications for delivery include rupture of membranes with labor, evidence of chorioamnionitis, intractable premature labor or fetal distress (after fetal viability is attained). Delivery almost always must be by Cesarean section for all subsequent pregnancies, since the fetal surgery incision is rarely in the lower uterine segment. Typically patients are discharged from the hospital one week after surgery. Outpatient tocolytics, monitoring and ultrasound examinations are continued until delivery.

By last report, there have been 42 open fetal surgeries performed at UCSF[75] and a few cases reported in other centers around the world. In the series at UCSF, there have been no maternal deaths; however, there has been significant maternal morbidity secondary to the tocolytic agents and their side-effects. The management protocol for congenital cystic adenomatoid malformations and congenital diaphragmatic hernias are presented as well as a brief overview of the results from open fetal surgery for urinary tract obstruction and sacrococcygeal teratomas.

Congenital cystic adenomatoid malformation

Congenital cystic adenomatoid malformation (CCAM) is a rare anomaly that is characterized by overgrowth of the terminal respiratory elements. The spectrum of disease presentation ranges from a child with recurrent respiratory infections to a hydropic, stillborn fetus. Prenatal diagnosis is possible by an ultrasound examination revealing a cystic mass within the thorax. This mass may result in a mediastinal shift and possibly hydrops. Hydrops is thought to be secondary to the cystic mass causing vena caval obstruction and/or cardiac compression. In a review of the natural history of twelve CCAMs diagnosed *in utero*, Adzick and associates[76] reported that the prognosis was dependent on the absence or presence of fetal hydrops. Six of the seven fetuses without evidence of hydrops survived, following neonatal surgery. Within this series there were five fetuses with hydrops; two pregnancies were terminated and three pregnancies were continued with no neonatal survivors.

In a recent review Kuller and associates[77] reported the outcome of 22 pregnancies complicated by prenatally diagnosed CCAMs managed at UCSF. Eighteen women continued their pregnancy after diagnosis. Serial ultrasound examinations were performed to evaluate signs of hydrops. Nine of the fetuses did not develop hydrops, and were delivered between 32 and 42 weeks' gestation; all survived. Surgical resection of the cystic lung mass was performed in four neonates. Evidence of hydrops developed in nine of the fetuses between 20–27 menstrual weeks. One patient declined fetal therapy, delivered at 33 weeks and the infant died of respiratory distress. In the remaining eight fetuses detailed examinations by ultrasound, echocardiogram and karyotyping were performed. Needle aspiration of the predominant cystic lesion was attempted in four fetuses. Preterm labor occurred in one patient approximately one week after the procedure and a viable infant was delivered. A very stormy neonatal course ensued and the child has bronchopulmonary dysplasia. Rapid reaccumulation of the fluid occurred in the other three fetuses. In two pregnancies, Harrison double-pigtail catheters were placed under ultrasound guidance. A non-viable fetus was delivered two days following placement of the catheter in one case, and in the other patient the catheter malfunctioned and she underwent fetal surgery. Open fetal surgery was performed on six patients (one patient had failed needle aspiration; one had failed needle aspiration and catheter placement). An intrauterine fetal demise occurred approximately 7 h following surgery in one case. Delivery for maternal indications 2 days following surgery occurred in another case and the neonate subsequently died. There were four neonatal survivors that were alive and well.

The management protocol at UCSF is shown in Figure 5. Fetuses with CCAMs are followed closely with serial ultrasound examinations and allowed to go to term with planned delivery at a tertiary care center for neonatal resuscitation and surgery. The development of hydrops in a fetus over 32 menstrual weeks with a CCAM is an indication for delivery (betamethasone is given if indicated). In the very preterm fetus with hydrops, the prognosis is very grim; the family is counseled and offered open fetal surgery. By last report, eight fetuses have undergone open fetal surgery for CCAM with hydrops[75].

Congenital diaphragmatic hernias

Congenital diaphragmatic hernias (CDH) have a birth incidence of 2–5 per 10 000[78] although the true incidence may be higher, because CDHs have been associated with stillbirths. Failure of the pleuroperitoneal canal to close properly results in the abdominal contents herniating into the thoracic cavity and compressing the fetal lung parenchyma. Stomach, bowel and liver may be found within the chest and may result in significant mediastinal shift (Figure 6). Neonatal correction is possible with replacement of the abdominal viscera and repair of the defect in the diaphragm. Unfortunately, the neonatal course is frequently complicated by pulmonary hypoplasia, which is secondary to compression of the lung

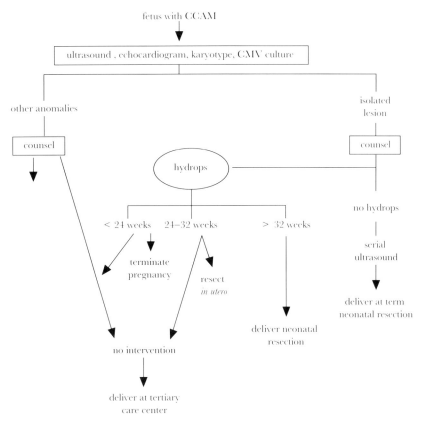

Figure 6 *Protocol of University of California, San Francisco for management of fetus with congenital cystic adenomatoid malformation (CCAM). CMV, cytomegalovirus*

parenchyma *in utero*. Survival for *neonates* diagnosed with CDH with appropriate neonatal resuscitation, surgical correction and extracorporeal membrane oxygenation has been reported to be as high as 70–80%[79]. In contrast, studies evaluating the outcome of *fetuses* diagnosed with CDH found the survival rate was less than 30%[80,81]. These studies excluded fetuses and neonates with associated anomalies and chromosomal aneuploidy. This wide disparity in survival rates has been attributed to stillbirth, early neonatal death or failed neonatal resuscitation at delivery, resulting in referral centers seeing a biased group. This has been coined the 'hidden mortality'[82]. More recent series suggest that the survival rate of fetuses prenatally diagnosed with CDH and delivered at tertiary centers is 40%.

A retrospective review of 94 cases of CDH diagnosed *in utero* was reported by Adzick and associates[80]. There were several important conclusions that became evident in that study:

(1) Prenatal diagnosis of CDH was accurate;

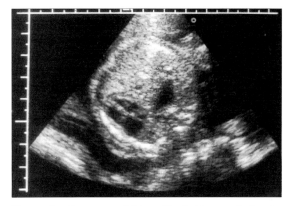

Figure 5 *Sonogram of fetus with diaphragmatic hernia, demonstrating stomach bubble in the chest*

(2) Despite conventional therapy, the neonatal prognosis was poor;

(3) Polyhydramnios was a common marker of CDH and was a poor prognostic sign; and

(4) Fetal CDH was a dynamic process, with the severity of the disease correlating with the size of the defect.

In this series, 16% of the fetuses had associated lethal anomalies and 5% had chromosomal aneuploidy.

In an elegant series of experiments in the pregnant ewe, Harrison and associates[83] have documented the pathophysiology of CDH, devised treatment plans and demonstrated that repair *in utero* can possibly avoid pulmonary hypoplasia. Inflation of a silastic balloon that had been placed within the fetal lamb thorax, stimulating the abdominal viscera to compress the lung, resulted in pulmonary hypoplasia. Deflation of the balloon, simulating *in utero* repair, allowed normal lung development and growth[84]. Further experiments revealed that creating a defect in the diaphragm of the fetal lamb allowed herniation of abdominal viscera into the thorax and resulted in pulmonary hypoplasia[85]. Replacement of the abdominal viscera with repair of the diaphragmatic defect avoided the development of pulmonary hypoplasia. A silastic silo to enlarge the abdomen and avoid increased intra-abdominal pressure was found to be beneficial in these experiments[85].

Pregnancies complicated by fetal CDH have a detailed examination by ultrasound, echocardiogram and karyotyping. During the ultrasound examination the position of the liver is determined by Doppler, locating the vessels within the liver. Vessels curving up into the chest have been found to be a fairly reliable sign that liver is herniated into the thorax. By last report, 20 pregnancies complicated by fetal CDH have undergone open fetal surgery. Four of the seven fetuses with no liver herniated into the fetal thorax survived and are doing well. None of the fetuses that had liver in the thorax have survived, and it is theorized that pushing the liver back into the abdomen causes compromised blood flow through the ductus venosus, which results in fetal demise. Overall survival has been 20%.

Recently, Harrison and associates[75] have been evaluating a different approach to CDH repair. Tracheal occlusion in fetal lambs obstructs the release of lung fluid into the amniotic fluid, the build-up of lung fluid slowly increases the lung size and gradually pushes the bowel, stomach and liver down. This therapy may offer a new treatment option to fetuses with liver herniation into the thoracic cavity. The UCSF management protocol for fetuses with CDH is presented in Figure 7.

Urinary tract obstruction

Open fetal surgery for urinary tract obstruction has been performed on eight fetuses at UCSF[86]. Seven fetuses had bladder marsupialization, while one fetus underwent ureteral marsupialization. Intractable preterm labor at 25 weeks resulted in a delivery of a non-viable fetus in one patient. A pregnancy was terminated during re-exploration for persistent oligohydramnios when multiple fetal anomalies were noted. Two neonates died from pulmonary hypoplasia and there were four neonatal survivors. Renal insufficiency has developed in one child requiring renal transplantation. We are not currently investigating the role of open fetal surgery in fetuses with urinary obstruction, because we believe placement of a Rocket catheter is a better alternative.

Sacrococcygeal teratomas

Teratomas are neoplasms that arise from pluripotent cells and are composed of a wide diversity of tissues. They are the most common neoplasm found in the newborn with an incidence of 1 in 35 000; over half are sacrococcygeal. These lesions are usually benign, but up to 18% may be associated with other anomalies of the musculoskeletal, renal or nervous systems. Prognosis is dependent on associated anomalies, pathology, location of the teratoma and the development of hydrops. Hydrops is thought to develop when an arteriovenous malformation

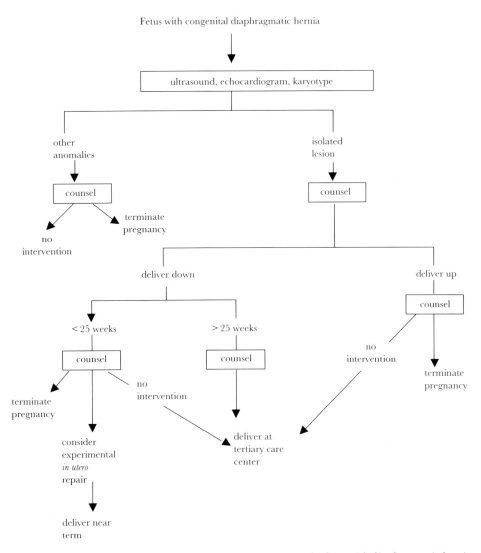

Figure 7 *Protocol of University of California, San Francisco for management of a fetus with diaphragmatic hernia*

within the mass results in high-output cardiac failure and is considered by many to be a preterminal event[87]. Two fetuses with sacrococcygeal teratomas and hydrops underwent open fetal surgery at UCSF; neither survived. We are no longer investigating open fetal surgery in fetuses with sacrococcygeal teratomas.

References

1. Liley, A. W. (1963). Intrauterine transfusion of foetus in haemolytic disease. *Br. Med. J.*, **2**, 1107–9

2. Fuhrmann, K., Reiher, H., Semmler, K. *et al.* (1983). Prevention of congenital malformations in infants of insulin-dependent diabetic mothers. *Diabetes Care*, **6**, 219–22

3. Molsted-Pederson, L. and Pedersen, J. F. (1985). Congenital malformations in diabetic pregnancies, clinical viewpoints. *Acta Paediatr. Scand.*, **(S320)**, 79–84
4. Scriver, C. R. and Clow, C. L. (1980). Phenylketonuria: epitome of human biochemical genetics. *N. Engl. J. Med.*, **303**, 1336–1400
5. Koch, R., Azen, C., Friedman, E. G. and Williamson, M. L. (1984). Paired comparisons between early treated PKU children and their matched sibling controls on intelligence and school achievement test results at eight years of age. *J. Inhert. Met. Dis.*, **7**, 86–90
6. Holtzman, N. A., Kronmal, R. A., vanDoornick, W., Azen, C. and Koch, R. (1986). Effect of age at loss of dietary control on intellectual performance and behavior of children with phenylketonuria. *N. Engl. J. Med.*, **314**, 593–8
7. Lenke, R. R. and Levy, H. L. (1980). Maternal phenylketonuria and hyperphenylalaninemia. *N. Engl. J. Med.*, **303**, 1202–8
8. Levy, H. L. and Waisbren, S. E. (1983). Effects of untreated maternal phenylketonuria and hyperphenylalaninemia on the fetus. *N. Engl. J. Med.*, **309**, 1269–74
9. Luke, B. and Keith, L. G. (1990). The challenge of maternal phenylketonuria screening and treatment. *J. Reprod. Med.*, **35**, 667–73
10. Buehler, B. A., Delimont, D., van Waes, M. and Finnell, R. H. (1990). Prenatal prediction of risk of the fetal hydantoin syndrome. *N. Engl. J. Med.*, **322**, 1567–72
11. MRC Vitamin Study Research Group (1991). Prevention of neural tube defects: results of the Medical Research Council Vitamin Study. *Lancet*, **338**, 131–7
12. Hurley, L. S. and Bell, L. T. (1974). Genetic influence on response to dietary manganese deficiency in mice. *J. Nutr.*, **104**, 133–7
13. Keen, C. L., Saltmann, P. and Hurley, L. S. (1980). Copper nitrilotriacetate: a potent therapeutic agent in the treatment of a genetic disorder of copper metabolism. *Am. J. Clin. Nutrition*, **33**, 1789–803
14. Evans, M. I., Chrousos, G. P., Mann, D. W. *et al.* (1985). Pharmacologic suppression of the fetal adrenal gland *in utero*: attempted prevention of abnormal external genital masculinization in suspected congenital adrenal hyperplasia. *J. Am. Med. Assoc.*, **253**, 1015
15. David, M. and Forest, M. G. (19984). Prenatal treatment of congenital adrenal hyperplasia resulting from 21-hydroxylase deficiency. *J. Pediatr.*, **105**, 799
16. Shulman, D. I., Mueller, O. T., Gallardo, L. A., Stiff, D. and Oster, H. (1989). Treatment of congenital adrenal hyperplasia *in utero*. *Pediatr. Res.*, **25**, 2
17. Pang, S. Y., Pollack, M. S., Marshall, R. N. and Immken, L. (1990). Prenatal treatment of congenital adrenal hyperplasia due to 21-hydroxylase deficiency. *N. Engl. J. Med.*, **322**, 111–15
18. Killeen, A. A., Seeling, S., Ulstrom, R. A. and Orr, H. T. (1988). Diagnosis of classical steroid 21-hydroxylase deficiency using an HLA-B locus-specific-DNA-probe. *Am. J. Med. Genet.*, **29**, 703–12
19. Nyham, W. L. (1975). Prenatal treatment of methylmalonic acidemia (editorial). *N. Engl. J. Med.*, **293**, 353–4
20. Ampola, M. J., Mahoney, M. J., Nakamura, E. and Tanaka, K. (1975). Prenatal therapy of a patient with vitamin B 12 responsive methylmalonic acidemia. *N. Engl. J. Med.*, **293**, 313
21. Packman, S., Cowan, M. J., Golbus, M. S. *et al.* (1982). Prenatal treatment of biotin-responsive multiple carboxylase deficiency. *Lancet*, **1**, 1435–8
22. Roth, K. S., Yang, W., Allan, L., Saunders, M., Gravel, R. A. and Dakshinamurt, K. (1982). Prenatal administration of biotin in biotin-responsive multiple carboxylase deficiency. *Pediatr. Res.*, **16**, 126–9
23. Davison, K. M., Richards, D. S., Schatz, D. A. and Fisher, D. A. (1991). Successful *in utero* treatment of fetal goiter and hypothyroidism. *N. Engl. J. Med.*, **324**, 543
24. Perelman, A. H., Johnson, R. L., Clemons, R. D., Finberg, H. J., Clewell, W. H. and Trujillo, L. (1990). Intrauterine diagnosis and treatment of fetal goitrous hypothyroidism. *J. Clin. Endocrinol. Metab.*, **71**, 618–21
25. Polin, R. A. and Fox, W. W. (1992). *Fetal and Neonatal Physiology*. pp. 1842–9. (Philadelphia: W. B. Saunders)
26. Brook, M. M., Silverman, N. H. and Villegas, M. (1993). Cardiac ultrasonography in structural abnormalities and arrhythmias: recognition and treatment. *West. J. Med.*, **159**, 286–300
27. Kleinman, C. S., Copel, J. A., Weinstein, E. M., Santrulli, T. V. and Hobbins, J. C. (1985). *In utero* diagnosis and treatment of fetal supraventricular tachycardia. *Semin. Perinatol.*, **9**, 113–29
28. Hill, L. M. and Malkasian, G. D. Jr. (1979). The use of quinidine sulfate throughout pregnancy. *Obstet. Gynecol.*, **54**, 366–8
29. Gembruch, U., Hansmann, M. and Bald, R. (1988). Direct intrauterine fetal treatment of fetal tachyarrhythmias with severe hydrops fetalis by antiarrhythmic drugs. *Fetal Ther.*, **3**, 210–15
30. Weiner, C. P. and Thompson, M. I. B. (1988). Direct treatment of fetal supraventricular tachy-

cardia after failed transplacental therapy. *Am. J. Obstet. Gynecol.*, **158**, 570–3
31. Gembruch, U., Hansmann, M., Redel, D. A. and Bald, R. (1988). Intrauterine therapy of fetal tachyarrhythmias: intraperitoneal administration of antiarrhythmic drugs to the fetus in fetal tachyarrhythmias with severe hydrops fetalis. *J. Perinat. Med.*, **16**, 39–44
32. Gembruch, U., Manz, M., Bald, R. *et al.* (1989). Repeated intravascular treatment with amiodarone in a fetus with refractory supraventricular tachycardia and hydrops fetalis. *Am. Heart J.*, **118**, 1335–8
33. Kleinman, C. S. and Copen, J. A. (1989). Fetal cardiac dysrhythmias. In Creasy, R. K. and Resnik, R. (eds.) *Maternal Fetal Medicine: Principles and Practice*, 2nd edn., pp. 344–56. (Philadelphia: W. B. Saunders)
34. Schmidt, K. G., Ulmer, H. E., Silverman, N. H., Kleinman, C. S. and Copel, J. A. (1991). Perinatal outcome of fetal complete atrioventricular block: a multicenter experience. *J. Am. Coll. Cardiol.*, **17**, 1360–6
35. Owen, R. D. (1945). Immunogenic consequencies of vascular anastomoses between bovine twins. *Science*, **102**, 400–1
36. Turner, J. H., Hutchinson, D. I. and Petricciani, J. C. (1973). Chimerism following fetal transfusion. *Scand. J. Haematol.*, **10**, 358–66
37. Fleischman, R. A. and Mintz, B. (1979). Prevention of genetic anemias in mice by microinjection of normal hematopoietic stem cells into the fetal placentas. *Proc. Natl. Acad. Sci. USA*, **76**, 5736–44
38. Harrison, M. R., Slotnick, R. N., Crombleholme, T. M., Golbus, M. S., Tarantal, A. F. and Zanjani, E. D. (1989). *In-utero* transplantation of fetal haemopoietic stem cells in monkeys. *Lancet*, **2**, 1425–7
39. Crombleholme, T. M., Harrison, M. R. and Zanjani, E. D. (1990). *In utero* transplantation of hematopoietic stem cells in sheep: the role of T cells in engraftment and graft versus host disease. *J. Pediatr. Surg.*, **8**, 885–92
40. Micklem, H. S. (1972). Cell proliferation in haematopoietic spleen colonies of mice: difference between colonies derived from injected adult bone marrow and foetal liver cells. *Cell Tissue Kinet.*, **5**, 159–64
41. Lucarelli, G., Izzi, T., Porcellini, A. and Delfini, C. (1979). Infusion of fetal liver cells in aplastic anemia. *Haematol. Blood Trans.*, **24**, 167–170
42. Diukman, R. and Golbus, M. S. (1992). *In utero* stem cell therapy. *J. Reprod. Med.*, **37**, 515–520
43. Touraine, J. L., Raudrant, D., Debaud, A. *et al.* (1992) *In utero* transplantation of stem cells in humans: immunological aspects and clinical follow-up of patients. *Bone Marrow Trans.*, **9**(S1), 121–6
44. Birnholz, J. C. and Frigoletto, F. D. (1981). Antenatal treatment of hydrocephalus. *N. Engl. J. Med.*, **303**, 1021–3
45. Clewell, W. H., Johnson, M. L., Meier, P. R. *et al.* (1982). A surgical approach to the treatment of fetal hydrocephalus. *N. Engl. J. Med.*, **306**, 1320
46. Manning, F. A., Harrison, M. R., Rodeck, C., Members of the International Fetal Medicine and Surgery Society (1986). Catheter shunts for fetal hydronephrosis and hydrocephalus – report of the International Fetal Surgery Registry. *N. Engl. J. Med.*, **315**, 336–40
47. Chervenak, F. A., Berkowitz, R. C., Tortora, M. *et al.* (1985). Management of fetal hydrocephalus. *Am. J. Obstet. Gynecol.*, **151**, 933–42
48. Hudgins, R. J., Edwards, M. S. B., Goldstein, R. *et al.* (1988). Natural history of fetal ventriculomegaly. *Pediatrics*, **82**, 692–7
49. Drugan, A., Drause, B., Canady, A. *et al.* (1989). The natural history of prenatally diagnosed cerebral ventriculomegaly. *J. Am. Med. Assoc.*, **261**, 1785–8
50. Reid, L. M. (1984). Lung growth in health and disease. *Br. J. Dis. Chest.*, **78**, 113–34
51. Thomas, D. F. M. (1984). Urological diagnosis *in utero*. *Arch. Dis. Child.*, **59**, 913–15
52. Holzgreve, W. and Evans, M. I. (1993). Nonvascular needle and shunt placement for fetal therapy. *West. J. Med.*, **159**, 333–40
53. Brock, D. J. H., Rodeck, C. H. and Ferguson-Smith, M. A. (1992). *Prenatal Diagnosis and Screening*. (New York: Churchill Livingstone)
54. Appleman, Z. and Golbus, M. S. (1986). The management of fetal urinary tract obstruction. *Clin. Obstet. Gynecol.*, **29**, 483–9
55. Mahoney, B. S., Filly, R. A., Callen, P. W., Hricak, H., Golbus, M. S. and Harrison, M. R. (1984). Fetal renal dysplasia: sonographic evaluation. *Radiology*, **152**, 143–6
56. Lipitz, S., Ryan, G., Samuell, C. *et al.* (1993). Fetal urine analysis for the assessment of renal function in obstructive uropathy. *Am. J. Obstet. Gynecol.*, **168**, 174–9
57. Holzgreve, W., Lison, A. and Bulla, M. (1989). SDS–PAGE as an additional test to determine fetal kidney function prior to intrauterine diversion of urinary tract obstruction. *Fetal Ther.*, **4**, 93–96
58. Crombleholme, T. M., Harrison, M. R., Golbus, M. S. *et al.* (1990). Fetal intervention in obstructive uropathy: prognostic indicators and efficacy of intervention. *Am. J. Obstet. Gynecol.*, **162**, 1239–44
59. Wilkins, I. A., Chitkara, U., Lynch, L., Goldberg, J. D., Mehalek, K. E. and Berkowitz, R. L. (1987). The nonpredictive value of fetal urinary electro-

lytes: preliminary report of outcomes and correlations with pathologic diagnosis. *Am. J. Obstet. Gynecol.*, **157**, 694–8
60. Muller, F., Dommergues, M., Mandelbrot, L., Aubry, M. C., Nihoul-Fekete, C. and Dumez, Y. (1993). Fetal urinary biochemistry predicts postnatal renal function in children with bilateral obstructive uropathies. *Obstet. Gynecol.*, **82**, 813–20
61. Holzgreve, W., Lison, A., Bulla, M. *et al.* (1991). Protein analysis to determine fetal kidney function (abstract). *Am. J. Obstet. Gynecol.*, **164**(S), 336
62. Longaker, M. T., Laberge, J. M., Dansereau, J., Langer, J. C., Crombleholme, T. M., Callen, P. W., Golbus, M. S. and Harrison, M. R. (1989). Primary fetal hydrothorax: natural history and management. *J. Pediatr. Surg.*, **24**, 573–6
63. Nicolaides, K. H. and Azar, G. B. (1990). Thoraco-amniotic shunting. *Fetal Diagn. Ther.*, **5**, 153–64
64. Bebbington, M. W. and Wittmann, B. K. (1989). Fetal transfusion syndrome: antenatal factors predicting outcome in 19 cases. *Am. J. Obstet. Gynecol.*, **160**, 573, 9B–19
65. Gonsoulin, W., Moise, K. J., Kirshon, B. *et al.* (1990). Outcome of twin–twin transfusion diagnosed before 28 weeks of gestation. *Obstet. Gynecol.*, **75**, 214–16
66. DeLia, J., Emery, M. G., Sheafor, S. A. and Jennison, T. A. (1985). Twin transfusion syndrome: successful *in utero* treatment with digoxin. *Int. J. Gynaecol. Obstet.*, **23**, 197–201
67. Wittmann, B. K., Farquarson, D. F., Thoman, W. D. S. *et al.* (1986). The role of feticide in the management of severe twin transfusion syndrome. *Am. J. Obstet. Gynecol.*, **155**, 1023–6
68. DeLia, J. E., Cruikshank, D. P. and Keye, W. R. (1990). Fetoscopic neodynium : Yag laser occlusion of placental vessels in severe twin–twin transfusion syndrome. *Obstet. Gynecol.*, **75**(6), 1046–53
69. Pinette, M. G., Pan, Y., Pinette, S. G. and Stubblefield, P. G. (1993). Treatment of twin–twin transfusion syndrome. *Obstet. Gynecol.*, **82**(5), 841–6
70. Moore, T. R., Gale, J. and Benirschke, K. (1990). Perinatal outcome of forty-nine pregnancies complicated by acardiac twinning. *Am. J. Obstet. Gynecol.*, **163**(3), 907–12
71. Robie, G. F., Payne, G. G. and Morgan, M. A. (1989). Selective delivery of an scardiac acephalic twin. *N. Engl. J. Med.*, **320**, 512–13
72. Fries, M. H., Goldberg, J. D. and Golbus, M. S. (1992). Treatment of acardiac–acephalus twin gestations by hysterotomy and selective delivery. *Obstet. Gynecol.*, **79**, 601–4
73. Harrison, M. R., Golbus, M. S., Filly, R. A. (eds) (1990). *The Unborn Patient: Prenatal Diagnosis and Treatment*, 2nd edn. (Philadelphia, PA: WB Saunders)
74. Jennings, R. W., MacGillevray, T. E. and Harrison, M. R. (1993). Nitric oxide inhibits preterm labor in the rhesus monkey. *J. Matern. Fetal Med.*, in press
75. Harrison, M. R., (1993). Fetal SUrgery. *West. J. Med.*, **159**, 341–9
76. Adzick, N. S., Harrison, M. R., Glick, P. L. *et al.* (1985). Fetal cystic adenomatoid malformation: prenatal diagnosis and natural history. *J. Pediatr. Surg.*, **20**, 483–8
77. Kuller, J. A., Yankowitz, J. Goldberg, J. D., Harrison, M. R., Adzick, N. S., Filly, R. A., Callen, P. W. and Golbus, M. S. (1992). Outcome of antenatally diagnosed cystic adenomatoid malformations. *Am. J. Obstet. Gynecol.*, **167**, 1038–41
78. David, T. J. and Illingworth, C. A. (1976). Diaphragmatic hernia in the southwest of England. *J. Med. Genet.*, **13**, 253–62
79. Heiss, K., Manning, P., Oldham, K. T. *et al.* (1989). Reversal of mortality for congenital diaphragmatic hernia with ECMO. *Ann. Surg.*, **209**, 225–30
80. Adzick, N. S., Harrison, M. R., Glick, P. L. *et al.* (1985). Diaphragmatic hernia in the fetus: prenatal diagnosis and outcome in 94 cases *J. Pediatr. Surg.*, **20**, 357
81. Benacerraf, B. R. and Adzick, N. S. (1987). Fetal diaphragmatic hernia: ultrasound diagnosis and clinical outcome in 19 cases. *Am. J. Obstet. Gynecol.*, **156**, 573
82. Harrison, M. R., Bjordal, R. F., Langmark, F. and Knutrud, O. (1978). Congenital diaphragmatic hernia. The hidden mortality. *J. Pediatr. Surg.*, **13**, 227–30
83. Harrison, M. R., Jester, J. A. and Ross, N. A. (1980). Correction of congenital diaphragmatic hernia *in utero*. I. The model: intrathoracic balloon produces fetal pulmonary hypoplasia. *Surgery*, **88**, 174–82
84. Harrison, M. R., Bressack, M. A., Churg, A. M. and deLorimier, A. A. (1980). Correction of congenital diaphragmatic hernia *in utero*. II. Simulated correction permits fetal lung growth with survival at birth. *Surgery*, **88**, 260–8
85. Harrison, M. R., Ross, N. A. and deLorimier, A. A. (1981). Correction of congenital diaphragmatic hernia *in utero*. III. Development of a successful surgical technique using abdominoplasty to avoid compromise of umbilical blood flow. *J. Pediatr. Surg.*, **16**, 934–42
86. Crombleholme, T. M., Harrison, M. R., Langer, J. C. *et al.* (1988). Early experience with open fetal surgery for congenital hydronephrosis. *J. Pediatr. Surg.*, **23**, 1114–21
87. Flake, A. W. (1993). Fetal sacrococcygeal teratomas. *Semin. Pediatr. Surg.*, **2**, 113–114

Therapeutic strategies in the management of intrauterine growth retardation

R. N. Pollack and M. Y. Divon

INTRODUCTION

Intrauterine growth retardation (IUGR) is one of the most common complications of pregnancy, and represents a major cause of perinatal morbidity and mortality. Birth weight remains the single most important determinant of perinatal outcome, and it is for this reason that the management of the growth retarded fetus continues to present the perinatologist with a daunting challenge[1]. Battaglia has highlighted the fact that infants of low birth weight may be categorized as being either preterm and appropriately grown, preterm and growth retarded, or term and growth retarded[2]. Williams and colleagues[3] have shown that within defined gestational age strata, the birth weight centile is inversely correlated with perinatal mortality. The diagnosis of IUGR has already been reviewed in this volume by Carrera and colleagues (Chapter 23). It is our intention to focus this review on the management of the growth retarded fetus.

Intrauterine growth retardation may result from a broad variety of etiologies. These etiologies may be classified as being related to either fetal, placental, or maternal factors[4]. It is obvious that the mechanisms which led to the development of IUGR may influence the choice of therapy for this condition. For this reason, the nature of the insult which led to impaired fetal growth must be considered when assessing the efficacy of treatments for IUGR.

Fetal causes of IUGR include karyotypic abnormalities, inborn errors of metabolism, and congenital anomalies or infections. Data from the Metropolitan Atlanta Congenital Defects Program have shown that 38% of all chromosomally abnormal infants are growth retarded[5]. Similarly, in that series, 8% of all growth retarded infants had a major congenital anomaly. The detection of major congenital anomalies is therefore a primary concern in the management of IUGR. The detection of such anomalies may seriously alter the management of the growth retarded fetus. When such anomalies are detected early in pregnancy, a termination may be offered to the parents. When such anomalies are detected late in gestation, intensive fetal monitoring and Cesarean birth should be avoided. Fetal assessment to rule out the presence of multiple anomalies or the presence of karyotypic abnormalities is crucial. This assessment may be based upon ultrasonographic and echocardiographic examination, as well as on invasive techniques including amniocentesis, cordocentesis, and placental biopsy. Depending upon the nature of the anomaly, the appropriate pediatric consultations should be obtained, and parents counseled as to fetal prognosis. In cases where the potential for fetal salvage exists, the planning for delivery assumes great importance. Infants should be delivered at centers that have experience in caring for the critically ill newborn, and that can provide ready access to neonatal surgical expertise. In cases where there is no potential for fetal salvage, the parents should be provided with the necessary support, and the delivery should be conducted as atraumatically as possible. The possibility of organ donation after the death of the newborn may be discussed with the parents prior to delivery, since this undertaking requires considerable logistical co-ordination. After the death of the anomalous newborn a full examination should be performed including a karyotypic evaluation. This information is important when the parents are counseled as to the recurrence risk of the anomaly.

Congenital infections also represent an important cause of IUGR[6]. The contribution of congenital infections to the overall burden of fetal growth is not known. Infection with the parasite *Toxoplasma gondii* has been associated with a variety of perinatal sequelae including IUGR, hydrocephaly, hydrancephaly, microcephaly, hepatomegaly, and non-immune hydrops fetalis[7]. Risk factors for infection with this organism include exposure to cat litter, as well as consumption of raw meat. Maternal infection may be heralded by the presence of a mononucleosis-like illness but is confirmed by the presence of an IgM response to *Toxoplasma gondii*. The diagnosis of congenital toxoplasmosis is based on isolation of the parasite from fetal tissues including blood or amniotic fluid. It may also be based on the demonstration of an IgM response to *Toxoplasma gondii* in fetal blood. Similarly, a biological response to fetal infection may be observed. This response may include anemia, thrombocytopenia, leukopenia, and elevations in liver enzymes. Although *Toxoplasma gondii* is one of many organisms which may result in perinatal infections with serious sequelae, it is the only organism for which *in utero* therapy is well established. Maternal treatment with spiramycin, a macrolide antibiotic, and drugs such as sulfadiazine, a sulfonamide, and pyrimethamine, a folic acid antagonist, have been shown to reduce the risk of congenital toxoplasmosis[7]. The role of these treatments in improving birth weight of fetuses at risk for congenital toxoplasmosis has not been explored.

The placenta is an organ which is responsible for the nutritive and respiratory functions which are required to sustain fetal life and adequate growth *in utero*. It is therefore not surprising that placental pathology can result in impaired fetal growth. Animal studies have shown that following placental embolization with microspheres, a 30% decrease in birth weight was observed[8]. Histologic evaluation of placentas in pregnancies complicated by IUGR usually fails to reveal a consistent pathological picture[9]. Abnormal cord insertions, placental infarctions, chorioangiomata, and abruptio placenta have all been associated with IUGR[4]. These processes are for the most part irreversible and are not amenable to therapy. Chazotte and colleagues[10] have recently described a case of hydrops fetalis associated with a placental chorioangioma. They observed resolution of the hydrops after spontaneous infarction of the chorioangioma. This observation suggests that, on occasion, placental pathological processes may be reversible. The possibility therefore exists that resolution of placental pathology may result in improved fetal growth.

THERAPY FOR IUGR

The growth of the fetus *in utero* reflects a delicate equilibrium between the mother, the placenta, and the fetus. Fetal growth depends on adequate maternal fuel supply, and a maternal vascular tree which can delivery these fuels to the feto-placental unit. As mentioned previously, intact placental function is also a prerequisite for adequate fetal growth.

Bed-rest

Bed-rest is probably the single therapy most commonly recommended for the treatment of fetal growth retardation. Theoretically, bed-rest results in decreased blood flow to the periphery, and an increase in blood flow to the utero-placental circulation. This increase in utero-placental blood flow supposedly contributes to improved fetal growth[11]. Interestingly, there is a striking paucity of data validating these assumptions.

Laurin and associates[12] have recently assessed the efficacy of bed-rest for the treatment of IUGR. A total of 107 patients with sonographic evidence of fetal growth retardation at 32 weeks of gestation were randomized to be treated with bed-rest in hospital or outpatient management. There was no difference in birth weight or perinatal outcome between the two groups. The authors concluded that bed-rest in hospital was not associated with any demonstrable benefit in this small sample.

Maternal nutritional supplementation

The provision of adequate fuels to the fetoplacental unit has long been a focus of research into fetal growth. Both observational and interventional studies suggest that maternal nutritional deprivation has a modest effect on fetal birth weight. The seminal studies into the impact of nutritional deprivation on fetal growth date back to the Dutch famine of 1944–1945[13]. During this period, severe caloric restriction to less than 1500 daily calories, was associated with a modest decrease of approximately 300 g in mean birth weight. These data eventually led to the first studies of therapies to improve the weight of growth retarded fetuses. In these studies, a modest increase in birth weight was associated with dietary supplementation to indigent mothers at risk of IUGR[14]. It should be noted that this modest increase in birth weight may be explained by the increased gestational period of fetuses born to mothers who received nutritional supplementation. Careful analysis of the data from such studies supports the hypothesis that prepregnancy nutritional supplementation to underweight mothers may have a greater effect on birth weight than supplementation during the index pregnancy[15]. Similarly, Caan and colleagues[16] have shown that in the Women, Infants and Children (WIC) program, interpregnancy food assistance had a greater effect on reproductive outcome than food assistance during pregnancy. These data suggest that nutritional supplementation in the form of orally administered caloric and/or protein supplements have, at best, a modest effect on increasing birth weight.

The effects of maternal parenteral nutritional supplementation on fetal growth in the setting of IUGR has also been studied. Experience with mothers suffering from malnutrition because of illnesses complicating pregnancy has shown that intravenous hyperalimentation is a treatment modality which can reduce the incidence of fetal growth retardation[17]. Mesaki and associates[18] administered solutions of 10% glucose and 12% amino acids to nine patients who had growth retarded fetuses. A control group of eleven patients with growth retarded fetuses did not receive nutritional supplementation. A significant increase in the birth weight of the treated fetuses was observed. The mean birth weight in the treated group was 2994 g, whereas that in the control fetuses was 2490 g. Beischer and colleagues[19] have reported on their experience with a large series of 473 patients who were identified on the basis of abnormal urinary estriol excretions. In the initial phase of the study, patients were treated only with bed-rest. Later in the study patients received parenteral supplements of carbohydrates, amino acids, and lipids. Although parenteral nutritional supplements did not increase fetal size, a decrease in perinatal mortality was associated with this treatment.

Maternal deficiencies in trace metals has also been associated with IUGR. Wells and associates[20] have observed that peripheral leukocyte zinc levels, a sensitive indicator of tissue zinc status, were decreased in mothers of growth retarded infants. Simmer and colleagues[21] have recently reported that zinc supplementation was found to significantly reduce the incidence of IUGR. In a randomized double-blind trial, 22.5 mg effervescent zinc citrate supplements were given to pregnant mothers at high risk for developing fetal growth retardation between 15 and 25 weeks of gestation. In the control group, 25% of the mothers had growth retarded infants (defined as a birth weight of less than the 10th percentile). None of the mothers who took the zinc supplement had infants who were growth retarded. If these data are indeed reproducible, this simple therapeutic approach may be useful in the prevention of fetal growth retardation in gravidas at elevated risk of developing this condition. It remains to be determined if this therapeutic approach has a role in the treatment of the fetus who already is suffering from impaired growth *in utero*.

The role of eicosanoids in reproductive biology has been the focus of extensive interest in recent years. The roles of these substances in the onset of labor, in the pathogenesis of pre-eclampsia, and in the pathogenesis of IUGR have all been explored. Idiopathic intrauterine growth retardation has been associated with reduced uteroplacental perfusion. This has been demonstrated using techniques such as dynamic placental scintigraphy[22], and Doppler velocimetry of the umbilical and uterine arteries[23]. The vasoactive properties of the eicosanoids thromboxane A_2 (TxA_2), and prostacyclin I_2 (PGI_2) have been explored as mediators of reduced uteroplacental flow seen in idiopathic fetal growth retardation. Prostacyclin is a powerful vasodilator, and thromboxane is a powerful vasoconstrictor. The balance between these two powerful substances contributes to the vascular tone of the uteroplacental bed. Dietary manipulation has been shown to alter the balance of TxA_2 and PGI_2. The principal marine n-3 fatty acid is eicosapentaenoic acid, which competes with arachidonic acid as a substrate for the cyclo-oxygenase enzyme. The consumption of fish oils is therefore thought to result in a net decrease in the synthesis of TxA_2, and an increase in the concentration of prostacyclin[24]. The changing ratio of these two vasoactive substances resulting from the consumption of fish oils is thought to result in vasodilatation.

Olsen and colleagues[25] have noted that the average birth weight in the Faroe Islands is greater than the average birth weight in Denmark. They have suggested that the diet of the Faroe Islanders which is rich in fish oils may contribute to this different in average birth weights. Andersen and co-workers[26] have hypothesized that the consumption of a diet rich in fish oils results in an alteration in the thromboxane : prostacyclin balance in favor of prostacyclin. This alteration leads to an increase in uteroplacental blood flow and therefore to an increase in birth weight. They suggest that dietary supplementation with fish oils may result in increased birth weight, and may be of use in the prevention and treatment of IUGR.

Sørensen and colleagues[27] have studied the effect of fish oil supplementation on both maternal and fetal eicosanoid production. Patients in the 30th week of pregnancy were randomly assigned to receive either 2.7 g n-3 fatty acid supplementation, or a control preparation. They observed a significant decrease in fetal blood TxA_2-generating capacity associated with the administration of fish oil supplements. These data support the hypothesis that consumption of fish oils alters the balance between TxA_2 and PGI_2 resulting in a relative increase in PGI_2. The physiological results of this phenomenon include vasodilatation, decreased blood viscosity, and improved oxygen delivery to fetal tissue. These data would suggest that consumption of fish oils may be an attractive therapeutic modality for the prevention and/or treatment of intrauterine growth retardation.

Oxygen therapy

Fetal growth and development is contingent upon a variety of factors relating to substrate delivery. Adequate perfusion of the uteroplacental bed and adequate delivery of amino acids, lipids, and carbohydrates are all conditions without which normal fetal growth cannot proceed. Oxygen delivery to fetal tissues is also crucial to the maintenance of normal growth. Medical conditions such as cyanotic heart disease and asthma, which impair maternal oxygenation are associated with IUGR[4]. Similarly, it has been observed that the mean birth weight at high altitudes is lower than the mean birth weight at sea level[28]. This difference in mean birth weights is felt to represent the net result of the decreased oxygen tension at high altitudes. This ultimately leads to diminished oxygen delivery to the developing fetus and to the impairment of fetal growth.

An appreciation of the centrality of oxygen delivery to the adequacy of fetal growth has led various investigators to study oxygen tension in the growth retarded fetus. Soothill and colleagues[29] have performed cordocenteses on 38 growth retarded fetuses, and have reported the umbilical venous oxygen tension. They noted that the oxygen tension in growth retarded fetuses was significantly lower than that observed in 150 gestational age-matched control fetuses. In 14 of the 38 fetuses (37%) studied, the umbilical venous oxygen tension was more than two standard deviations below the mean for gestational age-matched control fetuses. These data confirm that impairment in oxygen delivery to the fetus is associated with impaired fetal growth. These data also raise the intriguing possibility that improvement in fetal oxygenation may be of use in preventing or even reversing fetal growth retardation.

Based on these observations, Nicolaides and colleagues[30] have explored the role of maternal oxygen supplementation as a treatment modality for the growth retarded fetus. In a preliminary report[30] these authors have observed a significant decrease in fetal mortality associated with maternal oxygen supplementation when compared to historical controls. The fetal mortality in the historical controls was 85%, whereas the mortality rate in the growth retarded fetuses whose mothers received oxygen supplementation was only 20%.

Battaglia and co-workers[31] have recently reported the results of their trial of maternal hyperoxygenation in the treatment of IUGR. Thirty-six patients whose pregnancies were complicated by fetal growth retardation were randomly assigned to receive either bed-rest, or 55% oxygen administered at a rate of 8 l/min around the clock. The gestational ages of the fetuses studied ranged from 26–34 weeks. It should be noted that the inclusion criteria for this study were particularly rigorous. The fetuses studied all had oligohydramnios, abnormal umbilical artery Doppler flow velocity waveforms, and sonographic abdominal circumference measurement of less than the fifth percentile of the reference population. These authors noted that maternal hyperoxygenation was associated with a statistically significant improvement in umbilical venous blood gas parameters between the time of admission and the time of delivery. The pO_2 increased from 21.2 mmHg to 27.7 mmHg; the pCO_2 decreased from 43.7 mmHg to 38 mmHg; and the oxygen saturation increased from 57% to 71.8%. Likewise, the pH increased from 7.31 to 7.34 with maternal treatment. Although Battaglia and colleagues did not observe any difference in the birth weights of the two groups, they did observe a significant difference in perinatal mortality rates. The control group had a perinatal mortality rate of 68%, whereas the fetuses whose mothers received hyperoxygenation had a perinatal mortality rate of only 29%. These data suggest that maternal hyperoxygenation could be of use in the management of fetal growth retardation. However, Harding and associates[32] have recently reported that although this therapeutic modality is promising, there are risks that may theoretically be associated with maternal hyperoxygenation. Animal studies suggest that discontinuation of hyperoxygenation may be associated with a period of fetal oxygenation even worse than that observed prior to the institution of therapy[32]. For this reason, they advise against introduction of maternal hyperoxygenation until larger trials have been undertaken.

Pharmacological therapy

Aspirin and dipyridamole

The administration of a variety of pharmacological agents for the prevention and treatment of intrauterine growth retardation has been the subject of extensive investigation. The agents that have been studied include aspirin and dipyridamole. As discussed previously, blood supply to the uteroplacental bed is thought to reflect the balance between the vasoconstrictive properties of TxA_2 and the vasodilatory influence of PGI_2. The ratio between these two vasoactive compounds is subject to modulation by exogenous substances. These substances include fish oils and drugs such as aspirin. Aspirin (or acetylsalicylic acid) is an inhibitor of the cyclo-oxygenase enzyme. This action is mediated by the irreversible acetylation of cyclo-oxygenase[33]. Administration of aspirin in low doses of 1–2 mg kg^{-1} day^{-1} inactivates platelet cyclo-oxygenase and results in decreased synthesis of TxA_2. This effect, which is well described in the non-pregnant state, has recently been shown to occur in platelets of normal pregnant patients. Low-dose aspirin therapy has not been found to significantly alter the synthesis of PGI_2. Hence the net effect of the administration of aspirin in low doses is the alteration of the $TxA_2 : PGI_2$ ratio. This change probably results in vasodilatation of the uteroplacental bed. Administration of low-dose aspirin also exerts effects on platelet reactivity. Louden and colleagues[34] have recently demonstrated a significant decrease in collagen-induced platelet aggregation and serotonin release in the platelets of normal pregnant patients treated with low-dose aspirin. It is because of these important physiological effects that aspirin has been explored as a potential treatment for fetal growth retardation.

Wallenburg and co-workers[33] studied the effects of low-dose aspirin and dipyridamole for the prevention of idiopathic IUGR. In a small non-randomized study which utilized historical controls, they demonstrated a significant reduction in the incidence of fetal growth retardation in patients who received aspirin and dipyridamole. Dipyridamole was administered because it is a phosphodiesterase inhibitor, and as such delays the degradation of cyclic adenosine monophosphate (cAMP). This increase in cAMP concentration may render platelets more sensitive to the effects of prostacyclin and may also serve to stimulate prostacyclin synthesis. The incidence of fetal growth retardation defined as a birth weight of less than the tenth percentile was 61.5% in the group of historical controls. In contradistinction, the incidence of IUGR in the patients who received aspirin and dipyridamole was only 13.3%. This preliminary study, although encouraging, is hampered the lack of randomization and by the absence of an appropriate control group.

Interestingly, Wallenburg observed one fetal death in his study. This occurred in the treatment group where one patient had a stillbirth of an appropriately grown fetus at 27 weeks of gestation. The cause of this fetal loss was thought to be abruptio placenta. This observation is particularly intriguing in light of a recent study of low-dose aspirin in the prevention of pre-eclampsia in low-risk nulliparous women. In this recent study, Sibai and colleagues[35] found that although low-dose aspirin did bring about a modest reduction in the incidence of pre-eclampsia, its use was associated with a significant increase in the incidence of abruptio placenta. The significance of this association between low-dose aspirin and abruptio placenta remains to be determined.

The study of Wallenburg and Rottmans[33] explored the role of low-dose aspirin and dipyridamole in the prevention of IUGR in mothers at high risk for developing this condition. The utility of low-dose aspirin in the treatment of established uteroplacental insufficiency is a related issue which has been studied by Trudinger and co-workers[36]. In a randomized, controlled, double-blind trial, 150 mg/day of aspirin was administered to 22 patients who had abnormal umbilical artery flow velocity waveforms. The inclusion criteria for this study were the presence of an umbilical artery flow velocity waveform systolic/diastolic ratio above the 95th percentile of the reference population. This finding was taken as evidence of uteroplacental insufficiency, based on the data of Giles and colleagues[37] which showed the presence of an abnormal umbilical artery flow velocity waveform to be the physiological correlate of a pathological obliteration of placental tertiary stem villi. The control group consisted of 24 patients with abnormal umbilical artery flow velocity waveforms. The administration of low-dose aspirin was associated with a significant increase in mean birth weight of 516 g and a significant increase in placental weight. Although these data are of interest, it should be noted that the mean birth weight ratio in the untreated patients with abnormal umbilical artery fetal velocity waveforms was 21.5. This unexpected finding calls into question the presence of uteroplacental insufficiency in this patient population. A smaller birth weight ratio would have been expected in patients with evidence of uteroplacental insufficiency. Nonetheless, these data do support the ability of low-dose aspirin to increase birth weight in high-risk pregnancies.

Recently, larger scale trials which explore the role of aspirin and/or dipyridamole in the prevention of fetal growth retardation have been published. Uzan and associates[38] have reported the results of the EPREDA trial; a multicentred, randomized, controlled, double-blind trial which was undertaken in France. A total of 323 patients were randomized between 15–18 weeks' gestation. Patients were allocated to receive either a placebo or 150 mg/day aspirin, or 150 mg/day aspirin and 225 mg/day dipyridamole. Inclusion criteria were the presence of fetal growth retardation, stillbirth, or abruptio placenta in at least one prior pregnancy. Aspirin was found to have a significant effect on increasing birth weight in patients at risk of fetal growth retardation. A mean increase in birth weight of 225 g was associated with aspirin administration. The incidence of IUGR, defined as a birth weight of less than the 10th percentile, was 13% in the aspirin-treated patients, whereas that in the control population was 26%. No significant differences were noted between patients treated with aspirin alone vs patients treated with aspirin and dipyridamole. The authors concluded that aspirin is effective in increasing birth weight in patients at high risk of fetal growth retardation, and that the addition of dipyridamole to this treatment regimen confers no added benefit. The authors hypothesized that the mechanism of action of aspirin in increasing birth weight is related to its modulation of the balance between TxA_2 and PGI_2. Another possible mechanism which would explain these findings is the prolongation of the gestational period. The mean gestational period in the patients who received treatment was 264 days, whereas the mean gestational period in the control group was 258 days. This difference in the gestational period of 6 days can fully explain the observed increase in birth weight of the aspirin-treated patients. Nonetheless, when fetal birth weights were expressed as birth weight percentiles, a significant reduction in fetal growth retardation was noted in the aspirin-treated group. These data support the hypothesis that the administration of low-dose aspirin to patients at high risk of fetal growth retardation results in a modest increase in birth weight and a modest reduction in the incidence of IUGR.

The Italian Study of Aspirin In Pregnancy[39] did not support the use of aspirin in the prevention of fetal growth retardation. In this multi-centered trial, 1106 women at moderate risk of IUGR were randomized to receive either 50 mg aspirin daily, or no treatment. The inclusion criteria for the study were broad and included a history of chronic hypertension, nephropathy, pre-eclampsia, IUGR, age of less than 18 or greater than 40 years, or a twin gestation. Patients were randomized between 16 and 32 weeks' gestation and therapy was continued up to delivery. No differences between the control group and the aspirin-treated group were noted with respect to birth weight, incidence of fetal growth retardation, length of gestation, incidence of pre-eclampsia or perinatal mortality rate. When data were stratified by criteria of entry into the trial and patients with a history of IUGR were studied, aspirin was not found to exert any effect on birth weight or on the incidence of IUGR. The authors note that the negative result of their study contrast with the positive results of prior studies including that of Uzan and associates[38]. They suggest that the broad inclusion criteria adhered to may have been responsible for this negative result that may represent a type II error. The inclusion criteria employed resulted in a heterogeneous group of patients in whom an imbalance of eicosanoid production was not the sole predisposing factor for IUGR or pre-eclampsia. This may explain why aspirin administration did not result in an increased mean birth weight or a decreased incidence of fetal growth retardation in this study.

β-mimetics

The administration of β-adrenergic agonists as tocolytic agents is an accepted therapy in contemporary obstetrical practice. These agents have a number of effects on uteroplacental hemodynamics[10]. One of these effects is the stimulation of myometrial adenylate cyclase which results in myometrial relaxation. Myometrial relaxation consequently results in decreased resistance to uterine blood flow and increased uterine perfusion. Similarly, the direct vasodilatory effect on the uterine arteries of β-mimetics may result in increased uterine perfusion. This increase in uterine perfusion may be useful in the treatment of fetal growth retardation. In a recent study, Cabero and colleagues[11] administered β-adrenergic agents to a group of patients with sonographic evidence of IUGR. He was unable to demonstrate any benefit associated with β-agonist administration in this setting.

Atrial natriuretic peptide

Atrial natriuretic peptide (ANP) is an endogenous peptide synthesized in the right atrium which has diuretic, natriuretic, and vasodilatory properties[12]. The biological effects of ANP are thought to be mediated through the stimulation of guanylate cyclase, resulting in an increased intracellular concentration of cyclic guanosine monophosphate. ANP has been reported to dilate the placental vasculature in late pregnancy in several animal models[13,14]. The role of ANP in the pathogenesis of IUGR resulting from uteroplacental insufficiency has recently been studied. Should this substance be implicated in the pathogenesis of IUGR, administration of ANP may provide a novel therapeutic approach for treatment of the growth retarded fetus.

Jansson[15] has explored the implication of ANP administration in the animal model. He administered a continuous low-dose infusion of ANP to pregnant guinea pigs following the induction of fetal growth retardation by uterine artery ligation. He found that the administration of ANP resulted in an increase of 26% in the blood flow to the placentas of the growth retarded fetuses. Based on these data Jansson suggested that ANP infusion may have therapeutic value in pregnancies complicated by fetal growth retardation.

Kingdom and colleagues[16] have recently studied plasma ANP concentrations in human pregnancies complicated by IUGR. They found that the umbilical venous plasma concentration of ANP in growth retarded fetuses was significantly higher than that observed in fetuses exhibiting normal growth. The authors suggest that this may represent an adaptive response of the growth retarded fetus as it attempts to increase its blood supply.

The possibility that ANP receptor physiology is also disturbed in fetal growth retardation warrants careful consideration. McQueen and co-workers[17] have recently studied the characteristics of ANP receptors from the arteries of human placentas from normal pregnancies and pregnancies complicated by IUGR. They observed an 80% reduction in the number of ANP receptors in pregnancies complicated by IUGR, vs. control placentas. These data would support the hypothesis that perturbation of ANP receptor physiology may be associated with the pathogenesis of IUGR. Hopefully, further basic research into the role of ANP in normal fetal growth will help clarify its significance in fetal growth retardation.

Fetal nutritional supplementation

Normal fetal growth is contingent upon the adequacy of nutrient supply to the developing fetus. Impairment of this supply leads to the restriction of fetal growth. We have discussed various strategies for increasing nutrient supply to the fetus including maternal nutritional supplementation, maternal hyperoxygenation and pharmacological manipulations aimed at increasing uterine blood flow. The possibility of directly administering nutritional supplements to the fetus and by-passing the maternal circulation has also been explored by numerous investigators.

The amniotic fluid contains nutrients including sugars, proteins, amino acids, and lactate. These nutrients are swallowed, digested, and absorbed by the fetus *in utero*[48,49]. It has been estimated that the ingestion of amniotic fluid provides the fetus with 10–30 calories/day, and 0.2–0.3 g protein/kg/day in the third trimester[50,51]. It would therefore appear that it is physiological to administer fetal nutritional supplementation transamniotically. Experimental evidence also suggests that absorption of nutrients may also occur through the placenta, fetal membranes, and umbilical cord[52]. Transamniotic fetal feeding with a dextrose solution in a pregnant rabbit model resulted in an increase in fetal weight[53]. The evidence that substantiates the use of this approach in human pregnancy is entirely anecdotal and uncontrolled[52].

Direct nutritional supplementation of the fetus via the intragastric approach has also been attempted. In this experimental model, intragastric nutritional supplementation was capable of compensating for maternal dietary restriction and prevented fetal growth restriction[54]. Charlton and Johengen[55] studied the effects of direct intravascular administration of dextrose and amino acids to chronically catheterized fetal sheep. The sheep were subjected to placental embolization in an attempt to induce fetal growth retardation. Intravascular supplementation was shown to prevent the development of IUGR in this experimental model. These data support the efficacy of direct nutritional supplementation of the fetus either transamniotically, intragastrically, or intravenously in an attempt to prevent the development of IUGR. However, the relevance of these data to clinical practice remains to be determined.

Mechanical therapy

A novel approach for the prevention of IUGR was recently described by Shimonovitz and co-workers[56]. They described the pregnancies of three patients who were referred because of a history of severe IUGR. These patients had a history of pregnancies complicated by recurrent severe IUGR, despite treatment with low-dose aspirin and dipyridamole. All patients were admitted at 12–15 weeks' gestation and were treated with intermittent abdominal decompression using a Heyns suit. This apparatus consists of a plastic suit worn over a rigid frame which allows the pressure surrounding the abdomen to be reduced. Decompression is controlled by the patient who intermittently occludes tubing which leads from the suit to an exhaust pump[57]. A negative pressure of 70 mmHg was applied for 30 s every minute for 30 min twice a day. The technique of intermittent abdominal decompression is thought to result in increased blood flow to the placental intervillous space[56]. In all three cases this therapy was associated with a normally grown liveborn fetus.

Heyns[58] first suggested that abdominal decompression would be of use in improving fetal oxygenation and uteroplacental blood flow. Hofmeyer[59] has undertaken a meta-analysis of the three studies of this treatment modality. He found that a significant reduction in perinatal mortality was associated with abdominal decompression (typical odds ratio = 0.36, 95% confidence interval 0.19–0.67). Controlled trials of this modality for the prevention of IUGR appear to be warranted. This treatment may ultimately prove to be of use in the prevention of fetal growth retardation.

Induction of pulmonary maturity

Liggins and Howie[60] have observed that maternal administration of corticosteroids resulted in a significant decrease in the incidence of neonatal respiratory distress syndrome. Crowley and colleagues[61] have recently undertaken a meta-analysis of all trials of corticosteroid therapy for the induction of pulmonary maturity. Twelve trials involving more than 3000 patients were reviewed. These data have shown that this therapy is associated with a significant decrease in respiratory distress syndrome, necrotizing enterocolitis, periventricular hemorrhage, and perinatal mortality. There was no strong evidence suggesting any adverse effects of corticosteroid therapy.

The role of antenatal corticosteroid therapy for the induction of pulmonary maturity in the setting of intrauterine growth retardation has not been clearly delineated. It has been suggested that the incidence of respiratory distress syndrome is reduced in pregnancies complicated by IUGR and hypertensive disease[62]. The growth retarded fetus is thought to be 'stressed'. This 'stress' may result in secretion of endogenous corticosteroids which in turn enhance pulmonary maturity. Owen and associates[63] have recently re-evaluated this concept. They compared neonatal outcome in newborns delivered prematurely because of pregnancy complications which necessitated premature delivery, and newborns born prematurely because of spontaneous preterm labour. They concluded that there was no survival advantage associated with a 'stressed' pregnancy and that the morbidities seen in 'stressed' fetuses were similar to those seen in fetuses who were not 'stressed'.

Preterm delivery of the growth retarded fetus is usually advised when the benefits of prolonging the pregnancy are outweighed by the benefits of delivery. A crucial variable in this equation is the presence or absence of pulmonary maturity. In the setting of arrested fetal growth and documented pulmonary maturity, delivery of the fetus prior to term is recommended[11]. Clearly, respiratory distress syndrome is a significant complication which can only serve to jeopardize the health of the growth retarded newborn. Corticosteroid therapy may be of use in promoting pulmonary maturity in the immature growth retarded fetus. The prevention of this complication by administering corticosteroid therapy would appear to be warranted. However, this issue has yet to be investigated prospectively in pregnancies complicated by fetal growth retardation.

CONCLUSIONS

IUGR continues to represent a major cause of perinatal morbidity and mortality. It is for this reason that recent insights into the pathogenesis of this disorder have aroused much interest. These insights have indicated that fetal growth retardation is not a single disease entity, but rather a physical sign which may result from a broad variety of pathogenetic mechanisms. It therefore stands to reason that the treatment modalities proposed must be tailored specifically to the various disease states capable of causing fetal growth retardation.

Fetal causes of IUGR include congenital anomalies and congenital infections. Most congenital anomalies are not yet amenable to *in utero* therapy. Nonetheless, when these anomalies are detected, management must focus on arriving at an accurate diagnosis and on delivering the newborn as atraumatically as possible, in as supportive an environment as possible. Congenital infections are an important cause of fetal growth retardation for which treatment is available at present only in the case of congenital toxoplasmosis.

The most important cause of fetal growth retardation is impaired nutrient supply to the fetus. This may result from impaired maternal nutrition, a decrease in transfer of oxygen to the fetus, or a decrease in blood flow to the uterus or placenta. In these circumstances, treatment involves increasing nutrient supply to the fetus. This may require maternal nutritional supplementation, maternal hyperoxygenation, or pharmacological manipulations aimed at increasing blood flow to the fetus. Direct administration of exogenous nutrients to the fetus either transamniotically or parenterally has also been explored.

Large scale randomized trials have provided conflicting conclusions as to the efficacy of low-dose aspirin in preventing IUGR. Hopefully, studies in progress will help clarify this important issue. Maternal hyperoxygenation has also been shown in a small study to decrease perinatal mortality in the growth retarded fetus. These preliminary data are very promising and should be replicated. In the future, manipulation of vasoactive peptides such as ANP and its receptors, may prove to be useful in the treatment of IUGR. This will await further clarification of the role of ANP in the pathogenesis of fetal growth retardation. Hopefully, these new treatments will lead to a decrease in the morbidity and mortality which results from impairment of fetal growth. Finally, educating the public to abstain from smoking or abusing drugs during pregnancy will, no doubt, contribute significantly to decreasing the incidence of IUGR.

References

1. McCormick, M. C. (1985). The contribution of low birth weight to infant mortality and childhood morbidity. *N. Engl. J. Med.*, **312**, 82–90

2. Battaglia, F. C. (1970). Intrauterine growth retardation. *Am. J. Obstet. Gynecol.*, **106**, 1103–14

3. Williams, R. L., Creasy, R. K., Cunningham, G. C., Hawes, W. E., Norris, M. A. and Tashiro, M. S. (1982). Fetal growth and perinatal viability in California. *Obstet. Gynecol.*, **59**, 624–32
4. Pollack, R. N. and Divon, M. Y. (1992). Intrauterine growth retardation: definition, classification, and etiology. *Clin. Obstet. Gynecol.*, **35**, 99–107
5. Khoury, M. J., Erickson, J. D., Cordero, J. F. and McCarthy, B. J. (1988). Congenital malformations and intrauterine growth retardation: a population study. *Pediatrics*, **82**, 83–90
6. Knox, G. E. (1978). Influence of infection on fetal growth and development. *J. Reprod. Med.*, **21**, 352–8
7. Nies, B. M., Lien, J. M. and Grossman, J. H. (1992). Torch virus-inducted fetal disease. In Reece, E. A., Hobbins, J., Mahoney, M. and Petrie, R. H. (eds.) *Medicine of the Fetus and Mother*, pp. 349–52. (Philadelphia: J. B. Lippincott Company)
8. Creasy, R. K., Barrett, C. T., de Swiet, M., Kahanpaa, K. V. and Rudolph, A. M. (1972). Experimental intrauterine growth retardation in the sheep. *Am. J. Obstet. Gynecol.*, **112**, 566–73
9. Fox, H. (1978). *Pathology of the Placenta*, p. 248. (Philadelphia: W. B. Saunders)
10. Chazotte, C., Girz, B., Koenigsberg, M. and Cohen, W. R. (1990). Spontaneous infarction of placental chorioangioma and associated regression of hydrops fetalis. *Am. J. Obstet. Gynecol.*, **163**, 1180–1
11. Cunningham, F. G., MacDonald, P. C., Gant, N., Leveno, K. and Gilstrap, L. C. (1993). *Williams Obstetrics*, 19th edn., p. 881. (Norwalk, Connecticut: Appleton & Lange)
12. Laurin, J. and Perrson, P. H. (1987). The effect of bedrest in hospital on fetal outcome in pregnancies complicated by intrauterine growth retardation. *Acta Obstet. Gynecol. Scand.*, **66**, 407–11
13. Stein, Z. and Susser, M. (1975). The Dutch famine, 1944–45 and the reproductive process: I. Effects on six indices at birth. *Pediatric Res.*, **9**, 70–6
14. Villar, J., Khoury, M. J., Finucane, F. F. and Delgado, H. L. (1986). Differences in the epidemiology of prematurity and intrauterine growth retardation. *Early Hum. Dev.*, **14**, 307–20
15. Viteri, F. E., Schumacher, L. and Silliman, K. (1989). Maternal malnutrition and the fetus. *Sem. Perinatol.*, **13**, 236–49
16. Caan, B., Horgen, D. M., Margen, S., King, J. C. and Jewell, N. P. (1987). Benefits associated with WIC supplemental feeding during the interpregnancy interval. *Am. J. Clin. Nutr.*, **45**, 29–41
17. Lee, R. V., Rodgers, B. D., Young, C., Eddy, E. and Cardinal, J. (1986). Total parenteral nutrition during pregnancy. *Obstet. Gynecol.*, **68**, 563–71
18. Mesaki, N., Kubo, T. and Iwasaki, H. (1980). A study of the treatment for intrauterine growth retardation. *Acta Obstet. Gynecol. Jpn.*, **32**, 879–85
19. Beischer, N. A. (1978). Treatment of fetal growth retardation. *Aust. N.Z. J. Obstet. Gynecol.*, **18**, 28–33
20. Wells, J. L., James, D. K., Luxton, R. and Pennock, C. A. (1987). Maternal leucocyte zinc deficiency at the start of the third trimester as a predictor of fetal growth retardation. *Br. Med. J.*, **294**, 1054–6
21. Simmer, K., Lort-Phillips, L., James, C. and Thompson, R. P. H. (1991). A double-blind trial of zinc supplementation in pregnancy. *Eur. J. Clin. Nutr.*, **45**, 139–44
22. Lunell, N. and Nylund, L. (1992). Uteroplacental blood flow. *Clin. Obstet. Gynecol.*, **35**, 108–18
23. Divon, M. Y. and Hsu, H. (1992). Maternal and fetal blood flow velocity waveforms in intrauterine growth retardation. *Clin. Obstet. Gynecol.*, **35**, 156–71
24. Leaf, A. and Weber, P. (1988). Cardiovascular effects of n-3 fatty acids. *N. Engl. J. Med.*, **318**, 549–57
25. Olsen, S., Hansen, H. S., Sørenson, T. I. A., Jensen, B., Secher, N. J., Sommer, S. and Knudsen, L. B. (1986). Intake of marine fat, rich in (n-3)-polyunsaturated fatty acids, may increase birth weight by prolonging gestation. *Lancet*, **2**, 367–9
26. Andersen, H. J., Andersen, L. F. and Fuchs, A. R. (1989). Diet, pre-eclampsia, and intrauterine growth retardation. (Letter). *Lancet*, **1**, 1146
27. Sørensen, J. D., Olsen, S. F., Pedersen, A. K., Boris, J., Secher, N. J. and FitzGerald, G. A. (1993). Effect of fish oil supplementation in the third trimester of pregnancy on prostacyclin and thromboxane production. *Am. J. Obstet. Gynecol.*, **168**, 915–22
28. Cunningham, F. G., MacDonald, P. C., Gant, N., Leveno, K. and Gilstrap, L. C. (1993). *Williams Obstetrics*, 19th edn., p. 878. (Norwalk, Connecticut: Appleton & Lange)
29. Soothill, P. W., Nicolaides, K. H. and Campbell, S. (1987). Perinatal asphyxia, hyperlacticaemia, hypoglycemia, and erythroblastosis in growth retarded fetuses. *Br. Med. J.*, **294**, 1051–3
30. Nicolaides, K. H., Campbell, S., Bradley, R. J., Bilardo, C. M., Soothill, P. W. and Gibb, D. (1987). Maternal oxygen therapy for intrauterine growth retardation. *Lancet*, **1**, 942–5
31. Battaglia, C., Artini, P. G., D'Ambrogio, G., Galli, P. A., Segre, A. and Genazzani, A. R. (1993). Maternal hyperoxygenation in the treatment of intrauterine growth retardation. *Am. J. Obstet. Gynecol.*, **167**, 430–5

32. Harding, J. E., Owens, J. A. and Robinson, J. S. (1992). Should we try to supplement the growth retarded fetus? A cautionary tale. *Br. J. Obstet. Gynecol.*, **99**, 707–10
33. Wallenburg, H. C. S. and Rotmans, N. (1987). Prevention of recurrent idiopathic fetal growth retardation by low-dose aspirin and dipyridamole. *Am. J. Obstet. Gynecol.*, **157**, 1230–5
34. Louden, K. A., Pipkin, F. B., Symonds, E. M., Tuohy, P., O'Callaghan, C., Heptinstall, S., Fox, S. and Mitchell, J. R. A. (1992). A randomized placebo-controlled study of the effect of low-dose aspirin on platelet reactivity and serum thromboxane B_2 production in non-pregnant women, in normal pregnancy, and in gestational hypertension. *Br. J. Obstet. Gynecol.*, **99**, 371–6
35. Sibai, B. M., Caritis, S. N., Thom, E., Klenaboff, M., McNellis, D., Rocco, L., Paul, R. H., Romero, R., Witter, F., Rosen, M., Depp, R. and the National Institutes of Child Health and Human Development Network of Maternal–Fetal Medicine Units. (1993). Prevention of pre-eclampsia with low-dose aspirin in healthy, nulliparous women. *N. Engl. J. Med.*, **329**, 1213–18
36. Trudinger, B. J., Cook, C. M., Thompson, R. S., Giles, W. B. and Connelly, A. (1988). Low-dose aspirin therapy improves fetal weight in umbilical placental insufficiency. *Am. J. Obstet. Gynecol.*, **159**, 681–5
37. Giles, W. B., Trudinger, B. J. and Baird, P. J. (1985). Fetal umbilical artery flow velocity waveforms and placental resistance: pathological correlation. *Br. J. Obstet. Gynecol.*, **92**, 31–8
38. Uzan, S., Beaufils, M., Breart, G., Bazin, B., Capitant, C. and Paris, J. (1991). Prevention of fetal growth retardation with low-dose aspirin: findings of the EPREDA trial. *Lancet*, **337**, 1427–31
39. Italian Study of Aspirin in Pregnancy. (1993). Low-dose aspirin in the prevention and treatment of intrauterine growth retardation and pregnancy-induced hypertension. *Lancet*, **341**, 396–400
40. Lippert, T. H., DeGrandi, P. B., Roemer, V. M. and Fridrich, R. (1980). Hemodynamic changes in placenta, myometrium and heart after administration of the uterine relaxant ritodrine. *Int. J. Clin. Pharmacol. Ther. Toxicol.*, **18**, 15–20
41. Cabero, L., Cerqueira, M. J., Del Solar, J., Bellart, J. and Esteban-Altirriba, J. (1988). Long-term hospitalization and beta-mimetic therapy in the treatment of intrauterine growth retardation of unknown etiology. *J. Perinatal Med.*, **16**, 453–8
42. Goetz, K. L. (1988). Physiology and pathophysiology of atrial peptides. *Am. J. Physiol.*, **254**, E1–15
43. Chemtob, S., Potvin, W. and Verma, D. R. (1989). Selective increase in placental blood flow by atrial natriuretic peptide in hypertensive rats. *Am. J. Obstet. Gynecol.*, **160**, 477–9
44. Reid, D. L., Goodfriend, T. L., Hollister, M. C., Phernetton, T. M. and Rankin, J. H. G. (1989). Effects of atrial natriuretic factor on maternal ovine vascular resistance. *J. Dev. Physiol.*, **11**, 25–8
45. Jansson, T. B. (1992). Low-dose infusion of atrial natriuretic peptide in the conscious guinea-pig increases blood flow to the placenta in growth-retarded fetuses. *Am. J. Obstet. Gynecol.*, **166**, 213–18
46. Kingdom, J. C. P., McQueen, J., Connell, J. M. C. and Whittle, M. J. (1992). Maternal and fetal atrial natriuretic peptide levels at delivery from normal and growth retarded pregnancies. *Br. J. Obstet. Gynecol.*, **99**, 845–9
47. McQueen, J., Kingdom, J. C. P., Jardine, A. G., Connell, J. M. C. and Whittle, M. J. (1990). Vascular angiotensin II and atrial natriuretic peptide receptors in normal and growth-retarded human placentae. *J. Endocrinol.*, **126**, 341–7
48. Pitkin, R. M. and Reynolds, W. A. (1976). Fetal ingestion and metabolism of amniotic fluid proteins. *Am. J. Obstet. Gynecol.*, **123**, 356–63
49. Charlton, V. and Rudolph, A. M. (1979). Digestion and absorption of carbohydrates by the fetal lamb *in utero*. *Pediatric Res.*, **13**, 1018–23
50. Gitlin, D., Kumate, J., Morales, C., Noriega, L. and Arevalo, N. (1972). The turnover of amniotic fluid protein in the human conceptus. *Am. J. Obstet. Gynecol.*, **113**, 632–45
51. Lilley, A. W. (1972). Disorders of amniotic fluid. In Assali, N. S. (ed.) *Physiopathology of Gestation*, Vol. 2, pp. 157–206. (New York: Academic Press)
52. Harding, J. E. and Charlton, V. (1991). Experimental nutritional supplementation for intrauterine growth retardation. In Harrison, M. R., Golbus, M. and Filey, R. (eds.) *The Unborn Patient*, 2nd edn., pp. 598–613. (Philadelphia: Saunders)
53. Mulvihill, S. J., Albert, A., Synn, A. and Fonkalsrud, E. W. (1985). *In utero* supplemental fetal feedings in an animal model: effects on fetal growth and development. *Surgery*, **98**, 500–5
54. Charlton, V. and Johengen, M. (1985). Effects of intrauterine nutritional supplementation on fetal growth retardation. *Biol. Neonate*, **48**, 125–42
55. Charlton, V. and Johengen, M. (1987). Fetal intravenous nutritional supplementation ameliorates the development of embolization-induced growth
56. Shimonovitz, S., Yagel, S., Zacut, D., Ben Chetrit, A., Hochner Celnikier, D. and Ron, M. (1992). Intermittent abdominal decompression: an option for the prevention of intrauterine growth retardation. *Br. J. Obstet. Gynaecol.*, **99**, 693–5

57. Hofmeyr, G. F., Metrikin, D. C. and Williamson, I. (1990). Abdominal decompression: new data from a previous study. *Br. J. Obstet. Gynaecol.*, **97**, 547–8
58. Heyns, O. S., Samson, N. S., Graham, J. A. C. (1962). Influence of abdominal decompression on intra-amniotic pressure and fetal oxygenation. *Lancet*, **1**, 282–92
59. Hofmeyer, G. J. (1989). Abdominal decompression in pregnancy. In Chalmers, I., Enkin, M. and Keirse, M. J. N. C. (eds.) *Effective Care in Pregnancy and Childbirth*, pp. 647–52. (Oxford, New York, Toronto: Oxford University Press)
60. Liggins, J. C. and Howie, R. N. (1972). A controlled trial of antepartum glucocorticoid treatment for the prevention of respiratory distress syndrome in premature infants. *Pediatrics*, **50**, 515–25
61. Crowley, P., Chalmers, I. and Keirse, M. J. N. C. (1990). The effects of corticosteroid administration before preterm delivery: an overview of the evidence from controlled trials. *Br. J. Obstet. Gynecol.*, **97**, 11–25
62. Perelman, R. H., Farrell, P. M., Engle, M. J. and Kemnitz, J. W. (1985). Developmental aspects of lung lipids. *Ann. Rev. Physiol.*, **47**, 803–22
63. Owen, J., Baker, S. L., Hauth, J. C., Goldenburg, R. L., Davis, R. O. and Copper, R. L. (1990). Is indicated or spontaneous preterm delivery more advantageous to the fetus. *Am. J. Obstet. Gynecol.*, **163**, 868–72

Index

abdominal biomorphic data 242
abdominal measurements by ultrasound 138
    for IUGR diagnosis 264,266
abdominal palpation for amniotic fluid volume estimation 321
abdominal wall anomalies, transvaginal ultrasound for 130
abortion
    clinical, in ACT 11–12
    missed 444–6,447,448
    threatened 442–4
abruptio placentae *see* placental abruption
absent or reverse end-diastolic flow (ARED) 456
    neurological examinations and 467–8
    in umbilical artery 461–2,463
acardiac twinning 157,528
acetylcholine reactivity in afferent fibers of cerebral cortex 48,49
acetylcholinesterase in amniotic fluid 335
acetylsalicylic acid *see* aspirin
acid lipase deficiency 374
acid–base status correlated with IUGR 416–17
acoustic fetal stimulation 228–9
actocardiography for fetal well-being monitoring 225–30
    analysis 226
    principles 225
adrenocorticotropic hormone (ACTH) in amniotic fluid 341
adrenal hyperplasia, congenital 332
β-adrenergic agonists
    effects on uterine and fetal hemodynamics 394
    in IUGR 543
    in multifetal pregnancy 185
afferent growth in cerebral cortex 47–8
albinism 369–70
alcohol
    effects on uterine and fetal hemodynamics 394
    IUGR and 254
allocortex development 41–2
amniocentesis 331–43
    in multifetal pregnancy 188
amnioinfusion 343
amnionicity of multifetal pregnancy 152–6
amnioscopy 331
amniotic fluid
    analysis 317–57
        methods 320–43
            invasive 331–43
            non-invasive 321–31
        rationale for 317
        physiology 317–20
    blood in 332–3
    cell content 329,332–3
    culture 331,336–7
    cytokine inhibitors 340–1
    drugs in 342–3
    embolism 336
    endothelins 339
    esterase 337–8
    α-fetoprotein 335–6
    glucose 334,338
    glycoprotein levels for cystic fibrosis test 108
    growth factors 334–5
    immunosuppressive factors 340–1
    index (AFI) 323–7
    infection indicators 336–42
    ingestion 544
    interleukins 338–9
    meconium in 332
    metabolites 333–4
    particulates in 327,332–3
    pH 329
    phospholipids 329–30
    prostaglandins 339–40
    tumor necrosis factor 339
    visual inspection 328
    volume 232,238,242
        dynamics 326
        evaluation of PROM from 330
        intrapartum screening for 326–7
        IUGR and 267
        multiple gestation and 327
        vaginal collection for analysis of 328
    white blood cell count 338
analgesic effects on fetal hemodynamics 390–1
anemia
    Fanconi's 372
    in mother causing IUGR 255
anencephaly, transvaginal ultrasound for 129
anesthetic effects on fetal hemodynamics 390–1
aneuploidy detection 65
angiotensin
    effects on uterine and fetal hemodynamics 394
    sensitivity, pre-eclampsia and 492
angiotensin II, pregnancy-induced hypertension and 492
anhydrotic ectodermal dysplasia 368–9
anticardiolipin antibodies, fetal loss and 497
anticonvulsant therapy effects on fetus 517
antigen-specific receptors, diversity of 19
antihypertensive drug effects on uterine and fetal hemodynamics 389–90
antiphospholipid antibodies, fetal loss and 497
aortic artery blood flow velocity waveforms 440,441
    abnormalities 102
    classification 456
    fetal descending 457–8
    in fetal hypoxia 382,384
    in IUGR 301,304,305,306,415,416
    in SGA 463
Apgar score in ACT 15

aplasia cutis congenita 369
arachidonic acid cyclo-oxygenase pathways 492
archicortex development 42–3
arcuate artery blood flow velocity waveform analysis 460
    in IUGR 463
areal differentiation in cerebral cortex 46
arrhythmias 520
arterial circulation in fetal hypoxia 384–5
arterial perfusion syndrome, twin reversed 157
artificial ventilation, neonatal cerebral blood flow and 483
asphyxia
    fetal 89,93
    perinatal 483,484
aspirin therapy in pregnancy 491–503
    dosage 500
    effects in healthy nulliparous pregnancy 495–7
        on uterine and fetal hemodynamics 392
    pharmacology and kinetics 492–4
    prevention of hypertension 495
        of IUGR 494–5
        of pre-eclampsia 494
        of preterm labor 497–8
    rationale 491–2
    safety aspects 498–500
    treatment of pre-eclampsia 497
        of IUGR 541–3
assisted conception techniques (ACT), pregnancy outcome of 11–18
astroglia development 46
ataxia telengiectasia 371
atenolol effects on fetal hemodynamics 390
atrial contractions 520
atrial flutter/fibrillation 520
atrial natriuretic peptide role in pregnancy 544
atrioventricular block 520
atrioventricular blood flow velocity waveform 440
auditory evoked potentials in preterm infants 50
autoimmune disease
    blood flow velocity waveform analysis in 465–6
    in mother, causing IUGR 256
axodendritic synapse development in brain 37–8
axonal ingrowth in cerebral cortex 45

bed-rest
    for IUGR 538–9
    in multifetal pregnancy 185
beneficence-based obligations 3–4,5,6
bilirubin in amniotic fluid 333–4
biometric parameters 231–2
    for IUGR diagnosis 261
biophysical profile, fetal 187,213–50
    baseline 242
    clinical application 245–7
    factors influencing 235–7
    functional 243–4
    hemodynamic 244–5
    IUGR and 270
    Manning 237–9
    modifications to Manning 239–41
    progressive 241–7

biotin-responsive carboxylase deficiency 519
biparietal diameter for IUGR diagnosis 261–3
birth weights
    in ACT 15
    effect of ultrasound screening on 81,83
    low, definition 252
    in multifetal pregnancy 184,188
    very low, outcome of infants with 311
    see also intrauterine growth retardation
blighted ovum 444–6,447,448
blood
    assessment by ultrasound 401–2
    circulation in mother, IUGR and 256
    flow 245
        centralization, IUGR and 274–7
        classes 456
        decentralization, IUGR and 277–8
        sonography, follicular 161–3
        velocity waveform analysis 455–7
        for fetal hypoxia 381–3
        see mainly under specific vessels e.g. uterine
    gas analysis, in umbilical cord 201,202,462
        correlation with IUGR 417
blood–brain barrier destruction 100
bone marrow transplantation 521
    for Chediak–Higashi syndrome 370
brain
    death 277
    development pre- and perinatally 35–55
    functional morphology and pathology 91–2
    injuries, antepartum 209–10
    pathology 89–106
        perinatal 96–102
        postnatal 102–3
    vesicles ultrasonography 148
brain-sparing effect 302,304,393
breathing movements 233,237
    effects on BFWV 456–7
    IUGR and 267–8
bupivacaine effects on fetal hemodynamics 390–1
butyrylcholinesterase in amniotic fluid 335

Cajal–Retzius cell development 42,43
callosal afferent growth in cerebral cortex 48
callosal axons at birth 52
carbon dioxide effects in cerebral circulation 482
carboxylase deficiency 519
cardiac *see also* heart
cardiac blood flow, fetal, in IUGR 302
cardiac defects
    analysis by ultrasound 138
    aspirin and 498
cardiac output in IUGR 306
cardiopathy *see under* congenital
cardiopulmonary disease in mother, causing IUGR 254
cardiotocography
    automated analysis 402–5,406
    changes in recordings 234
    clinical applications 199–202
    Dexeus score 243
    evaluation 195–205

fetal heart rates 197–202
fetal movements 196–7
parameters, IUGR and 268–70
principles 196
cardiovascular system anomalies, transvaginal ultrasound for 131–2
carotid artery
common 479
blood flow velocity waveforms for fetal hypoxia analysis 384
internal, blood flow velocity waveform analysis in hydrocephaly 480–1
in IUGR 480
pulsatility index changes in IUGR 305
catechol estrogens in amniotic fluid 341
cell
death in brain 38
tolerance induction in utero 19–20
cell-packing density in cerebral cortex 47
celom solutes 317–19
central nervous system
anomalies, transvaginal ultrasound for 128–9
development, classification of stages of 147
fetal centers of 236
ultrasonography 141–50
cephalic area for IUGR diagnosis 263–4
cephalic biomorphic data 242
cephalocele, transvaginal ultrasound for 129
cephalometric parameters curve profile 265–6,267
cerebellar ultrasonography 149–50
cerebral artery
anatomy 477,478
anterior 479
blood flow velocity waveforms 406
for fetal hypoxia 382,384–5,386
in IUGR 302,305,463,479–80
during labor 482
in perinatal asphyxia 484
in polyhydramnios 481
middle 477–9
resistance indices 402
cerebral autoregulation 482,484,485
cerebral circulation 441
during labor 481–2
functional vascular morphology 483–5
in hydrocephaly 480–1
in IUGR 479–8
neonatal 482–3
in normal pregnancy 477–9
in other pregnancy complications 481
in perinatal period 477–88
cerebral cortex development pre- and perinatally 35–55
cerebral hemisphere ultrasonography 149
cerebral hemodynamic adaptation, postnatal 482–3
cerebral hemorrhage, aspirin effects on 498–9
cerebral metabolism increase 482
cerebral palsy
causes 209
incidence 208,311–12
cerebral vascular morphology, functional 483–5

cerebroplacental ratio 402
cervical *see* uterine cervix
Cesarean section
anesthetic effects on fetal hemodynamics during 391
in multifetal pregnancy 187
Chediak–Higashi syndrome 370
Chlamydia culture in amniotic fluid 337
chondrodysplasia punctata syndrome 365–6
chorioamnionitis 337
chorioamnionitis
hemorrhagic lesions association with 93,94,95
choriocarcinoma 448
chorionicity of multifetal pregnancy 152–6
choroid plexus
blood flow 441–2
cyst detection 66
Christ–Siemens–Touraine syndrome 368–9
chromosomal abnormalities
in blighted ova 444
causing IUGR 255,257
ultrasonic markers of 65–7
chromosomal instability syndromes 371–2
chronic disease in adulthood, risk of 73
Circle of Willis 477,*478*
cleft lip/palate
aspirin and 498
with ectodactyly – ectodermal dysplasia 369
clinodactyly detection 65
cobalamin therapy 519
cocaine exposure effects 343
Cockayne–Touraine epidermolysis bullosa 367
Cockayne's syndrome 371–2
collagen defect 373
colony-stimulating factor-1 in amniotic fluid 334–5
computer applications in fetal medicine 117–24
for fetal heart rate analysis 289–97
future trends 122–3
hardware 117–18
operating systems 118
perinatal applications 119–22
software 118–19
computerized tomography for amniotic fluid volume estimation 321
congenital adrenal hyperplasia 518,519
congenital anomalies
brain 210
cardiopathies, ultrasound screening of 61–3
cystic adenomatoid malformation 529–30
diaphragmatic hernias 530–2
ectodermal defects 368–9
heart disease risk 74
photosensitive porphyria 373
see also malformations
conjoined twins 157
connective tissue disorders, inherited 373
Conradi–Hunermann syndrome 365
Copenhagen trial of ultrasound screening 82
copper
excess 372
therapy in mother, effects on fetus 518

cord *see* umbilical cord
corpus luteum morphology, function and vascularization 163–5
cortical development 38–41
    staging system 39–41
cortical organization, transient 45–6
cortical plate development 42–3,44–5
cortical reorganization and initial areal differentiation 46–8
cortication, focal abnormal 95–6,97
cortico-cortical axon redistribution in cerebral cortex 52
corticosteroids
    effects on fetus 518–19
    for respiratory distress syndrome 545
corticotropin-releasing hormone in amniotic fluid 341
counseling of patient for fetal therapy 8
    see also genetic counseling
crinkled gene phenotype 518
crown–rump length for IUGR diagnosis 261
2CTG computer system for fetal heart rate analysis 289–97
CTT 2000 fetal heart monitor 214
cystic adenomatoid malformation, congenital 529–30
cystic fibrosis
    clinical picture 107–8
    diagnosis 107–8
        mid-trimester 108–10
        prenatal first trimester 111–12
    genetic counseling 107–15
    inheritance 108
    risk 74,109,112–13
    screening 108
cystic hygroma, transvaginal ultrasound for 127–8
cytokine inhibitors in amniotic fluid 340–1
cytokines, role of 20

delivery
    modes in ACT 14–15
        in multifetal pregnancy 186–7
    timing in IUGR 303
dendritic development in brain 37,46
dendritic maturation 51
developmental state at birth 51–2
dexamethasone effects on uterine and fetal hemodynamics 394
Dexeus score 234,244
    IUGR and 268–70
diabetes in mother
    blood flow velocity waveform analysis in 464–5
        causing IUGR 254–5
    fetal heart rate in 220
diaphragmatic hernias, congenital 530–2
dietary deficiencies, neural tube defects and 518
digital convergence in fetal medicine 123
dipyridamole therapy in pregnancy for IUGR 494,495,541–3
Doppler *see under* transvaginal sonography; ultrasonography
Dowling–Meara epidermolysis bullosa 366–7
Down's syndrome
    detection 65,66
    diagnosis 336
    hydronephrosis in 131
    hygroma in 128
    risk 73–74
drugs
    analysis in amniotic fluid 342–3
    effects on fetus 517–20
ductus arteriosus
    blood flow peak velocity correlated with IUGR 416
    effects of aspirin on 499
    patent, cerebral blood flow and 483
ductus venosus
    blood flow velocity waveforms 425–7,429–31
        in fetal hypoxia 386
    fetal behavioral states and 431–3
    role 425
dye dilution in amniocentesis 331
dyslexia in children, effect of prenatal ultrasound screening on 86

echocardiography for fetal screening 61
ectodactyly – ectodermal dysplasia and cleft lip/palate 369
ectodermal defects, congenital 368–9
ectopic pregnancy in ACT 12
Ehlers–Danlos syndrome 373
eicosanoid role
    in lung vascular relaxation 499
    in pregnancy 539–40
electrophysiological development 48–50
embolism, amniotic fluid 336
embolization syndrome in twins 157
embryogenesis sonography 165–8
embryoscopy 331
encephalopathy, prenatal hypoxic-ischemic 92–6
endometrial carcinoma analysis by ultrasound 138
endothelins in amniotic fluid 339
endothelium-derived relaxing factor 492
enteral feeds in premature babies 314–15
enzymatic assay of fetal tissue 360
ependymitis, granular 99,100
ephedrine effects on fetal hemodynamics 391
ephrine effects on fetal hemodynamics 391
epidermal growth factor in amniotic fluid 335
epidermolysis bullosa 366–8
    dermolytic 367–8
    epidermolytic 366–7
    junctional 367
epidermolytic hyperkeratosis 363–4
epidural analgesia effects on fetal hemodynamics 390–1
epidural hematoma, effects of aspirin on 500
erythropoietic porphyria 373
esterases in amniotic fluid 337–8
estriol, myoma and 47
ethics in fetal therapy 3–10
    concept of fetus as patient 4–5
    criteria for 7–8
    standard of care 6–7
evoked potentials development, changes in 50–1

exencephaly, transvaginal ultrasound for 129
experimental therapy
    for previable fetal patient 8
    for viable fetal patient 7–8
eye movement in fetus 48

Fabry's disease 372–3
facial analysis by ultrasound 136,137
Fanconi's anemia 372
fatty alcohol oxidoreductase deficiency 365
femoral artery blood flow velocity waveform analysis 458
femoral length for IUGR diagnosis 265
femoral shortening detection 65–6
ferning of amniotic fluid 329
fertility drug effect on outcome of triplet pregnancies 188–9
fertilization sonography 165–8
fetal/fetus *see mainly under specific subject e.g. malformations*
fetal alcoholic syndrome 254
fetal biochemical parameters, IUGR and 270–1
fetal biophysical profile 231–50
    IUGR and 270
fetal circulation *see* hemodynamics
fetal distress 102
    correlated with growth in utero 414–15
    in diabetes mellitus 465
    diagnosis by actocardiography 228
    uterine artery ultrasound and 420–1
fetal examination, routine 79–88
fetal loss
    early 442–50
    prevention by aspirin 497
    risk 73
        in multifetal pregnancy 189–90
fetal measurements, automatic capture 120
fetal monitoring by computer systems 119
    see also specific monitoring systems e.g. ultrasonography
fetal order at birth, IUGR and 255–6
fetal stimulation, acoustic and photic 228–9
fetal tone 233,238,244
fetal well-being assessment 226–7,267–71
    by actocardiography 225–30
    during late pregnancy 455–75
    in multifetal pregnancy 187–8
fetoplacental circulation in pre-eclampsia 464
α-fetoprotein in amniotic fluid 335–6
    as marker for chromosomal defects 65
fetoscopy 331
fibronectin in amniotic fluid 341
fillagrin analysis in skin samples 360–2
finger clinodactyly and hypoplasia detection 65
Finnish nephrosis 335
fish oil therapy in IUGR 540
flow cytometry for phenotypic analysis of fetal lymphocytes 21–2
folic acid therapy for neural tube defect prevention 335–6
follicle sonography, pre-ovulatory 161–3

α-galactosidase-A activity deficiency 372–3
gammaglobulin therapy in thrombocytopenia 512,513
genetic aspects of cystic fibrosis 111–12
genetic counseling
    for cystic fibrosis 107–15
    non-directive prenatal 71–7
genetic disease
    diagnosis 72–3
    prenatal diagnosis 75
    prognosis and therapy 73
    risk 73–4
    screening 71
genotype analysis from amniocentesis 331–2
germinal matrix hemorrhage 93,98
gestational age at delivery
    in ACT 15
    in multiple pregnancy 14
gestational sac size sonography 168
gestational trophoblastic disease 448–9
Glasgow trial of ultrasound screening 81
gliogenesis in brain 38,46
gliosis 90,94,99,100,101,103
glucose in amniotic fluid 334,338
glycoprotein in amniotic fluid, test for cystic fibrosis 108
goiter 519
graft vs. host disease following transplant in fetus 521
gravidin in amniotic fluid 341
great vessel Doppler ultrasound in IUGR 413–18
Griscelli syndrome 370
growth
    characteristics 251
    correlated with fetal distress in utero 414–15
    discrepancy in twins 156
    potential, decrease in intrinsic 256–7
    rate, sonography of 166–7
growth factors
    in amniotic fluid 334
    role 20
Gunther's disease 373

Hallopeau–Siemens epidermolysis bullosa 367–8
handedness in children, effect of prenatal ultrasound screening on 85
Harlequin fetus 364–5
head circumference for IUGR diagnosis 263–4,266
health of children following ACT 15–16
heart
    examination by ultrasound 137
    failure, venous signs of 275,276
    malformations *see* cardiac defects; congenital cardiopathies
    rate
        analysis 207,233–4,238,440
        analysis by cardiotocography 196
            baseline 197
            accelerations and decelerations 197–8
            limits of normality 198–202
            variations 198,201,202

analysis by computerized system, in normal and IUGR fetuses 289–97
    assessment of reproducibility 291–2
    baseline determination 290
    accelerations and decelerations 290–1
    normal ranges in third trimester 292–3
analysis by Doppler ultrasound 401–2
analysis by telephone 213–23
    acceptability and psychological impact 217
    acceptance rate 215–16
    clinical case presentation 217–20
    economics 217
    transmission of traces 217
    trials 220–2
elevation 219
hypoxia and 401
    Porto system 403,404,405
indications 221
IUGR and 293–4,480
relationship to BFWV 457
sinusoidal 227
sounds, auscultation of 207
Helsinki trial of ultrasound screening 82,86,87
hematocrit analysis from vaginally collected sample 329
hemodynamic profile in fetus 255
    Doppler ultrasound 271–2,273,274
    in early pregnancy, transvaginal sonography in 435–53
    effect of maternal vasoactive agents on 389–98
    in hypoxia 399–401
    in IUGR 299–309
hemorrhagic lesions at fetal post-mortem, cerebral 93,94,95
hemostasis
    fetal, aspirin effects on 498–9
    maternal, aspirin effects on 499–500
hepatic vein blood flow velocity waveforms 427,429,430
heredopathia atactica polyneuritiformis 365
hernias, congenital diaphragmatic 530–2
herniation, midgut, transvaginal ultrasound for 130
heroin addiction, IUGR and 254
Heyns suit 545
hiccuping, fetal 226,227
histogenetic events of fetal brain development 36–8
    of cerebral cortex 38–48
histological examination of fetal brain 90
HPA-A1 antigen 511
ß-human chorionic gonadotropin marker for chromosomal defects 65
human immunodeficiency virus (HIV)
    in amniotic fluid 337
    thrombocytopenia and 506
humeral shortening detection 65–6
hydrocephaly
    blood flow velocity waveform analysis and 480–1
    shunting 522–3
    transvaginal ultrasound for 129,130
hydronephrosis 523
    transvaginal ultrasound for 131
hydrops fetalis 526,529,533
    polyhydramnios and 328–9

hydrothorax 525–7
21-hydroxylase deficiency 518
hypertension in pregnancy
    blood flow velocity waveform analysis 481
    causing IUGR 254
    fetal heart rate in 218
    prevention by aspirin 495,496
    prostaglandin role in 491–2
    uterine artery ultrasound velocimetry 420–3
hypoxemia
    fetal response to 383–5
    neonatal, aspirin and 499
    umbilical artery blood flow velocity waveform analysis in 462,463
hypoxia
    assessment, blood flow velocity waveform analysis in 479–80
    prenatally 381–8
    with color Doppler and automated heart rate analysis 399–411
    definition 399
    effects on fetal centers of CNS 236

ichthyoses 362–3
    autosomal recessive 364
    rare syndrome associated with 364–8
    X-linked 363
immune disorders 370–1
immune system, fetal 313
immune thrombocytopenias *see* thrombocytopenias, immune
immunoglobulin G (IgG) therapy in premature babies 313–14
immunosuppressive factors in amniotic fluid 340–1
implantation sonography 165–8
in vitro embryo as patient 6
in vitro fertilization
    effect on outcome of triplet pregnancy 188–9
    psychomotor development in fetuses following 15
indomethacin effects on uterine and fetal hemodynamics 392
infantile polycystic kidneys, transvaginal ultrasound for 131
infection
    causing IUGR 255,257,538
    in premature babies 313–14
inherited diseases causing IUGR 255
inhibin in amniotic fluid 342
insulin-like growth factor in amniotic fluid 334
insulin-like growth factor-binding protein-1 in amniotic fluid 334
intelligence quotient, effects of aspirin on 499
interleukin-1 in amniotic fluid 340–1
interleukins in amniotic fluid 338–9
intermediate zone development in brain 37,42
intermittent abdominal decompression 545
intracranial blood volume monitoring 210
intracranial circulation 441
intracranial hemorrhage in thrombocytopenia 509,510–11
intrapartum external monitoring 207–11

intrauterine fetal brain death 277
intrauterine growth retardation (IUGR) 251–87
    analysis 405
        by actocardiography 227–8
        by blood flow velocity waveform 413–18,459–64
            carotid artery 479
            cerebral arteries 479
            uterine artery 419–24
    analysis by cardiotocography 202
    analysis by fetal heart rate 289–97
    antenatal diagnosis 260–71
    brain pathology and 101–2
    classification 258–60
    definition 252–3
    delivery timing 278
    effects of maternal oxygenation on 393
    in diabetes mellitus 465
    etiology 253–6
    fetal hemodynamics 299–309
    incidence 253
    natural history of fetal compromise in 271–8
    neonatal cerebral blood flow 483
    pathogenesis 256–8,259
    pathophysiology 299–300
    prevention by aspirin 494–5,496
    risk diagnosis 260
    screening 57,67
    therapeutic management 537–49
    type diagnosis 265–7
intraventricular hemorrhage 93
ischemic-hemorrhagic lesions of placenta 419–24

karyotype analysis from amniocentesis 331–2
keratin analysis in skin samples 360–2
kidney, multicystic dysplastic, transvaginal ultrasound for 131
Koebner epidermolysis bullosa 366

labetalol effects on fetal hemodynamics 390
labor
    cerebral blood flow velocity waveform analysis 481–2
    induction, effect of ultrasound screening on 81
    problems in ACT 14–15
lactate concentration correlated with IUGR 417
lambda sign in placental ultrasound 156
learning problems following prematurity 312
legal intervention in fetal therapy 8
legal standard of fetal care 7
leukomalacia, periventricular 95,96,98–9,100
    detection of 210
limb defects analysis by ultrasound 138
liver
    transplantation in fetus 521
    volume measurement by ultrasound 138
    see also hepatic vein
London trial of ultrasound screening 79–80
lung maturation evaluation 329–30
lupus anticoagulant, fetal loss and 497
lymphatic system malformation, transvaginal ultrasound for 127–8
lymphocyte
    B-cell lineage 23–4,25–8
    culture *in vitro* from neonates 22
    differentiation antigens 20
    expression of activation antigens in cord blood 24–5,28
    ontogeny during intrauterine life 19–32
    phenotype analysis in utero 20–2
        change *in utero* 22–4
    role in fetal immune system 313
    T-cell lineage 22–3,25–8
lymphopoiesis, fetal 19

magnesium effects on uterine and fetal hemodynamics 394
magnetic resonance imaging for amniotic fluid volume estimation 321
malformations
    in ACT 12–13
    aspirin and 498
    detection 537
    effect of ultrasound screening on 83
    risk 73,74
    screening for 57,58–61
    surgery for 522–7
    transvaginal ultrasound detection of 127–34
malnutrition causing IUGR 258
manganese therapy in mother, effects on fetus 518
marginal zone development in brain 36–7,41–2,47
masculinization of female fetuses 518–19
maternal factors in IUGR 254–5
Meckel–Gruber syndrome, transvaginal ultrasound for 131
meconium
    in amniotic fluid 332
    grading 328–9
    obstruction in cystic fibrosis 107
membrane-attack-complex inhibitory protein in amniotic fluid 341
membranes, artificial rupture of 343
    see also premature rupture of membranes
Menkes' syndrome 372,518
mental retardation
    brain pathology in 91–2
    risk 73
meta-analysis on ultrasound screening trials 83–4,86
metabolic disorders in fetus 334,372–3,518–19
metabolites in amniotic fluid 333–4
metal deficiency, IUGR and 539
methoxamine effects on fetal hemodynamics 391
methylmalonic acidemia 519
metoprolol effects on fetal hemodynamics 390
β_2 microglobulin assessment 524–5
microvillar enzymes test for cystic fibrosis 109
milk feeds in premature babies 314–15
miscarriage, uterine malformations and 172
    see also fetal loss
mole 448
monosomy X, hygroma in 128
moral status for fetus 4
mortality *see* neonatal; perinatal; prenatal mortality
movements in fetus 233, 237–8,243,244

analysis by cardiotocography 196–7, 200
IUGR and 267–8
mucopolysaccharidoses, genetic counseling in 72
multifetal pregnancy 183–94
   amniotic fluid volume and 327
   antenatal assessment of fetal well-being in 187–8
   birth weights 184
   chorionicity and amnionicity 151–9
   complications 156
   fetal outcome in 13–14
   growth discrepancy 156
   incidence 151, 183
   IUGR and 255–6
   management 184–5
   mode of delivery 186–7
   perinatal mortality 184
   reduction in 189–91
   scanning 152
   survival rates 155
   treatment strategies 185–6
   vanishing twin syndrome 156
   see also specific types e.g. twins
muscular dystrophy, genetic counseling in 72
myoma 447

naproxen effects on uterine and fetal hemodynamics 392
natural killer cells, fetal 24
neocortex development 41–3
neonatal brain
   pathology 101
   circulation 482–3
neonatal hemostasis, aspirin effects on 498–9
neonatal hypoxemia, effects of aspirin on 499
neonatal intensive care
   admission rate for multiple pregnancies 14
   outcome following 311–12
neonatal lymphocyte culture *in vitro* 22
neonatal mortality
   for multiple pregnancy 14
   risk 73
neonatology advances 311–15
networked imaging system 122
neural tube
   defects
      from diet 518
      folic acid therapy for 335–6
   development 36
   ultrasonography 148, 150
neurological examinations, ARED flow and 467–8
neurological function of children, effect of prenatal ultrasound screening on 85
neuron
   migration 37, 43, 45, 51–2
   peptidergic 47
   pyramidal 46
neuropathology, developmental 89–91
nifedipine therapy in multifetal pregnancy 185
non-conjugated estriol marker for chromosomal defects 65
non-stress test 187, 225, 268

false-positive 226–7
Norwegian trials of ultrasound screening 80–81
nuchal fold detection 65
nuchal translucency detection 66
nuclear medicine for amniotic fluid volume estimation 321
nutritional supplement therapy
   fetal 544–5
   maternal, for IUGR 539–40
nylidrin effects on uterine and fetal hemodynamics 394

obstetric complications in ACT 14
oligodendroglia development 46
oligohydramnios 322–5
   assessment 232
   transvaginal ultrasound 131
   in twin 327
   uterine artery ultrasound 420–1
omphalocele, transvaginal ultrasound for 130
ontogeny of human lymphocytes during intrauterine life 19–32
osmotic gradient between maternal serum and amniotic fluid 319–20
ovarian transvaginal sonography 161–5
ovarian volume measurement by ultrasound 137
ovum
   blighted 444–6, 447, 448
   dangers on journey through Fallopian tube for 171–2
oxygen
   tension in IUGR 540–1
   therapy for mother, effects on uterine and fetal hemodynamics 393
      in IUGR 540–1
oxygenation of fetus correlated with IUGR 416–17

paleocortex development 42–3
Pasini epidermolysis bullosa 367
peak-systolic velocity 444
perinatal asphyxia 483, 484
perinatal brain pathology 96–102
perinatal mortality
   aspirin and 499
   blood flow velocity waveform analysis and 466–7
   effect of ultrasound screening on 82, 86–7
   incidence 207, 208, 238
   in multifetal pregnancy 13, 184
      triplets 190
      twins 527
periventricular leukomalacia detection 210
phenotype
   analysis of fetal lymphocytes 20–2
   changes of lymphocytes *in utero* 22–4
phenylephrine effects on fetal hemodynamics 391
phenylketonuria in mother, fetal effects of 517
phenytoin therapy, maternal, 517
phospholipids in amniotic fluid 329–30
photic fetal stimulation 228–9
pigmentary disorders 369–70
pindolol effects on fetal hemodynamics 390
placental abruption

aspirin therapy and 542
blood flow velocity waveform analysis 466
effects of aspirin on 499–500
placental anatomy 435–40
placental counting by ultrasound 155
placental grading 232–3,239–40,242
IUGR and 268
placental infarction 421
placental ischemic lesions 93,419–24
placental morphology in hemorrhage 421
placental mosaicism causing IUGR 256
placental problems in multifetal pregnancy 157
placental volume measurement by ultrasound 138
platelet
count in fetus, prediction of 509–10
dysfunction in pregnancy-induced hypertension 492
transfusion in thrombocytopenia 512,513
polyhydramnios 327–8
amniocentesis and 336
blood flow velocity waveform analysis in 481
in twin 327
porphyria 373
post-term pregnancy blood flow velocity waveform analysis 465
postnatal brain pathology 102–3
postsynaptic site development in brain 37–8
pre-eclampsia
aspirin prevention of 494,496
therapy for 497
blood flow velocity waveform analysis 464,481
prostaglandin role in 491
precursor cells, fetal 24,29
pregnancy
complications in ACT 11
Doppler ultrasound prediction of 449–50
ectopic, in ACT 12
loss see abortion; fetal loss; miscarriage
loss see fetal loss
multiple see multifetal pregnancy; triplets; twins
outcome of assisted conception techniques 11–18
termination counseling 71
testing counseling 71
pregnant woman's autonomy 5–6,8
premature rupture of membranes (PROM) 327,328–33
amniotic fluid volume for evaluation of 330
pulmonary hypoplasia and 330–1
prematurity
analysis by TVS 178–9
brain pathology in 96–101
enteral feeding 314–15
infection 313–14
multifetal pregnancy 184
outcome following intensive care 311–12
surfactant therapy 312–13
survival rates 311
prenatal diagnosis, genetic counseling for 71
prenatal mortality
due to infection 93
rate in triplets 188–9
presubplate development in cerebral cortex 43

presynaptic axonal development in brain 37
preterm labor prevention by aspirin 497–8
prolactin in amniotic fluid 341
proliferating cells, fetal 24,29
prostacyclin role in pregnancy 491,492,540
prostaglandins
in amniotic fluid 339
for pregnancy termination, cerebral hemorrhagic lesions associated with 93
role in ductus arteriosus patency 499
in maternal and fetal adaptation during pregnancy 491
synthetase inhibitors effects on uterine and fetal hemodynamics 392–3
protein electrophoresis 525
protein-C absence in amniotic fluid 336
psychomotor development of IVF fetuses 15
pulmonary artery blood flow velocity waveforms 440
peak velocity correlated with IUGR 416
pulmonary hypoplasia, PROM and 330–1
pulmonary maturity induction 545
pulmonary valve peak velocities in IUGR 306
pulsatility index 235,243,245,381–2,456
carotid artery 479
in fetal hypoxia 384
in hydrocephaly 480
cerebral arteries 384–5,478,479
in polyhydramnios 481
in subdural hematoma 481
cerebral vessels in IUGR 302
descending aorta 457–8
in IUGR 301
femoral artery 458
IUGR and 274
renal artery 458
subchorionic hematoma 447
umbilical artery 457
uteroplacental circulation 459
umbilical artery in fetal hypoxia 383
in IUGR 301,304,305
umbilical-placental vessels 439,444
pyelectasis
detection 66
transvaginal ultrasound for 131

quadruplets 154,155
incidence 183

radiography of amniotic fluid 321
RADIUS trial of ultrasound screening 82–3,86,87
reflex activity score 243
Refsum's disease 365
relaxin in amniotic fluid 341
renal anomalies 523–4
renal artery blood flow velocity waveform analysis 458
in IUGR 302,304,305,463
renal disease in mother causing IUGR 254
resistance index 401,402,438,456
perinatal asphyxia 483
subchorionic hematoma 447
umbilical artery 457

umbilical-placental vessels 439,444,445
respiratory distress syndrome
    neonatal cerebral blood flow 483
    in premature babies 312
    therapy for 545
respiratory tree fluids 319
ritodrine effects on uterine and fetal hemodynamics 394

sarcococcygeal teratomas 533
schizophrenia, neuropathology of 103
separating membranes analysis 155
sex
    determination of twins 155
    ratio in ACT 15
sextuplets 154
shunt placement in utero 522–7
Sjögren–Larsson syndrome 365
skeletal dysplasia, transvaginal ultrasound for 132
skeletal system anomalies, transvaginal ultrasound for 132
skin
    as source of amniotic fluid 319
    biopsy 359–62
    development 361
    disease, prenatal diagnosis of 359–77
skull decompression during birth 482
small-for-gestational-age (SGA)
    blood flow velocity waveform analysis 460,461
        cerebral artery 479–80
    definition 252,266
smoking effect
    on birth weight 81
    on uterine and fetal hemodynamics 394
    on IUGR 254
sonoembryology see transvaginal sonography 141
spina bifida, transvaginal ultrasound for 129
spinal anesthesia effects on fetal hemodynamics 391
stem cell transplantation 520–2
steroid hormones in amniotic fluid 342
Stockholm trial of ultrasound screening 81–2,86
streptococcal infection in premature babies 314
stress in fetus 545
    see mainly fetal distress
stuck-twin phenomenon 327
subchorionic hematoma 442–4,447
subdiaphragmatic venous vestibulum, venous Doppler assessment and 427–8
subdural hematoma blood flow velocity waveform analysis 481
subplate zone development in cerebral cortex 44–5,47,51–2
subventricular zone development in brain 37,42
sudden infant death syndrome, neuropathology of 102–3
sulindac effects on uterine and fetal hemodynamics 392–3
supraventricular tachycardia 520
surfactant therapy for premature babies 312–13
surgical intervention to fetus 520–33
    open 528–33

symphosis fundal height measurement for IUGR diagnosis 260–1
synapse
    development in brain 37–8,43–4
    functional activity 50
syphilis, congenital 336–7
systemic lupus erythematosus, blood flow velocity waveform analysis in 465–6
systolic-to-diastolic ratio 456
    inferior vena cava 458
    uteroplacental circulation 459

tachyarrhythmias 520
tachycardia, fetal heart rate monitoring 219,221
telemedicine 123
teratogenic effects of aspirin 498
teratomas, sarcococcygeal 533
terbutaline effects on uterine and fetal hemodynamics 394
thalamic ultrasonography 149
thalamocortical axon development 50–1
thrombocytopenia
    in mother, fetal heart rate in 220
    immune
        alloimmune 511–15
            diagnosis 512
            fetal management 512–15
            neonatal management 512
        differential diagnosis 505
        gestational 506–8
            diagnosis and management 507–8
            incidence 506
            pathogenesis 506–7
        incidence 505
thrombocytopenic purpura, immune
    incidence 508
    management 510
    maternal management 508–9
    pathophysiology 508
    prediction of fetal platelet count 509–10
thromboxane
    role in pregnancy 491,492,540
thyroid abnormalities 519
thyroxine therapy for goiter 519
tissue characterization 120–1
TMF fetal heart rate monitor 213–14
tocolysis
    in IUGR 543
    in multifetal pregnancy 185–6
toe clinodactyly and hypoplasia detection 65
Toxoplasma gondii, IUGR and 538
transabdominal ultrasound for fetal screening 64
transforming growth factor β_2 in amniotic fluid 341
transfusion
    syndrome in twins 157
    therapy 520
translucency detection, first-trimester 66–7
transvaginal sonography (TVS)
    advantages 179
    color Doppler, of fetal first three weeks 161–74

fertilization, embryogenesis and implantation 165–8
ovary 161–5
ovum journey dangers 171–2
uterine environment 168–70
uterine perfusion changes with placentation 170–1
for early pregnancy hemodynamics 435–53
of fetal central nervous system 141–50
for fetal screening 63–5
in multifetal pregnancies 152–6
for uterine cervix evaluation in pregnancy 175–80
for uterine circulation studies 300
of venous return in fetus 425–34
see also ultrasound
trehalase test for cystic fibrosis 109
treponemes in amniotic fluid 336–7
trichothiodystrophy 373–4
triplets
    biophysical score 188
    cervical cerclage 186
    effect of fertility drugs and IVF on outcome 188–9
    incidence 183
    mode of delivery 186–7
    perinatal mortality 190
    reduction to twins 189
trisomy causing IUGR 255,257
trisomy 13 detection 66
trisomy 18 detection 65
trisomy 21 *see* Down's syndrome
trophoblastic cell failure in pregnancy 299
tumor
    size analysis by ultrasound 138
    surface tissue by ultrasound 136
tumor necrosis factor in amniotic fluid 339
twin-to-twin transfusion syndrome 157,527
twins
    acardiac 528
    amniotic fluid volume 327
    cervical cerclage 186
    conjoined 157
    cord entanglement 157
    dichorionic-diamniotic 153,155
    embolization syndrome 157
    embryology 152
    incidence 151,527
    IUGR and 255
    malformations and aneuploidies 156
    monochorionic-diamniotic 153,155
    perinatal mortality 527
    reversal arterial perfusion syndrome 157
    sex determination 156
    survival rates 155
    types 151
    vascular anastomosis 157

ultrasonographer skill 138–9
ultrasonography 57–69,79
    for amniotic fluid volume analysis 322–8
        1-cm pocket 323
        2-cm pocket 323
        8-cm pocket 323
        clinical outcome after normal of low AFI 325–6
        comparison of maximal vertical pocket with AFI 324–5
        cord or limb-containing pockets 324
        correlation of AFI with clinical oligohydramnios 325
        dynamics of 326
        four-quadrant sum of pockets 323–4
        intrapartum screening for 326
        subjective 322–3
        variability in AFI measurements 325
    costs 84–5
    Doppler, for assessment of fetal heart rate 399–411
        of cerebral circulation in perinatal period 477–88
        effect of maternal vasoactive agents on uterine and fetal hemodynamics in 389–98
        for fetal hypoxia assessment 381–8
        for hemodynamic profiles 235
        for IUGR 413–18
    for diagnosis of IUGR 261–5,267–8,271–2,273,274
    false-negatives 59–61,62,64
    false-positives 62,63
    for fetal tissue characterization 120–1
    for fetal well-being monitoring during late pregnancy 455–75
        complicated pregnancy 459–66
        follow-up studies 467–8
        randomized controlled trials 466–7
        uncomplicated pregnancy 457–9
    markers of fetal chromosomal defects 65–7
    perinatal 119–20
    randomized controlled trials 79–84
    requirements 58
    safety aspects 85–6,450
    three-dimensional 122,135–40
        clinical application 136–9
        technique 135–6
    uterine artery, ischemic-hemorrhagic lesions of placenta and 419–24
    see also transvaginal sonography
umbilical artery
    absent end-diastolic blood flow correlated with IUGR 415–16
    blood flow velocity waveform analysis 235,244,457
        for fetal hypoxia analysis 381,382,383–4,403,405
        in IUGR 270,272–4,275,277,301,542
        in post-term pregnancy 465
        in SGA 460,461,463
        see also under pulsatility index
    resistance indices 402
umbilical cord
    blood gas values 201,202
        lymphocyte expression of activation antigens 24–5,28
    entanglement in twins 157
umbilical vein
    blood flow velocity waveforms 425–7
        for fetal hypoxia analysis 384
umbilical-placental circulation 438–40

underachievement following prematurity 312
urinary tract
    anomalies, transvaginal ultrasound for 131
    infection in mother causing IUGR 255
    obstruction 532
        bilateral 525,526
urine
    contribution to amniotic fluid 319
    measurements for renal function 524
    production in fetus, IUGR and 267
uropathy, obstructive 523–5
uterine artery
    blood flow velocity waveform analysis 168–70,460
        in ischemic-hemorrhagic lesions of placenta and 419–24
        in IUGR 300–1,463
        in pre-eclampsia 464
        in pregnancy complications 450
uterine cervical cerclage 186
    in multifetal pregnancy 186
uterine cervix
    evaluation by TVS 175
        anatomy 176–7
        length 176,178
        wedging 178,179
uterine contraction
    analysis 291
    cerebral blood flow and 481
uterine environment sonography 168–70
uterine fibroids 446–7
uterine hemodynamics, effect of maternal vasoactive agents on 389–98
uterine perfusion changes with placentation 170–1
uterine shape definition 176
uterine volume for IUGR diagnosis 264
uteroplacental circulation analysis 436–8,458–9
    in gestational trophoblastic disease 448–9
    in missed abortion and blighted ovum 444–6
    in threatened abortion 444
    in uterine fibroids 446–7
uteroplacental factors causing IUGR 256,257
uteroplacental insufficiency pathophysiology 299–300

vaginal collection of amniotic fluid following spontaneous rupture of membranes 328–33
vanishing twin syndrome 156
vascular anastomosis in twins 157
vascular changes in uterus, sonography 168–70
vascular resistance, silent stage of increase in 271–2
vasoactive agent effect on uterine and fetal hemodynamics 389–98
vasodilatation in perinatal asphyxia 484
vasopressor effects on fetal hemodynamics 391
vena cava
    inferior, blood flow velocity waveform analysis 425–7,428–9,430,458
        in IUGR 306,463
venous blood flow velocity waveform analysis 458
    in IUGR 303,463
venous circulation in fetal hypoxia 385
venous infarction, periventricular 97–8
venous return in fetus 425–34
    in second half of pregnancy 428–31
ventricular zone development in brain 36–7,41,45
ventriculomegaly 522–3
viability of fetus 5–6
vibroacoustic stimulation 229,234
videoconferencing in fetal medicine 123
virtual reality systems in fetal medicine 123
vitamin supplement therapy in mother
    B_{12} therapy 519
    fetal effects of 518
volume measurements by ultrasound 137–8,139

Weber–Cockayne epidermolysis bullosa 366
white blood cell count in amniotic fluid 338
Wiskott–Aldrich syndrome 370–1
Wolman's disease 374

xeroderma pigmentosum 371

zinc supplement therapy for IUGR 539
Zwa antigen 511